Dilemmas in Otorhinolaryngology

Dilemmas in Otorhinolaryngology

EDITED BY

D.F.N. Harrison MD MS PhD FRCS (Hon) FRACS (Hon) FRCS (Ed)

Professor of Laryngology and Otology,
University of London;
Senior Consultant Surgeon,
The Royal National Throat, Nose and Ear Hospital,
London

CHURCHILL LIVINGSTONE
EDINBURGH LONDON MELBOURNE AND NEW YORK 1988

CHURCHILL LIVINGSTONE
Medical Division of Longman Group UK Limited

Distributed in the United States of America by Churchill
Livingstone Inc., 1560 Broadway, New York, N.Y. 10036,
and by associated companies, branches and representatives
throughout the world.

First published 1988

ISBN 0 443 03554 7

British Library Cataloguing in Publication Data
A CIP Catalogue record for this book is available from the
British Library.

Library of Congress Cataloging in Publication Data

Dilemmas in otorhinolaryngology.

   1. Otolaryngology. I. Harrison, D. F. N.
[DNLM: 1. Otorhinolaryngologic Diseases. WV 100 D576]
RF46.5.D55 1988 617'.51 87-31975

Printed and bound in Great Britain at The Bath Press, Avon

Preface

As an enthusiastic solver of crossword puzzles, I have recourse to a wide variety of reference books and other valuable sources of information. Although providing excellent word interpretation they rarely assist in word usage. Such is the case of the noun which occupies such a prominent position in the title of this volume. Dilemma originates from the Greek prefix di(two) plus lémma(premis) and may be literally defined as 'choosing between two equally undesirable alternatives or propositions'.

> 'The doctor's dilemma was whether he should tell the patient the truth or risk his refusing the treatment.'
> (G.B. Shaw, 1906)

But, in this book, experienced and talented doctors have been given the task of expressing their opinions on selected ear, nose and throat problems over which there is considerable confusion. Since each chapter has at least two contributors and there are certainly several options—dilemma may be considered an acceptable title!

In order that the reader shall not necessarily be left with only a wealth of information without any conclusion, senior members of the specialty have been persuaded to write a short critique of papers and—in many instances—their own view of the problem. Contributors have originated from many parts of the world and apart from minor corrections of expression, no editorial pruning has been applied. Each essay stands on its own merit under the banner of its author. However, responsibility for choice of topic is mine but I am sure that the considerable thought and effort which has been put into this volume will be amply rewarded by its contribution to the practice of what is now the foremost of the surgical specialties.

The burden of assembling the manuscripts, retyping and generally keeping a wary eye on the whole project has fallen on my invaluable aide Shirley Player. Without such assistance few of us would achieve anything!

London, 1988   D.F.N.H.

Contributors

P.W. Alberti MB BS PhD FRCS FRCS(C)
Professor and Chairman,
Department of Otolaryngology,
University of Toronto;
Otolaryngologist-in-Chief,
Mount Sinai and Toronto General Hospitals,
Toronto, Ontario, Canada

R.R. Alford MD
Distinguished Service Professor,
Olga Keith Wiess Professor and Chairman,
Texas Medical Center, Baylor College of
Medicine,
Houston, Texas, USA

B.J. Bailey MD FACS
Wiess Professor and Chairman,
Department of Otolaryngology,
University of Texas Medical Branch;
Galveston, Texas, USA

J. Ballantyne CBE FRCS Hon FRCS(I)
Consulting Ear, Nose & Throat Surgeon,
The Royal Free Hospital, London;
Consultant Ear, Nose & Throat Surgeon,
King Edward VIIth Hospital for Officers,
London, UK

J.D. Baxter MD CM MSc FRCS(C)
Professor & Chairman, Department of
Otolaryngology,
McGill University, Montreal, Canada

H.A. Beagley MB ChB FRCS DLO
Late Consultant Audiological Physician,
The Royal National Throat, Nose & Ear Hospital,
London, UK

H.F. Biller MD
Professor & Chairman,
Department of Otolaryngology,
Mount Sinai Medical Center,
New York, NY, USA

D.A. Bowdler FRCS
Department of ENT, University of Liverpool,
Liverpool, UK

D.E. Brackmann MD
Clinical Professor of Otolaryngology,
University of Southern California School of
Medicine, Otologic Medical Group, Inc. and
House Ear Institute, Los Angeles, CA, USA

D.J. Brain FRCS
Senior Surgeon, Birmingham and Midland Ear,
Nose & Throat Hospital;
Senior Clinical Lecturer in Oto-Rhinolaryngology
at the University of Birmingham,
Birmingham, UK

R.L. Brubaker MD
Department of Otolaryngology,
Washington University School of Medicine,
St Louis, MO, USA

P. Clifford MD MCh FRCS
MD (Hon. Karolinska Inst)
Honorary Consultant Otolaryngologist,
King's College Hospital, London, UK;
Formerly Chairman, South East Cooperative
Oncology Group (SECOG)

J. Conley MD
Professor of Clinical Otolaryngology—
Head and Neck Surgery (Emeritus),
Columbia-Presbyterian Medical Center,
New York, NY;
Chief of the Head & Neck Service (Emeritus),
St Vincent's Hospital, New York, NY, USA

C.B. Croft FRCS FRCS(Ed)
Consultant Ear, Nose & Throat, Head and Neck
Surgeon, The Royal National Throat, Nose &
Ear Hospital, London, UK

W.S. Crysdale MD, FRCS(C)
Associate Professor, Department of
Otolaryngology, University of Toronto;
Otolaryngologist-in-Chief, The Hospital for Sick
Children; Attending Staff, Wellesley Hospital;
Consultant Staff, Hugh MacMillan Medical
Center, Toronto, Ontario, Canada

B.J. Cummings MB ChB FRCPC FRCR FRACR
Department of Radiation Oncology,
The Princess Margaret Hospital, Toronto;
Associate Professor of Radiology, University of
Toronto, Ontario, Canada

V.M. Dalley MB BS FRCR
Honorary Consultant Radiotherapist,
Royal Marsden Hospital, London,
King's College Hospital, London, and
Royal National Ear, Nose & Throat Hospital,
London, UK

H. Diamant MD
Formerly Professor and Head of the Department
of Otorhinolaryngology, University of Umea,
Sweden

A.B. Drake-Lee FRCS
Consultant ENT Surgeon,
Royal United Hospital, Bath, UK

B. Drettner MD
Professor of Otolaryngology,
Karolinska Institute, Stockholm;
Head of The Department of Otolaryngology,
Huddinge Hospital, Huddinge, Sweden

S. Edström MD
Assistant Professor and Reader,
Department of Otolaryngology
Gothenburg University, Gothenburg, Sweden

J.M. Fredrickson MD FRCS(C) FACS
MD(Hon.)
Lindburg Professor and Head, Department of
Otolaryngology,
Washington University School of Medicine,
St Louis, MO, USA

A.P. Freeland FRCS
Consultant in Otolaryngology, Radcliffe
Infirmary, Oxford;
Clinical Lecturer, University of Oxford, UK

P. Freeman FRCS FRACS DLO
Consultant Otolaryngologist,
Alfred Hospital,
Melbourne, Victoria, Australia

G.A. Gates MD FACS
Professor and Head, Otorhinolaryngology,
The University of Texas Health Science Center,
San Antonio, Texas, USA

W.P.R. Gibson MB BS FRCS(Otol.) MD(Lond.)
Professor of Otolaryngology, The University of
Sydney; Head of Department of Otolaryngology,
The Royal Prince Alfred Hospital, Sydney,
NSW, Australia

M.E. Glasscock III MD
Clinical Professor of Surgery (Otology and
Neurotology), Vanderbilt University School of
Medicine, Nashville; Clinical Professor of
Otolaryngology, University of Tennessee College
of Medicine, Memphis, TN, USA

V. Goodhill MD FACS
Otology, Neuro-otology, Otological Surgery,
Division of Head & Neck Surgery,
UCLA Medical Center, Los Angeles, CA, USA

D.J. Hare LLB
Solicitor of the Supreme Court (England & Wales),
Partner in Wilkinson & Durham, Surrey, UK

D.F.N. Harrison MD MS PhD FRCS
(Hon.)FRACS (Hon.)FRCS(Ed)
Professor of Laryngology & Otology, University
of London; Senior Consultant Surgeon, The
Royal National Throat, Nose & Ear Hospital,
London, UK

R. Hinchcliffe MD PhD FRCP
Professor of Audiological Medicine,
Honorary Consultant to The Royal National
Throat, Nose & Ear Hospital, London, UK;
Honorary Consultant to the Sixth People's
Hospital, Shanghai, China

D.J. Howard FRCS FRCS(Ed)
Deputy Director, Professorial Unit, The Institute

of Laryngology & Otology, University of London;
Honorary Consultant Surgeon, The Royal
National Throat, Nose & Ear Hospital, London,
UK

W.M.S. Ironside FRCS
Consultant ENT Surgeon (retired)

A.G. Kerr FRCS
Consultant ENT Surgeon,
Royal Victoria Hospital, Belfast, N. Ireland, UK

S.C. Levine MD
Assistant Professor,
Department of Otolaryngology
(Otology/Neurotology),
University of Minnesota, Minneapolis, MN, USA

W.S. Lund MS FRCS
Consultant ENT Surgeon,
The Radcliffe Infirmary,
Oxford, UK

B.F. McCabe MD
Professor and Head, Department of
Otolaryngology—Head and Neck Surgery,
The University of Iowa, IA, USA

P. McKelvie MD ChM FRCS DLO
Consultant Surgeon, The Royal National Throat,
Nose & Ear Hospital, London;
Dean, The Institute of Laryngology and Otology,
University of London, UK

Kevin X. McKennan MD
Private Practice—Otology/Neurotology,
Sacramento ENT Surgical and Medical Group,
Sacramento, CA, USA

A.G.D. Maran MD FRCS FACS
Head of Department of Otolaryngology,
University of Edinburgh;
Consultant Otolaryngologist, Royal Infirmary,
Edinburgh, UK

J. Marquet MD
Head of the ENT Department, University of
Antwerp, Belgium

J.A.M. Martin MB BS FRCS
Director, Nuffield Hearing & Speech Centre,
Consultant in Audiological Medicine,
Professor Associate, Brunel University;

Honorary Senior Lecturer, Institute of
Laryngology & Otology; Honorary Lecturer,
Department of Phonetics & Linguistics, University
College London, UK

A.R. Maw MB BS FRCS
Consultant Otolaryngologist,
Bristol Royal Infirmary, Bristol, UK

H.S. Millar FRCS FRACS DLO
Senior Otologist,
Royal Melbourne Hospital,
Melbourne, Victoria, Australia

A.W. Morrison MB ChB FRCS DLO
Consultant Otolaryngologist,
The London Hospital;
Lecturer in Otolaryngology,
University of London, UK

I.P. Munro ChB FRFPS(G) FRCS(Ed)
Consultant ENT Surgeon, Glasgow, UK (retired)

E.N. Myers MD FACS
Professor and Chairman, University of Pittsburg
School of Medicine, Department of
Otolaryngology; Professor, Department of
Diagnostic Services, University of Pittsburg
School of Dental Medicine; Chief, Department of
Otolaryngology, Eye and Ear Hospital of
Pittsburg, PA, USA

T. Palva MD D Med Sci
Professor of Otorhinolaryngology,
University of Helsinki, Finland

W.R. Panje MD
Professor and Chairman, Otolaryngology—Head
and Neck Surgery Department, University of
Chicago Medical Center,
Chicago, IL, USA

R. Parish MD
Head & Neck Fellow, Memorial Sloan-Kettering
Cancer Center,
New York, NY, USA

B.W. Pearson MD FRCS(C)
Associate Professor of Otolaryngology,
Mayo Medical School, Rochester, Minnesota;
Consultant in Otolaryngology, Mayo Group
Practice, Jacksonville, FL, USA

S. Peeters MD
ENT Department, University of Antwerp, Belgium

H.J. Pelzer Jr DDS MD
Department of Otolaryngology, Northwestern
University, The Medical School, Chicago, IL,
USA

C.R. Pfaltz MD
Head of the Department of ORL,
University Hospital, Basel, Switzerland

R. Pracy MPhil MB FRCS (Hon.)FRCSI
Formerly Dean, The Institute of Laryngology &
Otology; Consultant Otolaryngologist, The Royal
National Throat, Nose & Ear Hospital, and The
Hospital for Sick Children, Great Ormond Street,
London, UK

J.L. Pulec MD
Clinical Professor of Otolaryngology,
The University of South California;
President, Ear International, Los Angeles,
CA, USA

R.B. Sessions MD FACS
Associate Attending Surgeon, Memorial
Sloan-Kettering Cancer Center, New York;
Professor of Otorhinolaryngology—Head and
Neck Surgery; Attending Otorhinolaryngologist,
New York Hospital, NY, USA

O.H. Shaheen MS FRCS
Consultant ENT Surgeon, Guy's Hospital,
London, and The Royal National Throat, Nose
& Ear Hospital,
London, UK

H.J. Shaw VRD FRCS
Chairman—Head and Neck Unit,
Royal Marsden Hospital, London, UK

G.A. Sisson MD
Department of Otolaryngology,
Northwestern University, The Medical School,
Chicago, IL, USA

C.W. Smith MB FRCS DLO
Consultant Otolaryngologist, York Hospitals,
York, UK

G.D.L. Smyth MD FRCS
Consultant ENT Surgeon, Royal Victoria
Hospital, Belfast, N. Ireland, UK

G.B. Snow MD PhD
Professor and Chairman, Department of
Otolaryngology—Head and Neck Surgery, Free
University Hospital, Amsterdam, The Netherlands

M.F. Spittle MB BS MSc DMRT FRCR
Radiotherapist and Oncologist,
Meyerstein Institute of Radiotherapy and
Oncology, The Middlesex Hospital, London, UK

P.M. Stell ChM FRCS
Professor of Otolaryngology,
University of Liverpool, Liverpool, UK

S.D.G. Stephens MPhil MRCP
Physician in Charge, Welsh Hearing Institute,
University Hospital of Wales, Cardiff, UK

M.S. Strong MD FRCS
Professor, Department of Otolaryngology,
Boston University School of Medicine, Boston,
MA, USA

J. Thomsen MD PhD
University ENT Department, Gentofte Hospital,
Hellerup, Denmark

J.P. Tonkin AM MB BS(Syd.) DLO(Lond.)
FRCS(Eng.) FRACS
Chairman, Department of Otolaryngology,
St Vincent's Hospital, Sydney, NSW, Australia

M. Van Durme
Speech Therapist, University of Antwerp, Belgium

P.H. Ward MD FACS
Professor of Surgery and Chief, Division of Head
and Neck Surgery (Otolaryngology), UCLA School
of Medicine, Los Angeles, CA USA

Contents

1

What is informed consent?

B.J. Bailey

INTRODUCTION

The profession of medicine has changed dramatically during the first 85 years of this century. We often tend to focus upon the technological changes that have taken place, because they are quite dramatic and because they are constantly in the public spotlight. During the past decade, physicians in the United States have become acutely aware of the impact of economic, legal and political changes upon their personal medical practices.

Physicians are also acutely aware of the medical-legal crisis that has come to pervade our thinking and our actions in the course of daily medical practices. In fact, professional liability concerns are repeatedly ranked at the top of the list in surveys of physicians when they are asked to indicate the most serious problems they face in their professional lives. In spite of this concern, there is sometimes a lack of understanding with regard to the fundamental issues that underlie the specific circumstances that bring physicians to the courtroom.

Informed consent is one of the concepts about which physicians must become thoroughly informed. This is a welcome opportunity for me to express my personal opinions on this important topic and I want to make it clear that, in this essay, my views will be originating from the perspective of a surgeon who practises otolaryngology-head and neck surgery. I intend the information to be applicable to all physicians.

Informed consent is a new, revolutionary and very powerful concept. The fact that it has the potential to be a very positive force is often overlooked because of its frequent association with allegations that it has not been adequately provided to a particular patient.

In this essay, the goal will be to attempt to answer nine relevant questions:

1. Informed consent—what is it?
2. What are the origins and evolution of informed consent?
3. What are the basic elements of informed consent?
4. How does a physician accomplish it?
5. What are the obstacles to informed consent?
6. Why is informed consent necessary?
7. Why is there such ambiguity and inconsistency?
8. In what ways does it sometimes go astray?
9. Are there some special circumstances?

Informed consent—what is it?

Like so many phrases, the term informed consent sounds deceptively simple. It is the act of patient consent for a diagnostic or therapeutic intervention by the physician that is given after the patient has been informed about the event and its associated risks. The complex interaction between the professions of medicine and law has introduced a number of subtle, but extremely important additional stipulations that have transformed a simple act into a complex process.

In fact, it has become so complex that I sometimes wonder if we have forgotten about informed consent. Because informed consent has become such an operationally problematic issue, because it may be harmful to doctors and patients and because it may be harmful to the relationship between the two, it is seen by some physicians as a negative factor in their practice. The facts suggest, however, that if an individual physician (or if the profession generally) should attempt to discard the concept of informed consent, it would simply have to be re-

1

invented and re-established, because it is fundamental to the *trust* which underlies all interactions
between doctors/teachers/healers and their patients/
students.

The recent medical literature dealing with
informed consent has been enriched by contributions from many disciplines—physicians, nurses,
attorneys, legislators, ethicists, philosophers and
others. In their writings, they have often tried to
capture the essence of informed consent by means
of a term or phrase and there is great diversity in
the wording that has been used.

Informed consent has been referred to most
frequently as a *legal requirement/legal doctrine*
(Andrews 1984, Annas 1984, Cassell 1978, Gerber
1984, 1985, Healey 1984, Koopersmith 1984, Miller
1981, Pulmeri 1984, Redden & Baker 1984, White
1983). This designation refers to the legal force of
informed consent and has evolved through a series
of court decisions that have shaped and transformed
those features of informed consent that pertain to
the law.

The second most common designation for
informed consent is as an *obstacle/threat* to the
development of clinical research and such specialized
surgical areas as the implantation of prosthetic
devices (Cancer Research Campaign Working
Party in Breast Cancer 1983, Dudley 1984, Monaco
1983, Neville-Smith 1984, Reed & Camille 1985).
Many authors are quite impatient with the restric-
tions that are imposed by informed consent as it
relates to the impossible task of fully informing
individuals who might wish to consent to participate
in a clinical trial, or who might wish to have a
prosthetic device implanted, but who cannot be
fully informed of all of the potential risks because
these remain to be determined. Neither can the
physician clearly describe the relative advantages
or disadvantages compared to other forms of therapy
when that is precisely the reason for which the
investigation is being conducted.

The third most common term associated with
informed consent relates to it as a *document* or a
contract between a physician and a patient (Golan
& Ben-Hur 1983, *Hospital Progress* 1983, Klein
1984, Weaver 1984). While this might be considered
to be a narrow view, the practical matter is that
there are many specific features that are of great
importance to hospitals and hospital administrators.

This is also the mechanism by which documentation of informed consent has been obtained, and it
is the point at which the physician becomes vulnerable if it is not accomplished adequately.

Informed consent has also been described as a
mechanism or process (Lennox-Smith 1983, Macklin
1977), a medical-legal issue (Northrop 1985, Redden
et al 1985), a subject of widespread public interest
(Chalmers 1983, Lennox-Smith 1983), an ethical
principal (Chuang & Man 1983, Donagan 1977), a
constitutional right in the United States (Monaco
1983), a double-edged sword (The New England
Journal of Medicine 1984), an option rather than a
requirement for clinical research (*Lancet* Editorial
1984), and a consumerism issue that requires legis-
lative regulation (Berman 1984).

The more we learn about informed consent, the
more apparent it becomes that it is a multifaceted
concept. There is no doubt that it has become a
fundamental doctrine in the USA. Beyond that, it
is also a basic bioethical imperative and is the
foundation of the relationship of trust that must be
an integral part of the physician–patient relationship. It is necessary for patients to be fully informed
of all of the material facts in a medical decision
situation if they are going to have a real choice
among various options and if they are going to
participate actively in their own care, which is to
say in the determination of their fate.

Informed consent is the process of interaction
between a doctor and a patient that *must* take place
in order to generate the information that *both parties*
need in order to reach a rational decision about
therapy, in order to plan for the future, and in order
to maintain their relationship beyond the early
evaluation period and into the phase of treatment
and long-term management. The way in which this
process unfolds frequently foretells the degree of
success that will be achieved in the treatment or
management of the entire illness, and in that regard
informed consent may serve as a 'marker' or pre-
dictor of the therapeutic outcome.

Informed consent is a very strong concept, and
in spite of its many imperfections, it will endure.
As noted by Cassell (1978):

> That patients forget things or may deny unpleasant
> realities in no way detracts from their right to exercise
> choice or participate in their own care to the degree
> that they can and wish or do not wish. It should always

be remembered that informed consent is a concept whose force should come not primarily from its legal necessity, but rather from its enhancement of good medical care. The needs of the patient should dictate its form and content.

Origins and evolution of informed consent

The past 85 years have been a period of remarkable transition in society with regard to all of its traditional institutions. Medicine has not been isolated from these events, and during this century there has been a great emphasis upon the rights of the individual and the importance of involving individual patients in all medical decisions. Informed consent is simply one small part of the transition from a *paternalistic* approach to medicine, in which the physician functioned as a parent might in the course of advising a child, to a new concept of *autonomy* in which the patient is responsible for all major decisions.

If we focus upon the legalistic aspects of this transition, we note that there are many courts and many cases in various geographical locations that have influenced the shape and appearance of this doctrine. From an analysis of many of these cases we have drawn six that serve as examples of landmark changes in the legal doctrine of informed consent.

The first case we should examine is *Mohr* v. *Williams* (Koopersmith 1984), which was the first judicial decision in the USA to recognize the existence of the tort concept in recovery for medical misadventures through a suit filed against a physician. This was the case of a surgeon practising in the State of Minnesota who obtained the patient's consent for an operation on the right ear, but who performed the actual operation on the patient's left ear, presumably because it was the site of more serious disease. The Minnesota court held that the 'the act of the defendant (physician) amounted at least to a technical *assault and battery*' and that 'a citizen's first and greatest right is the inviolability of his person'.

The case of *Mohr* v. *Williams* in 1905 truly marked the end of an era and opened the doors for today's tensions between the professions of law and medicine.

Nine years later, in 1914, the case of *Schloendorff* v. *the Society of New York Hospitals* (Koopersmith 1984) took the process further. This was a case in which a patient thought she was undergoing a diagnostic abdominal surgical procedure. The surgeon removed a fibroid tumour and acknowledged that he had performed a therapeutic operation because it was in the best interest of the patient even though he had not obtained consent for that. The court ruled that this operation, without the patient's consent, amounted to a situation in which the surgeon has committed '*trespass*'. The judge's statement in this case could be viewed as the second cornerstone of the concept of autonomy as opposed to paternalism. The judge stated:

> . . . every human being of adult years and sound mind has a right to determine what shall be done with his own body, and a surgeon who performs an operation without his patient's consent commits an assault, for which he is liable in damages. . . . This is true except in cases of emergency where the patient is unconscious and where it is necessary to operate before consent can be obtained.

In spite of such a remarkable start, the revolution from paternalism to autonomy was delayed, perhaps because there was no 'grass roots' sentiment for this transition. It may well be that patients felt that the change was unnecessary, or perhaps that they were not ready to handle the responsibility for life and death decisions that was being offered to them. One might well imagine that there would be some scepticism among patients during the first half of this century with regard to whether or not the new system would be better for them.

In any event, there was little substantive change for almost 50 years. There were relatively minor adjustments in the relationship between physician and patient, physician and attorney, and physician and liability insurance carrier. There was a trickle of 'malpractice' litigation, but still, most patients tended to place themselves into the hands of their personal physician with a general attitude of 'do what you feel is best for me, you understand the complexities of medical decisions, and I do not'.

The second round of change actually began at the end of World War II in 1945. The years between 1945 and 1960 saw three major trials that affected the concept of informed consent. These three trials were the *Nuremberg Trials* (resulting in the (*Nuremberg Code*), *Salgo* v. *Stanford*, and *Natanson* v. *Kline*.

Let us look first at the issue around the Nuremberg Trials and the Nuremberg Code. At the end of World War II, people were shocked to learn of the 'brutal medical experiments' that had been conducted within Hitler's Third Reich. Those responsible for these travesties were brought to trial and the results of multiple trials, involving many types of offences and occurring over many years, were the basis for several modifications of legal doctrine as embodied in the Nuremberg Code. The strategy of the defence in these trials was limited for obvious reasons. The defence attorneys were unable to claim that the subjects had benefited from these 'experiments'. There certainly had been no effort made to obtain subject consent, so the defence attorneys had no option other than an argument 'that consent is not legally essential'.

That defence was actually rather interesting and its believability (limited though it is) rests on three points that the defence had to establish:

1. That the State has the right to demand of its individual citizens that they make certain sacrifices for the greater good of the total community, and that the State alone may decide the nature and degree of those sacrifices,

2. That there is no real distinction between the conscription of citizens to serve in the military, to drop an atomic bomb on an enemy city, or to submit to medical experimentation. The ultimate goal is the best thing for the community.

3. That there were many historical precedents for medical experimentation being conducted without the informed consent of the subjects (e.g. prisoners, inmates of mental institutions, etc.) and that the word 'volunteer' was often a camouflage and a hypocrisy.

The above arguments failed in the Nuremberg Trials and the outcome was formalized in the Nuremberg Code. Its basic theme was that the rights of the individual were declared to be paramount. Henceforth, experimentation would not be permitted without the *informed consent* of the subjects. In a larger context, the concept of a greater common good became subordinate and the era of rugged individualism became dominant.

But we are ahead of ourselves in the story, because the phrase 'informed consent' was used for the first time in the 1957 case of *Salgo* v. *Leland Stanford Jr, University Board of Trustees*. In this case, the patient suffered paralysis following diagnostic aortography and sued on the basis that there had been no disclosure of the risks of this diagnostic procedure. The court ruled that failure to inform the patient adequately is a form of *negligence*, and went on to state:

> . . . a physician violates his duty to his patient and subjects himself to liability if he withholds any facts necessary to form the basis of an intelligent consent by the patient to the proposed treatment. Likewise the physician may not minimize the known dangers of a procedure or operation in order to induce his patient's consent.

The introduction of the concept of *negligence* has turned out to be quite important. No longer is it necessary for the physician to simply stay within the bounds of what he has contracted with the patient; now the validity of the contract itself is being questioned. If the outcome of either a diagnostic or a therapeutic intervention is harmful to the patient, the focus of the court centres upon whether or not the contract between the patient and the physician was flawed.

The next important event occurred three years later, in 1960. One might assume that if a recommended treatment is entirely conventional or standard (e.g. radiation therapy) and if that treatment is undertaken to cure a life-threatening condition (such as cancer), that there would be little likelihood of the physician being sued successfully by a patient.

It turns out that one would be incorrect in making such an assumption. In the case of *Natanson* v. *Kline*, a patient was treated for breast cancer by a series of cobalt radiotherapy treatments. Subsequently, the patient suffered soft tissue and bone damage and brought suit against the radiotherapist. The court heard the facts and then held that, in the absence of an emergency, the physician has a duty to disclose *all* of the known risks of the treatment to the patient. Failure to do so places the doctor in a position of personal liability.

These last two cases were the prototypes for the most common form of contemporary professional liability suits—namely, the allegation that the treating physician was negligent in his duty to inform the patient of *all reasonable risks* according to a presumed standard of disclosure.

But what is the nature of the presumed standard

of disclosure and what efforts have been made to assure that it is *reasonable* in terms of both the physician and the patient? What is the yardstick by which our disclosure to our patients is to be measured.

The answers to these questions have been variable, ambiguous and changing. The case of *Canterbury* v. *Spence* (Klein 1984, Koopersmith 1984) is one of the most famous landmark cases of the 1970s that served to determine the nature of both the yardstick and how it is to be used. The patient developed paralysis after a laminectomy and subsequently alleged that certain *material* facts were not disclosed and that, had these facts been disclosed, consent for the surgery would not have been granted. The new twist in *Canterbury* v. *Spence* was the decision by the court to forego reliance upon the testimony of expert medical witnesses to establish whether or not the facts were indeed material (or integral) to the concept of an informed consent. In essence, the court made the transition from a 'professional' basis for the yardstick (having physician expert witnesses questioned about what would be expected of reasonable physician practitioners) to a 'lay' basis for the yardstick. The new point of reference was based upon what a reasonable patient would consider or judge to be *material* information in the sense of being a necessary consideration for arriving at a position of understanding sufficient to generate an informed consent. To a degree, *Canterbury* v. *Spence* delegated the concept of 'expertness' in medical litigation to a secondary position. Expert witnesses could provide explanations, perspectives and opinions, but they were no longer *essential* to the legal process.

There have been other cases that have made specific technical contributions to the movement of informed consent from the background to the forefront of medicolegal activity, but these six landmark trials have provided the stepping-stones for the journey across the legal stream.

The transition has been only one small segment of the larger movement within society from paternalism to autonomy. Unless it is viewed within this context, it is difficult to interpret the unfolding of events.

The contemporary interface between medicine and law can be characterized as it pertains to the concept/legal doctrine of informed consent. This can be accomplished only when the physician and the patient have met the following requirements:

1. The physician discloses all of the material information regarding the procedure. This must include the nature of the procedure, along with material risks, complications and options that are known.

2. The patient must be competent and must understand the disclosure that has been made. After an appropriate period of discussion and consideration, the patient shall decide voluntarily to accept or refuse that which is proposed.

As Redden & Baker (1984) point out, the system can break down at any of several points, leading to a potential for litigation. Patients may bring suit against the physician for performing an operation without their consent (battery), or when consent was given, but the patient had not been informed adequately (negligence). Most of the cases in the USA at present are filed on the basis of negligence. This requires the plaintiff to prove that an injury has been sustained. In addition, it must be established that (1) there was a reasonably foreseeable risk that the injury would occur, (2) the risk was not disclosed to the patient, and (3) the procedure would not have been accepted by the patient if the risk had been disclosed.

What are the rules and elements of informed consent?

In a practical sense, informed consent was first articulated forcefully in the Nuremberg Code, and it is the basic points of this Code that constitute its framework. During the course of its evolution, many organizations have endorsed informed consent as a part of the individual human rights movement and several organizations, such as the American Medical Association, the American Psychological Association and the American Hospital Association, have endorsed the principles in general and have modified the details to reflect their particular perspectives. The United States Department of Health, Education and Welfare (DHEW), which is now the Department of Health and Human Services, issued a definition of informed consent in 1975 which included the following:

The knowing consent of an individual or her legal representative, so situated as to be able to exercise free power of choice without undue inducement or any element of force, fraud, deceit, duress, or other forms of constraint or coercion. The basic elements of information necessary to such consent include:

1. A fair explanation of the procedures to be followed, and their purposes, including identification of any procedures which are experimental.

2. A description of any attendant discomfort and risks reasonably to be expected.

3. A description of any benefits reasonably to be expected.

4. Disclosure of any appropriate alternative procedures that might be advantageous for the subject.

5. An offer to answer any inquiries concerning procedures.

6. An instruction that the person is free to withdraw and discontinue participation in the project or activity at any time without prejudice to the subject.

Chuang & Man (1983) provide an excellent discussion of some of the rules for obtaining informed consent that have resulted from some of the lawsuits pertaining to informed consent.

There is the question, 'Who is responsible for obtaining the informed consent?'. It is clear that the primary responsibility rests with the physician who is in charge of the patient. However, it has been found acceptable in several recent court cases for the actual obtaining of the consent to be performed by clinical staff members, as long as they are adequately trained for the task. In view of the fact that a great deal of time may be required to obtain informed consent, it is reassuring that several studies have indicated that the quality of the informed consent is not diminished when designated individuals are utilized. My personal preference for obtaining informed consent is to accomplish the task in three steps. In the case of a proposed operation, the first discussion takes place in the outpatient setting when the operation is proposed. We take as much time as is necessary to exchange information with each other and, when the patient consents to admission to the hospital for surgery, I still view this as only a tentative consent. After admission to the hospital, I engage in a review of what I consider to be the most important information and answer any questions that may have occurred to the patient since our first conversation. If a general consent to proceed is obtained at that point, I then ask one of our senior residents to discuss all of the details of the risks, complications and alternatives with the patient, without being

present myself. Nursing personnel are often involved as well in this third step.

There are also certain rules with regard to the method of obtaining informed consent and these rules vary from state to state in this country (USA). In many settings, the surgeon will employ standardized consent forms in order to be in compliance with the law. This form was developed in order to be in compliance with the laws of the State of Texas in regard to informed consent. While this approach is taken in only a few states at the present time, it is likely that the number will increase over the next decade. Regardless of the document itself, Chuang & Man feel that the following three elements are essential if the requirements for informed consent are to be met:

. . . (a) the method of communication must be comprehensible to the patient, (b) the patient must be given an adequate opportunity to ask questions, and (c) the communication must be recorded so that its existence as well as appropriateness is documented for future examination.

As mentioned previously, there are a number of inconsistencies with regard to the standard that is applied to judge informed consent. While there is a variable application of assessment of the adequacy of informed consent, the two types of standards that are employed are the 'community standard' (or professional standard) and the 'material risk standard'. The community standard is a requirement that the physician in charge disclose information in the manner and to an extent that other similar physicians in the community would disclose under the same circumstances. The material risk standard shifts the focus to the patient, rather than the physician. It requires the physicians to disclose information that would be considered material or significant by a 'reasonable patient' who is confronted with the need for a specific diagnostic or therapeutic intervention. Obviously, both of these standards are open to very wide differences of interpretation. It may be helpful at this point to comment briefly on what the informed consent is *not*. The concept of informed consent is not the same as an 'educated consent' and it never can be. An educated consent would be a standard of information exchange which permitted the patient to know and understand everything that the physician knows and understands. When these cases are held up for close scrutiny and criticism in the legal courts, patients frequently claim that they recall hearing all of the words, but that they did not understand fully what was meant and, on this basis, they challenge the validity of the consent obtained. This the 'twilight zone' that forms the basis for most of the litigation with which we are confronted. Even when patients indicate that they understand fully the information that has been provided, we must remember that this understanding is on a very superficial level and that we eventually reach a point beyond which the patient cannot progress further in terms of understanding. At this point, the decision becomes a matter of faith and this may be the most important value associated with our efforts to obtain informed consent. The fact that we are working diligently to explain as much to every patient as they can possibly understand, leads most of them to sense that they are placing their trust in an individual who is truly concerned about their welfare. If there were no reason for informed consent other than this one, it would be sufficient to justify our continuing efforts.

How does the physician obtain informed consent?

There are some 'dos' and some 'don'ts' in regard to the obtaining of informed consent. The responsibility for completing the task successfully rests with the physician and, therefore, it is the physician's responsibility to initiate the dialogue. The conversation must be established in the tone and at the level most clearly comprehensible to the patient.

The discussion usually begins with a description of the facts as they relate to the disease process and is usually a clear listing of the facts that are known in each of the areas to be covered. Having completed this and answered any questions the physician begins to interpret the facts and to explain what has been said until the patient can either paraphrase or begin to ask questions that indicate a level of comprehension of what is being discussed.

It is advisable to project the situation into the future in a manner that is understandable without being overly threatening to the patient. The physician must explain what will happen if nothing is done and how the absence of the proposed action will

affect the patient, the family, ability to work and other related issues. At this point it is usually logical to bring things back to the present and to explain objectively the therapeutic options that are available and their relative probabilites of being successful. There should be a discussion concerning the risks, the costs, the discomfort, the inconvenience, the timing, the sequence of events and as much material information as is reasonable and *appropriate* to the situation and the personality of the physician, the patient, and the patient's family.

Obviously, this takes a long time and this is further support for the position that informed consent must be done in stages, with time for the patient to absorb the information and the impact of the information upon their lives. Many patients are unable to ask any questions at the time of the initial discussion, but come back with a long list of questions subsequently.

In summary then, obtaining informed consent in the ideal circumstances will involve an exchange of information through the process of rational discourse and is likely to facilitate the care and management of the patient by building an environment of trust while simultaneously complying with the legal requirements that have been imposed. As pointed out by Cassell (1978) one must avoid such pitfalls as hiding or shading the truth and must keep the discussion free of extraneous personal bias and motivations. At the same time, it is important to avoid an overemphasis on the negative side of the picture which might result from an encyclopaedic and graphic list of all possible known risks and hazards. This is such a formidable task that it is unlikely that it is ever accomplished with perfection, but both the physician and the patient should gain from the effort that is made.

What are the obstacles to informed consent?

There are many explanations for the imperfection that creeps into the process of obtaining informed consent. In this section, we shall comment upon a dozen of these obstacles, while acknowledging that there are probably at least as many that we have overlooked.

1. First and foremost is the patient's lack of medical knowledge. In spite of our best efforts to

present information clearly and understandably, it must be acknowledged that there is always some degree of limitation in the understanding of the issues. The physician must be alert to the signs and symptoms of misunderstanding, just as he/she is alert to medical signs and symptoms.

2. Beyond the specific shortcomings in medical knowledge, patients are generally naive in a scientific sense. Patients often realize that they do not understand 'doctor talk', but may be unaware of their deficits in comprehending scientific fundamentals. Generally, they are unused to dealing with the abstract concepts of mathematical probability, with decision sequences and with uncontrolled variables. It is important to review all of these issues as they pertain to specific medical and surgical problems, but it is equally important to avoid conveying the impression that so much is unknown that the entire therapeutic process is just a matter of luck.

3. The emotional state of the patient may be a serious obstacle and the level of anxiety and fear must be considered as the discussions progress.

4. The discussion may be impeded by a patient bias that is secondary to some powerful prior life experience. For example, in discussing chemotherapy with patients, they may have a strong reaction on the basis of their observation of a relative who had chemotherapy many years ago and who became extremely ill. There are also certain religious doctrines that bias the discussion; for example, the prohibition of blood transfusion by the beliefs of Jehovah's Witness patients without regard to any mitigating factors or consequences.

5. The discussion may be blocked by impaired cognition on the part of the patient. This may be the result of the disease process itself or may be secondary to educational or language deficits. It is also clearly a factor in regard to these discussions when they are conducted with children.

6. Patient defence mechanisms may be excessively developed so that they will simply refuse to believe that any of this is happening to them. Others may be unwilling to engage in the discussion because of an overdeveloped sense of *fatalism*, and the feeling that the outcome is predetermined and 'what will be, will be'.

7. The emotional background and feelings of patients may inhibit their comprehension of the issues that must be faced. Excessive amounts of guilt, grief, hostility, or suspicion may prevent their participation in a discussion that must be based on logic and rational considerations.

8. There may be problems with informed consent when the communication with the patient involves physicians from several disciplines. At times, we have noted confusion and conflict when several different individuals are involved in the obtaining of informed consent. This is a particular problem in the case of randomized clinical trials (Cancer Research Campaign Working Party in Breast Cancer 1983) and may become a major obstacle in the contemporary health science centre where great pains have been taken to organize activities so that they are in compliance with a 'team health care' concept. Well-intentioned medical students, nurses, social services staff and others each make an effort to deal with the patient's problems independently. In the worst possible circumstance, there may be actual open competition between disciplines as they compete for the patient's decision in regard to therapy. This invariably results in serious conflict and in a breakdown of patient trust with regard to the entire institution and must be avoided.

9. The law itself may become a problem, especially when it is misunderstood or misinterpreted. The zealous pursuit of informed consent may result in unreasonably explicit or detailed descriptions of the risks and complications that could occur, for example, following any surgical procedure. Commonsense and compassion for patient feelings must be balanced against full disclosure of all material information.

10. The pressure of time and schedules can be an obstacle on the part of the physician or the patient. Time pressures cause two problems. The first is the problem of a discussion that is unreasonably short. There might be a temptation on the part of either party to abbreviate areas of discussion that are necessary for a full exchange of information. The second problem that can arise is the perception on the part of the patient that the physician is in too much of a hurry to conduct the discussion properly. The relationship is definitely 'off on the wrong foot' when the patient concludes that other things are more important to the physician than the best interest of the patient.

11. Informed consent can be subverted when-

ever elements of coercion begin to intrude into the process. Coercion may be overt or covert and may arise from any of a variety of factors. The problem of 'leaning too hard' on the patient must be kept clearly in mind at all times so that individual patients have autonomy that is complete in regard to the decisions that affect them. These issues of coercion become complicated when they involve strongly held religious beliefs on the part of the patient, or rigid views of parents when there are decisions involving the care of their children. Macklin (1977) addresses this subject from both perspectives and concludes with the following comment:

> I have argued that the autonomy of patients, as rational persons, ought to be respected. But this autonomy implies a responsibility for one's decisions—a responsibility that entails acceptance of the consequences. And these consequences include the right of physicians to reject a treatment regimen proposed by the patient, which is contrary to sound medical practice. . . . the risks are indeed great in the cases we have been discussing. But the sorts of risks to health or life a person may take, in the interest of something he considers worth the risk, appear to know no bounds. If an adult agent is rational and competent to make decisions, the risks are his to take.

12. Ambiguity is an ever present phenomenon in the course of all human communication. In spite of all of our efforts to speak clearly and understandably, we, as physicians, frequently fall short in our efforts to communicate with precision. Another source of ambiguity can arise when we fail to listen. Monaco (1983) emphasizes this when she states the following in regard to obtaining informed consent from parents of children who need therapy:

> Quality in, quality out. The consent process can be complete and realistic, or it can be a sham. The key is in whether physicians listen to parents' questions and answer them. It must be certain that information is given on what is happening, that the parent is told what could happen in the specific treatment involved, and that the information given is up-to-date.
>
> A parent's decision as surrogate for a child can only be as good as the information that physicians provide.

What are the sources and types of ambiguity in informed consent?

There are a number of points during the course of obtaining informed consent where ambiguity may become a problem for either the physician or patient. This ambiguity may be conscious or subconscious on the part of either participant in the discussion.

The physician may express himself ambiguously with regard to the relative importance of a long list of benefits when they are compared with a long list of risks. It is difficult for both the physician and the patient to process this information intellectually when there are emotional overtones of anxiety and confusion. Having been informed of some 'bad news' in regard to a disease, one should expect that the patient and the patient's family will be worried, frightened and somewhat confused. Many thoughts and concerns will be running through their minds, particularly in the time immediately after they have been informed that there is a problem that requires treatment. At the other extreme one occasionally finds patients and families where there is an unrealistic degree of hopefulness, wishful thinking and optimistic expectation. Patients and families with a pre-existing prejudice in either direction tend to hear and remember only the most positive or the most negative aspects of the discussion.

Another area where the process of informed consent begins to be threatened by ambiguity lies in the language that is often used by physicians. When we describe complex disease processes and our intervention for them, whether it be in verbal communication or in scientific articles, the language used is often rich in adjectival and adverbial adornment and, therefore, carries a great temptation to 'tilt' the discussion in a more positive direction. For example, a surgeon may view surgery as the most effective modality in most instances of a particular illness that is amenable to surgical intervention, and may have held that view since his days as a medical student. That may be the reason for seeking surgical training and for pursuing a career as a surgeon. It is very difficult for such an individual to present advice that is entirely free of bias.

Another source for the introduction of subtle bias arises when it is almost certain that the patient will require surgery if a healthy state is to be restored. As paternalistic as it may be, it is also an act of human kindness to emphasize the positive possibility of a successful outcome and to minimize the risks and complications. Similarly, it would be unkind to be totally comprehensive and explicit in describing every conceivable risk and complication associated with the surgical procedure.

Most physicians have a tendency to be slightly optimistic or slightly pessimistic as a part of their general personality. That particular subjective personality tilt may creep into the language that is used and may cause phrases like 'most of the time' to begin to blend into the phrase 'usually' as the discussion progresses and perhaps to even shift gently to a point of 'almost always' by the time the description and the interaction between physician and patient have been concluded.

Ambiguity may arise out of the aura of physician authority (or even infallibility in the extreme case) that may be excessively formed in the mind of either the patient or the physician. When these authoritarian characteristics exert their influence on the informed consent communication, the process may indeed become paternalistic, rather than participatory.

There may be ambiguity based on the failure of the physician to converse on the proper level for full and complete understanding on the part of the patient. This may be associated with a considerable amount of non-verbal communication on the part of either party, the mannerisms of the physician may interject strong and persuasive accents on top of very objective speech without the physician even being aware of the impact of his body language. The patient may engage in body language that is equally destructive to a full and comprehensive exchange. This may take the form of head nodding which the physician interprets as full and complete understanding, while the patient may be nodding, only as a sign of respect for the physician or for other inappropriate reasons.

In addition to the ambiguity that arises in individual discussions, there is a further ambiguity in regard to discussions that deal with the concept of informed consent. Legal interpretations and requirements are different, not only in different geographic locations around the globe, but even in different states within this country. Beyond that, there are extreme variations in the receptivity of the concept of informed consent by society generally in different countries and by different professions. In fact, the concept is not at all welcome in many parts of the world, as emphasized by Gerber (1984) who states the following:

> . . . it seems that, on present indications, the strict informed consent doctrine first enunciated in the USA,

is unlikely to take root in Australia. The American doctrine, clearly formulated in *Canterbury* v. *Spence* affirmed that it was for the *law*, not for *medicine* to determine the standard of care which a physician owes to his patient in the area disclosure. . . . This case highlighted a shift in emphasis away from what a careful doctor ought to *tell* to what a prudent patient ought to *know*. . . . The Australian position is vastly different. What constitutes reasonable disclosure is, it would seem, a matter left largely to the good sense of the medical profession.

How did informed consent get such a tarnished image?

It would seem that, on balance, there are many more good features than bad to the process of informed consent. If that is true, why do we find so much opposition to this doctrine and why do so many physicians view the process negatively? There appear to be several related answers to these questions, and half a dozen of these answers will be noted and discussed briefly in the remainder of this section.

Firstly, in the education of the present generation of physicians, there was an overemphasis on the concept of 'high-tech' and an underemphasis on 'high-touch'. Sophisticated technology has enabled the medical field to diagnose and treat patients more effectively and precisely than ever before, but it has extracted in return a high price. It has taken some of the personal touch and some of the art away from medicine and has replaced it with expensive machinery. Many physicians view informed consent as the equivalent of a signed operative or diagnostic procedure consent form. In some situations, informed consent even became a responsibility handled by a brochure or video tape. On an intermediate level, there are situations in which the entire process of informed consent is the responsibility of a nurse, medical student or resident physician in training. Informed consent continues to be the responsibility of the most senior or responsible physician on the treatment team and, because it is time consuming and these individuals tend to be inordinately busy, informed consent has become a nuisance and a time drain for many physicians.

Informed consent underwent a negative transition during the time that it was subtly evolving from a positive role in the doctor–patient interaction and bond toward a new position where it is seen as a legal threat to the practice of medicine. It may not be overly critical to state that certain opportunistic attorneys have exploited the flaws in the process to infer that some degree of physician negligence is always present in these situations so that a patient may claim a *lack of understanding* of the disease process, the evaluation, or the treatment. As a major part of the malpractice crisis of the past decade, 'the informed consent controversy' was launched and underway.

Subsequently, the physician/explainer developed a more defensive posture and tried to avoid any area of patient misunderstanding through the use of longer, more detailed, more explicit, more frightening communications with patients. The objective seemed to be an *educated consent*, but that was a concept that was unattainable by definition. There simply is not enough time to accomplish an educated consent, a condition in which everything that is discussed is fully understood by the patient. There have been instances of consent forms of more than 15 pages for some complex surgical procedures, such as the implantation of an artificial heart. Excessive attention to the legal aspects of informed consent are simply another stimulus that moves things in the direction of depersonalization of medical practice.

The subtleties of the shift of informed consent from a process designed to meet valid patient needs to a process designed to protect the physician or the hospital from litigation were not lost on either party. It became a negative experience for both parties, something to be tolerated and endured, but not enjoyed.

Donagan (1977) comments upon this transition in the following manner:

> . . . the truth appears to be that, before the public at large thought of it at all, the problem of informed consent became a matter of controversy in the medical profession because of changes in the relations of physicians to patients, and of experimental medicine to clinical medicine, of which physicians naturally became conscious before the public. The contribution of laymen to defining some of the issues cannot be denied. But the doctrine of informed consent as we now have it is principally the achievement of the medical professional: lawyers and politicians entered the field late, and their contribution has been secondary. Philosophers, in good Hegelian fashion, for the most part arrived to take stock after the work had been done.

It became a popular topic for the bioethical community and a popular topic for medical authors. It became an appropriate subject for experimentation and innovation. It has even become an important philosophical item in the human rights movement of this past century. To the degree that a process, which was heretofore a personal dialogue between physician and a patient, has become the property of so many interests outside of medicine, it has come to be viewed less positively by the medical profession. We seem to have many individuals very interested in our activities and it seems to us that it sometimes goes beyond the valid point of physician accountability. Perhaps we are becoming somewhat paranoid about such matters, but, if the threat to the practice of medicine at a level of high quality and compassion is not imaginary, our concern should not be termed paranoia.

Patients, attorneys, judges and philosophers have been influential in stimulating and shaping many fundamental changes in the *concept* of informed consent. It is a very uncommon event for a physician to be accused of providing treatment without the patient's consent. It is even quite uncommon for physicians to be accused of obtaining consent by misrepresentation. The usual assertion is that important facts never came up for discussion, and thereby the patient was pre-empted from exercising a personal right to participate in an informed decision. It is then asserted that the physician is not competent if he is unable to describe in words that can be understood everything that could matter to the individual as a patient in the course of the treatment that is being proposed. It is little wonder that with the frequency of the allegations, many of which take the form of frivolous legal suits, that physicians are developing some adverse behaviour in regard to informed consent.

Are there special circumstances regarding informed consent?

There are a number of situations in which the usual guidelines and methodology for obtaining informed consent may be modified.

1. *Clinical research* often contains a mixture of research and medical treatment. For example, when one is evaluating the therapeutic safety and effectiveness of a new operation, there are many

unknown risks and complications and it becomes difficult to compare the unknown outcome of the new procedure with the known outcome of existing operative techniques. The modified guidelines for conducting clinical research must always contain certain key elements.

a. There must be a full explanation of all that is known at the time in regard to risks, complications and alternative therapy.

b. There must be a complete understanding of the proposed intervention by the patient.

c. The patient's consent must be freely given.

d. The element of therapy must be primary and the element of research must be secondary.

Clinical medicine always contains some elements of novelty or experimentation. Problems arise when these are not presented in the form of a controlled clinical investigation, but are simply interjected casually into the practice of medicine without the patient's awareness of the element of experimentation.

As noted by Donagan (1977) the existing laws permit the concept of an individual becoming a 'volunteer' and placing himself in a dangerous situation where harm could result from a new treatment (or where there could be less good obtained than from standard treatment). The Nuremberg Trials and the subsequent Nuremberg Code raised a challenge to the traditional concept of 'volunteers' and started a new trend that makes it much harder (in some instances nearly impossible) to conduct research involving potentially coercible subjects such as prisoners, soldiers, or children.

This tightening of the clinical research system was increased by the case involving the Jewish Chronic Diseases Hospital (1963), in which an experiment was conducted that involved patients at that institution. The director of JCDH allowed physicians from an outside cancer research institute to inject suspensions of cultured human cancer cells into 22 patients in order to study the mechanism and rate of rejection of the injected material. Suit was brought against the medical director who asserted that he had obtained verbal consent from the subjects, but that they had not been told that cancer cells would be injected, because that information would generate too much fear. Ultimately, the medical director and the principal investigator were found to be guilty of fraud and deceit in the

practice of medicine. The defence was that the full extent of the information was withheld 'for the good of the subjects' so that they would not become unreasonably anxious about the possibility of 'getting cancer' when there was no known risk of that possibility.

The Helsinki Declaration in 1963 further clarified some of the ambiguities in regard to clinical research. All of us who engage in clinical investigation are well aware of the safeguards, checks and balances, and complexities of obtaining institutional, peer-reviewed, approval for the work that needs to be done. There is an attitude of negativity with regard to these 'obstacles' to the conduct of clinical research, but, upon reflection, one realizes that without these safeguards, a few individuals would engage in practices that would jeopardize the entire enterprise of clinical investigation and perhaps create a situation in which it truly does become impossible.

For philosophers, there is less interest in these practical problems and more interest in some of the fascinating arguments that can be raised. If there is a greater good for society (in the form of the new information that will be derived from the research), then it may be argued that individual rights are secondary to the more important rights of the group (society at large). It might, therefore, be permissible to proceed with research on the basis of govermental conscription or the lawful compulsion of research subjects as was debated in the Nuremberg Trials, or by deceitful or incompletely obtained informed consent as in the case of the JCDH investigations.

The special nature of clinical investigation, in regard to informed consent, is that it must be imperfect by definition. While this creates certain challenges for the investigators, these hurdles are not insurmountable.

2. The second area of controversy and deviation from the standard guideline for informed consent involves those patients who *refuse lifesaving treatment*. The classic example of this patient group is the individual who is a member of the religious faith known as Jehovah's Witnesses. It is a tenet of their faith that they may not receive blood or blood products from other individuals, even if it is needed under lifesaving circumstances. There are court cases in which adult individuals and children (whose refusal is being managed by adults) were coerced

into accepting transfusions by a court order. These complex issues are reviewed by Mackland (1977) and by Miller (1981) in review articles that provide an in-depth look at the issues that are involved.

Equally fascinating are the issues in regard to decisions to refuse lifesaving treatment by individuals who are not refusing on religious grounds. An example might be an elderly, educated, terminal cancer patient who has suffered a myocardial infarct and has been resuscitated successfully following cardiac arrest but who now insists, in the event of a subsequent cardiac arrest, that there be no effort made for further resuscitation.

A slightly different set of circumstances and factors for consideration would be raised by a nonpsychotic individual who has suffered organic brain effects from disease or medication and who now insists irrationally upon refusing all further appropriate care. Other examples might include the suicidal patient, or the incompetent patient who refuses medical care.

These are examples of patients who are expressing their individual autonomy as patients to be in complete command of their fate. The reaction of individual physicians and of specific courts has been variable, but one has no difficulty observing a legal trend in the direction of greater patient autonomy.

3. Chuang & Man (1983) have noted that there are a number of legal precedents in regard to situations in which physicians, as defendants, have won lawsuits in the absence of documented informed consent:

a. Treatment or tests under police order or court order.

b. When there is a risk that exists only when an operation is performed improperly.

c. When the procedure involves minor or remote risks.

d. When the risks and alternatives are not known to the medical community at the time of the treatment.

e. When the risks, benefits, discomfort and alternatives are common knowledge.

f. When it can be shown that the patient was aware of the risks.

g. When the physician can prove that the patient's behaviour indicated 'implied consent'.

h. When the patient might experience undue distress or stress in the process of disclosure.

i. When the patient has requested not to go through the process of informed consent and has waived his or her right without encouragement from the physician.

Some of these items described above have been discussed in the pertinent literature under the headings of *therapeutic privilege*, which is a vague, but implied, right of the physician in some instances to withhold informed consent because of his very strongly held feeling that it would have a powerful, negative impact on the treatment programme in process.

The matter of waiver of informed consent as a patient option is certainly a controversial concept. The waiving of informed consent, when suggested by the physician, or the decision to exercise therapeutic privilege, would certainly be circumstances that would suggest a high degree of paternalism on the part of the patient.

CONCLUSION

Informed consent is a multifaceted concept. Like a chameleon, it changes its appearance when placed on different backgrounds, or when seen in a different light. It is particularly susceptible to differences in perception that are dependent upon the eyes of different beholders.

Pragmatically, informed consent is an essential element of surgical practice whose force is derived from what it can do to improve the quality of the physician–patient relationship by showing the patient that the doctor cares for the patient as a person. Secondarily, it is a legal doctrine that can be ignored only at great peril to the physician or clinical investigator.

Methodically, it is an intellectual, dialogue-based process of explanation, discussion and feedback that moves the decision and consent objectives from the older, paternalistic position to a point of greater patient autonomy.

Philosophically, it is the mechanism by which individual physicians translate the general body of medical morality into moral medical action.

Ethically, it is the medical portion of the centuries-long emergence of individual freedom, being part of the marching parade that includes the Magna Carta, the Declaration of Independence and the

Emancipation Proclamation. Whether we like it or not, the forces at work in society invariably produce changes within medicine. The rights and authority of the individual are increasing and the rights and authority of governments, social institutions (churches, schools, etc.) and healers are decreasing. Patients may vary considerably in their desires for detail in the information that is presented to them, but they do wish to know about what is being proposed and to participate in important medical decisions.

Metaphorically, informed consent is a double-edged sword (The New England Journal of Medicine 1984). One edge is the positive effect of information in reassuring the anxious patient who is facing the unknown and strengthening the doctor–patient bond. The other edge is the negative effect of frightening to patients with complicated and pessimistic information. The objective nature of unbiased, scientific communication usually carries a distant, dispassionate and uncaring flavour that is the opposite of the needed physicians' compassion.

Informed consent can be a heavy burden for the physician. It thrusts upon a surgeon a major responsibility that is above and beyond diagnosis and treatment. It drains time and energy from a doctor's day, while adding medical legal risks to the practice of medicine. In spite of this, it carries potential for great good. Arising as an outgrowth of the larger social movement for greater individual freedom and self-determination, it has become an important focal point in the doctor–patient decision-making partnership. The challenge for each of us is to take informed consent seriously and to develop the mature judgement that is necessary to limit the potential for harm and to exploit the opportunities for improved patient care.

The physician must have at his command a certain ready wit for dourness is repulsive to both the healthy and the sick.

(Hippocrates)

Answering the question, 'What is informed consent?' may provide the lawyer with a dilemma but not the doctor. The Nuremberg Code sets out the circumstances in which the medical profession can experiment on human beings, but it is equally appropriate to apply it to the daily care of the sick. If the word treatment is substituted for experiment the code reads as follows:

The voluntary consent of the human subject is absolutely essential. This means that the person involved should have the legal capacity to give consent; should be so situated as to be able to exercise free power of choice, without the intervention of any element of force, fraud, deceit, duress, over-reaching or other ulterior form of constraint or coercion, and should have sufficient knowledge and comprehension of the elements of the subject matter involved as to enable him to make an understanding and enlightened decision. This latter element requires that, before the acceptance of an affirmative decision by the patient, there should be made known to him the nature, duration and purpose of the treatment; the method and means by which it is to be conducted; all inconveniences and hazards reasonably to be expected. The duty and responsibility for ascertaining the quality of the consent rests upon each individual doctor who initiates, directs and engages in the treatment. It is a personal duty, the responsibility for which may not be delegated to another with impunity.

This counsel of perfection must be our goal. The dilemma is how to put it into practice. Many otolaryngologists would echo Calnan's assertion (Calnan 1983) that informed consent is impossible. They would probably agree with him that 'assisted consent' is the only realistic goal and that even this is likely to be 'given more on the basis of trust than understanding'. Few would go as far as those who maintain that informed consent is a myth and a fiction and that patients do not understand, cannot understand and do not want to be told (Meisel 1981a).

It is not my purpose to discuss the legal niceties of informed consent. That is for the lawyers to do. I am concerned with those matters which affect the clinician day by day as he practises medicine in the UK in an environment singularly free from the threat of litigation. I will try and provide answers to questions such as:

What rights has the patient to information?
What information should he be given?
How is this to be transmitted?
What is the value of the consent form?
When does lack of information constitute negligence?

It will not be possible to comment on special problems, such as obtaining informed consent for the treatment of the mentally ill, prisoners-of-war, Jehovah's Witnesses, or for removing organs for transplant, specimens at autopsy and for carrying out research.

The principles that have to be applied are common to all these.

What right has the patient to information?

The arguments in favour of keeping patients informed about their treatment are legal, religious, moral and philosophical. Legally, a patient's consent must be obtained before any examination or treatment is undertaken. Many actions on the patient's part are taken to indicate implicit consent to what is to take place. The arrival at the outpatient department with the doctor's letter, or move to occupy a seat in front of (or more often facing) a bull's eye lamp, are accepted. Baring the arm gives implicit consent to take a blood sample, and lying on the couch permission to carry out an examination, but no more.

Explicit or expressed consent is required before an operation and can be obtained orally or in writing. There is no legal requirement to obtain the consent in writing but, because it can more easily be proved in evidence should there be a dispute, it is highly desirable.

The view of the Roman Catholic Church is expressed by Pope Pious XII in his remarks to an audience of anaesthetists in 1957 (*British Medical Journal* 1986):

The rights and duties of the doctor are correlative to those of the patient. The doctor in fact has no separate or independent right where the patient is concerned.

In general he can only take action if the patient explicitly or implicity, directly or indirectly, gives him permission.

Raanan Gillon (1986b) has outlined the standard moral obligations that men and women have to one another in this way:

Our general duty not to harm others requires that for the most part we try our best to obtain their willing consent to what we propose. Respect for the autonomy of the patient has numerous implications: the patient should be given adequate information; he should not be lied to (unless this is deliberately chosen for humane purposes); should have strategic control over the course of action to be pursued, that is that the patient, having been given advice by the doctor, is then given the opportunity to decide whether to accept or not. Furthermore, and this is the real test, the patient's rejection of medical advice should not lead to a shrugging of the shoulders, a cooling of attitude and, 'if you cannot trust my advice perhaps you had better find another doctor you can trust'. What should follow instead is a genuine attempt to understand the patient's reasons for rejecting the advice and searching for the best option. He would argue that respect for autonomy even provides a prima facie case for punctuality.

Hippocrates did not mention the need to obtain the patient's consent before attempting examination or treatment, but as Dunstan (1983) says: 'The modern doctor practising anywhere in Western Europe or North America today, and increasingly elsewhere, even in such authoritarian countries as Japan, has to work within the principles of consent'. Paloni (1983), also writing in the above publication, maintains with others that, 'The indissoluble bond to both the concept and the practice of consent is "informed consent"'.

However, it is not necessary to concentrate entirely on the philosophical, religious and legal arguments in favour of obtaining informed consent from patients. Ordinary commonsense and humanity will persuade the doctor to keep his patients informed and there is increasing evidence that surgical and medical treatment is often ineffective if it is not backed up by adequate information. It can succeed without them, but it is likely in these circumstances that, although the operation is successful, the patient will be less than satisfied.

What information has to be transmitted?

Many patients have decided long before they reach the consulting room that if their particular complaint can be cured by surgery they will undergo any reasonable operation that is recommended. They give the impression that, even if they were told that there was a risk of death or mutilation, they would not demur. This blind faith is a measure of the trust that patients still have in the medical profession.

The reputation for reliability and concern for the patient's best interest has been won by several generations of doctors whose dedication and commitment have given the medical profession the position it now enjoys. It is enhanced in the 20th century by the importance given in a materialistic western society to physical health. Greater knowledge of medical matters, awareness of the side effects of drugs and the complications of surgery, criticisms in the media, reaction against authoritarianism and paternalism, and the move to look upon misfortune as being 'somebody's fault' have undermined some patients' faith in the medical profession. Fewer will be prepared to rely in the future on uninformed consent and whether they will be any happier as a result is immaterial. There is no turning back.

Despite a more questioning approach to the prospects of surgery, most patients are prepared to accept that there must be some risks and are not deterred by them. Alfidi (1971) attempted to assess this in patients who were about to undergo arteriography. In a very detailed description of the nature of the procedure and its complications, he made it quite clear that this could be fatal and that there had been four deaths in 6500 arteriograms that he had been involved with. Only one or two patients out of 100 questioned refused to undergo the arteriogram as a result, although as this was about to take place when they were given the questionnaire, it was rather late for them to change their minds. Eighty-nine per cent said that they thought the information they had been given was useful, but only three-quarters thought that all patients should receive it and none but a handful wanted to know anything more about complications. However, 27% said that the knowledge made them less comfortable about undergoing the procedure and it is this significant percentage that most surgeons in Great Britain have in mind when they decide what and what not to tell their patients. A further study by Alfidi (1975), in which patients were questioned some time before the arteriogram was to take place, produced similar results.

A decision about which risks to mention to the patients and which to emphasize varies in different circumstances. It is of less importance in an emergency than in a planned procedure. It can have greater significance before an elective operation designed to improve the quality of life than before an operation for cancer or some disease that could be life-threatening. Claims for negligence are much more common following stapedectomy than laryngectomy.

Fine judgement is required when deciding what information needs to be transmitted to the patient. For instance, it is not the general practice in the UK to warn patients undergoing middle ear and mastoid surgery that the facial nerve may be damaged. I must confess that, having acted as the expert witness for the defendant in a week-long trial in which a claim for negligence was made because of a postoperative facial palsy, I determined in future to warn all my patients of this risk:

> The defendant was a recently appointed consultant who had initially begun training as a general surgeon and then turned to otolaryngology. He was described by an eminent consultant, under whose eagle eye he had trained, as one of the best technicians he had ever come across. The plaintiff was a middle-aged divorcee who had suffered a partial but permanent facial palsy following stapedectomy. It was the third stapes operation that the surgeon had performed since becoming a consultant. There was no suggestion that there had been any lack of care or high-handedness by the surgeon, who was an honest and straightforward, slightly shy man. He acknowledged that he must have damaged the nerve but none of the suggested ways in which this might have occurred could be proved. The case went against him. It was thought that the judge was considerably influenced by the surgeon's answer to one of the questions put to him when being cross-examined by the plaintiff's counsel: 'Mr B, you have accepted that you are responsible for the very unsightly and permanent disability that this lady has suffered. At the moment that your knife came near to the nerve, or your drill became overheated and caused damage in this way, or the small hook that is used in the operation became trapped in the congenitally exposed portion of the nerve—we do not know which if any of these is the right explanation—were you competent or incompetent? After a moment's thought the quiet reply came, 'Incompetent'.

It has been said that incompetence is not necessarily negligence, but in this instance it appears that

it was. There may be many reasons why I still do not warn my patients of the possibility of a facial palsy following middle ear and mastoid surgery. One important one must be the desire to avoid causing them unnecessary anxiety. If accidents for negligence began to equal those that take place in North America, otologists would certainly have to increase the preoperative anxiety of patients by telling them of this risk. Facial palsy occurs in less than 1 in 100 mastoid operations and, even then, is usually only temporary; so many hundreds of patients would suffer unnecessarily because of the individual doctor's fear of legal action. Nevertheless, there are those who insist that all material risks should be revealed to the patients however distant and alarming. The Association for the Victims of Medical Accidents (1984) would put it this way: 'It is no argument that some people do not want to know—the rest of us do'. They go further than many courts in the USA who apply the ruling that rejoices under the name of 'The Prudent Patient Test', or 'The Reasonable Person's Standard'. This states that a risk is material when a reasonable person, in what the physician knows or should know to be the patient's position, would be likely to attach significance to the risk or cluster of risks before deciding whether or not to forego the proposed therapy. Even then the doctor is given the 'therapeutic privilege' of withholding information which would pose a threat of psychological detriment to the patient (Hawkins 1984, Medical Protection Society 1984).

How is the information best transmitted?

It is appropriate under this heading to say something about the problems of communication in hospitals and the difficulties of ensuring that patients are able to make a knowledgeable evaluation of recommended treatment. According to Sir James Spence, 'The real work of the doctor is only faintly understood by many people—this is a consultation and all else in the practice of medicine derives from it'. If this is true, and I believe it is, what takes place between the doctor and the patient is all important. Communication by word of mouth, gesture or facial expression can have lasting effects. It is doubtful whether words spoken by anyone else, even a spouse, are so readily retained. The surprising thing is, despite this, doctors still have a reputation for being bad communicators. This received official acknowledgement when, in 1963, the Central Health Services Council felt it necessary to establish a special Commission of Inquiry, chaired by Cohen, into communications between doctors, nurses and patients (Central Health Services Council 1973). In their report they recommended that, when patients were admitted to hospital, a named person should be identified as their personal doctor. This recommendation was not implemented and years later patients can leave hospital after lengthy stays without knowing the names of any member of the medical or nursing staff who looked after them. Cohen and his collaborators also said, 'It is self-evident that the thinking and practice of doctors is greatly influenced by their experience in training, and many of them aspire for the rest of their lives to reproduce a pattern of care which they saw as students'. The neurosurgeon who was defended in the Sideaway case was described by the plaintiff as a 'man of few words' and the trial judge referred to him as an 'obsessively particular surgeon and a reserved, slightly autocratic man of the old school' (Schwartz & Grubb 1985). Although a highly distinguished and expert clinician, it seems likely that those who modelled themselves on a personality of this sort would have difficulty in communicating satisfactorily with patients, especially anxious and timid ones. Hopefully, no student these days would come under the influence of the consultant who, whilst visiting a patient in bed, was faced with a number of questions and as a result turned to the group of students accompanying him and said: 'This patient asks so many questions he must want to be a medical student'. Sadly, consultants can still be described as 'hurdles which have to be overcome' rather than sources of information and counselling.

Most claims for negligence against doctors are the result of failures in communication. The doctor may be ignorant, idle, indifferent, inaudible, or incomprehensible. The patient may be deaf, uninterested, incapable of understanding and impatient. Differences in language, culture and education do not help. Patients and doctors may fail to communicate because they are temporarily disturbed by emotions, such as anxiety and fear on the patient's side, or resentment and pride on the doctor's. The most common cause of failure in the UK is probably

lack of time. Judge Kirby suggests that it is difficult in 30 minutes to translate into lay terms what the surgeon has taken 15 years or more to learn (Kirby 1983). How much more difficult in the 5 or 10 minutes that is usually available in the average ENT outpatient department. I shall not forget the occasion when, in what I thought was a leisurely fashion, with the help of a diagram, I described the nature of a submucus resection operation to a patient who seemed more intelligent than the average and anxious to be informed, only to hear the following conversation take place when she returned to her friend in the waiting room: 'How did you get on then?' 'Oh, he was very nice but he doesn't half talk a lot'.

There are various ways of trying to get around the problem. Simple diagrams are readily available and can be of considerable help. Some surgeons have descriptions of operations reproduced in a simplified form to hand to patients. Extracts from lay journals, publications such as *Self Health* produced by the College of Health, can be used. Pre-admission classes for parents and children not only help to allay anxiety about details of hospital admission, but also give an opportunity for parents to ask questions about routine procedures. The use of videos and tape recorders for more complicated procedures can be tried. The fact remains that, despite repeated efforts to inform patients of the nature of the operations they are to undergo, or have undergone, their first question on attending a follow-up clinic is often, 'What exactly did you do, doctor?'. This ties in with American experience, and Robinson & Merav (1985), investigating the success of providing informed consent to patients prior to heart surgery, concluded that their patients had 'generally poor retention in all categories of informed consent some six months after surgery'. Meisel (1981a), reviewing the many investigations that had been undertaken to try and assess patients' understanding of information they have been given, concluded, 'What we find is very little wheat and much chaff . . . whether informed consent is feasible is still an open question'.

Consent forms

As we have seen, there is no legal obligation to obtain a signed consent form prior to surgery. Even when one is obtained it has no magical properties, but it does protect the surgeon and employing authority from being sued for assault and battery. Such claims will only succeed when there has been, as Ian Kennedy puts it, 'wholly unconsented touching' (Kennedy 1983). Unless obtained by false pretences, or forgery, a signed consent form makes nonsense of a claim based on this premise. The occasion where a patient denied having signed the form and a handwriting expert was called in to give evidence must be a rarity.

The consent form plays a very small part in the defence of a claim for negligence. Like baptism, it is intended to be an outward and visible sign of something much more important. This is the careful explanation of all that the Bench of Judges in Great Britain believe is necessary before the patient can be said to know enough to allow the consent, alluded to in the form, to receive the added lustre of becoming 'informed'. In malpractice cases, the courts will be very interested in evidence that it is not only the habit of the doctor concerned to explain the nature and purpose of operations to his patients, but that he has done so in the case under scrutiny. In my experience, when there is a conflict of evidence between the plaintiff and the defendant, the doctor is usually given the benefit of the doubt.

Nurses are not generally called to substantiate or refute a patient's claim that he was not informed. Although it is common in Canada and the USA to obtain a witness to the signing of the consent form, this appears to be little more than icing on the legal cake rather than an attempt to provide an observer to act as a policeman, or to see that the doctor does his informing properly. Nevertheless, there are a few occasions where it is wise to consider obtaining the signature of a witness to conversations undertaken with patients. This is particularly so when it is felt that they may be litigation minded.

Apart from a few exceptions, such as termination of pregnancy and sterilization, the practice in the UK is to use a simple consent form which is based on that recommended by the Department of Health and Social Security in a circular issued in 1975 (Department of Health and Social Security 1975). This contains reference to three matters relating to the operation:

1. That the nature and purpose has been explained.
2. That further alternative operations and anaesthetics may, if necessary, be used.

3. That there is no guarantee that a particular practitioner will perform the operation.

Until 1957 the form said that the nature and purpose (or effect) and *risks* of the operation had been explained. Rather surprisingly, the word 'risks' was then dropped; This followed an action by *Bolam* v. *Friern Barnett Hospital* after a patient had suffered a fractured leg during electroconvulsive therapy (*Bolam* v. *Friern Hospital Management Committee* 1957). The defence societies still support the use of the simple consent form and there is little enthusiasm for the very elaborate and detailed ones commonly used in North America. There is much evidence that these are not read properly or understood and may discourage the much more effective exchange of information by word of mouth, which is the hallmark of the British system.

Clifford Hawkins has recently suggested that some indication of the common risks of a particular operation should be included on the consent form with an indication of the chance of these occurring (Hawkins 1985). Thus, for sterilization by tubal ligation, the figure of 1 failure in 250 would be included. I personally believe this information would be better provided in a simple explanatory note of the type which I have already described and which I know is used by some urologists and gynaecologists.

When does lack of information constitute negligence?

In 1974, a senior consultant neurosurgeon performed a laminectomy and facetectomy on Mrs Sideaway for the relief of pain (Medical Protection Society 1984). She became seriously disabled due to interference with the blood supply to the spinal cord. She sued the hospital and the executors of the surgeon (who had died before the issue of the writ) claiming that he had been negligent in failing to warn her of the risk that materialized. The trial judge dismissed the plaintiff's case, as did the Court of Appeal. Their opinion was based on the Bolam decision, that a doctor was not guilty of negligence, 'if he has acted in accordance with practices accepted as proper by a responsible body of medical men skilled in that particular art'. Mrs Sideaway was given leave to appeal to the House of Lords but was unsuccessful yet again. However, despite dismissing the appeal unanimously, there were considerable differences in the opinions expressed by the five Law Lords, which are likely to have significantly changed the attitude of trial judges faced with actions brought by aggrieved patients because of failure to obtain informed consent before operations. Only one of the noble Lords accepted the Bolam doctrine unmodified. The others judged that this needed modifying to give patients a greater opportunity to make a decision based on adequate information about risks. Lords Bridges and Keith said, 'When questioned by a patient of apparently sound mind about risks involved in the particular treatment, the doctor's duty was to answer both truthfully and fully as the questioner required'. In my experience, this is already expected by many trial judges and, furthermore, most otologists realize this. The information given to the patient prior to stapedectomy can be used as an example. The patient will be told that there is a small risk of losing all the hearing in the operated ear. It will not be enough to rely on the practice of a much loved senior otologist who, in a brief handout, warned, 'that the hearing might suffer following the operation'. The temptation to minimize the disability resulting from a dead ear will be resisted. When the patient is told that his hearing may get worse and is inclined to accept the risk because 'I have nothing to lose', he will be told that he has: namely, the ability to use a hearing aid in the ear concerned. I have little doubt that the patient who loses all his hearing following stapedectomy and can show that he was not warned in this way could mount a successful claim for negligence based on lack of informed consent.

What criteria will be used in the future for deciding what material risks should be shared with patients is still to be discovered. Will it be the prudent patient, doctor, or judge that decides? We may have to resort yet again to the man on the front seat of the London passenger omnibus. Hopefully, it will be a long time before lack of informed consent becomes a major cause of litigation in the UK. The unsatisfactory state of affairs in the USA came to a head in 1978 as a result of the increasing number of claims for negligence against doctors, many of which were based entirely on the supposed lack of informed consent. This led to a spiralling of the insurance premiums which had to be paid and these often exceeded $20 000 per annum. The antagonism felt by some doctors is illustrated by the graffiti that was often to be seen in New York: 'Support the legal profession. Send your son to medical school'.

SUMMARY

It is clear that the patient is entitled to as much information as he requires to make a balanced decision about whether to go forward with the treatment that has been recommended. The consultation should ideally be leisurely and as informal as possible, allowing the patient the opportunity to ask the questions that he feels needs answering so that he can make knowledgeable evaluation of the procedure proposed. Information is more likely to be effective if given by word of mouth, but visual aids and explanatory notes can help. Complicated consent forms are more likely to confuse the patient than to provide a clear account of the nature of an operation and its risks. The British patient is as well informed as those cared for by other health systems and is as likely to receive unbiased advice. Failure to warn patients of material risks associated with elective operations may lead to litigation, and claims for negligence can succeed on these grounds alone. Actions for negligence are more often a result of the consultant's attitude to the patient than to his failure to warn of particular risks. We must remember that, in common with other physicians, the otolaryngologist's role is, 'above all to care (curare): and only in caring can he hope sometimes to cure (sanare)'.

INTRODUCTION

A reading of these two interesting and informative chapters seems to me to raise a supplementary question—not only, 'what is informed consent?' but also, 'why do we need to know?'. There is much in common in the approach of the two distinguished contributors to the concept of informed consent. But what is our object in raising the question? Is it so that, in applying his own interpretation of informed consent, each doctor can be sure that he is fulfilling a duty to his patient, which he recognizes exists independently of extraneous considerations? Or is the question raised in order to avoid a lawsuit? The latter consideration is naturally of some concern to both writers and, whilst I hope to comment on the humanitarian aspect, I propose to concentrate mainly on legal considerations.

The humanitarian approach

Mr Smith points out that answering the question, 'What is informed consent?' may provide the lawyer with a dilemma but not the doctor. Both authors refer to the Nuremberg Code which, albeit produced in exceptional circumstances, is taken, correctly in my view, as applying to therapeutic as well as experimental techniques. Professor Bailey analyses the application of the Code in research matters in the lucid manner which is a feature of both essays. Bailey regards informed consent as a multifaceted concept and, as such, it can hardly be capable of a cryptic definition. Maybe informed consent is like the elephant—we may not be able to define it, but we can recognize it when we see it. Need we then go further?

The legal approach

Certainly, notwithstanding the dilemma which Smith recognizes as affecting the lawyer, the latter must try to go further—or at least consider the difficulties. Before this, two preliminary points should be mentioned. First, it is necessary to distinguish between a claim against a surgeon based on a lack of informed consent (by whatever name called) and a claim based on some other alleged shortcoming.

Smith refers to a case in which he acted as expert witness; however, the matters related seem to imply that the admitted incompetence was in the conduct of the operation and not in the information given leading to the patient's consent. Similarly, in the Jewish Chronic Diseases Hospital case referred to by Bailey, the shortcoming of those concerned was by way of fraud or deceit; there could be no true consent involved. Secondly, the doctrine of informed consent as a legal concept is limited to certain States of North America; it does not enjoy universal approval and has been specifically rejected as a legal concept, for example, by the Courts of England.

The differences in approach between the Courts of England and those of some States in North America are particularly significant. How far would those differences in approach lead to differing results in any particular set of circumstances? Both writers draw attention to the 'milestone' cases in their respective countries: *Sideaway* v. *Board of Governors of the Bethlem Royal Hospital and the Maudsley Hospital* (Law Reports UK 1985) in England, and *Canterbury* v. *Spence* (Law Reports USA 1972) in the USA. The facts are given by Smith and Bailey and I need not repeat them. Mrs Sideaway failed to make out her case against Mr Falconer. The case is somewhat unsatisfactory in that the trial judge did not have the benefit of evidence from the consultant, who had died after the operation was performed. He did not accept Mrs Sideaway's evidence in toto and found the following:

> . . . the probabilities are . . . that [Mr Falconer] explained the nature of the operation . . . in simple terms . . . I think it is probable that he mentioned the possibility of disturbing a nerve root and the consequences of doing so: but I am satisfied that he did not refer to the danger of cord damage or to the fact that this was an operation of choice rather than necessity.

Smith also refers to the earlier English case of *Bolam* v. *Friern Hospital Management Committee* (Law Reports UK 1957), which was considered by the court in *Sideaway*. The well-known *Bolam* case, put briefly, applied the standards of professional practice to determine the doctor's duty. Despite the differences of emphasis between the judges in the case, to which Smith refers, *Sideaway* must be taken as having modified *Bolam*; whilst rejecting the informed consent concept as having a place in English law, the court analysed the doctor's duty to disclose information to the patient in considerable detail. It must now be accepted in English law that the doctor has a duty to disclose, which goes further than had been thought to be the case before *Sideaway*. In the particular circumstances of *Sideaway*, the end result was that Mr Falconer's omission to warn his patient of the risk of injury to the spinal cord did not constitute negligence.

Does the duty to disclose go further in the 'informed consent' jurisdictions than elsewhere? Would Mrs Sideaway have been more successful had she been claiming in an American jurisdiction? Let me try to measure her case against the four propositions of *Canterbury* v. *Spence*, viz:

1. The root premise is the concept that every human being of adult years and of sound mind has a right to determine what shall be done with his own body.

2. The consent is the informed exercise of a choice and that entails an opportunity to evaluate knowledgeably the options available and the risks attendant upon each.

3. The doctor must therefore disclose all 'material risks'; what risks are 'material' is determined by the 'prudent patient' test, i.e. '[would] a reasonable person in what the physician knows or should know to be the patient's position . . . be likely to attach significance to the risk . . . in deciding whether or not to forego the proposed therapy'.

4. The doctor, however, has the benefit of an exception to the general rule of disclosure. This exception enables the doctor to withhold from his patient information as to risk if sound medical judgement shows that communication of it would present a threat to the patient's well-being.

It seems at least possible that Mrs Sideaway would have been equally unable to establish her claim had her accident occurred in Washington DC. The actual decision in the *Canterbury* case in the Court of Appeals was that a new trial was ordered because the relevant issues were required to be put before a jury. Basing themselves on the approach of the courts which heard *Sideaway*, in relation to the facts as opposed to the law, the jury may well have concluded that either the prudent patient would

have regarded the risk which materialized in Mrs Sideaway's case as too remote, or that the surgeon may have been justified under the exception mentioned above from referring to the risk.

Conversely, what of *Canterbury* in England? The Court of Appeals referred the case for the jury's decision on the facts. In practical terms, identical questions on the facts would have arisen for the Court to determine had the case taken place in England, but on the basis of a duty to disclose, not a doctrine of informed consent.

As a legal concept, the term 'informed consent' does seem to be flawed. Bailey points out that 'the concept of informed consent is not the same as an "educated consent" and it never can be'. What, therefore, is meant by 'informed'? How much information should (or can) the patient absorb before he can be said to have become 'informed'? English law would say that 'a doctor cannot set out to educate the patient to his own standard of medical knowledge of all the relevant factors involved' (Lord Bridge of Harwich in *Sideaway*). Bailey draws attention, as the principal obstacle to informed consent, to the patient's lack of medical knowledge. Smith refers to Calnan's assertion that 'informed consent is impossible'. As indicated above, the *Canterbury* approach to informed consent does not find universal favour, even in North America whence it sprang. Mr Gerald Robertson, writing in Law Quarterly Review (1981), pointed out that only a minority of States in the USA have chosen to follow *Canterbury* and that since 1975 'there has been a growing tendency for individual States to enact legislation which severely curtails the operation of the doctrine of informed consent'. The *Canterbury* approach was accepted in Canada in *Reibl* v. *Hughes* (Law Reports Canada 1978, 1980), but again, one feels that the same result could have been reached by different means. In that case a successful action was brought against a surgeon, arising out of a brain operation to avert a threatened stroke. The patient was not warned of the attendant risk that the operation might precipitate the stroke, or even cause death. It is likely that an English Court would have reached the same conclusion without the aid of a doctrine of informed consent. There was clearly a material risk which the patient did not have the opportunity to evaluate.

In another Canadian case, *Schintz* v. *Dickinson*

(Law Reports Canada, British Columbia 1985), the Court was concerned with an action against a dentist. The facts very briefly were that for the purposes of the extraction of a fourth wisdom tooth a local anaesthetic by mandibular block was administered requiring six injections. The operation was performed without negligence but the injections caused the patient to suffer nerve damage of the lingual nerve, leaving part of her tongue permanently numb. Paraesthesiae in her jaw, teeth and cheek were resolved in about a month. The expert evidence was that the risk of this damage was below 1% and the risk of permanent damage less than that. Since there were no special or unusual elements concerned, the fact (as found by the court) that the dentist gave no explanation or advice to the patient as to the possible risk of any damage resulting from the operation did not give the patient a cause of action; the trial judge could properly conclude that a warning would have been counter-productive. Again, a similar result in England or in most of the States of the USA seems probable. The percentage risk was, interestingly, about the same as in *Sideaway*.

To revert to my supplementary question, Why do we need to know, maybe—at least so far as concerns decisions of the courts which have not accepted the *Canterbury* view—we do *not* need to know. Where legal responsibility is concerned, those jurisdictions which have eschewed the 'informed consent' approach have avoided the very dilemma to which Smith draws attention in his opening sentence. In the 'informed consent' jurisdictions, the exceptions to the doctrine recognized by the courts can lead one to doubt the validity of the doctrine itself. The physician's obligation seems to be comprehended more easily in terms of his duty to give information relevant to the particular patient's circumstances—a duty recognized in somewhat different ways in both *Canterbury* and *Sideaway*.

Research

Do different considerations apply in the case of research? It is submitted that the considerations are the same but that the application of them may differ. I found Professor Bailey's commentary on the problems of research particularly helpful; Mr

Smith specifically excludes research from his analysis. Whether one takes the *Canterbury* line on informed consent or the *Sideaway* line on the duty to disclose, the significance of the risk involved to the individual patient is a factor in determining the information to be given. It may be logical to assume that, if a perfectly healthy volunteer attends at a Cold Research Station, he should know of all the risks involved and be given the opportunity on a purely subjective basis of deciding whether he wishes to submit himself to them. In the case of a clinical trial, however, the considerations may be different. Given that the patient is in need of some treatment in any event, then the difficulties, dangers, or discomforts of option A (perhaps an experimental technique) compared with option B (for this purpose taken as the standard technique) need to be alluded to. On the basis of *Sideaway* the courts in England would be reluctant to adopt any approach that could be seen to encourage 'defensive medicine', and one would not expect North America to be behind in the way of research. We are faced by a question of degree—how informed is 'informed'— and clinical judgement has in the past been generally a reliable guide as to what is necessary. The works of the ethical committees having jurisdiction over medical trials provide an adequate safeguard in humanitarian terms, but the law is concerned in this context with the instances which inevitably arise of failure to adhere to the proper course. Unfortunately, the proper course to which one should have adhered is sometimes charted only after the event. It seems inevitable that over the next few years the courts on both sides of the Atlantic will have to pronounce on events arising from clinical trials. Taking account of the differing approaches in different States of the Union, we may well find a difference of approach between the 'informed consent' jurisdictions and the 'duty to disclose' jurisdictions. Whether these divergent approaches will lead to similar conclusions remains to be seen.

CONCLUSION

The effect of the doctrine of informed consent in matters of medical negligence should be seen in the context of claims for negligence and related claims in general. Whilst this may not be of immediate interest to doctors in the exercise of their day-to-day duties and responsibilities, nevertheless it can possibly give a guide to the way in which the legal scene may develop in the future. It is a natural and inevitable human reaction that, if one suffers damage, there should be a remedy and compensation. In certain fields on both sides of the Atlantic a move can be detected towards 'no fault liability'. The developing approach of Courts and legislators to product liability of manufacturers both in North America and in Europe presents many problems to manufacturers and they are having to learn to live with the problems. Liability is, in some instances, absolute and it is at least arguable, if one can be sufficiently detached about such things, that where there is suffering there should always be recompense and society at large should bear the cost. To some extent, this is a practical approach where the level of damages is, broadly speaking, compatible with the economic loss. It is here that the widest divergence between Europe and North America is to be found. The levels of damages awarded by North American Courts dictate the level of premiums to be paid there for the corresponding insurance cover, whether for medical negligence, product liability insurance or any other form of third party cover. These levels of awards do affect the corresponding premiums in Europe but it seems unlikely that in England, for example, it would be necessary for an insurance fund to have to meet the level of damages that it may have to meet for a corresponding claim in North America, even though the decision of the Court on the question of liability may be the same.

Mr Robertson, in the article referred to, said that, 'The doctrine of informed consent, expanding as it does the liability of the medical profession, is the servant of judicial policy regarding such expansion'. Judicial policy in North America, in some States at least, has developed 'informed consent' as a legal concept; judicial policy in England has rejected it. But although informed consent may not have been universally accepted as a legal doctrine, its place in matters of medical ethics is secure. In practice, those whose approaches to the problem are as prudent and caring as those of both Bailey and Smith should find themselves reasonably well defended against negligence claims arising from any alleged lack of information, whether on the basis of informed consent or the duty to disclose.

REFERENCES

B J Bailey

Andrews J D 1984 Informed consent statutes and the decision-making process. The Journal of Legal Medicine 5: 163–217

Annas G J 1984 Why the British courts rejected the American doctrine of informed consent (and what British physicians should do about it). American Journal of Public Health 74 (no 11): 1286–1288

Berman M 1984 Informed consent: The case for legislation. Michigan Medicine (Special report) November: 556

Cancer Research Campaign Working Party in Breast Cancer 1983 Informed consent: ethical, legal and medical implications for doctors and patients who participate in randomised clinical trials. British Medical Journal 286: 1117–1121

Cassell E J 1978 Informed consent in therapeutic relationships: Clinical aspects. Encyclopedia of Bioethics. New York p 767–769

Chalmers G A 1983 Fraud in science. British Medical Journal 287: 616

Chuang M Y, Man P L 1983 Informed consent—ethical considerations. Medicine and Law 2: 19–25

Donagan A 1977 Informed consent in therapy and experimentation. The Journal of Medicine and Philosophy 2 (no 4): 307–329

Drane J F 1984 Competency to give an informed consent. A model for making clinical assessments. Journal of American Medical Association 252 (no 7): 925–927

Dudley H A F 1984 Informed consent in surgical trials. British Medical Journal 289: 937–938

Gerber P 1984 Informed consent. The Medical Journal of Australia 140: 89–94

Gerber P 1985 Informed consent—the last of Mrs Sideaway? The Medical Journal of Australia 142: 643–645

Golan J, Ben-Hur N 1983 Informed consent in plastic surgery Medicine and Law 2: 113–115

Healey J M 1984 Connecticut's informed consent case II. Connecticut Medicine 48 (no 1): 59

Hospital Progress 1983 Case example. March: 78

Klein C A 1984 Informed consent. Nurse Practitioner May: 56–60

Koopersmith E R G 1984 Informed consent: The problem of causation. Medicine and Law 3: 231–236

Lancet Editorial 1984 Consent: How informed? i: 1445–1447

Lenox-Smith I 1983 A question of consent. Practitioner 227: 18

Macklin R 1977 Consent, coercion, and conflicts of rights. Perspectives in Biology and Medicine 360–371

Miller B L 1981 Autonomy and the refusal of lifesaving treatment. The Hastings Center Report, August, p 22–28

Monaco G P 1983 Informed consent: Does the consent process reflect the realities of current treatment, procedures and side effects? The American Journal of Pediatric Hematology/Oncology 41: 401–407

Neville-Smith C H 1984 How informed are patients who have given informed consent? British Medical Journal 289: 558

The New England Journal of Medicine 1984 Informed consent and the therapeutic alliance. 311 (no 1): 49–51

Northrop C E 1985 The ins and .outs of informed consent. Nursing 61: 9

Pulmeri P A 1984 Informed consent—beware. Journal Clinical Gastroenterology 6: 471–475

Redden E M, Baker D C 1984 Coping with the complexities of informed consent in dermatologic surgery. Dermatology and Surgical Oncology 10 (no 2): 111–116

Redden E M et al 1985 The patient, the plastic surgeon and informed consent: New insights into old problems. Plastic and Reconstructive Surgery 75: 270–276

Reed M E, Camille A O 1985 Implant manufacturer and physician: Must both warn the patient of a product's risks? American College of Surgeons' Bulletin. 70 (no 5): 19–21

Weaver J P 1984 The problem with the operative patient. Surgery, Gynecology and Obstetrics 159: 579–580

White W D 1983 Informed consent: Ambiguity in theory and practice. Journal of Health Politics, Policy and Law 8 (no 1): 99–119

C Smith

Action for the Victims of Medical Accidents 1984 Annual report, p 1

Alfidi R J 1971 Informed consent Journal of the American Medical Association 216: 1325

Alfidi R J 1975 Controversy, alternatives and decisions in complying with informed consent. Radiology 114: 231–234

Bolam v. Friern Hospital Management Committee [1957] All ER 118: 1, Weekly Law Reports 582

British Medical Journal 1986 Doctors and patients. 292: 259–261

Calnan J 1983 Talking with patients. Heinemann, London, p 77

Central Health Services Council 1973 Communications between doctors, nurses and patients. HMSO, London, p 6

Dunstan G R 1983 In: Dunstan GR, Seller MJ (eds) Consent in medicine. King Edward Hospital Fund, Oxford, p 17

Department of Health and Social Security 1975 Circular, vol 15. HMSO, London, p 117

Gillon R 1986a Ordinary and extraordinary means. British Medical Journal 292: 259

Gillon R 1986b Doctors and patients. British Medical Journal 292: 467

Hawkins C 1985a Mishap or malpractice. Blackwell Scientific Publications, Oxford, ch 7, p 190, 197

Kennedy I 1983 In: Dunstan G R, Seller M J (eds) Consent in medicine. King Edward Hospital Fund, Oxford, p 86

Kirby Hon Mr Justice M D 1983 Informed consent, what does it mean? Journal of Medical Ethics 9: 69–75

Medical Protection Society 1984 Annual report, p 18

Meisel A 1981a The exceptions to informed consent. Conn. Med. 45: 27–32

Meisel A 1981b What do we know about informed consent? Journal of the American Medical Association 246 (no 21): 2476

Paloni P E 1983 In: Dunstan G R, Seller M J (eds) Consent in medicine. King Edward Hospital Fund, Oxford, p 78

Robinson G, Merav A 1976 Informed consent: recalled by patients tested postoperatively. Annals of Thoracic Surgery 22: 210

Schwartz R, Grubb A 1985 Why Britain can't afford informed consent. Hastings Center Report, August. New York, p 20

D J Hare

Law Reports (United Kingdom) 1985 Vol 1. Appeal Cases, p 871

Law Reports (USA) 1972 Vol 464. Federal Reporter 2nd series, p 772

Law Reports (United Kingdom) 1957 Vol 1. Weekly Law Reports, p 582

Law Reports (Canada) 1978 Vol 89. Dominion Law Reports 3rd series, p 112

Law Reports (Canada) 1980 Vol 114. Dominion Law Reports 3rd series, p 1

Law Reports (Canada, British Columbia) 1985 Vol 2. British Columbia Court of Appeal. Western Weekly Reports, p 673

Robertson G 1981 Law Quarterly Review 97: 102

2

Evaluation of noise induced hearing loss—a medicolegal dilemma

P.W. Alberti

It has been known for several centuries that exposure to high levels of sound can damage hearing and, indeed, the deafening effects of naval gunfire were commented upon during the Napoleonic wars (Parry 1825). With progressive industrialization came greater amounts of an unwanted byproduct of power—noise—and, by the latter part of the 19th century, boilermakers' deafness was so well recognized that it was described as having reached epidemic proportions (Barr 1886). With the advent of workers' compensation in the early part of this century, hearing loss caused by acute trauma at work, which prevented a worker from earning his living, became compensable. Hearing loss from prolonged exposure to noise was also recognized as an industrial injury, but was not compensated because no loss of earnings could be demonstrated. Deafness from military noise exposure was compensated in both world wars and the first modern comprehensive system of assessment and rehabilitation for noise-induced hearing loss was introduced by the American Department of Veterans' Affairs specifically for injured World War II veterans. In the civil arena, the first tentative steps towards compensating hearing loss caused by prolonged exposure to noise occurred in the late 1940s and did not become widespread until the social changes which swept the Western world in the 1960s took up the cause of safety, health and freedom from injury in the workplace as a right for each worker.

Noise is the most ubiquitous of industrial pollutants. However, there is no clear indication of either the incidence nor of the prevalence of hearing loss that is caused by prolonged exposure to it, although the numbers of compensation claims which are made are exceedingly high. For example, in the province of Ontario, Canada, with a population of 9 million people, approximately 3500 new claims for noise-induced hearing loss are processed annually by the compensation board, of which 40% are severe enough to be compensable. The numbers rose steadily during the 1970s. The total number of claims received between, 1 January 1970 and 31 December 1985 is 27 763, and the number compensated is 13 906. These figures are in line with those in many other industrialized communities.

Prevention, management and evaluation of noise-induced hearing loss has become a major task for a wide range of disciplines, including engineering, industrial hygiene, audiology, occupational health and otolaryngologists. This chapter concerns itself with one facet of the problem, the medicolegal evaluation of noise-induced hearing loss claims, with specific emphasis on the role of the otologist. The emphasis will be on the assessment rather than details of legal minutiae. These are more properly dealt with under the heading forensic audiology; a good introduction is provided by Hinchcliffe (1981).

The task of the medical assessor, when faced with a patient presenting for evaluation of a potential industrial hearing loss claim, is to quantify accurately the hearing loss and ascribe to it a cause. These tasks may be difficult. The claimant who has worked in high levels of sound for some time and who has a hearing loss may well be convinced that noise is the cause of the impairment. To accept this on face value is to accept that working in noise protects a person from all other causes of hearing loss. The prevalence of other ear disease causing both conductive and sensorineural hearing loss, such as otosclerosis, chronic otitis media, Ménière's syndrome and sudden hearing loss, is likely to be similar in a noise-exposed population as in the population at large. This is one of the reasons why a medical, as opposed to only an audiological, evaluation is an essential part of the assessment of such a claim. In our own series of compensation board assessments, in 1222 consecutive claimants, other ear disease was found to be the primary cause of the hearing loss in 5% (Alberti & Blair 1982). From the medical standpoint, an accurate history, complete otolaryngologic examination and full audiological assessment are an essential first step of such an evaluation.

The history can present difficulties. It is the writer's experience that the average person does not remember nondescript medical events that occurred more than 10 years previously. Thus, a 50-year-old claimant is unlikely to remember childhood ear disease and may indeed even forget operations that took place 25 or 30 years earlier. Knowledge of the onset of hearing loss is rarely accurate. The writer has seen many claimants who date the onset of the problem about 10 years earlier, who have been re-evaluated 8 or 10 years later and who still date the onset of their problems 8–10 years ago, sometime after the previous evaluation! With an increasingly mobile workforce there may be great difficulty in communicating with a patient because of language problems. In Ontario, 36% of the workforce have as their native language neither English nor French, the official Canadian tongues, and in approximately 14% of claimants for industrial hearing loss there is a major communication gap caused by lack of a common language (Alberti & Blair 1982). It is probable that this is also a problem in other jurisdictions. If translation is required, the services of a professional translator are much to be preferred to those of a family member who, in the writer's experience, both interpolate so many of their own views and fail to understand the questions being put that such consultations are unlikely to provide accurate information. History of ototoxic drug use is extremely difficult to obtain, family histories of hearing loss are frequently unavailable, confusion appears to abound about the date of onset of aural discharge, and the history of military noise exposure is difficult to unravel. It is clear that many veterans wished one thing only, to be discharged from the service, and that formal hearing testing did not occur prior to the demobilization process in many armies.

Accurate recording of a work history is also frequently extremely difficult. Workers do not remember where they were employed or, if they do, frequently have an inaccurate record of actual length of employment at a given work site or job. The writer has been impressed by the lack of correlation between the worker's memory of jobs and those submitted by companies concerning the same worker. Thus, 5 years on a drilling machine in a mine may in fact be documented as 5 or 6 months a year drilling over a 6-year period. Examples abound in all industries. Overwhelmingly, in the writer's opinion, the claimants are not deliberately dissembling. What is being described is what the worker remembers. None the less, it makes the task of the otologist attempting to analyse one of these cases extremely difficult.

AUDIOLOGICAL ASSESSMENT

The degree of accuracy required for hearing measurement in a medicolegal assessment is greater than that required for diagnostic testing. Matters are compounded by more frequent dissembling in hearing tests when the results are potentially translatable into money. In our own experience the audiogram with which an industrial claimant arrives is on average almost 10 decibels worse than our final product. This has been evaluated on two separate occasions against different cohorts of 500 claimants each (Alberti & Hyde 1983, unpublished). The reasons for this are varied and include the presence of temporary threshold shift in some first audiograms, inappropriate instruction, failure to understand the test and sometimes deliberate exaggeration. A medicolegal evaluation must be carried out with the subject free of temporary threshold shift. In our opinion, after chronic noise exposure, the claimant should be out of noise for a minimum of 48 hours prior to the test. If the claimant has been deafened by a single loud bang then a period of at least one month should elapse before medicolegal testing— something which usually happens anyway. The audiologist should acquire skill in forensic testing and be alert to incongruities in results.

Our standard test battery includes pure-tone air and bone conduction thresholds at 250, 500, 1000, 2000, 3000, 4000, 8000 Hz (and mid frequencies too, if there is a great slope), speech reception threshold (SRT), speech discrimination tests, tympanometry and stapedius reflex estimations. We look carefully for agreement between the SRT and puretone thresholds and feel that the SRT should be ± 5 dB of the average of the better two of the three pure-tone frequencies (PTA), 500, 1000, 2000. In an uncomplicated noise-induced hearing loss, air and bone conduction thresholds should be similar. Likewise, in a pure noise-induced loss, it is unusual to have a 500 Hz threshold markedly depressed. We use 500 Hz threshold of worse than 35 dB as one of the triggers for repeated and additional testing, as we do discrepancy between the SRT and PTA (Alberti et al, 1978). Stapedius reflex thresholds, particularly at the frequencies 500 and 1000 Hz, 30 dB or closer to the admitted pure-tone threshold are also a major warning signal of an inaccurate threshold. It is often appropriate to start at this type of test with impedance audiometry, particulary if there is an automatic strip chart write out which the patient can see, for it persuades them that some form of automatic testing is underway.

Many tests have been described to identify exaggerated hearing loss but relatively few to quantify it. Suspicion is raised by the audiometric criteria suggested earlier and by the patient's behaviour during the testing. This includes extreme hesitancy in responding during audiometric tests, the ostentatious use of a hearing aid often with a cupped hand, a quavering finger in response to tones and inappropriate, but meaningful responses in speech audiometry such as north-east for north-west and good girl for cowboy.

The quantification of exaggerated hearing loss is more difficult. If there is a gross discrepancy between the ears or if there is an unilateral loss, the pure-tone Stenger test is a valuable tool. In our own practice, if there is any doubt, we move on to evoked response audiometry and, in neurologically normal adults as most of these claimants are, we place great emphasis on the use of slow vertex responses. These were amongst the first of the evoked responses to be described and commercial machines to test them were introduced in the 1960s. Although originally designed to test infants and children, they have become the standby for adult medicolegal audiometry because pure-tones can be used as stimuli and thus a pure-tone audiogram can be approxi-

mated. Our own experience with this test in industrial claims is now in excess of 4000 subjects. The overwhelming majority of patients can be tested, although there are some, less than 5%, in whom strong alpha rhythms or excessive myogenic action makes testing difficult (Hyde & Alberti 1986). Those with the strong alpha rhythms can be tested by the middle latency responses although our experience here is smaller.

There is much recent emphasis in the literature about the use of auditory brainstem responses (ABR) and electrocochleography (ECoG) in the evaluation of difficult to test hearing losses. These tests are helpful in establishing an overall hearing level, but are difficult tools to use in attempting to obtain a tonal audiogram. Even more than SVR, they are epiphenomena of hearing and, in a standard testing format, utilize click stimuli which evoke a response from large parts of the cochlea. While good tools for detecting the presence of hearing in difficult-to-test infants, they are inappropriate tools for quantification of hearing loss in adult medicolegal examinations.

It should be emphasized that it is extremely risky to give a medicolegal opinion on the outcome of one test. If there is a difference between tests, the patient should be reinstructed and a genuine attempt made to reconcile the differences. There may be anatomical causes for incongruities, such as ear canals collapsing under the pressure of a headset, as well as exaggeration. The patient should be given a gracious way out, reinstructed and encouraged. Confrontation is less effective than cajoling in producing an accurate threshold. If there is a genuine unilateral loss without good cause, the patient must be investigated for acoustic neuroma or other non-industrial cause. In our own experience we have now found nine patients with acoustic neuroma presenting as industrial hearing loss pension claimants. The physician evaluating such claims should remember that he has a prime responsibility to the patient.

Having assessed hearing accurately, the otolaryngologist now must attempt to ascribe a cause to the hearing loss. In a patient with the classical audiogram and history, this is easy, but there are many exceptions. Matters of concern include the audiometric configuration, the history of noise exposure, and the relative weighting to be placed upon other ear disease as a cause of hearing loss in the presence of a history of noise exposure. It is true to say that there are very few audiometric configurations which are exclusively caused by specific aetiologies. In the case of a sensorineural hearing loss the audiogram reflects the end result of a potentially wide range of factors which share a common target organ, the cochlea. Thus, ototoxic drugs destroy hair cells, hair cells may degenerate as a result of ageing, as a result of certain childhood infections, as a result of noise exposure, or as a result of genetic factors, to name but a few. Moreover, in the case of noise exposure, the cochlea certainly does not distinguish between sounds that the recipient is paid to listen to and those which are adventitious. The common end product of most of these lesions is a non-specific sensorineural hearing loss, usually with emphasis on the higher frequencies.

The initial hearing loss from noise exposure is classically a notch or dip occurring between 2000 and 6000 Hz, characteristically described as occurring at 4000 Hz. However, as has been shown, with enough sound for a long period, the hearing loss extends over a broader range of frequencies and after a prolonged exposure to high levels of industrial noise the loss may be a straight line slope or even be fairly flattish. The question is occasionally raised whether excessive exposure to sound can produce predominantly low frequency hearing losses or ones with a dip centred elsewhere than a 3–6 kHz. This is certainly evidence in the literature that the major effect in the cochlea of a high energy pure-tone sound is produced half an octave above the centre frequency of that sound (Moddy et al 1976) and, indeed, a quite early paper on hearing loss sustained by jet engine mechanics (Dickson & Watson 1949), who were wearing hearing protectors, demonstrated predominantly low frequency hearing loss, it being hypothesized that hearing protectors protected the ears from the higher frequency sound. Thus, the writer is prepared to accept that in certain industrial situations where the frequency spectrum of the sound is known and found to be low frequency, that an atypical audiogram, with either a flattish shaped spectrum or even a dip in lower frequencies may result. The author's own experience is with workers in the abrasive industry where the refractories used to produce the abrasive, emit an intense low frequency should centred between 200 and 400 Hz, and where hearing losses are severe at the 500 Hz range.

A particular knotty problem in the assessment of potentially noise-damaged ears is to obtain an idea of the amount of the radiated toxin, i.e. noise, to which they have been exposed. Industries change, machinery is renewed and memories are capricious. Even if sound level measurements are available from the industrial plant where the claimant is employed, their worth is usually not great. Many claimants come after 25 or 30 years of industrial noise exposure, in the early years of which no protection was used, and when the machinery may have been different from that which has been recently tested. In some instances it became louder and others quieter. The ship-builder of 40 years ago riveted whereas the shipbuilder of today welds and is exposed to less sound. The paper maker of 40 years ago was exposed to less sound than the paper maker of 20 years ago because the newer machines are quicker, faster and very much noisier. There are remarkably few plants where the machinery and noise level remain constant over the working life of an employee.

Detailed sound surveys, if available, may bear little relationship to the actual noise exposure of an employee. In a telling experiment at one steel plant in Ontario, three workers in a boiler house were fitted with individual noise dosimeters and the sound exposure computed over a working day. Jobs were supposed to be identical but their time-weighted 8-hour sound exposure differed by 5 dB. One worker had reason to spend some time in the steel mill where the sound intensity was higher and another spent a significant time in the office complex. In the writer's experience it is extremely difficult to obtain really accurate figures of sound exposure and most estimates are crude.

Tables of risk based on 8 hours exposure per day, 5 days a week for 10 years and more, are often quoted in attempting to devise regulations. In the writer's opinion they have little part to play in regulations nor in the assessment of a single case. They are statistical tables based on whole populations, without, however, taking into account individual susceptibility. It is also extremely difficult to relate an individual noise exposure to an 8-hour period. Few workers spend 8 hours in noise—the average workshift in the writer's country is $7\frac{1}{2}$ hours and when work breaks such as lunch and tea are removed the exposure is less. Alternatively, if overtime is regularly worked it is greater than 8 hours. More than this, noise levels are rarely constant and may vary cyclically throughout the working day. More recently, matters have been compounded (fortunately) by the introduction of personal hearing protection.

Even when sound levels are assumed to be known and equal, the reaction of individuals vary greatly. There are tough and there are tender ears. Melnick (1978) shows for populations who have spent 40 years in a 95 dBA environment the average hearing loss at 0.5, 1 and 2 kHz is 3dB for the 10th percentile and greater than 11 dB for the 90th percentile. A similar, but grosser, example by the writer shows a 45 dB frequency hearing loss (0.5, 1, 2 and 3 kHZ) in one 53-year-old miner with a 25-year work history of hard rock drilling, whereas a fellow miner of the same age who had a similar job, had an average hearing loss of 10 dB. The only difference between the two is that the claimant with normal hearing had also been a tank driver in World War II!

Matters are further confused by controversy over trading relationships between length of noise exposure and intensity. European writers use an equal energy concept Leq and thus 3 dB halving and doubling, i.e. a 93 dB, 4-hour exposure is exactly equivalent to 90 dB 8-hour exposure and 87 dB 16-hour exposure (Leq 8 90 dB), whereas US authorities by and large have adopted a 5 dB halving and doubling relationship (L OSHA) in which case a 95 dB exposure for 4 hours is equivalent to 90 dB for 8 hours and 85 dB for 16 hours (L OSHA 8 90 dB). As Mills & Going (1982) have cogently argued, it is unlikely that any single value for halving and doubling is universally applicable.

Attempts to measure individual sound level exposure by means of personal dosimeters is also fraught with difficulty. The earlier dosimeters only measured the period of time which the worker was exposed above a baseline level. Later instruments do integrate the exposure over the equivalent of an 8-hour work day. Nevertheless, the microphones and electronics of these devices falls short of class A sound level meters. Matters are compounded by the fact that wherever companies are anxious enough to provide dosimeters to measure sound level

exposure, they are also almost certainly now providing hearing protection. The number of studies which have evaluated the sound level pressure within the ear canal of a protected worker over the working day, is small.

There is also no good rule for the interrelationship between sound exposure for longer than average working days with longer than average gaps between exposure, as for example in offshore oil drilling rigs where workers may spend 12 hours a day for 10 days then have 10 days rest and quiet afterwards. The petrochemical industry in North America has adopted 12-hour work shifts with 3 or 4 days off in between. What the appropriate trading relationship is here is quite unknown. A further confusing factor is the effect of additional non-occupational noise. A worker with a marginal noise exposure at work who is exposed to 2 hours of the intense transportation noise daily may show more hearing loss than a worker who lives close to the plant.

The cumulative effect of lifetime noise exposure is difficult to assess. Much is made of social noise exposure and the popular press is replete with articles about the hazards of portable radios. When these claims are examined they are not found to be based on fact—indeed very careful reviews and studies have failed to find harmful effects of such devices (Davis et al 1984). In the writer's opinion, they have little part to play in current noise claims, because the total social noise exposure, when compared with a lifetime total of occupational noise exposure, is relatively modest. More study is required. Personal radios are only one cause of confusion in medicolegal claims. Most North Americans use small arms for hunting, many use power tools for hobbies, or chain saws for wood cutting. The miner who works 8 hours a day drilling, wearing protectors and even so exposing his TMs to an L (OSHA) 8 of 91 dB, and then spends a further 2 hours at home, using a radial arm saw, not using protectors, at 96 dB, adds significantly to his daily noise exposure. It should be emphasized, however, that the exposure must be prolonged over many months or years to have a significant effect. The literature really does not help in quantifying the deleterious effect of what is known as sociocusis. The occasional exceptional case is, however, noteworthy. A high school crafts teacher claimed for industrial hearing loss caused by power tools used to instruct his pupils. Neither he nor his pupils used protective devices. Nevertheless, the total daily exposure seemed low to produce the fairly typical (although originally exaggerated) notched audiogram. Detailed questioning revealed that he worked harded and longer at a 'recreational' task of home building, using many more power tools than at teaching. The total daily noise exposure was thus enough to produced the loss, although the claim was denied as not being occupational in origin.

A further difficulty in medicolegal evaluation of noise-induced hearing loss is the relative weight to be placed upon the effect of noise and other ear disease. What is the interaction between treated and untreated otosclerosis and occupational hearing loss? Certainly the conductive loss is not due to sound exposure. What of the sensorineural loss? It is known that many otosclerotics show a Carhart notch which classically shows a 5 dB bone conduction loss at 500 Hz, a 10 dB loss at 1000 Hz and a 15 dB loss at 2000 Hz before reverting back to normal in the higher frequencies. Should all industrial claimants with presumed otosclerosis have the Carhart notch corrected before evaluating the noise-induced component of their hearing loss? In truth they probably should, but the writer's experience is that legislators, jurists and others evaluating occupational losses have the greatest difficulty in comprehending this correction, and from a pragmatic standpoint it has been abandoned. It is also clear that as otosclerosis may only develop in the third or fourth decade of life, significant sound exposure may have taken place for years prior to this and that an otosclerotic may also show noise-induced hearing loss. The writer knows of no rule which helps to sort this out. Likewise, the susceptibility of a stapedectomized ear to high levels of sound compared to a non-stapedectomized ear is moot. Indeed, there is some evidence that suggests the progress of sensorineural hearing loss in non-noise-exposed otosclerotic ears is more rapid in the unoperated than in the operated side. Our own evidence (Alberti et al 1980) suggests that stapedectomy has no effect on the susceptibility of the ear to noise exposure. Similar arguments apply to ears afflicted by chronic otitis media.

The writer's practice in evaluating such claims, crude though it appears, is as follows. Sound level measurements or estimates of sound exposure are required and, in the knowledge that some ears are unusually susceptible to sound, levels of 85 dB and above for a work day, with exposure for 5 or more years, are considered potentially hazardous. The exception is exposure to a sudden intense sound or explosion, such as a warning signal to which the claimant was too close, a sledge hammer hitting a boiler close to the claimant working inside or an accidental blast exposure while mining. Only bone conduction thresholds are assessed for noise loss but then the total bone loss is almost always allowed, even in the presence of an added conductive component produced by middle ear disease. In asymmetrical sensorineural loss a major effort is made to determine whether there is a cause for the additional loss. If so, this is diagnosed and the case adjudicated as if both ears were like the one which was only suffering from noise damage. If no other cause is found, and if the shape of the audiograms are the same with only minor degrees of difference, the asymmetry is also allowed as due to occupational cause.

Old audiograms may be of great help. Many industries have a programme of screening audiometry covering many years. Access to these data is helpful for several reasons. If there is a pre-employment or early audiogram showing a hearing loss, it can limit the current employer's liability. Conversely, a normal early audiogram and a slowly progressive loss may serve to attribute cause to the current workplace. Signs of sudden change, for example a bilaterally symmetrical, slowly progressive loss, showing rapid unilateral deterioration, makes noise an unlikely cause of the worsening. The writer has identified several 'sudden' hearing losses in this way that were initially referred as noise induced, and where the acute episode had been forgotten in the original history.

Presbycusis corrections vary throughout the world and depend to some extent on the level at which pensions begin and the frequencies which are compensated. If only lower frequencies (500, 1000 and 2000 Hz) are compensated then presbycusis corrections are less rational than if only higher frequencies are compensated (1000, 2000 and 3000 Hz). The effect of presbycusis is also varied and inexorably confused with genetic changes. In the writer's opinion the paper by Corso reviewing the various corrections is a landmark in this area.

This chapter will not address the correlation between hearing loss, handicap and disability which are variably legislated throughout the world.

The following case history illustrates some of the difficulties in this type of assessment.

Case report

ML, a 75-year-old man of Yugoslav origin who spoke little English and who was accompanied by his grand-daughter who acted as a translator, was evaluated for an industrial hearing loss claim. He had migrated to Canada and worked as a gold miner, drilling underground from 1930 to 1937. He was involved in a blasting accident in 1936 when a shot detonated prematurely, severely injuring his left arm, and tattooing the left side of his face with stone chips. Following multiple operations he ultimately made a good recovery. The compensation file of that era included a photocopy of a referral letter to an otolaryngologist because of an intermittent right side aural discharge, the side opposite to the blast injury. He returned to Yugoslavia where he remained during the war and, once again, in 1953, returned to Canada as a gold miner. He sustained an appalling injury shortly thereafter when his head was squashed between a rock wall and the tow motor which he was driving underground. This aggravated his right-sided ear disease and, in addition, he developed a transient facial paralysis. He was treated on an in-patient basis in a Toronto teaching hospital for his right-sided aural discharge, by means of topical therapy and the then popular antibiotic mixture Dichrystamycin, which is a mixture of dihydrostreptomycin and penicillin. No radiological evidence of fracture of the temporal bones were found. His facial palsy recovered as did he and he returned to mining. In 1977, now aged 75, he laid a compensation claim for occupational hearing loss resulting from noise, the blasting accident and the head injury. The local otologist, who first saw him, found a bilateral mixed deafness with a discharging ear on the right side and an intact tympanic membrane on the left. He diagnosed otitis media, otoslcerosis and presbycusis. Referred for further evaluation, the claimant was adamant that his left-sided hearing was due to the blasting accident in 1936 and the right-sided discharge due to the head injury in 1953. He also complained bitterly of steady hissing tinnitus which had been present for many years. He had never worn ear defenders, had not been in the armed forces, had not used guns for hunting, had not used snowmobiles, chainsaws, nor did he give any other history of noisy hobbies. There was no family history of hearing loss. It

was almost impossible to communicate with him directly but his grand-daughter was an adequate translator. His complaint was of sounds not being loud enough and, even when loud enough, not being clear. He had never worn a hearing aid. Examination of the right ear showed a healed, distorted middle ear compatible with a long-standing, but now healed, otitis media plus a posterior canal wall fracture line. The left tympanic membrane was normal and showed no evidence of prior injury. It was mobile. The rest of his ear, nose and throat examination was normal. He had a significant left-sided conductive hearing loss plus a predominantly high frequency sensorineural loss. The middle ear compliance was low. There was no evidence of an ipsilateral stapedius reflex. In the right ear his initial thresholds were highly unreliable, but ultimately, with evoked response audiometry, cajoling and repeated testing, demonstrated a mixed hearing loss. The opinion forwarded to the compensation board was that the left-sided hearing loss was totally unrelated to industrial causes and almost certainly due to otosclerosis. Unfortunately, I was unable to agree that the right-sided hearing loss was due to the 1953 injury because of the record of a discharging ear in 1937. It was probable, however, that the fracture was due to the 1953 injury and, at most, the bone conduction loss in the right ear could be attributed to that incident. Some of his bone conduction loss might have been due to ototoxic drugs. The dosage of the dihydrostreptomycin used was not known. In the event, with a combination of old chronic ear disease, probable otosclerosis, exposure to ototoxic drugs, a severe head injury, extreme industrial noise exposure drilling as a miner, and advancing years, it was remarkable that his bone conduction hearing was as good as shown (Alberti 1982).

This case, although unusual, does illustrate the wide range of potential problems facing the otolaryngologist.

CONCLUSIONS

The evaluation of hearing loss, produced by noise, for medicolegal purposes is an art as well as a science. The quantification of hearing loss is relatively easy, but the attribution of cause of hearing loss is difficult and depends a great deal on individual judgement based upon an excellent history, and requires a degree of factual information which is usually not available.

INTRODUCTION

Patterns of forensic audiology which have developed in the various countries of the world reflect, to a great degree, the cultural, legal, political and socio-economic systems which obtain in those countries. This is merely a specific instance of Weber's (1912) concept that, in general, systems of law reflect economic, political and social factors, a concept that was reaffirmed by the American jurist Cardozo in 1921. Thus, what, for example, Sulkowski might have to say for forensic audiology in Poland and even, perhaps, Alberti for forensic audiology in Canada, might not be applicable to the scene in England. But then, as David & Brierley (1968) point out, the Law of England is not that of either the Isle of Man or of Scotland.

Because of this difference in legal systems, the author will confine himself to a discussion of this topic as it applies to the English legal system, with which he has had the most experience.

In England there is essentially a dual system of law, i.e. the common law and the statute law. Moreover, there are broadly two aspects of statute law which relate to the topic under discussion, i.e. occupational hygiene provisions (specifically, the 1961 Factories Act and the 1974 Health and Safety at Work Act) and social security provisions (specifically, the 1975 Social Security Act, under which noise-induced hearing loss is a prescribed occupational disease).

In 1974, noise-induced hearing loss became a prescribed disease under the 1965 National Insurance (Industrial Injuries) Act (the Social Security Act's predecessor).

In a 1978 judgment (*McIntyre* v. *Doulton*), the judge said (after referring to a Scottish case), 'I hold, therefore, that section 29 (of the Factories Act) does cover the dangers created in a place of work by excessive noise'. The same opinion was expressed by the judge in *Kellett* v. *British Rail Engineering Ltd* 1984, although the judge in *McGuinness* v. *Kirkstall Forge* 1978 and the judge in *Thompson and others* v. *Smiths Ship Repairers* 1984 did not find, on the facts in those cases, any breach of the statutory duty.

Claims that defective hearing is attributable to an employer's negligence (blameworthiness) are therefore usually based on the dual claim that: (a) the employer is in breach of a Common Law duty, and (b) he is in breach of a statutory (section 29 of the Factories Act) duty.

Consequently, individuals may claim compensation for damage to their hearing by actions for negligence as well as under social security legislation. (Under social security legistation, i.e. State insurance, the need to prove negligence or other default is removed.) In addition there are a number of compensation schemes for out-of-court settlements. These schemes are based on agreements between insurers and trade unions. Such agreements are, of course, governed by contract law.

(Contract law is essentially the law relating to agreements. Together with the law of tort (under which the Law of Negligence comes), contract law broadly covers the law of rights and obligations. Apart from drawing on common law, contract law also draws on equity and statute law.)

The rules under which individuals may claim compensation for occupational or other damage to hearing will therefore depend upon which approach is being made. These differences also encompass differences in the nature and extent of the medical examination, although this is not often appreciated. Under the social security legislation, conditions are more circumscribed. There is, therefore, not much latitude for differences in medical examination procedure in respect of Department of Health and Social Security claims. Moreover, under union/insurers agreements, the standard of proof required is fixed by agreement between the parties. According to Chuang Wei Ping (1985), this standard of proof may be virtually non-existent.

In common law actions, the medical practitioner may be called upon not only to examine a claimant, but also to give evidence on the state of, say, preventive occupational audiology since its inception. Moreover, a reading of Chuang's monograph would indicate that there is anything but a smooth running of common law procedures in this matter.

'To be involved' or 'not to be involved' in these common law actions is thus now said to be the greatest dilemma of ear specialists in Britain. But, used in that sense, the term 'dilemma' has a more colloquial connotation since the word is defined as 'a logical or actual position presenting only a choice between two or more unwelcome alternatives' (Oxford English Dictionary). There may well be no 'unwelcome alternatives' in forensic audiology. As was pointed out by Sir Roger Ormrod (1972), law, medicine and science have in common the search for the truth. Thus, if there are any dichotomous choices it is between the welcome truth (or methods on searching for the truth) and the unwelcome untruth.

Nevertheless, in this particular field, with particular reference to common law actions, one can define a progressive series of what might be termed *pseudodilemmas*.

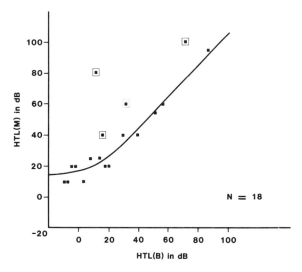

Fig. 2.1 A comparison of the hearing threshold level reported for one particular frequency (1 kHz, right ear) for 18 consecutive plaintiffs who had been seen by the same two medical examiners. One of these had used manual audiometry, which gave reported thresholds indicated by HTL (M), the other used self-recorded audiometry, which gave reported thresholds indicated by HTL (B). The figure reflects two major sources of error associated with manual audiometry as it is frequently used in medicolegal work, i.e. the failure to detect exaggeration and its use in inadequately sound-treated test rooms. The values enclosed in squares refer to plaintiffs where exaggeration was established by ERA.

THE CASCADE OF PSEUDODILEMMAS

To accept?

Thus the *first pseudodilemma* is whether or not to *accept* instructions from a solicitor to examine his client and make a report on that examination. One reason for a doctor declining could be on the grounds that he is fully committed to, for example, the surgical management of auditory disorders and he would rather leave the assessment of occupational hearing disorders to those members of the medical profession with a special interest and training in such matters.

Another reason for declining to accept a solicitor's instructions would be that one does not have the necessary experience and expertise to comply with instructions. Figure 2.1 shows a series of measurements of a particular hearing level reported by one medical examiner and compared with the measurements found by another medical examiner using a more sophisticated procedure. Clearly, the first medical examiner would be able to claim, with all justification, that, if he were to accept instructions, the hearing levels that he would report would, more likely than not, be spurious.

A third reason could be that the doctor does not wish to put himself at risk of being discredited. In British court actions, expert evidence is dealt with under what is termed an adversarial system (as opposed to the Continental inquisitorial system). As Havard (1984) points out, the success of the adversarial system depends to a large extent on the

degree to which the expert witness for one side can be discredited by the other side.

In the case of *Thompson and others* v. *Smiths Ship Repairers*, this approach went even further. There was an attempt to discredit the broad base of relevant scientific knowledge. For example, there was an attempt to nullify the scientific evidence which had been accepted by the judge in *McIntyre* v. *Doulton*, i.e. that 'the loss of hearing (in occupational noise-induced hearing loss) is apparently faster in the earlier stages'. (This is implicit in Robinson and Shipton's NPL tables.) Had this antagonistic approach succeeded it would have left the running in future cases entirely to the lawyers.

Unfortunately, in forensic audiology, attempts to discredit the other side's expert witnesses have not been confined to the courtroom, nor have such attempts been kept within the limits that the law allows. Exemplifying this was the attempted character assassination of the doctor who would be the defendant's principal expert medical witness in the 1983 ONIHL (occupational noise-induced hearing loss) trials. The libellous attack using television was merely the tip of an iceberg. The political machine was also brought into the attack. This tarnished not only the Reithian image of British broadcasting but also the Citrinian image of British trade unionism as well as the Fabian image of the British Labour Party. The attack introduced the most sordid era in the history of personal injuries litigation in Britain.

Clearly, however, a medical examiner cannot decline cases from defendant's solicitors on these grounds and yet accept cases from plaintiff's solicitors. To show impartiality he would have to decline cases from both sides. Such an action would mean a halt to the litigation process and not be in the interest of justice. The number of solicitors that can be troublesome is, however, less than a handful of the solicitors (about 165) who are involved in litigation in this area. All doctors who agree to become medical examiners (and, therefore, potentially expert witnesses) should therefore also accept cases from defendant's solicitors.

How to elicit the anamnesis?

The *second pseudodilemma* relates to taking the *history* from the plaintiff. As Rosenberg (1972) points out, 'the case history is the first test'. The pseudodilemma is how this should be elicited. The use of standardized questionnaires eradicates many of the sources of error inherent in conventional history taking (Cochrane et al 1951).

Since the common law compensates for loss of amenity, it is important to ascertain the impact which any alleged damage to hearing has had on the individual. Thus, the use of questionnaires based upon Noble and Atherley's work (Noble & Atherley 1970, Atherley & Noble 1971, Noble 1978) would appear to possess obvious advantages. Lutman and his colleagues (1986), however, argue that, for the assessment of disability and handicap, performance measures are to be preferred to questionnaires. The latter are more 'prone to bias from extraneous factors such as exaggeration, personal opinion and inappropriate self-perception'. In particular, questionnaires, because of their very nature, contain leading questions. This can lead to uncertainties regarding the severity, or even the existence, of a symptom. For example, in one case heard in court, there was a dispute over whether or not the plaintiff

suffered from tinnitus. The dispute had clearly arisen because of the use, by one doctor, of a questionnaire with leading questions. Moreover, it would appear that, over the years, the pattern of response to questionnaires has changed. A response pattern which is favourable to plaintiffs has been emerging. Paradoxically, some solicitors acting for plaintiffs have opposed the use of questionnaires. Nevertheless, what the law compensates is a plaintiff's loss of amenity. Only the plaintiff can know in what way, and to what extent, his quality of life has been affected by virtue of defective hearing. The doctor will also require the answers to certain questions that are relevant to causation. It would thus behove him to use the system of eliciting the medical history which is more akin to that used by lawyers in eliciting evidence. The doctor then records the actual questions which are posed and the actual answers which are given. He can start the questioning by asking, 'What is the problem?'. This method gives the plaintiff the opportunity to give a full account of his auditory handicaps, aspects of which may not have been highlighted by conventional questionnaires. An alternative approach could be to use Barcham & Stephens (1980) open-ended problems questionnaire. However, this questionnaire would still need to be supplemented by additional questions.

It should be noted that nowhere else in clinical audiology is the distinction between semeions and symptoms (Wilbush 1984) so important. Symptoms are those sensory experiences which are spontaneously reported to the doctor; semeions are those which are elicited only by direct questioning.

Request other medical records

The *third pseudodilemma* is whether or not to request *records* from the plaintiff's family doctor and from hospitals which he may have attended. Many medical examiners do not take the trouble to consult these records, but they can be immensely valuable when one furnishes one's report. Indeed, Lord Denning (1984) advised these doctors to 'collect the attendance records made by all the doctors who had examined and treated the patient and all the notes made by the nurses and doctors in every hospital where he was'. He then goes on to say, 'At one time it was thought that these were confidential and could not be disclosed without the consent of the patient himself and the doctors and nurses and hospital concerned. But that notion is gone, because their disclosure is necessary in the interests of justice'. The principle was stated in *Attorney General* v. *Mulholland* (1963). It is usual, however, for a form of authority to be signed by the plaintiff to facilitate the release of records. Indeed were such records to be released to someone other than the patient without his consent and without a court order, then he might have a right of action at law for breach of confidence (Medicolegal 1985). Section 31 of the Administration of Justice Act 1970 empowered the courts to make an order that any person likely to be made a party to an action should produce for inspection any documents in his possession or power that were likely to be relevant. Sections 33 and 34 of the Supreme Court Act 1981 enacted that production of such documents might be limited to the applicant's legal, medical or other professional adviser. Thus, the plaintiff might be advised to agree to a settlement for reasons which his advisers do not disclose to him.

Information contained in these reports can affect not only the diagnosis but also the assessment and apportionment. Sometimes the information contained in the records is not to the advantage of the plaintiff. This explains the obstacles that solicitors for plaintiffs may sometimes put in the way of the acquisition of copies of these records. If there is any tardiness an application for a court order invariably produces the required result.

Most family doctors are quite helpful in the matter of having sight of their records on a plaintiff once they have the signed form of authority. A small minority express some reluctance, saying that one should apply to the appropriate family practitioner committee (FPC). It is correct that the medical notes of NHS general practice patients are the property of the Secretary of State and, through him, of the FPCs, although the notes are in the actual possession and custody of the family practitioner. However, as Palmer (1980) points out, the FPCs are generally content to leave it to the individual family doctor concerned. If there are any delays and a form of authority has been signed, the solicitors for the plaintiff will then write to the family practitioner pointing out that this is a perfectly usual practice.

In respect of hospital notes, the legal rights of the Secretary of State are vested in the district health authorities. Thus, an application for hospital notes should properly be directed to the appropriate health authority. There are, however, delays so that if copies of the required notes are not received by the time the doctor furnishes his report, he should make it quite clear that his report is contingent on nothing being noted in the family doctor's or the hospital's records which might require him to modify his opinions.

Examine?

The *fourth pseudodilemma* relates to *whether or not properly to examine* the plaintiff.

A number of laymen labour under the delusion that 'if a man has worked in noise all his life, how can there be anything else which has affected his hearing?'. There is, however, no evidence that the development of an ONIHL either cures preceding hearing disorders or 'immunizes' an individual against the development of subsequent non-noise-induced hearing defects.

Not only is there ample evidence that occupational noise-exposed individuals suffer from auditory disorders other than those due to noise, but the chances of finding a non-noise-induced auditory disablement may even be greater than that of finding a noise-induced one.

The term disablement is used here in the sense accorded to it by Wood (1980), i.e. 'a collective descriptor referring to any experience identified variously by the terms impairment, disability and handicap'. As McGinnis (1982) points out, these three terms roughly correspond to 'bits that don't work', 'activities that can't be carried out' and 'roles that can't be performed'. Unfortunately, the term disablement has already been defined legally. In *Hudson* v. *Secretary of State for Social Services* [1972], disablement was defined as the sum of disabilities which, when compared with the powers of a normal person, can be expressed as a percentage. There is, therefore, still the need to find a suitable term, which has not already been defined, to cover impairment, disability and handicap. Nevertheless, for the purposes of this paper, the term will be used in the sense accorded to it by Wood.)

As an example, in his 1926 study of 1011 English weavers, McKelvie (1933) observed that 68 suffered from 'nerve deafness' and 178 suffered from 'other forms of deafness'. Chronic otitis media, or sequelae, was present in 7.5% of the weavers. Subsequent studies in England and other parts of the world have indicated that surdogens (factors which impair hearing) other than noise may account for an appreciable proportion of auditory disorders in occupational noise-exposed subjects. Precise figures are, however, often not available. For example, in reporting a study of Scottish jute weavers, Taylor and his colleagues (1965) said, 'of the 401 weavers and retired weavers examined, the audiometric data on 150 were eliminated because of failure to satisfy the criteria for inclusion'. Previously the authors had listed a number of rejection criteria. These criteria were based upon a clinical aural examination. In another hearing study of Scottish jute weavers, Kell and his colleagues (1971) reported that 21 out of 88 subjects who had agreed to take part in the research were rejected for medical or noise exposure reasons. In the Joint Medical Research Council/National Physical Laboratory's Survey of Hearing and Noise in Industry (Burns & Robinson, 1970), a clinical aural examination resulted in the elimination of 11% of subjects. At the 1970 Occupational Hearing Loss Conference held at the British National Physical Laboratory, Raber (1971) reported the Austrian experience:

Out of the bulk of nearly 30 000 mass audiometric data on workers exposed to continuous noise, only 600 cases were without otological abnormalities, personal history of ear disease, gunfire experience, etc. When we examined the audiograms meeting these stipulations, we found relatively mild cases of noise-induced hearing loss. In our opinion this means that there are many other factors influencing the degree of hearing loss in noise-exposed people.

Where borderline noise hazardous conditions are concerned, the predominance of other auditory disorders is even more apparent. El Alami (1981) reported a 1979 study in a London factory where the workers in the 'noisy' area were exposed to average noise levels around 86 dB(A). A sample of 28 men was examined from each of two factory areas which had been designated either as 'noisy' or 'non-noisy'. There were 8 abnormal audiograms in the 'noisy area' group and 11 abnormal audiograms in 'the non-noisy area' group. Moreover:

(a) The 'very severe cases of deafness' (2) were not attributable to noise exposure.

(b) Conditions other than ONIHL accounted

for the majority of abnormal audiograms in the factory.

(c) None of the abnormal audiograms attributed to noise exposure alone were from the men who worked in the 'noisy' area.

Point (a) is merely one instance of a general finding in people exposed to occupational noise hazards, i.e. severe hearing impairments indicate the influence of factors other than occupational noise. For example, in a study of steel workers aged 55 to 64 years, Howell (1975) found that 'mild' or 'marked' impairment of hearing (according to 1964-based American Academy of Ophthalmology and Otolaryngology criteria) was more than six times as common in the men who had clinical evidence for aural pathology (i.e. other than that to be attributed to ageing or to noise exposure).

The above-mentioned studies which have shown the importance of factors other than noise have almost exclusively been based upon a clinical aural examination. There is increasing evidence not only that systemic disorders can influence the hearing but that the effect can be appreciable (Lim & Stephens 1985).

In 1974, Alberti, an otologist working in Canada, summarized his own experience and sentiments based upon the examination of more than 700 individuals claiming in respect of ONIHL:

It is a common fallacy to accept that, because a man has been exposed to high sound levels and is hard of hearing, the two are inevitably related. This study has demonstrated, once again, that workers in high sound levels are no different from the population at large in the incidence of other ear disease which may produce hearing loss of a variety of types, including those in which the audiometric configuration is similar to that produced by noise; therefore, it is incumbent upon otologists to insist upon full otological history and examination prior to awarding a pension for occupational hearing loss.

British audiological physicians are clearly alive to the importance of extra-aural factors. For example, Coles (1981) has said, in respect of the investigation of auditory disorders, 'we do a full range of haematological tests . . .'. His concern for a subject's haematological status was amply justified by his Institute (of Hearing Research) subsequently discovering the immense importance of blood viscosity (Browning et al 1986).

Further confounding factors are introduced into

clinical forensic audiological practice. Many subjects, quite naturally, exaggerate their hearing losses and their auditory handicaps. Alberti and his colleagues (1974) reported that, in their series, 20% of claimants exaggerated the loss. More recently, Rossi and his colleagues (1985) reported that exaggeration was present in 45% of 257 claimants who had been examined in Turin in the first half of 1985. Moreover, for the group of claimants showing exaggeration, the average difference between the ERA (electric response audiometric) threshold and the pure-tone threshold was 45 dB at 3 kHz. The magnitude of this difference is that it is the difference between having, for DHSS purposes, an 80% disablement assessment and not reaching a compensable level at all. At the moment it is not clear whether the differences in the data reported by Alberti and his colleagues and by Rossi and his colleagues can be accounted for by cultural differences, or whether they indicate an increase in the prevalence of exaggeration.

An examination of claimants will greatly reflect the experience and expertise of the doctor. Thus a primary physician might content himself with a single test—the therapeutic test of ear syringing. If the individual had worked in a noise-hazardous occupation and the hearing did not improve with syringing, then the impairment might well be attributed to occupational noise damage. An ENT surgeon would probably content himself with an otoscopic examination together with air and bone conduction audiometry using manual techniques. This is quite understandable in view of his role in health care in endeavouring to alleviate impaired hearing that is amenable to surgical intervention, i.e. the conductive auditory disorders. (However, reliance on these three methods only to assess the aural condition has resulted in otosclerosis being wrongly diagnosed. This is because a spurious air–bone gap has gone undetected. Had tuning fork tests and/or acoustic impedance studies been done, a false diagnosis of otosclerosis would not have been made.) The audiological physician will (or should) want to conduct a more extended examination of the plaintiff. The results of such an examination frequently bring to light the existence of other surdogens. These may or may not be playing a part in the plaintiff's hearing impairment, let alone his auditory handicap. Consequently, some solicitors

acting for plaintiffs have endeavoured to restrict the examination as much as possible. The maximum constraints that have been imposed on a medical examiner occurred when one union was preparing for litigation in connection with claims in respect of ONIHL. In these examinations, the medical examiner acting for defendants was constrained from using even an ear speculum. Thus, even the traditional method of examining the ear which was introduced by von Tröltsch in the 19th century was denied to that examiner.

Nowadays, many doctors would wish to conduct an otomicroscopic examination of the ear since, as Lundborg & Linzander (1969) pointed out, with conventional examination techniques using ear specula without magnification, even experienced otologists may overlook clinically important middle ear details. Ingelstedt and Flisberg's modification of Siegle's speculum using plain glass without magnification is a very useful otomicroscopical accessory. It makes it easy to observe the mobility of different parts of the drum and malleus as well as the movements of the latter bone. However, even with the use of an ear microscope, the configuration of the external acoustic meatus and the presence of the associated hairs are such as to prevent a view of the eardrum in the majority of adult British men unless an aural speculum is used.

These obstacles should not deter the medical examiner. Data are available which can be used to assess the probabilities of hearing impairment due to cerumen and to ear disease. Nevertheless, such hindrance of the medical examination is contrary to a 1983 interlocutory judgment in Holt v. British Aerospace. The plaintiff's solicitors had endeavoured to constrain the medical examination which two medical examiners instructed by the defendants had proposed to conduct. It was a case of alleged noise-induced hearing loss. The case was heard before the district registrar who ruled, 'So long as the defendants choose a professional man with obviously good qualifications, then it seems to me that he should be given the right to make the decision (regarding which tests to do)'. The Registrar distinguished this case from the one of Prescott v. Bulldog Tools 1981 on the grounds that in Holt, 'nothing is really known about the plaintiff's deafness'. In Prescott, the plaintiff had an asymmetrical hearing loss with a total loss on one side. The judge who heard the interlocutory appeal in this case, was faced with affidavits provided by the plaintiff's solicitors which portrayed a horrendous nature for the tests which the medical examiner instructed by defendants proposed to do. In any event, the judge said that,

> . . . the court imposes no restrictions on such examinations of any kind. If defendants go to a particular expert and if he says he will only carry out an examination in a particular way, it is for those defendants to decide whether to request a plaintiff to be examined on those terms, and if the question arises and if the plaintiff objects to those terms it is for the Court to weigh the reasonableness of the objection against the reasonableness of the defendant's request for that examination . . . . All it is necessary for me to determine is the reasonableness of the defendant's request as reasonably seen by them, and the reasonableness of the plaintiff's objections as seen by him (by which, of course, I mean as reasonably seen by him), and then to compare the weight of the reasonableness of the request with that of the reasonableness of the objection. For that purpose it does not seem to me (at any rate, in this case) to be necessary to resolve such conflicts as there are between the various deponents.

In the absence of the results for a medical examination, the doctor may still be able to make an assessment as to whether or not the plaintiff's hearing has been damaged by noise (provided, of course, that data on audiometric thresholds are not available). After the audiogram has been inspected (with regard to general configuration—pattern of impairment, degree of loss, symmetry), the National Physical Laboratory Tables (Robinson & Shipton 1977), which relate hearing levels to noise-emmission levels, should be consulted. The occupational history will give some idea of the noise exposure which an individual would have sustained. The tables will also give some idea of the extent to which the measured thresholds are compatible with the occupational history.

More recently, Robinson (1985) has published a step-by-step procedure to test the probability that factors other than noise exposure have been implicated in a hearing impairment. Other data (e.g. Alberti et al 1978, 1979, Chung et al 1981, 1983, Klockhoff et al 1974) are also available, and can be used to assess the probability that factors other than the alleged occupational noise have been involved.

How is the hearing to be measured?

The fifth pseudodilemma relates to the method of *hearing measurement.* For the various claims which might arise under social security law provisions, various methods have been laid down. For example, with regard to hearing assessments in respect of the severe disablement allowance, the Department of Health and Social Security requires the claimant to be tested using a live conversational voice test (DHSS 1985). The same procedure is adopted for both war pension and industrial injury claims. For assessments under the prescribed occupational disease provisions, a manual pure-tone audiogram is required. Under that scheme, preference is given to using a manual pure-tone audiogram for assessment since the scheme was set up in consultation with ENT surgeons for a scheme to be implemented by ENT surgeons. For claims under the common law, no system is laid down. Nevertheless, attempts have been made, and continue to be made, to have self-recording audiometry (Bekesy 1947) excluded. Self-recording audiometry (SRA) has picked up too many cases of exaggeration.

Clinical tests for hearing assessment are at present being contested by the Royal National Institute for the Deaf on the grounds of their imprecision and unreliability. As Figure 2.1 indicates, the accuracy of manual audiometry is also to be questioned. Indeed, having regard to Figure 2.1, it may well be argued that conventional manual audiometry should now be abandoned for all medicolegal purposes. In its review of the first 586 ONIHL claims cases who were reassessed after a 5-year period, the DHSS (1982) expressed surprise that 31% showed an apparent improvement in hearing of at least 10 dB and 13% of cases appeared no longer to satisfy the minimum hearing loss requirements. The DHSS attributed the findings to 'lack of experience on the part of consultants and technicians . . . faulty testing equipment . . . non-organic hearing loss'.

If SRA is not available for medicolegal hearing assessments, then exceptions to the non-use of manual audiometry might be made provided

1. The ambient sound levels in the test room did not exceed specified values, e.g. as given in the draft International Standard ISO/DIS 8253.

2. There was employed, in addition, a test to detect exaggeration, e.g.

(a) the modification of Harris' (1958) test by Kerr and his colleagues (1975),

(b) the combination of manual pure-tone audiometry with speech audiometry (Alberti et al 1978) (although this combination seems to work for some examiners, e.g. Taylor (1986) —from personal communication—it does not seem to work for others), or

(c) the modification of Theodor and Mandel-corn's (1973) technique by Haughton and his colleagues (1979).

3. The testing was conducted by a qualified individual.

The Health and Safety Executive's Discussion Document on Audiometry in Industry (1978) recommended discrete frequency pulsed-tone air-conduction SRA for routine use in industry. The document points out that SRA has a number of advantages:

1. Virtual elimination of bias due to the audio-metrician.

2. The unambiguous nature of the subject's response.

3. The provision of a permanent record without a possibility of transcription errors.

4. A visible indication of the quality of the sub-ject's test performance.

Sweep frequency SRA has the additional advantage that it can detect incipient, or other, noise-induced notches when discrete frequency audiometry, whether manual or self-recording, has failed to do so.

The use of continuous test-tone sweep frequency audiometry, in addition to pulsed test-tone sweep frequency audiometry, considerably enhances the possibility of detecting spurious thresholds. Thus, the preferred method for measuring the threshold of hearing for medicolegal purposes is sweep frequency combined pulsed and continuous test-tone SRA. If necessary, sweep frequency SRA can be backed up by fixed frequency SRA, e.g. if, at any frequency, there is some uncertainty about the true threshold measured by sweep frequency testing.

SRA also has the advantage in that it is the same type of audiometry that was used in the Medical Research Council/National Physical Laboratory's Survey of Hearing and Noise in Industry (Burns & Robinson 1970). Robinson and Shipton's tables are based upon that study. SRA was also the type of audiometry used by Robinson and his colleagues (1984) to determine the hearing disability threshold level.

There have been suggestions that some individuals might find SRA difficult. It would appear that there is a general tendency of doctors to under-estimate the intellectual capabilities of the proletariat (e.g. Evans 1986). In any case, SRA can be performed satisfactorily by subjects with a mental age of 7 years (Price & Falck 1963).

Delegate the testing?

The *sixth pseudodilemma* concerns whether or not any part of the tests should be *delegated* to others. On occasion, solicitors acting for plaintiffs have endeavoured to make a point that some doctors delegate testing (or some of the tests) to other audiological, or para-audiological, personnel. Apart from making a nuisance of themselves, it is not quite clear why this should be done. Nevertheless, the examining consultant should point out that para 4 of the DHSS Report of the Working Party on the Responsibility of the Consultant Grade points out that 'the clinical responsibility of the consultant includes the personal execution or, where possible and appropriate, the delegation and subsequent supervision, of all items of the medical care of patients in his charge'. Some examiners make a point not only of delegating certain tests to others but of actually naming the person who did the particular test.

Which disablement scales to use?

The *seventh pseudodilemma* concerns the choice of *disablement scales*.

A number of scales have been, or are, in use to assess auditory disablement. Frequently, the medical examiner does not know which scales are being used by his instructing solicitor. In that event, it would be prudent to indicate the claimant's position on a number of scales. Thus in addition to indicating whether or not the claimant reaches Robinson's (1984) hearing disability threshold level, one can report where the claimant would be on the DHSS scale for assessing percentage disablement for ONIHL as a prescribed occupational disorder.

The Dundee Index (Kell et al 1971) was one of

the first experimental attempts to relate the degree of hearing impairment in people working in noise-hazardous occupations to the degree of social disability/handicap. Although the calculation to obtain the index involves subtracting a value for the hearing level at 4 kHz, the resulting index shows a good correspondence with the hearing threshold level at 2 kHz. The balance of scientific evidence indicates that measures of auditory disability probably correlate better with losses at this frequency than with those at any other frequency.

At least one audiological physician (Coles 1975) has voiced the sentiments of others regarding which method to use for rating handicap: 'It could be that the measured impairment is in fact a better guide to the true social handicap than the patient's description of his hardships'. Coles drew attention to Acton's (1973) finding that one of the best correlations ($r = 0.643$) was between the hearing threshold level averaged over 1, 2 and 3 kHz and the results obtained from the questionnaire used by Kell and his colleagues. Nevertheless some workers, e.g. Salomon & Parving (1985), are making attempts to get away from the tonal threshold as a basis for disability and handicap assessments. These workers base assessments on self-assessments of speech perception which also includes the ability to perceive visual clues.

A *Method for Assessment of Hearing Disability* (the so-called 'Blue Book') which had been proposed jointly by the British Association of Otolaryngologists and the British Society of Audiology (British Journal of Audiology 17:203-212) has failed to secure endorsement by the courts. It is now in abeyance pending further deliberations, but this time in conjunction with the British Association of Audiological Physicians and the British Association of Audiological Scientists.

To apportion?

The *eighth pseudodilemma* relates to *apportionment*. Apportionment has been defined as the dividing of a legal right into its proportionate parts, according to the interests of the parties concerned (Saunders 1970). In the field of ONIHL, apportionment refers to recognizing and quantifying various components in a hearing disablement. Since there is, as yet, no agreed scale for either auditory disability or auditory

handicap, this leads us to considering auditory impairment when attempting apportionment.

The medical examiner might be asked by the instructing solicitor as to whether or not he can conduct an apportionment exercise on a plaintiff's hearing loss. The answer must be in the affirmative. The principle of apportionment was accepted in *Thompson and others* v. *Smiths Ship Repairers*. Apportionment for hearing loss may be in respect of

1. Apportionment between different causes of the hearing loss.
2. Apportionment between different employment sources (including both civilian and military occupational noise exposure) of a noise-induced hearing loss.
3. Apportionment between different periods in the same employment.

The third type of apportionment may be necessary because the law recognizes that an employer may be negligent over a certain period only of a plaintiff's employment. It is held, for example, that, prior to a certain date in the 1950s or 1960s (depending on the nature of the industry), an employer cannot be held to be negligent in respect of his employee sustaining occupational noise damage to his hearing. The date on which an employer becomes negligent is termed the date of guilty knowledge (DGK). For British Rail Engineering Ltd, it has been held to be 1955. For other parts of British industry, 1963 appears to apply (e.g. in *McGuinness* v. *Kirkstall Forge* and in *Thompson and others* v. *Smiths Ship Repairers*). The period of presumed negligence (PPN) would end when protection from exposure to hazardous noise was provided (if at all).

The starting point for calculations of apportionment is the application of the results of Burns and Robinson's (1970) study.

The results are available in tabular form, i.e. the tables for the Estimation of Noise-induced Hearing Loss by Robinson and Shipton (see References), frequently referred to as the NPL tables. 'They are the only comprehensive source of data currently available' (Mustill in *Thompson and others* v. *Smiths Ship Repairers*); 'The authority of the tables is in my judgment not in dispute, they are of the highest authority' (Popplewell in *Kellett* v. *British Rail Engineering Ltd*).

These research workers quantified noise-exposure and derived an equation which related measured hearing levels to noise-exposure, expressed in terms of what they termed the noise immission level (NIL) and to age.

Although Burns and Robinson studied workers who had been exposed to noise of an essentially continuous character, it has since been shown that this type of analysis can also be applied to intermittent/impulsive noise (Atherley & Martin 1971, Martin & Atherley 1973).

To provide numerical values on which to base apportionment in respect of periods of time, it is necessary to conduct what has been termed a *retrodictive* exercise. This involves working back from a known threshold of hearing. It is essentially a reconstruction of the curve of an ONIHL based upon measurement of the plaintiff's hearing at one or other point in time. In this reconstruction of the course of the ONIHL, cognisance is taken of any changes in levels of noise exposure. There is now a large body of information available on noise levels

which obtain, or have obtained, in the various noise hazardous occupations.

For the purpose of calculating the hearing-damaging effect of noise, noise levels are expressed as equivalent continuous sounds levels (*Leq*). The *Leq* is given in decibels on the A weighting scale of the sound level meter, i.e. in dB(A). When the *Leq* value is combined with the duration of noise exposure it produces a figure termed the noise immission level (NIL) which is expressed in dB (NI).

A comparison of the inferred noise-induced hearing loss (INIHL) (inferred from the total noise immission level) with the measured thresholds of hearing will indicate whether or not the degree of measured hearing loss is commensurate with the occupational history given by the plaintiff. A lesser degree of hearing loss than anticipated would indicate a hyposusceptible individual; a greater loss than expected would indicate a hypersusceptible

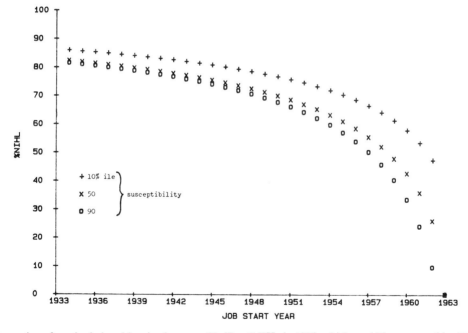

Fig. 2.2 Proportion of a noise-induced hearing loss, e.g. 24 dB at 2 KHz in 1985, which would have accured by 1963 (a year which is frequently taken as the date of guilty knowledge, i.e. the start of negligent periods of occupational noise exposure), according to the year when the job was started. For the purposes of this analysis, it has been assumed that no hearing protection has been used and the job has been equally noisy between the time when the job was started and 1985. In practice (a) noise levels have fallen with the passage of time, and (b) hearing protection has been afforded sooner or later. Thus the proportion of NIHL which would have accrued before the DGK is frequently even greater than this figure indicates. The 10%ile, 50%ile and 90%ile can be equated with individuals whose ears are very susceptible 'normally' susceptible and very resistant, respectively, to noise damage. The figure was constructed using formula (4) in Robinson and Shipton's NPL Acoustics Report Ac 61, 1977.

individual. The NPL tables quantify the degree of susceptibility in terms of noise susceptibility percentiles (NSP). Thus, if one knows the value of two of the three measures, ANIHL (adduced noise-induced hearing loss—adduced from the measured hearing threshold levels), TNIL (total noise immission level) and NSP (noise susceptibility percentile), then one can infer the third measure. The degree of certainty in the calculations will hinge on the accuracy of estimating the TNIL. However, in practice, when it comes to calculating percentage apportionment in respect of DGK, these uncertainties are not critical (see Fig. 2.2).

Some confusion has been generated by misinterpretation of the caveat in the preface to the NPL tables, i.e. 'prediction for the individual remains impossible'. This caveat applies to calculating what a measured threshold ought to be at a given point in time when one has information only on what the CNIL (cumulative noise immission level) might be by that date. In clinical forensic audiological practice, the starting point is always at least one audiogram.

Prognosis?

The *ninth pseudodilemma* relates to *prognosis*. An examiner might be asked by instructing solicitors to make a prediction of the *future course* of a plaintiff's hearing. The prefatory caveat mentioned above has also been used by some plaintiff's solicitors to argue against the possibility of making such a forecast. Again, the picture in clinical practice is different from that envisaged by the caveat. As mentioned under 'apportionment', one or more audiograms are available on which to base a prediction. Knowledge of the noise levels to which a subject has been exposed taken in conjunction with the measured threshold of hearing at a particular frequency will indicate a particular NSP at that frequency. For this exercise, the National Physical Laboratory Tables, or Robinson's specific equations, on which the tables are based, are used for calculations. The accuracy of the predictions, will, of course, be governed by any uncertainty in the adduced TNIL.

The doctor should point out that the principle of prediction is merely a special case of *prognosis*. He should further emphasize that making a prognosis is an everyday occurrence in medical practice—and has been from time immemorial. Edelstein (1967)

pointed out that Littre and Daremberg reached the accepted conclusion that the establishment of the concept of prognosis constituted one of the scientific achievements of ancient medicine.

Advise on quantum?

The *10th pseudodilemma* relates to *quantum*.

The examiner may be invited to make observations on *quantum* (how much money should the plaintiff be given?). There is no reason for him not to accede to this request. Legally, an assessment of quantum will hinge on an assessment of the loss of amenity. Perhaps the nearest medical concept for this is the degree of handicap.

In the Court of Appeal in *Robinson* v. *British Rail* 1982, it was held that the audiogram was not to be used as the sole arbiter in quantifying a plaintiff's handicap ('a mere comparison of decibel loss can be very misleading' per Lord Justice Kerr). Thus, one man may have less hearing impairment than another man and yet suffer a greater handicap. But this concept enunciated by the Court of Appeal, i.e. the limitations of audiograms in determining loss of amenity, is adhered to by audiological physicians. Indeed, it is these doctors who, having regard to the total medical, psychological and sociological picture, are perhaps best able to provide a global assessment of handicap.

Advise on rehabilitative measures?

The *11th pseudodilemma* relates to advice about, or action on, the audiological *rehabilitation* of plaintiffs.

Affidavits have been produced by solicitors acting for plaintiffs in an endeavour to defeat any attempts to institute (or improve) audiological rehabilitation. The purpose is absolutely clear—to increase quantum. But, as at least one plaintiff has said, 'What is money if I cannot have my hearing back!' It can, in fact, be questioned as to whether or not money can compensate for anything other than actual monetary loss—and this applies not only to physical damage (personal injury) but also to psychological damage (defamation).

Worse, many plaintiffs are told by doctors, including ear specialists who have examined them, that 'there is nothing we can do for you. A hearing aid will not help you'. This must surely be a reflection on the inadequacy of the audiological training provided for ENT specialists.

It is now abundantly clear, e.g. from Lund & Hoyvik (1979) and others, that individuals with noise-induced hearing loss can derive appreciable benefit from hearing aids. Attention, however, needs to be given to the type of aid and the earmould engineering. Hearing aid provision is, indeed, a most sophisticated clinical science (Stephens 1984).

If a plaintiff has a hearing disability and does not have a hearing aid he should be told that such an instrument will help him. If he does have a hearing aid, then he should be assessed as to the adequacy and appropriateness of the auditory rehabilitative measures adopted in his case. The majority of the plaintiffs seen by the author have inadequate hearing aid systems, inclusive of the hearing aid itself and the earmould engineering.

The number of claimants who have environmental hearing aids is abysmally poor. Claimants should be advised regarding the approach to be made to obtain such aids, if they are indicated.

Unfortunately, there is, as yet, little or no legal support for such attempts to improve the audiological rehabilitation of plaintiffs. In the judgment given in the interlocutory appeal in *Prescott* v. *Bulldog Tools*, the judge said, 'I would be surprised if any medical man would seek to treat, or even examine for the purpose of treatment, a person who was not his patient'. Perhaps the judge had in mind medical or surgical treatment, and not rehabilitative measures. Or is it because, as Lord Gifford (1984) has claimed, the legal profession has failed to respond to the needs of people? Certainly, it could be argued that the provision of a hearing aid, and the response to its fitting, formed an essential component in the assessment of disability. In any case, it is extremely doubtful whether any medical practitioner could be found in this country who would be willing to say in the witness box that he did not wish his patient to have a hearing aid (or provided with a better one).

Comment on other reports?

The *12th pseudodilemma* relates to *comment on other reports.*

A doctor may be asked to comment on other medical reports. There is again no reason for him refusing to accede to this request.

The comment may be in respect of, for example:

1. The medical, occupational and family history elicited by other doctors.
2. The medical examination.
3. The audiogram.
4. The conclusions (including diagnosis and prognosis) reached regarding the auditory disablement.

For example, the history-taking may have failed to elicit the fact that the plaintiff had formerly served in the armed forces or had used a 12- bore gun. The failure of both medical examiners instructed by the plaintiff's solicitor to elicit the fact that the plaintiff had used a 12-bore gun paved the way to the collapse of the plaintiff's case in *McIntyre* v. *Doulton*.

All too frequently the doctor has restricted his examination to an otoscopic examination to exclude the presence of cerumen and to ensure that the ear drum shows no gross pathology. Indeed, in view of the rhetogenic anxiety that has been generated in plaintiffs, it is extremely doubtful as to whether or not a doctor is now able to conduct more than a superficial examination without alarming the plaintiff. In his report, however, the doctor should make this quite clear. He should state that it is a provisional report based upon a preliminary examination.

Some reports show audiograms which may be suspiciously spurious, e.g. not showing a traumatic notch but conforming to an equal loudness contour, or they may be unquestionably spurious, e.g. showing the recorded air conduction and bone conduction hearing levels to be identical at all test frequencies in both ears.

(NB Notches may be obscured by exaggeration/or ageing changes. Coles (1981) says that a useful trick is to subtract the average hearing level appropriate to the man's age (Table 4 of Robinson and Shipton's NPL Tables) from the measured hearing levels. This will often reveal a notch.)

The conclusions (including diagnosis and prognosis) may not be based upon the actual findings. Medical examiners have been known to exaggerate as much as plaintiffs.

Should the doctor tell?

The *13th pseudodilemma* relates to '*should the doctor tell?*'

An increasing number of plaintiffs are now appearing with normal audiograms. Although it has been stated that other psycho-acoustic measures would be abnormal, such defects will need to be demonstrated in these cases. A more likely diagnosis in these cases is cophophobia (Gk: fear of deafness). This condition is the result of a number of factors, but principally it is a result of the adverse effects of the well-intentioned health education programmes— noise awareness campaigns—which have been instigated by the Health and Safety Executive.

Should such plaintiffs be allowed to persist in their misconceptions or should they be reassured that their hearing is essentially normal? The medical profession is becoming increasingly aware of the malefficient effects of *labelling*, i.e. all the consequences, medical and social, which occur when an individual is informed, rightly or wrongly, that he has some disease or other body abnormality (Haynes et al 1978).

Amend the report?

The *14th pseudodilemma* relates to *amending a report*.

The medical examiner may have sent in a report on a plaintiff to the instructing solicitor who has then returned it requesting an amendment. The amendment will invariably be from a plaintiff's solicitor who wishes the report to present his client's case in a more favourable light.

The rights of such a request have previously been subject to a court hearing. A firm of solicitors was endeavouring to enforce their requested amendment by withholding payment of fees to the medical examiner. The court held that an expert medical report is meant for the impartial assistance of the court and not simply to buttress one party's case. The doctor was right in refusing to amend his report (Medicolegal 1979).

Slant the evidence?

This, the *15th pseudodilemma*, is related to the previous pseudodilemma. It concerns any active or passive action by an examiner to colour his evidence to promote one or other side in a case. It is almost certainly due to the fact that many doctors see themselves as acting for one or other side, and not for the court. A doctor's report should be the same no matter which side has instructed him. Indeed, in *Thompson and others* v. *Smiths Ship Repairers*, most of the proof that the plaintiffs' hearing loss

was due to occupational noise damage was provided by the expert witnesses called by the defendants. Paradoxically, the plaintiffs' lawyers attempted (unsuccessfully) to rebut the proof. This puzzling feature was most probably due to the fact that acceptance of the proof would have implied acceptance of the method of proof. The method was based upon Robinson and Shipton's NPL tables and these tables were then used when apportionment was under discussion. This involved the retrodictive exercise mentioned previously and showed that very little ONIHL had accrued since the DGK. There was therefore the danger that the court could have used the *de minimis* principle to reject the claims.

Brownlie (1984) has discussed the matter of slanted evidence with particular reference to the criminal law. There have been recent cases where the expert witness' evidence has 'lacked the objectivity which it should have exhibited'. There are fears that some of this bias may be intruding into the forensic audiological scene. For example, to describe a claimant with normal hearing as being 'nowhere so deaf as to require a hearing aid' can surely be for no other purpose than to convey the impression that the claimant has other than normal hearing. It should also be noted that the term 'deafness' should now be restricted to individuals whose hearing is so impaired that they are unable to communicate by acoustic means (WHO 1980). Thus the term 'occupational deafness' is a misnomer.

This bias has also been observed in unsolicited reports from family doctors in response to requests from medical examiners to provide copies of medical records that they hold on claimants. For example, along with copies of a claimant's medical records, one family doctor forwarded a report to the effect that the claimant had 'over the past years, become more and more deaf. I am in no doubt that the deafness is due to noise at the workshops. I would class his case as industrial deafness'. The accompanying medical records did indeed show that the claimant had consulted his family doctor about his ears on several occasions over the previous 20 years or so. However, on each occasion a middle ear condition had been diagnosed!

In addition, concern has been expressed in recent times regarding the manner in which expert evidence comes to be organized by lawyers. Comments have been made both in the Court of Appeal and in the House of Lords. In the House of Lords judgment, Lord Wilberforce has said that, 'while some degree of consultation between experts and legal advisers was entirely proper it was necessary that expert evidence presented to the Court should be, and should be seen to be, the independent product of the expert, uninfluenced as to form or content by the exigencies of litigation' (*Whitehouse* v. *Jordan and another* 1980).

Doctors engaged in any aspect of forensic medicine should endeavour to maintain an impartial presentation of their evidence.

Teaching?

The *16th pseudodilemma* concerns resistance to the use of medicolegal case material for *teaching* purposes. Here there can be no dilemma. A commitment to teaching and the dissemination of knowledge form integral parts of the Hippocratic Oath. If one does not teach, how can one pass on knowledge of this subject to others? Moreover, the abysmally poor standard of forensic audiological medical practice in Britain demands a greater teaching allocation than at present. At the moment teaching in forensic audiology in Britain is limited to short components in the audiological courses at the universities of Manchester and of Southampton.

Research?

The *17th pseudodilemma* relates to *research*.

Plaintiffs' solicitors have previously issued affidavits endeavouring to prevent medical examiners conducting research. If doctors accept, as part of their moral purpose, not just responsibility for the health of 'my patients' but the health of all sick people, including future sick people, then medical research is ethically justified (Gillon 1985). British audiological physicians and scientists, e.g. Coles & Mason (1984), have clearly indicated that they are not to be constrained in pursuing research on claimants in respect of 'alleged noise-induced hearing loss'. It would, however, be of interest to know of the observations made by the relevant ethical committees in such cases.

This restriction on research is clearly one which plaintiffs' solicitors impose on medical examiners

instructed by defendants' solicitors, but not on examiners instructed by themselves. For example, one plaintiff said, 'Doctor X asked me to do some extra tests since he was doing research on tinnitus'. Dr X had been instructed by the plaintiff's solicitor.

Although probably more is known about the effects of noise on hearing than the effects of any other surdogen, there are still large gaps in knowledge. For example, why is there apparently so much individual variability in respect of (a) the effects of a given noise exposure on hearing impairment, and (b) the effect of a given hearing impairment (or none at all) on auditory handicap? More research is also needed on the early detection of ONIHL and of the mechanism of this disorder. This, however, can only be achieved by collective involvement and co-operation which, as has been mentioned in connection with another occupational disorder, is surely a fundamental prerequisite for success in this field.

It is unfortunate that the insurers have a better image in promoting research into this occupational disorder than do the trade unions. One group of insurers provides a substantial covenant to promote research into the early detection of noise-induced hearing loss. Although the TUC (Trades Union Congress) supports an occupational health research unit, there is no remit for this to do research on noise-induced hearing loss, despite efforts to convince the TUC that this is the most prevalent occupational disorder.

Inform on unrelated matters?

The *18th pseudodilemma* relates to requests from solicitors to medical examiners to provide *information* on matters other than those directly related to the forensic theme. It is abundantly clear from affidavits issued by solicitors that examiners have been asked for, and have passed on, information on the roles and probable nature of employment contracts, of other medical examiners. Such actions can only merit disapproval.

Discuss with media?

The *19th pseudodilemma* relates to dialogues with the *media*.

As paragraph 7.1 of the British Medical Association's (1984) *Handbook of Medical Ethica* states, 'increasing, public interest in health matters has brought doctors more and more in contact with the media. It is therefore essential that doctors should be aware of the ethics involved in dealing with the media'. Disparaging remarks about other medical examiners can amount not only to professional misconduct but also to defamation.

Paragraph (iv)(b) of part II of the General Medical Council's (1983) *Professional Conduct and Discipline: Fitness to Practise* states that, 'The Council also regards as capable of amounting to serious professional misconduct: (i) The depreciation by a doctor of the professional skill, knowledge, qualifications or services of another doctor or doctors'.

Publish?

The *20th pseudodilemma* concerns whether or not to *publish* articles in the field of forensic audiology, or on a topic related to that field. The more one commits oneself in print, the more one is constrained in what one might or might not say in giving evidence, much to the chagrin of some doctors in the past. Publications such as this can, however, be considered as part of the teaching process.

CONCLUSIONS AND RECOMMENDATIONS

It is sad that the aforegoing is a reflection of perhaps the most sordid aspect of forensic medicine in Britain. In seeking reasons for this depressing state, one might find explanations some of which are particular to forensic audiology, whilst others relate more generally to law and medicine. Similarly, in seeking remedies, there are those which concern forensic audiology in particular; there are others which have a more general application.

With regard to more general explanatory factors, there are, as was mentioned previously, problems created by the British adversarial system.

In the particular context of common law actions in forensic audiology, there appears to have been a failure to grasp that what the law is *primarily* concerned with is negligence and not ONIHL. Moreover, as Munkman (1985) has pointed out, 'negligence as the criterion of liability involves the further test of reasonable foreseeability, which has been shown up as vague, capricious and subjective when applied to anything more complex than bows and arrows, or horses and carts'.

The work of Burns and Robinson, whilst providing the necessary knowledge for noise-induced hearing loss to become a prescribed occupational disease under statute law (as well as the knowledge on which to base a code of practice), paradoxically provided the knowledge to jeopardize many common law actions. This is because the common law recognizes that an employer may have been negligent over a certain (later) period only of an employee's employment. As was mentioned previously, the date (DGK) on which an employer became negligent is frequently taken to be 1963. Thus a large part of the British workforce in noise-hazardous jobs would have worked initially during a period of non-negligent exposure. Taken in conjunction with the Burns and Robinson data (rapid development of noise-induced hearing loss in the earlier years), this would mean that much (for many people, most) of the noise-induced loss would have occurred during a non-negligent period. Indeed, for men who have been in the noisiest jobs and who are now on the verge of retirement, a negligible loss only would have occurred during a negligent period. Moreover, analysis of the Burns and Robinson data indicates that those who are more susceptible to noise-damage would show a much greater loss in the earlier years. Thus, those who appeared to be more deserving (older men who had the noisiest jobs and were more susceptible, and so had the greater hearing losses) would receive the least compensation at common law. It was the failure to appreciate this that led to a number of not wholly successful litigations. The extent of legal, medical and scientific ignorance on this matter is indicated by Hazards Bulletin 40 of the British Society for Social Responsibility in Science (1984). The Bulletin referred to 'derisory payments' in *Thompson and Others* v. *Smiths Ship Repairers* and the fact that the insurers demanded their legal costs. The derisory payments were because there had been relatively little change in the noise-induced hearing loss over the negligent period. The insurers demanded their legal costs because the court had awarded costs to them. This was not surprising since the insurers had, before the trial, paid into court sums which were greater than those which the court had subsequently awarded the plaintiffs. Payments into court are based upon an estimate of what plaintiffs might receive based upon current legal, medical and scientific knowledge of the subject.

It was thus the treble failure, i.e. failure to recognize that exposure to noise did not make a man immune to other aural disorders, failure to recognize the implications of Robinson's hyperbolic tangent/logarithmic function taken in conjunction with a step function (specifically, that of the DGK), and failure to recognize the uncertainties of tortious law—which Ison (1967) appropriately described as the forensic lottery—which inevitably led to the failure to achieve the total aims of a series of litigations. The frustrating effects of these experiences inevitably led, as both Freud and the Yale School of Psychology (Dollard et al 1939) would have predicted, to the aggressive behaviour which followed. These particular psychological reactions were probably also compounded by a guilt complex. The USSR recognized noise-induced hearing loss as an occupational disease in 1929. No British trade union backed a legal action in respect of the disorder until about 40 years later (Coles 1969).

The several ways in which the present situation might be *remedied* can be classified into six groups, i.e. educational, ethical, psychological, legal, political and technological.

There should be an expansion of *educational* courses, not only for medical practitioners engaged in forensic audiological work, but also for the other skill groups involved in forensic audiology and audiological jurisprudence. The instruction for medical people could be in the form of extending lectures, courses, to provide a formal forensic audiological programme.

Reminders might be sent out to doctors of the ethical codes which they should try to follow. Although Sir David Napley (1985), a past president of the Law Society, has claimed that the ethical standards which are required of lawyers are greater than those which are required of other professions, because of their obligation to inform a client if they have acted negligently, it would appear there is still room for changing the content of those ethical standards. As the MORI (Market and Opinion Research International) survey commissioned by the National Consumer Council (News item 1985a) indicated, there is considerable public concern about the solicitors' profession and a majority of the public favour an independent legal council to handle complaints against solicitors. The need for a reform of this profession has also been indicated by Joseph (1985) in his book *Lawyers can Seriously Damage your Health*. As Aris (1985) has pointed out, both the integrity and competence of members of that profession are now being questioned. The President of the Law Society has endorsed the establishment of a neutral body to handle complaints of negligence against solicitors (News item 1985c). The introduction of appropriate ethical standards for members of the mass media, particularly interviewers, investigating journalists and producers, would also seem appropriate. The Code of Conduct for Psychologists (1985), which has been adopted by the British Psychology Society, could well serve as the model for a code of ethics for these various other skill groups.

It might well be desirable to have an ethical code for claimants based on the proposed empiric oath (Young 1983) for patients.

(Sextus Empiricus was an outstanding Greek physician and philosopher about the year 200 AD. He was insistent that all people are different and need to be treated as such. Young's proposed empiric oath contains the words, 'When I am ill . . . I will tell the truth about my condition and expect that in return the truth will be told to me about the diagnosis and the prognosis in language that I can understand'.)

Psychological testing in the pre-employment selection of solicitors and members of the mass media could help to sift out those who were temperamentally unsuitable for those occupations.

Legal reforms comprise those that can be achieved in the short term, those that could be achieved in the intermediate term, and others which could be achieved in the long term. In connection with short-term measures, one might well follow Brownlie's (1984) recommendations in respect of improving the expert evidence in criminal cases. He suggests three points. The first is that an expert should not agree to give evidence if the instructing solicitor requires the expert to avoid discussing his evidence in advance with the opposing expert. The second point is that the expert should pay particular attention to the language in which he expresses his evidence so that it is readily understandable to a lay man with average intelligence. The third point is that there should always be a consultation at which the expert can assure himself that his evidence is understood by the counsel and solicitor who are to present the case in Court. As Brownlie points out, these at least are steps towards avoiding tragic situations where evidence of experts is needlessly devalued and the expert joins the ranks of the discredited and the rejected.

An even better practice that could be achieved in the short term would be for there to be a joint medical examination and, if it can be agreed, a joint report by the medical examiners instructed by the two sides (Denning 1984).

In the intermediate term, one could adopt a new legal procedure (Medicolegal 1986) which has been suggested. This procedure could not only avoid what Gudjonsson (1985) calls the ordeal of expert witnesses, but also the unacceptable delays and expenses in litigation. The suggested new procedure would be in every case where a plaintiff claims damages for personal injuries and the parties did not agree to the other side's medical reports. The papers, including the medical reports, would be referred to a medical committee which would specify the specialty of the referee required to decide the matter. The court would then select a referee from the list of referees qualified to consider the evidence. There would then be a hearing before the selected medical referee (or referees) chaired by a Queen's counsel to make recommendations as to the decision for the medical issues in the case. The hearing would be entirely informal and no shorthand notes would be taken. However, medical witnesses would give evidence and would be liable to cross-examination. Nothing said at the hearing would be admissible in evidence at any subsequent trial; should a trial follow. A similar scheme has been in operation in New York on an experimental basis and, despite receiving a mixed reception, appears to have been operating successfully (Anon 1956).

In the long term, one might hope that Britain would adopt a no-fault system, similar to New Zealand's no-fault accident compensation, and extend it to disease as the Government in New Zealand had considered doing in 1978 (Palmer 1979).

In the more distant future, one might foresee that the English adversarial system, which has sought to polarize British audiology, might well be replaced by the inquisitorial system of other EEC countries. Under the inquisitorial civil law system operating in most other European countries, expert witnesses are not subjected to destructive examination, cross-examination and re-examination.

There are, however, limits to the law (e.g. as illustrated by Allott 1980) in coping with change in social thought and forces. This is perhaps not because the law itself is to blame. Accepting the arguments of Kelsen and his school (Friedmann 1944), the system of law is determined by the *Grundnorm* of the State. And the forces that influence the nature of the State are the very factors which, as was pointed out in the introduction, determine the system of law. We have thus come full circle. But can the circle be broken? Perhaps only by the institution of *political* reforms. These may have to be far reaching. We may well pose the most fundamental of all political questions, i.e. the one posed by Kropotkin (1897): 'Do we really need the State?'

With the knowledge that is now available on the adverse effects of noise on hearing, and on measures which can now be taken to obviate such effects, *technology* has the means to implement effective programmes in this specific situation to ensure that hearing is protected. Indeed, many industries in Britain have had such hearing conservation programmes for a number of years. Thus, one would hope that occupational noise-induced hearing loss would largely disappear from the scene in less time than it would take for some of the other changes envisaged above to take effect.

SUMMARY

Thus the evaluation of noise-induced hearing loss has ramifications extending far beyond the functional assessment of a microscopic strip of acoustically sensitive neuroepithelium. But then, as Adam Politzer, the founder of otology, is reputed to have said, 'Everything is related to everything'.

I enjoyed reading the papers by Peter Alberti and Ronald Hinchcliffe. Each has written competently, from a wealth of experience, on the evaluation of noise-induced hearing loss. In many ways, they are in broad agreement, although there is a marked difference of tone in the two papers. Alberti has written in a concise, down to earth, pragmatic tone, setting out the position as he sees it. Hinchcliffe, on the other hand, reveals a deep involvement, introduces words which appear to be of his own making (Hinchogenic), indulges in coat trailing and frequently appears to have his tongue in his cheek.

Together, they highlight some very important areas in this field: first, the history, both medical and occupational; secondly, the accuracy of the audiogram; thirdly, the possibility of other aetiological factors in the deafness; and fourthly, the contribution of noise to the deafness. Throughout all the discussion, there is the impression that Alberti has his feet firmly on the ground and that Hinchcliffe, wanting to provide controversy, is being deliberately provocative. Despite being an ENT surgeon, I shall take a generous view of Hinchcliffe's controversy and comment with, perhaps, my own tongue just a little in my cheek.

The history

Alberti highlights something which has been the experience of all clinicians—patients forget. They have great difficulty in remembering the onset of their hearing loss and, consequently, their estimate of when they first had a hearing problem is often of little value. Hinchcliffe suggests that the first question ought to be, 'What is the problem?'. This is an excellent opening question because, as he indicates, sometimes there isn't a problem!

Hinchcliffe refers to questionnaires, stating that they have advantages, but appears, overall, to come down against them. Alberti makes no reference to questionnaires, but, in his last paragraph, refers to the evaluation as being an art as well as a science. In my view, questionnaires are rather like painting by numbers. It is true that one does get a picture, but one does not get the impressions that come from original art. Not only do questionnaires pose leading questions, but one does not have an opportunity of

assessing the plaintiff's reaction to the question. Providing that one is pleasant and sympathetic in taking a history, much more can be learned from a few direct questions and the spontaneous replies, than from pages of a questionnaire. The ring of truth that can come from a face-to-face history, and is so important in these cases, rarely comes from a questionnaire.

All plaintiffs are human; most would be pleased to have some extra money; many have been briefed beforehand about the answers which may prejudice their case, and a few are prepared to be blatantly dishonest. Consequently, one must continually be on one's guard about the manner in which a question is answered. When asking a question such as, 'Does anyone in your family have any problems with the ears or hearing?', if the plaintiff answers 'No' before one has finished the question, one must have a high index of suspicion about his negative answers. Herein lies part of the art.

Alberti draws attention to the plaintiff's acknowledgement of a sudden onset, or sudden acceleration, of his hearing loss. In the absence of a specific acoustic incident, this may well identify a cause not related to exposure to noise.

Hinchcliffe appears to assume that it is possible to have a reasonable idea of the noise exposure which any individual has had, simply by knowing his occupation. However, Alberti highlights the problem of the accuracy of the occupational history and illustrates this by the marked difference in the levels recorded by a dosimeter in two individuals who, on the face of it, had identical jobs. Not only do many plaintiffs have difficulty in remembering where they were employed, or for how long, but also have difficulty in recalling the time spent in noisy areas in specific jobs. This problem cannot be eliminated, even when one knows exactly the nature of the work, and the problem is even greater in someone who has worked in many different noisy jobs. Careful questioning is the only way to reduce the problem, although it still remains. I recently reported on an honest and straightforward plaintiff who stated that in his work in a boilerhouse verbal communication was impossible, even by shouting, because of the noise from the generator. He stated that he had to go outside to talk. It took quite a few questions to elicit that the generator runs only for routine testing and during power failures. Testing takes less than 1 hour each week, and there had been four power failures, averaging less than 1 hour each time, in the previous 5 years. Questionnaires, or aggressive questioning, will fail to elicit this type of situation. Gentle and sympathetic handling is what is required.

One's attitudes to occupational hearing loss, and its compensation, tend to be coloured by one's general background, social and political convictions and acceptance of the law of the land, whether or not one sees it as reasonable! Currently, the law of the land states that anyone who suffers injury at work due to failure of the employer to take reasonable precautions to protect him, is entitled to monetary compensation. In any particular case, it is not the role of the expert medical witness to make the laws but to act impartially within them. A specific medicolegal report ought to be similar, whether written on behalf of the plaintiff or the defendant. At the end of the examination, the plaintiff, who is usually unsophisticated in these matters, should not be able to tell from the attitude of the examiner whether he was being examined on his behalf, or for the defendant. When there is any aggression on the examiner's part, he usually has failed.

Audiological assessment

Alberti is once again down to earth and explicit in his description of his approach to this problem. There is a lot of science but, once again, art is added to it. Two of his sentences, in relation to difficult plaintiffs, bear repetition: 'The patient (plaintiff) should be given a gracious way out . . . .' and 'Confrontation is less effective than cajoling . . .'.

One can only hope that Hinchcliffe's tongue is in his cheek when he describes the three levels of experience and expertise of the expert medical witness: the primary physician, the ENT surgeon and the audiological physician. Excellent though many of them are, one cannot reasonably assume that the primary physician is an expert medical witness in this field. I would question Ron Hinchcliffe's image of the average ENT surgeon; it seems to be badly distorted. Although most of the surgery which I perform is for conductive hearing loss, my role in

health care is very much wider and I see many more patients with sensorineural than with conductive impairment.

Hinchcliffe is quite dogmatic about self-recording audiometry. Undoubtedly, a good sweep frequency self-recorded audiogram has much merit. However, although the wildly swinging audiogram of the malingerer may confirm exaggeration of the hearing loss, it still leaves one in doubt about the actual level of hearing. The direct involvement of an experienced audiological technician will, in most instances, give a closer approximation to the plaintiff's true hearing than the more extreme self-recorded audiograms.

Alberti discusses the problem of correcting for the Carhart notch and takes the pragmatic position that, since juries do not understand it, it is simpler to ignore it! Presumably he takes the same view of the impaired bone conduction responses due to the alteration of the middle ear mechanics in chronic suppurative otitis media.

Alberti accepts the position of slow vertex responses in evoked response audiometry, although Hinchcliffe makes no mention of these. However, Hinchcliffe emphasizes the point that there is much more to the problem than simply getting an accurate estimation of the audiogram.

Apportionment

Both authors indicate that two different types of apportionment are necessary. First, one must apportion between noise exposure and other causes of hearing loss. Secondly, one must apportion between different employment sources. Although both papers give guidelines, there is still a major problem. Noise at work does not protect against other causes of deafness and a fully resolved acute otitis media in childhood does not protect against noise-induced hearing loss. Although the National Physics Laboratory tables may be of help, Alberti points out that an accurate assessment of the noise emission level is very difficult. Many claimants have changed jobs on a few occasions and even the same job varies in its noise levels, depending on the nature of the work being done and the number of other noise-creating employees working nearby.

Alberti refers to exposure to non-occupational noise and gives particularly good guidance on it.

We are again dependant on the integrity of the plaintiff and the art of the history taking in identifying these non-occupational sources. Both emphasize the value of previous audiograms in determining the amount of deafness caused by noise, although neither makes reference to the possibility of the earlier audiogram being spurious, especially if it had been done by an untrained person in a screening programme.

Treatment of plaintiffs

The foundation of British medicine is that a request for specialist treatment is initiated by the family doctor. Consequently, even though the defendant may instruct the expert witness only to assess the plaintiff and not to treat, this applies only to that consultation. As I understand the law, there is no future binding on either plaintiff or specialist. If the expert medical witness feels that his department has something to offer the plaintiff in the way of treatment, and the plaintiff wishes to be treated, all that is required is that the plaintiff ask his family doctor to make the necessary referral.

To take a more dramatic example, if one has reasonable doubt about the possibility of an acoustic neuroma, one has a moral duty to take some action. One need simply to advise the plaintiff to see his family doctor with a view to referral for specialist assessment, diagnosis and treatment.

Other considerations

Hinchcliffe's paper covers a wider area than Alberti's. Hinchcliffe starts by defining the term dilemma, from the Oxford English Dictionary. Perhaps, as an aside, I could express the desire that he had checked all his words in the Oxford English Dictionary as I was unable to find surdogen, semeion, rhetogenic or cophophobia!

I do not have either a dilemma or a pseudo-dilemma when asked to submit a medical report on someone who has been a patient in the past. I see this as an obligation to my patient. Consequently, I find myself involved in this work as a matter of principle. However, having become involved in it, I have not come across some of the problems described by Hinchcliffe. Some of these result from

his prominent position and expertise in this field. Most of those involved in this type of medicolegal work will not have any problems with the media. However, unless they are experienced in this respect, they ought to hesitate before agreeing to give any interviews.

As far as I am concerned, there is no question of giving an opinion without examining the plaintiff. If such permission is refused and the case comes to a hearing, I do not think that it would be difficult to brief the defence in such a manner that those responsible for refusing permission to examine the plaintiff would regret this, and be unlikely to do it again.

I am tempted to overlook the implication that audiological physicians set higher standards of examination than ENT surgeons. The outstanding audiological physician would be expected to have higher standards than the average ENT surgeon, but there is no reason, of which I am aware, to suggest that the average audiological physician would have a higher standard than the average ENT surgeon. It has not been my experience. Indeed, my limited experience and my reasoning suggest that it is otherwise. The average ENT surgeon, by his training and everyday work, spends much more time using the microscope than the average audiological physician. He has the further advantage of operative confirmation, or refutation, of his conclusions. In any event, it is likely that in the majority of situations, microscopic examination of the tympanic membrane is unnecessary. As Walby et al (1983) have shown, even gross middle ear disease rarely leads to significant inner ear pathology; a little scarring of the tympanic membrane, visible only under the microscope, must only exceptionally be of practical significance in noise-induced hearing loss, in the absence of an air–bone gap on the audiogram.

I agree with Hinchcliffe that it is entirely reasonable to comment on the report of other specialists and that, unless some misunderstanding has been brought to light, one ought to be reluctant to amend one's own report, especially if, in the amending, the tone of the report is altered.

I am in full agreement that medicolegal work provides an excellent basis for both teaching and research and that the profession should not be denied this.

CONCLUSIONS

In conclusion, these are two stimulating and informative papers that will help to widen the horizons of all who read them. It has been a pleasure to have had the task of commenting on them. None the less, one wonders what would happen to works like these if Hinchcliffe's suggestion of pre-employment psychological tests for solicitors and members of the mass media were extended to audiological physicians and ENT surgeons. Surely the world would be a duller place.

REFERENCES

P W Alberti

Alberti P W 1982 The clinical assessment of industrial hearing loss—a case report and discussion. Journal of Otolaryngology 11: 94

Alberti P W, Blair R L 1982 Occupational hearing loss: An Ontario perspective. Laryngoscope 92: 535

Alberti P W, Morgan P P, Czuba I 1978 Speech and pure-tone audiometry as a screen for exaggerated hearing loss in industrial claims. Acta Otolaryngologica 85: 328

Alberti P W, Hyde M L, Symonds F M, Miller R B 1980 Effect of prolonged exposure to industrial noise on otosclerosis. Laryngoscope 90: 407

Barr T 1886 Enquiry into the effects of loud sounds upon the hearing of boilermakers and others who work amid noisy surroundings. Transactions of the Philosophy Society of Glasgow 17: 223–239

Corso J F 1980 Age correction factor in noise-induced hearing loss: a quantitative model. Audiology 19: 221

Davis A L, Fortnum H M, Coles R R A, Haggard M P, Lutman M E 1984 Damage to hearing arising from leisure noise: a review of the literature. MRC Institute of Hearing Research, Nottingham

Dickson E D D, Watson N P 1949 A clinical survey into the effects of turbo-jet engine noise on service personnel. Journal of Laryngology and Otology 63: 276

Hinchcliffe R 1981 Forensic audiology. In: Beagley H A (ed) Audiology and audiologic medicine. Oxford University Press, Oxford

Hyde M L, Alberti P W 1986 Auditory evoked potentials in audiometric assessment of compensation and medical-legal patients. Submitted for publication

Melnick W 1978 In: Lipscomb D (ed) Noise and audiology. University Park Press, Baltimore, ch 3

Mills J H, Going J A 1982 Review of environmental factors affecting hearing. Environmental Health Perspectives 44: 119

Moody D B, Stebbins W C, Johnson L-G, Hawkins J E 1976 Noise-induced hearing loss in the monkey. In: Henderson D, Hamernick R P, Dosanjh D S, Mills J H (eds) Effects of noise on hearing. Raven Press, New York

Parry C H 1825 Collections from the unpublished writings of the late C H Parry, vol 1. Underwood, London, p 544

R Hinchcliffe

Acton W I 1973 Hearing handicap Measures. Proceedings of Meeting of British Society of Audiology, London, 15 June

Alberti P W, Morgan P P, Le Blanc J C 1974 Occupational hearing loss—an otologist's view of a long-term study. Laryngoscope 84: 1822

Alberti P W, Morgan P P, Czuba I 1978 Speech and pure-tone audiometry as a screen for exaggerated hearing loss in industrial claims. Acta Otolaryngologica 25: 328–331

Alberti P W, Symons F, Hyde M L 1979 Occupational hearing loss. Acta Otolaryngologica 87: 255–263

Allott A 1980 The limits of law. Butterworths, London

Anon 1956 Impartial medical testimony: a report by a special committee of the Bar of the City of New York on the Medical Experts Testimony Project. Macmillan, New York

Aris S 1985 Solicitors who settle for a quiet life. The Times, London

Atherley G R C, Martin A M 1971 Equivalent continuous noise level as a measure of injury from impact and impulsive noise. Annals of Occupational Hygiene 14: 111, 28

Atherley G R C, Noble W G 1971 Clinical picture of occupational hearing loss. In: Robinson D W (ed) Occupational hearing loss. Academic Press, London

Barcham L J, Stephens S D G 1980 The use of an open-ended problems questionnaire in auditory rehabilitation. British Journal of Audiology 14: 49–54

Barr T 1886 Enquiry into the effects of the loud sounds upon of the hearing of boiler makers and others who work amid noisy surroundings. Proceedings of the Glasgow Philosophical Society 17: 223–239

Bekesy G von 1947 A new audiometer. Acta otolaryngologica 35: 411

British Medical Association 1984 The handbook of medical ethics. BMA, London

British Society for Social Responsibility in Science (1984) What price deafness? Hazards Bulletin 40. British Society for Social Responsibility in Science, PO Box 148, Sheffield S1 1FB

Browning G G, Gatehouse S, Lowe G D O 1986 Blood viscosity as a factor in sensorineural hearing impairment. The Lancet i: 121–123

Brownlie A R 1984 How often are experts right? In: Brownlie A R (ed) Crime investigation, art or science? Scottish Academic Press, Edinburgh

Burns W, Robinson D W 1970 Hearing and noise in industry. Her Majesty's Stationery Office, London

Cardozo B N 1921 The nature of the judicial process. Yale University Press USA

Chuang Wei Ping 1985 Forensic audiology. North Riding Infirmary, Middlesbrough, Cleveland, UK

Chung D Y, Mason K, Gannon R P, Willson G N 1983a The ear effect as a function of age and hearing loss. Journal of the Acoustical Society of America 73: 1277–1282

Chung D Y, Willson G N, Gannon R P (1983b) Lateral differences in susceptibility to noise damage. Audiology 22: 199–205

Cochrane A L, Chapman P J, Oldham P D 1951 Observers' errors in taking medical histories. The Lancet i: 1007–1009

Code of Conduct for Psychologists (1985) Bulletin of British Psychology Society 38: 41–43

Coles R R A 1969 A legal action for noise deafness. Annals of Occupational Hygiene 12: 223–226

Coles R R A 1975 The relationship between noise-induced threshold shifts, morphological change and social handicap. In: Bench R J, Pye A, Pye J D (eds) Sound reception in mammals. Symposia of the Zoological Society of London, no 37. Academic Press, London, p 107

Coles R R A 1981 In: Tinnitus. Ciba Foundation Symposium 85. Pitman, London, p 30, 31

Coles R R A, Mason S M 1984 The results of cortical electric response audiometry in medicolegal investigations. British Journal of Audiology 18: 71–78

David R, Brierley J E C 1968 Major legal systems in the world today. Stevens, London

Denning Lord 1984 Doctors and the courts. BMA News Review 10: 12–13

Department of Health and Social Security 1969 The responsibility of the consultant grade. Report of a working party. Her Majesty's Stationery Office, London

DHSS 1982 Occupational deafness, Cmnd 8749. HMSO, London

DHSS 1985 Severe disablement allowance: handbook for adjudicating medical authorities. DHSS, London

Dollard J, Miller N E, Doob L W, Mowrer O H, Sears R R 1939 Frustration and aggression. Institute of Human Relations, Yale University, USA

Duckworth D 1983 The classification and measurement of disablement. DHSS Research Report no. 10. HMSO, London

Edelstein L 1967 Ancient medicine. Johns Hopkins Press, Baltimore

El Alami A M 1981 Study on hearing ability and its relationship to noise levels in an East London factory. Journal of the Society of Occupational Medicine 31: 27–30

Evans R 1986 Letter to the Editor. The Guardian, 27 June

Friedmann W 1944 Legal theory. Stevens, London

General Medical Council 1983 Professional conduct and discipline: fitness to practise. GMC, London

Gifford A 1984 Talks to Sian Edwards. Radical Wales no. 4, p 8–9

Gillon R 1985 Beneficence: doing good for others. British Medical Journal 291: 44–45

Gudjonsson G H 1985 Psychological evidence in court: results from the BPS survey. Bulletin of the British Psychological Society 38: 327–330

Habib R G, Hinchcliffe R 1978 Subjective magnitude of auditory impairment. Audiology 17: 68–76

Hallam R S, Rachman S, Hinchcliffe R 1984 Psychological aspects of tinnitus. In: Rachman S (ed) Contributions to medical psychology. Pergamon, Oxford

Harris D A 1958 Rapid and simple technique for detection of non-organic hearing loss. Archives of Otolaryngology 68: 758–760

Haughton P M, Lewsley A, Wilson M, Williams R G 1979 A forced-choice procedure to detect feigned or exaggerated hearing loss. British Journal of Audiology 13: 135–138

Havard J 1984 No justice within the limit of the law. BMA News Review 10: 14

Haynes R B, Sackett D L, Taylor D W, Gibson E S, Johnson E L 1978 Increased absenteeism from work after detection and labeling of hypertensive patients. New England Journal of Medicine 299: 741–744

Health and Safety Executive 1978 Audiometry in industry. HMSO, London

Hinchcliffe R, Gordon A 1980 Subjective magnitude of

symptoms and handicaps related to hearing impairment. Proceedings of the Third International Congress on Noise as a Public Health Problem, Freiburg, 1978. ASHA Reports 10. American Speech-Language-Hearing Association, Rockville, Maryland, USA

Howell R W 1975 Ear pathology: its role in hearing impairment. Journal of the Society of Occupational Medicine 25: 28–32

International Standards Organization. Pure-tone audiometric test methods. Draft International Standard ISO/DIS 8253

Ison T G 1967 The forensic lottery. Staples, London

Joseph M 1985 Lawyers can seriously damage your health. Michael Joseph, London

Keatinge G F, Laner S 1958 Some notes on the effects of excessive noise on the hearing of a group of workers. British Journal of Industrial Medicine 15: 273–275

Kell R L, Pearson J C G, Acton W I, Taylor W 1971 Social effects of hearing loss due to weaving noise. In: Robinson D W (ed) Occupational hearing loss. Academic Press, London, p 179

Kerr A G, Gillespie W J, Easton J M 1975 Deafness: a simple test for malingering. British Journal of Audiology 9: 24–26

Klockhoff I, Drettner B, Svedberg A 1974 Computerised classification of the results of screening audiometry in groups of persons exposed to noise. Audiology 13: 326–334

Kropotkin P 1897 L'etat—Son role historique.

Lim D, Stephens S D G 1985 Hearing in the elderly. Paper given at the Annual Meeting of the British Society of Audiology, Hull

Lund O, Hyvik H 1979 Binaural hearing spectacles with no mould by acoustic trauma. Acta Otolaryngologica, suppl 360: 113–115

Lundborg T, Linzander S 1969 The otomicroscopic observation and its clinical application. Acta Otolaryngologica suppl 266

Lutman M E, Brown E J, Coles R R A 1986 Self-reported disability and handicap in the population in relation to pure-tone threshold, age, sex and type of hearing loss. British Journal of Audiology. (In press)

McGinnis B 1982 Foreword to Duckworth 1983

McKelvie W B 1933 Weavers' deafness. Journal of Laryngology and Otology 48: 607–608

Martin A M, Atherley G R C 1973 A method for the assessment of impact noise with respect to injury to hearing. Annals of Occupational Hygiene 16: 19–26

Medicolegal 1979 Medical reports not to the lawyers' liking. British Medical Journal ii: 1376

Medicolegal 1985 Disclosure of documents by doctors. British Medical Journal 290: 1973–1974

Medicolegal 1986 Legal delays and experts: a new proposal. British Medical Journal 292: 610–611

Munkman J 1985 Employer's liability at common law. Butterworths, London, p 24

Napley D 1985 The ethics of the professions. The Law Society's Gazette 82: 818–825

National Consumer Council 1985 In dispute with a solicitor. National Consumer Council, London

News item 1984 Lord Chancellor blames critics for hounding judge to death. The Times, September 22

News item 1985a Independent body for complaints against solicitors. The Times, April 11th.

News item 1985b Doctor's libel action over That's Life costs BBC more than £1m. The Times, 24 April

News item 1985c Law Society chief backs neutral body to handle complaints of negligence. The Times, 25 October

News item 1985d Outrageous conduct by BBC. Daily Mail, 6 December

Noble W G 1978 Assessment of impaired hearing. Academic Press, London

Noble W G, Atherley G R C 1970 The hearing measurement scale: a questionnaire for the assessment of auditory disability. Journal of Auditory Research 10: 229–250

Ormrod R F G 1972 Evidence and proof: scientific and legal. Medicine, Science and Law 12: 9–20

Palmer G 1979 Compensation for incapacity: a study of law and social change in New Zealand and Australia. Oxford University Press, Wellington

Palmer R N 1980 Consent, confidentiality, disclosure of medical records in the course of litigation. Medical Protection Society, London

Price L L, Falck V T 1963 Bekesy audiometry in children. Journal of Speech and Hearing Disorders 6: 129–133

Raber A 1971 In: Robinson D W (ed) Occupational hearing loss. Academic Press, London, p 159

Robinson D W 1985 The audiogram in hearing loss due to noise: a probability test to uncover other causation. Annals of Occupational Hygiene 29: 477–493

Robinson D W, Shipton M S 1977 Tables for the Estimation of noise-induced hearing loss. NPL Acoustic Report Ac 61, 2nd edn. National Physical Laboratory, Teddington, Middlesex

Robinson D W, Wilkins P A, Thyer N J, Lawes J F 1984 Auditory impairment and the onset of disability and handicap in noise-induced hearing loss. ISVR Technical Report no. 146, University of Southampton UK

Rosenberg P E 1972 Case history: the first test. In: Ketz J (ed) Handbook of clinical audiology. Williams & Wilkins, Baltimore, ch 4

Rossi G, Sulkowski W, Olina M, Avolio G, Giordano C 1985 Malingering and occupational hearing loss. Audiologia Italiana 2: 469–476

Salomon G, Parving A 1985 Hearing disability and Communication handicap for compensation purposes based on self-assessment and audiometric testing. Audiology 24: 135–145

Saunders J B 1970 Mozley and Whiteley's law dictionary, 8th edn. Butterworths, London

Smith R 1985 Occupationless health. British Medical Journal 291: 1024, 1338, 1409, 1563, 1707

Stephens S D G 1981 Auditory rehabilitation. In: Beagley H A (ed) Audiology and audiological medicine, vol 1. Oxford University Press, Oxford

Stephens S D G 1984 Hearing-aid selection: an integrated approach. British Journal of Audiology 18: 199–210

Taylor W, Pearson J, Mair A, Burns W 1965 Study of noise and hearing in jute weaving. Journal of the Acoustical Society of America 38: 113–120

Theodor L H, Mandelcorn M S 1973 Hysterical Blindness: a case report and study using a modern psychophysical technique. Journal of Abnormal Psychology 82: 552–553

Weber M 1912 Rechtssoziologie. In: Grundriss der Social-Oekonomik, part III, vol 2. Luchterhand, Neuwied World Health Organization 1980 International classification of impairments, disabilities and handicaps. World Health Organization, Geneva

Wilbush J 1984 Clinical information—signs, semeions and symptoms: Discussion paper. Journal of the Royal Society of Medicine 77: 766–773

Wood P H N 1980 The Language of disablement: a glossary related to disease and its consequences. International Rehabilitation Medicine 2: 86–92

Young M 1983 Hippocratic oath for doctors, empiric oath for patients. Self-Health 1: 35

A G Kerr

Walby A P, Barrera A, Schuknecht H F 1983 Cochlear pathology in chronic suppurative otitis media. Annals of Otology, Rhinology and Laryngology 92, supplement 103

3

Is there a future for cochlear implants?

J. Marquet, S. Peeters, M. Van Durme

INTRODUCTION

From recent reports from The World Health Organization we learned that, of the 4800 million peoples in the world, there are 308 million (6.4%) suffering from hearing impairment, of which 17.2 million (0.4%) represent the group of total or severe sensorineural hearing loss. Faced with the permanent improvement of middle ear surgery one of the main preoccupations of the otologist has been to find a solution for those for whom hearing aids are insufficient, using artificial hearing stimulation.

Attempts at electrical stimulation of the auditory apparatus were made by Alessandro Volta in 1800; he inserted metal rods in each ear and attached them to a circuit containing 30 or 40 electrolytic cells. His sensation, when closing the circuit, was like a blow on the head followed by a sound like the boiling of a viscid liquid.

The first attempt at a systematic investigation of electrical stimulation of the auditory system was published, as reported by Simmons (1966), in 1868 by R. Brenner of Leipzig. He used condenser discharges with a negative electrode applied to saline in the ear canal and the positive electrode to a distant part of the body. The auditory sensations were different in various observers and resembled hissing, ringing and buzzing at various pitches. All effects of this electrical stimulation were attributed to the excitation of the eighth nerve.

Modern interest in artificial auditory stimulation dates from 1930 when Wever & Bray (1930) discovered the cochlear electrical potentials. The cochlea was found to be a transducer of acoustical signals to electrical signals, although this electro-phonic hearing has to be differentiated from direct electrical stimulation of the cochlear nerve, which is the intention of cochlear implantation.

The first attempt to stimulate a totally deaf patient by a direct stimulation of the auditory nerve, was realized in 1957 by Djourno and Eyries, although it was only in the 1960s that the first therapeutical attempts to treat sensory deafness were made by different pioneer surgeons in this field: William F. House, Simmons and Michelson in USA as well as Chouard in France. In the 1960s and 1970s, single-channel and multichannel devices were developed and implantation programmes were set up with totally deaf people.

These implant programmes were experimental and have resulted in considerable scientific controversies. It appears that every possible theory on electrical stimulation has been tried out and has resulted in different kinds of experimental devices. All of them are based on the principle of bypassing the functional aspects of the inner ear and aim to be a crude replacement of the cochlear processing of sound. Some totally deaf patients with sensorineural hearing loss should benefit from such an artificial stimulation, since destruction of haircells is not necessarily followed by destruction of the nerve fibres and neural degeneration (Nadol 1984, Hinojosa et al 1985).

In recent years a great number of devices has been developed and even become commercially available. To straighten out this confusing amount of different kinds of cochlear implants from exhaustive descriptions already being reported (Ballantyne et al 1978, Brackmann 1976, Finkenzeller 1982, Gray 1985), the basic principles behind their development will be explained.

Parameters of sound perception

Two important parameters of sound perception are pitch and loudness.

The first one, pitch, is decoded in the cochlea because each nerve fibre is well tuned to a certain frequency and is connected to a specific part of the cochlea. This is called the tonotopic organization of the cochlea. From psychoacoustic tests it is clear that for low frequencies there is also a time coding mechanism, which means that, for these frequencies, pitch can also be determined by the time structure of the signal. Any device trying to replace cochlear function probably has to cope with both these coding mechanisms in order to make speech discrimination possible (Sachs et al 1983). Place coding can be approximated by electrical stimulation of various discrete areas of the cochlea. This advocates the use of multichannel bipolar stimulation. Time coding can be replaced by the rate of stimulation.

The second parameter is loudness, which is partially related to the neural activity in one nerve fibre and most likely the frequency selectivity of the neural tuning curve is also involved. In electrical stimulation, broad tuning curves are obtained and the dynamic range, expressed in minimal audible current steps, shows a serious reduction.

Electrode design

Extra- or intracochlear electrode

There is a controversy over whether the contact points should be very near to the surviving nerve fibres or not. This accounts for the basic difference between extra- and intracochlear devices.

The *extracochlear electrode* can be a single-channel monopolar or bipolar electrode, which is placed on the round window, or it can be a multichannel electrode, which is fixed in the promontory outside the cochlea. The advantage of this system is the decrease of risk of cochlear damage. A disadvantage is the large distance from the nerve fibre endings through which bipolar stimulation becomes less effective.

The *intracochlear electrode* is mostly placed in the scala tympani and stimulates a part of the cochlea.

Single-channel versus multichannel stimulation

Single-channel stimulation can transmit information on time coding, loudness and low frequency pitch, but the question is whether real speech intelligibility can be achieved. Most investigators agree that there is no reason to insert a single-channel electrode into the cochlea since it doesn't increase speech intelligibility.

It is a simple and less expensive device and is suitable for patients with a poor number of surviving nerve fibres, or for those whose cochlea is not accessible for an intracochlear electrode.

A *multichannel implant* is formed out of multiple pairs of bipolar electrodes spread throughout the cochlea. This electrode can stimulate discrete groups of nerve fibres, in their specific frequency range. The system potentially allows an increase of speech intelligibility, but in order to benefit from this sophisticated system the implanted patient must have a sufficient number of nerve fibres more or less uniformly distributed throughout the cochlea. Insertion, fixation or stimulation should not result in destruction of the surviving fibres.

Until now multichannel implants should be viewed as experimental devices and discussed as such with the potential patient. Not all patients will get benefit from a multichannel implant.

Monopolar versus bipolar stimulation

The injection of current from an active electrode towards a remote ground electrode is called *monopolar stimulation*. The current density is only high around the active contact surface and spreads in a uniform way in all directions. In this way a large number, if not all, of the surviving nerve fibres are stimulated simultaneously and the control of selectivity becomes difficult (Tonndorf 1977). This stimulation mode supplies information on pulse rate and intensity of the stimulus. The question remains whether such systems will achieve any speech discrimination in future.

Bipolar stimulation uses two electrode contact surfaces very near to each other and current is injected in between. The current density is high between the contact points but there is minimal spread. This means that only nerve fibres near to the contact points are stimulated. This mechanism allows simultaneous and successive stimulation of the discrete parts of the cochlea in different places, but it is only effective when the contact points are near to the nerve fibre endings.

Transmission

Transcutaneous versus percutaneous stimulation

When *percutaneous stimulation* is used the patient is provided with a plug through the skin. In the past this plug often had to be removed because of infection. Sometimes the percutaneous connection is used temporarily for several months, which gives an opportunity to conduct psychophysical studies without imposition of any of the limits of a telemetry system (Merzenich 1985, Banfai et al 1984).

In *transcutaneous stimulation* the signal is transmitted by an infrared or radiofrequency link with direct coupling. Most telemetry devices rely on simple induction coupling or on an amplitude modulated carrier, which provides essentially only voltage control of their output. Other groups use a more sophisticated system, which allows current control, or they use implanted electronics.

Speechprocessing

The speechprocessor is one of the main parts of the artificial electrical stimulating device. Its task is to decode the incoming speech signal and to translate it into meaningful electrical pulses. In future, progress will be made in the development of adequate speechcoding schemes. Up to now we can distinguish two general speechcoding strategies. The first one uses feature extraction. The second strategy is based on analogue processing schemes or filterbank processing. The combination of both strategies is even possible.

The stimulation modes are summarized in Figure 3.1.

What about the practical realization?

All this theoretical knowledge has led to the development of different commercial devices. Since it is

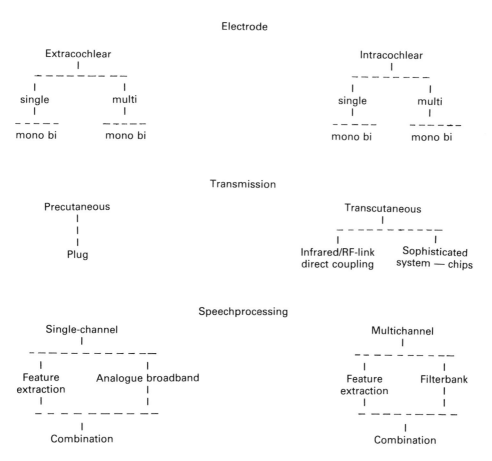

Fig. 3.1 Stimulation modes.

impossible to explain and describe all of them in detail, we will place a specific cochlear implant in our classification and, in order to avoid any misinterpretation, refer to the original articles.

The *3M-House implant system* is an intracochlear, single-channel, monopolar electrode. It is an insulated ball-tipped platinum wire of which approximately 6 mm is uninsulated. This uninsulated part passes through the round window. The system uses a magnetic coupling which holds the receiver and external transmitter coil in close proximity. The signal processor uses an analogue signal processing scheme. The information is bandpass filtered and transmitted to the internal part by 16 kHz amplitude modulation (House 1984, Bushong 1985). This single channel implant provides environmental sounds and improves lipreading and voice control.

The *3M-Vienna multifrequency device* has been developed by Prof. K. Burian, Dr I. Hochmair and Dr E. Hochmair. The extracochlear single-channel, monopolar electrode is placed in the recess of the round window. They also developed a 4-channel, bipolar intracochlear scala tympani electrode connected to an implantable receiver/stimulator circuit (Hochmair et al 1985, Burian et al 1984). Both of these implants are complemented by the same type of sound processor, which implements a single-channel, full bandwidth analogue sound signal processing scheme. In the case of the 4-channel intracochlear implant, the external portable sound processor is fitted to the one of the four channels best suited for speech understanding. Proper frequency equalization over the whole frequency range has proved to be very important. The device is called a multifrequency device because it amplifies various frequency bands individually and differently, as determined by the tested needs of each patient.

The same principle is used in the *Graigwell-Finetech cochlear implant system*, which is implanted at the University College Hospital (London—Fraser, Graham, Hazell). The speech processing strategy uses twin-channel compression, which is frequency dependent. The implant is an extra-cochlear round window single-channel, monopolar electrode. Trancutaneous transmission is executed using an amplitude modulated 12 MHz carrier wave (Dettmer 1984, Rosen & Ball 1986).

An example of a single-channel, extracochlear device which uses speech pattern extraction is the *EPI-device* (London—Douek, Fourcin). The goal of this group is optimal speech reception with lipreading. They only transmit the fundamental frequency of the voice (Moore et al 1984, 1985). The electrode is placed on, or near, the round window. To date, the group has concentrated on patients with 'open' ears allowing the electrode to be introduced via the ear canal without need for surgery. For patients with an intact eardrum, a tympanopexy is required. A gold platinum earmold serves both as an electrical earth and as a means of positioning the ball-tipped electrode. The stimulator is linked to the laryngeal frequency extractor by an infrared link and the microphone, which drives the frequency extractor, can either be worn by the patient or by his partner (Douek et al 1984).

The implant from Zurich (Spillman & Dillier 1985) is a round window, 2-channel, bipolar electrode, which uses analogue broadband speech processing and pulsatile stimulation. Their experiments with hardwired percutaneous connectors were not very encouraging (removal of the plug) and therefore they decided to use transcutaneous inductive coupling systems.

Other examples of single-channel, extracochlear implant systems are the *PRELCO-prosthesis* (Cazals et al 1984) and the one of J. Bosch et al (1985) (Barcelona—Spain), which is still experimental.

The Cochlear Prosthesis Group at Stanford has been engaged for several years in the development of an implantable multichannel receiver/stimulator and an external speech processor and transmitter. They fabricated rigid modiolar and flexible scala tympani electrode arrays. They tested an 8-channel monopolar pulsatile system using all custom integrated circuits in a welded titanium can and, at the present stage, they are trying to develop an 8-channel system with greater flexibility in its timing parameters and current waveforms. They compared different speech processing strategies, e.g. a formant tracking vocoder and an analogue single-channel processing strategy with amplitude compression and high frequency emphasis. Up to now a definite conclusion on an optimal speech processing strategy for the multichannel implant is not achieved.

The Stanford group concluded that the optimal multichannel cochlear prothesis is still a few years away and they co-operated with Biostim to produce a safe and commercially available single-channel cochlear system of reasonable speech discrimination potential. The electrode is placed 3 mm into the round window. The stimulator has an electronic circuit which allows different waveforms to be generated. The device is called the *Bioear cochlear implant* (Simmons 1984, White 1985).

At the university of Melbourne an intracochlear, multichannel implant was developed by Prof. Clark et al and at present it is distributed by Nucleus Limited. An intracochlear array of 22 electrodes is inserted up to 25 mm through the round window. It is connected to a receiver/stimulator implanted in the mastoid, which delivers charge balanced, biphasic current pulses to pairs of electrodes. The speech processor is based on feature extraction (f_0/f_2). It uses the acoustic signal amplitude, the signal periodicity and the frequency of the mid-range spectral peak (f_2) to determine stimulus amplitude, rate and which bipolar pair of electrodes to stimulate at any time (Patrick et al 1985, Mecklenburg et al 1985).

The *UCFH (Storz)* implant is provided with a 16-electrode intracochlear insert, which is designed for insertion 23–25 mm into the scala tympani. It is designed for either bipolar, monopolar or common ground plane operation. An implantable connector system provides replacement of defective receiving electronics without disturbing the functioning electrode. Receiving electronics are coupled in the connector to both receiving coils and electrode array. A percutaneous cable is used temporarily for 3–4 months in patients in the experimental series. At the end of this period the patient receives a permanent radiofrequency receiver.

The present system uses four channels, which are entirely independent, allowing simultaneous transmission to all four channels. The speech processor is based on a baseband vocoder system with four operating channels (Merzenich et al 1984, 1985).

The *Inneraid* implant, manufactured by Symbion, is the result of research at the University of Utah by Eddington (1983). It is a percutaneous multichannel electrode device. The implanted electrode has eight electrodes of which six are intracochlear and two are remote ground. Four of the intracochlear electrodes are selected to be used by the 4-channel sound processor, which is based on bandpass filtering. The stimuli are simultaneously transmitted.

A similar cochlear implant project is developed in the Republic of China. European multichannel devices are found in Germany. The *Implex* device of Hortmann is an extracochlear 8-channel system. It was originally developed by Prof. Banfai of Duren. The implant consists of a contact plate on which eight electrodes are fixed and two electrodes are free. The electrodes are positioned in exact correspondence to the projection of the cochlea. The two free electrodes are placed in the round window and in the tube. The speech processor is based on the principle of the vocoder. The electrode system is suitable for both percutaneous connection and for transcutaneous transmission. After the electrical measurements and thresholds are stabilized, the switchover to transcutaneous transmission is effected (Banfai 1984, Hortmann 1984).

Since January 1985 a completely novel extracochlear 16-channel system has been used by Prof. Banfai in which 14 electrodes are firmly fixed. In this implant the speech processing strategy takes into consideration the time resolution as well as the tonotopy. By means of a new wiring technique, simultaneous stimulation of several electrodes is excluded. All stimulus parameters are controlled by an 8-bit microprocessor (Banfai et al 1985).

In France the *Chorimac 12* channel cochlear implant was designed in co-operation with the Societé Bertin (Chouard et al 1984, MacLeod et al 1985). An electrode carrier is inserted through the round window into the first 18 mm of the scala tympani. In cases of congenital malformation, several cochlear fenestrations are performed on the promontory and the 12 monopolar electrodes are implanted one by one. The speech processor is based on filterbank processing.

A multichannel array with 12 bipolar channels, developed at the University of Copenhagen (Lauridsen et al 1983), is made by using thin-film production techniques.

Our last example is a bipolar intracochlear, multichannel implant *LAURA* (Forelec), which was developed at the Universities of Antwerp and Leuven and is still seen as an experimental device (Peeters et al 1985). The major advantage of this prosthesis is the development of a microprocessor, allowing extreme flexibility in the control of complex current wave forms of pulsetrains to the 8-channel bipolar intracochlear electrode array. The electrode impedance for each of the 16 contact areas can be checked at any moment by means of the implanted microprocessor controlling the implanted transmitter. Transcutaneous coupling is used with two separate inductive links for power and information transmission. The recently developed speech processor is based on the principle of a filterbank in combination with pitch extraction. The output of the speech processor is scanned by a low power 8-bit CMOS microprocessor. The processor can be fitted to the patient, not only for threshold and pain level but also for speechprocessing algorithm. This is possible since the internal device is flexible and allows the use of different kinds of speechprocessing strategies.

DISCUSSION

Describing the results and comparing the benefits and the extent of auditory information provided by different kinds of implants is almost imposssible, because the parameters are so different. Each team reported results of different measurements and developed their own tests, or used other languages. Nevertheless, we would like to refer to a comparative study and the measurements of the IOWA cochlear implant clinical project. Gantz et al (1985) compared three different kinds of cochlear implants of which two were single-channel and one multi-channel. All three of the cochlear implants evaluated were found to improve the communication skills of postlingually deafened adults. The implants provide a sound awareness and, in some circumstances, this is sufficient for identification of environmental sounds. One of the most important benefits of cochlear implants is their ability to supplement lip-reading. When contextual cues were available to the patient, a dramatic improvement in open-set performance was nóted. Familiarity with the speaker enhances speech understanding. The test battery documented the effect that mode of presentation of the test material has on the results.

A factor that may explain the differences in patient performance is the higher level top-down processing and cognitive skills of some patients. A correlation was found between those with a good lip-reading ability, reflecting high-level cognitive skills necessary to synthesize the limited information

provided by the present generation of cochlear implants.

From these considerations we strongly believe that techniques for artificial hearing stimulation have to be recognized as having important but restricted futures.

One should never forget that the main aim is to help the hearing impaired patient and never to use him just to realize surgical performance. While neural survival is the primordial and most significant factor regarding the success of such procedures, one has to keep in mind that the optimal and honest selection of the patient remains essential. First the candidate is to be informed of the actual pros and cons of the procedure. Four points are prominent:

1. There is a need for techniques that measure the amount and localization of auditory surviving neurons. Figure 3.2 summarizes the selection programme (Van Den Heyning et al 1985).

2. Psychological requirements must never be overlooked including strong motivation from the patient regarding rehabilitation.

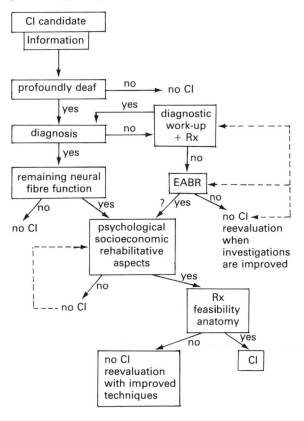

Fig. 3.2 Scheme of selection.

3. The social and economical aspects must be fairly discussed.

4. Modern rehabilitation must be provided to all operated patients.

Once the patient is implanted the role of rehabilitation will become prominent because it is proved that most of the learning occurs within the first several months. Strategies that supply the patient with the most efficient training sessions and techniques should be implemented.

CONCLUSION

We believe that, in the coming years, cochlear implants may be optimized and miniaturized and they will become a realistic and alternative hearing aid for the profoundly deaf. Nevertheless, we have to emphasize the experimental nature of the concept and the surgical techniques of cochlear implants. Therefore, we strongly advice restriction of these techniques to adults with postlingual total deafness. The adult prelingual group will be the next population. At present, we do not believe that children should be operated upon. Indeed, long-term follow-up of the first group of patients is to be studied regarding the real functional and social aspects, long-term tolerance and biocompatibility of the intra-auricular and intracochlear introduced devices.

INTRODUCTION

There is a simple one-word answer to this question on which all but the Luddites would agree, and that is 'yes'. This said, the orientation of the present chapter will be to look at cochlear implants as they are at present and as they are being implemented, then ask what is their real and realistic role.

All clinicians dealing with the completely deafened patients who have seen the benefits which some may derive from a cochlear implant will agree that they do have a present, and are bound to have a future, role. The particular question which I propose to examine concerns the potential clientele for such approaches, both from a quantitative and from a qualitative standpoint; the question of how and by whom they should be provided, the types of implants which should be used and the resource implications of such provisions.

At the present time, the approach of many otologists to cochlear implants has been similar to a mountaineer finding a new peak: 'We must go for it because it is there'. The aim of this chapter is to provide some degree of perspective and caution. To quote a well-known cochlear implant researcher at a cochlear implant meeting (Rosen 1984), 'We must make haste slowly'.

What is a cochlear implant?

A cochlear implant is a means of electrically stimulating the cochlear nerve, bypassing the transduction process of the cochlea. As such, from a functional point of view it may be regarded as a sophisticated hearing aid offering a way of overcoming dysfunction peripheral to it in the auditory pathway and, in particular, in the cochlea. It may be regarded, superficially, as being analagous to a hearing aid with a bone conduction transducer bypassing dysfunction in the middle and outer ear. The similarity is, however, limited in that both that and a standard air conduction transducer provide the same waveform to the oval window and hence to stimulate the cochlea. The nature of what is required to stimulate the cochlea optimally is well known and can be relatively well provided.

However, the exact nature of what is, or should be, optimally stimulating the dendritic receptors of the afferent fibres of the cochlear nerve, or the neurones themselves are not known. The electrical activity and selectivity of individual cochlear nerve fibres is well documented (e.g. Kiang 1965), but little useful information is available as to which is the optimal way of imparting frequency and intensity-specific information to all or part of the surviving cochlear nerve fibres. Certainly, the complexity of the coding which takes place in the cochlea is such that there is no reason to suppose that an electrical analogue of the acoustical signal is the optimal means of achieving such stimulation.

However, it must be admitted that workers using a variety of approaches, including such analogue stimulation, can provide for quite reasonable psychoacoustical discriminations (or psychoelectroauditory) between different signals (e.g. Foucin et al 1979). The more subtle electroauditory discriminations, or even relatively crude auditory discrimination or recognition of speech, have been consistently achieved only with multichannel implants, which, to some extent, may stimulate different parts of the cochlea (e.g. Tyler et al 1984).

We are thus left eventually with a device which may offer some degree of crude auditory sensation to an auditory system with a non-functional cochlea. It has been described by certain authors as the cochlear nerve's equivalent of a very crude hearing aid, although certain studies comparing cochlear implant effectiveness with that of standard hearing aids have compared it with even cruder aids! Certainly the signal processing incorporated in a number of cochlear implant input devices is far more sophisticated than anything included in any hearing aid. However, in terms of the sensation which it imparts to the stimulated individual, it remains extremely crude.

In addition to providing any meaningful electroauditory input, which certainly the single-channel devices do not, the implant does provide a variety of other useful information to the implantee. The three main areas of help in this respect are from the standpoint of providing timing and pitch cues to facilitate speechreading (lipreading), providing an awareness of environmental sounds and offering the listener some ability to monitor his/her own voice. In addition, in certain patients electroauditory stimulation may provide the patient with relief from distressing tinnitus. All these may also be provided by a hearing aid to an individual with any significant residual hearing so that the close analogy with hearing aids remains. A number of audiologists have thus been tempted to remark on the interest shown by some of their otological colleagues in implants when the same individuals had never shown any interest in hearing aids! The situation of the implant in the overall rehabilitative programme may be seen within the context of the management model of the audiological rehabilitative process, which we have developed elsewhere (Goldstein & Stephens 1981).

Who are the potential implantees?

Potential candidates for implantation can be considered on the basis of the aetiology of their hearing loss, site of the lesion, severity and psychoacoustics of the hearing loss, and a variety of other factors including patient attitudes and support, other health conditions, cognitive factors, etc.

As the prime aim of the implant is to bypass the non-functioning cochlea, the ideal candidate for cochlear implantation must, by definition, be one who has a non-functioning cochlea, but absolutely normal auditory neural pathways from the cochlear nerve to the auditory cortex. Unfortunately, such an ideal situation never exists, for in the absence of functioning hair cells there is always some degree of neural degeneration (Spoendlin 1971). However, in a number of conditions with complete loss of hair cells, a large number of the afferent fibres in the cochlear nerve survive, at least for a considerable length of time. Ideal candidates in this respect are patients with deafness related to aminoglycoside antibiotics and certain other ototoxic drugs and patients with a hearing loss stemming from bacterial meningitis. This last condition, whilst largely destroying the hair cells, generally leaves the auditory neural pathways intact. Other forms of infectious labyrinthitis may also have the same effect.

While a number of successful implants have been carried out on patients with more generalized causes of hearing loss and systemic disorders, these must be viewed with caution and each individual case considered on its merit, with careful assessment of the function of the more central pathways. This applies particularly in conditions such as syphilitic deafness and deafness arising from impairment of the blood flow to the cochlea.

Few people would contest the foregoing discussion. What is more contentious are the questions of the severity of the hearing loss and the age of the patient and how these relate to any criteria for implantation.

The more conservative groups concerned with cochlear implants, including all those currently active in the UK, implant only patients with no 'aidable' hearing, i.e. patients with a total hearing loss. At this stage, questions of definition arise with little agreement as to what total hearing loss actually is. A useful step in this direction has come with the recent work of Martin (1986) who defines total hearing loss in patients with normal middle ear function as when a 'valid auditory response cannot be elicited at 130 dB Hz in the range 500 to 4000 Hz or at the maximum output of the same audiometer at lower frequencies'.

This, by definition, excludes those patients with an additional conductive component to their hearing loss which could mean that they have air conduction thresholds in the order of 150 dB or more, but still useful cochlear reserves with potential bone conduction thresholds of some 90–100 dB, were it possible to adequately measure such thresholds. It is notable that a number of the 'star patients' described in the literature did have chronic middle ear disease or otosclerosis and the question remains as to whether electrical stimulation is activating the cochlear nerve directly in these cases, or indirectly via stimulation of the surviving hair cells. At the present time this is a dilemma difficult to resolve because of limitations of the output of currently available acoustical transducers.

Such considerations aside, and restricting further discussion to patients with sensorineural, indeed cochlear, hearing loss, we must consider how severe a hearing loss a patient should have before being regarded as a candidate for implantation. As mentioned above, a number of groups restrict candidature to those with a total hearing loss, much of the consensus here being compatible with Martin's (1986) definition. Other groups, however, implant ears with varying degrees of useable hearing, sometimes as good as 90 dB HL across the mid frequencies. The question which must be posed here is whether or not this is justified on ethical, auditory perceptual, or on economic grounds.

Let us consider first the ethical aspects. If an intracochlear implant is being introduced to a cochlea with useful residual hearing, this is basically destroying that cochlear function and denying the patient the potential benefits of more sophisticated orthodox amplification in the form, of, for example, signal processing hearing aids. The rationale maintained by those performing such implantation is the claim that the patient may obtain more useful amplification from an implant than from hearing aids. In many such cases a careful comparison has not been performed and, indeed, even where it has been performed the implant has usually been compared with fairly banal linear amplification hearing aids. It appears to be exceptional for a department interested in cochlear implants also to be interested in sophisticated hearing aids.

Such an argument on the basis of the irreversibility of changes resulting from implantation does not apply to the extracochlear electrodes, such as those used by the EPI group in London (Fourcin et al 1979) or the Hochmair group in Vienna (Hochmair & Hochmair Desoyer 1985), provided that no significant permanent damage to the middle ear results from the surgical procedure which could make any subsequent orthodox amplification more difficult.

From an auditory perceptual standpoint, it is apparent that a few patients with significant residual hearing have such severe auditory distortions stemming from their cochlear pathology that they may derive a more meaningful input from electrical stimulation. This said, it is important that appropriate signal processing techniques applied to acoustical amplification be considered and evaluated initially in such patients before irreversible implantation is performed. Indeed application of the implant signal processing in terms of fundamental frequency extraction has been successfully applied by one group (e.g. Rosen & Fourcin 1983).

Other approaches include frequency transposition, multichannel compression speech envelope enhancement and should be considered and, if relevant, evaluated before a patient with significant residual hearing is considered for an implant. The benefits which such patients might get from an implant to compare with those from the relevant hearing aid should not then be based on the 'star' patients, but rather upon the median results obtained with the particular device. In the case of single-channel implants, a trial of the implant signal processing system using promontory stimulation, although not without its limitations, should be considered for comparative purposes. It is obviously not possible to evaluate the potential benefit of multichannel implants in the same way.

The third consideration, and one which is becoming increasingly important under situations of limited resource availability, is that of cost/benefit. If, from a benefit standpoint, there is little to choose between the use of a sophisticated hearing aid and the implant, the former may be justified on a cost basis alone. In terms of hardware it is possible to purchase about 20 sophisticated hearing aids or more than 200 basic aids for the price of 1 cochlear implant system. In addition, there are the costs of hospital admission and indeterminate costs for the services of the surgeon, anaesthetist and other supporting staff. It is becoming inevitable, with limited resources, that such factors will play a part in the decision as to which approach is pertinent for a patient with residual hearing.

Finally we come to more psychological and general health matters, when a patient may not feel that surgical intervention with some inevitable risks is justified when they can obtain as much or almost as much benefit from a hearing aid. Furthermore, the individual's state of general health may be such as to preclude surgery.

In the USA there has been an extension of cochlear implants to children often with prelingual hearing losses (e.g. Ear and Hearing 1985). In most other parts of the world, the approach has been more circumspect, being restricted to postlingually deafened adults. Furthermore, the implant used with such children has been a fairly basic single-channel system.

Such implantation of children raises questions on ethical, linguistic and prognostic grounds. From an ethical standpoint, there is no question of a deaf child being able to give informed consent to such a procedure. With increased emphasis on children's rights taking place and likely to continue, this exposes those responsible to subsequent litigation, apart from the ethical fact that the child has generally played little part in the decision affecting his or her own future.

The second point concerns the effect of the implant on the child's speech and language development. While information is slowly being acquired as to the possible effects of implantation on speech conservation and rehabilitation in patients who had already acquired speech and language before losing their hearing (e.g. Abberton et al 1985, Waters 1986), the potential influence on the child endeavouring to acquire speech language presents a completely different set of problems. A description of results obtained in implanted children has been given by Kirk & Hill-Brown (1985) and these results are not encouraging. This is further compounded by the difficulty in obtaining appropriate control subjects. Indeed, the question of whether any benefit comes from the stimulation per se, as apart from the general rehabilitative procedures, has proven problematical even with adults (Waters 1986).

The prognostic implications concern both the aetiological factors and the possibilities of long-term damage. While the majority of children (98/164) implanted in the major programmes (Berliner & Eisenberg 1985) had deafness secondary to bacterial meningitis, 55 of the others suffered from a variety of forms of congenital deafness with possible implications for the intactness of the neuronal connections. Some of the possible risks from a prognostic standpoint have been discussed by Simmons (1985) and include increased dangers arising in middle ear infections and, more particularly, the risks of precluding more sophisticated implantation at a later date.

How many potential implantees are there?

The question of the numbers of potential implantees depends on the definition of what is a potential implantee. This has been considered by Thornton (1986), who shows that probably the most important criterion influencing the potential numbers is the hearing loss severity criterion adopted. Secondly, there is the question as to whether or not the patient has a prelingual hearing loss—a group which many workers still consider inappropriate. Furthermore, limitations may occur when considering the general health of the individual, i.e. whether the individual

can or should be submitted to the surgery necessary for implantation. This is particularly important, as the majority of individuals with profound or complete hearing loss are elderly. Any further considerations come with the psychological state and attitude of the patient together with the support which she/he may have from spouse, parents or children.

A final consideration relates to the attitude of the patient towards the implant. This is alluded to by Thornton, who found that there were only some 600 appropriate candidates in the UK (from a population of 56 million). From these, it seems reasonable to suppose that a significant proportion will not wish to have implants. They may prefer a vibrotactile approach, or feel 'deafness is insufficient reason for surgery', being resigned to their silent world. A number of postlingually deafened individuals have effectively integrated into the deaf community and have adopted sign language.

This final figure of some hundreds of potential cochlear implantees compares with the 8 million individuals in the UK who are potential candidates for hearing aids (Haggard et al 1981).

Which implants for whom?

As alluded to earlier, cochlear implants may range from a fairly basic single-channel device to very sophisticated multichannel implants. Certain more sophisticated extracochlear devices are also available, the sophistication initially introduced by their exponents to overcome the electrical problems, secondary to not having intracochlear stimulation.

Intuitively one's reaction is that, as far as possible, extracochlear devices should be favoured over intracochlear devices as their potential damage to surviving inner ear structures will be less. They do not preclude a sophisticated intracochlear implantation at a later date. However, there is increasing evidence (e.g. Tyler et al 1984) that more speech information may be discriminated by individuals with multichannel than with single-channel devices. Indeed, throughout the world, the majority of implanted patients who are able to recognize words auditorily are those fitted with the more sophisticated multichannel implants developed by the Melbourne and Utah groups.

Who then should have what? This question is further complicated by the suggestion derived from their findings (Tyler et al 1984) that those patients who do well with implants also do well with vibro-tactile stimulation. Presumably they are the individuals with the skills to extract the relevant speech information no matter in which modality it is presented.

As a rough rule of thumb, the author would argue that, if patients with residual hearing are to be implanted, they should have extracochlear implants to minimize the likelihood of destruction of this surviving function.

Among the totally deaf it might be reasonable to consider whether or not the individual is likely to have much surviving neural function, particularly in the middle and basal turns of the cochlea. If there is good neural, but no hair cell, survival the indications support a sophisticated multichannel implant. Ideally a device should be chosen which has the potential for upgrading as the signal processing system becomes more sophisticated.

If the evidence of neural survival is limited and generally restricted to the more apical part of the cochlea, emphasis should be on single-channel stimulation, using as sophisticated signal processing system as possible. The system will depend on the abilities and needs of the patient and Rosen & Ball (1986) have illustrated some of the differences which may be obtained in the same subjects using two different modes of stimulation. It is arguable that an intracochlear single-channel electrode can no longer be reasonably justified.

If preimplant electrical stimulation shows no response, or the patient either does not wish to have surgery or is likely to be put physically at risk by surgery, a sophisticated vibrotactile system should be used. Such systems are becoming increasingly sophisticated as a result of interest in the problems of the completely deaf, largely as a result of the enthusiasm for cochlear implants.

Who should be performing cochlear implantation?

Despite what the American Food and Drug administration may have decided, cochlear implants remain very much at an experimental and developmental stage. It is therefore important that implantation should be performed by teams who possess all the necessary skills to provide the appropriate rehabilitation for the patient, and who are able to evaluate the patient effectively with and without their implant. Such evaluation is particularly important as it is certain that future implants will be based on the better aspects of several existing implants coupled with new developments. All existing implants and their coding systems have a number of weaknesses and some of these have been highlighted by the recent studies of Tyler et al (1985, unpublished) and of Rosen & Ball (1986), who show that different aspects of different multichannel and different single-channel systems respectively may be valuable for coding different components of speech. It is imperative to ensure that, by implanting a crude system, the team is not precluding later implantation of a more sophisticated system and one of far greater benefit to the patient.

The important of having a comprehensive rehabilitative team able to help the patient obtain optimal benefit from his implant and to provide backup and support when problems arise is paramount. The surgical technique of implanting the electrode and receiver system is relatively simple for any competent otological surgeon. What is far more important is training the patient to derive maximum benefit from his implant with ongoing monitoring of his performance. Merely implanting the device and sending the patient away with a minimum of instruction is equivalent to giving the patient a hearing aid and telling him to go away and use it. It is likely to have equally ineffectual results, with the majority not being used, or certainly not being used to anything approaching full advantage.

Implantation should therefore be restricted to centres where, in addition to surgical expertise, there should be dedicated staff with sufficient experience to deal with any technical and electrical problems arising with the implant system, to provide the patient with high level training in audiovisual communication skills and to provide similar expertise in speech conservation and amelioration. In addition, staff expert in psychoacoustical and electro-physiological evaluation of the patient both pre- and postimplantation are necessary.

At the present time, when the procedures are still at an experimental level, it is recommended that cochlear implantation should be restricted to one or two centres in each country where the teams involved can slowly build up such expertise as to be of greatest benefit to the individual.

Can we afford cochlear implants?

In his recent article 'Straight thinking about cochlear implants', Haggard (1986) has raised the question of the resource implications of cochlear implant programmes. It is reasonably agreed that, for such devices to be most effective, they must be optimally used by the patient with the appropriate rehabilitative backup and training. That is to say that, if £5000–£10 000 is to be spent on each device, a considerable sum should be spent on the salaries of the rehabilitative professionals to ensure that such optimal use occurs. For the employment of these individuals to be worthwhile, there is the implication that they should be part of a team regularly performing implants. With the small number of potential candidates within the population this supports restriction of implantation to a few specified centres.

While the market economy applies to the health care in the USA, with implants being performed on those able to afford them, within the UK and most European countries a more reasonable egalitarian policy exists. Such a policy of 'to each according to his needs' was built into the health care systems of most European countries following the traumas of World War II (Stephens 1982). Within these countries, continuous economic growth with increasing resources can no longer be taken for granted and, particularly when much of the national product continues to be spent on armaments, the limits of health resources become apparent. This has been highlighted by the question of heart transplants.

While most members of society will accept the priorities of patients with greater disabilities, it is important to ensure that what is done for these individuals should be optimally effective. It is also important to ensure that it is not done at the expense of other services in an already poorly funded service. For example, a recent survey by the Royal National Institute for the Deaf indicated that, in certain ORL departments, the waiting time for a routine hearing aid fitting could be as long as 2 years. It would obviously be ludicrous for surgeons at such a centre to devote resources which could be offered to a large number of needy patients with moderate disability to a very few with severe disabilities. Apart from anything else, an appropriate professional infrastructure is necessary before cochlear implants can be introduced to the rehabilitative programme.

In order not to compromise existing facilities, it is also important that new resources should be made available. The case made by their enthusiasts should be sufficiently strong to convince governmental bodies as to their merit when a clear presentation of all relevant factors is made.

What good has come from cochlear implants?

In this final brief section I shall exclude the undoubted benefit which individual patients have derived from implants and concentrate on benefits in terms of increased knowledge and improved services.

A major benefit to emerge from the development of 'cochlear implant mania' has been a more serious appraisal of the problems and needs of patients with profound or complete hearing loss. Previously, work had largely been restricted to a few enthusiasts and charity-based establishments using techniques based on lipreading, manual communication and a few rather crude vibrotactile approaches. With the development of cochlear implantation programmes, more resources and interests have been applied to these problems. This has led to the development of test materials and approaches to evaluate the patients more effectively and a better acceptance of their global problems and needs by professionals. In addition, there have been important technological developments. Such developments have included the application of signal processing techniques used in implants, to hearing aids for patients with a minimal degree of residual hearing at the lower frequencies (Rosen & Fourcin 1983). In addition, there has been more general consideration of other signal processing approaches and the needs of such individuals with profound hearing losses. For patients with no hearing, more emphasis and interest has been applied to developing sophisticated vibrotactile systems.

The approaches have been developed partly in response to providing more help for individuals assessed for cochlear implantation and found unsuitable, and also perhaps by those professionals with a jaundiced view of cochlear implants and keen to prove an alternative approach. Whatever the motivation, such developments can only be good for our patients with total or subtotal hearing losses.

The contributions on this subject by Stephens and by Marquet et al are well written and very adequately address the 'state of the art' for cochlear implants, as it is known today. Each author has reviewed the theoretical considerations that pertain to extra-cochlear and intracochlear auditory nerve stimulation techniques and the limitations of today's technology. Both Stephens and Marquet et al stress that, in view of our understanding of auditory neurosystem stimulation today, the stage of development of existing cochlear implant devices should be considered as experimental in nature and that there is more technological development to be expected. Each contribution points out that cochlear implants are reasonable as alternative hearing aids for the profoundly deaf who otherwise cannot be helped with existing types of aids. Stephens emphasizes that, short of implantation of a device, profoundly deaf patients may benefit from signal processing hearing aids and vibrotactile devices.

Both authors comment that patients with some residual hair cells in the cochlea, in addition to large numbers of viable neurons, probably benefit most from cochlear implants. Yet it is to be noted that these same individuals, if sufficiently motivated and given the same intense rehabilitation attention might do as well with alternative means. This is a particularly important point as resources become more limited. Stephens and Marquet et al emphasize the importance of the postimplantation rehabilitation programme. It is clear that teams of individuals are needed to maximize the benefits of the biotechnology, bioengineering, implantation and physiological potential, as well as for the maximum utilization of the device.

Stephens and Marquet et al provide a rather complete and comprehensive overview of the principles behind the use of single-channel versus multi-channel electrodes and Marquet et al in particular, provide an historical perspective with respect to cochlear implants and a detailed description of the various devices known to exist today.

Both authors address the important considerations that the cochlear implant technology is providing. Both contributions point out the limited benefits to be obtained by single-channel devices and each one addresses the pros and cons of extracochlear versus intracochlear implants.

They emphasize that the rationale and/or justification for implantation of prelingually deaf children is as yet unproven. They are correct in questioning the use of implants in children on a scientific and ethical basis, especially in view of the evidence to date that speech-language acquisition in the implanted prelingually deaf child poses special challenges as compared to implanting postlingually deafened adults.

The selection of patients for cochlear implantation is addressed by both Stephens and Marquet et al. The importance of preimplantation cochlear stimulation, however, has yet to be proven as a reliable measure for predicting success with a cochlear implant. Both authors have stressed the limited speech processing capability of cochlear implants, so far as excellent, otherwise unassisted, speech reproduction and speech understanding is concerned.

Stephens and Marquet et al have answered the question posed as the title of their presentations in the affirmative, i.e. that there is a future for cochlear implants. The overall patient population for which the devices in their present stage of technological development have application, especially when strict criteria for their use are applied, is probably less than the enthusiasm for their use suggests. Both authors seem concerned about the over-utilization of the implant; the fact that injury to viable structures undoubtedly occurs as a consequence of the implantation and that this injury and the prior implantation may, in fact, preclude later implantation of more sophisticated devices. It is apparent in reading their two contributions that there is a need for data comparison and a need for standardization, not only in the selection of patients for implantation but in the definition of what devices are most appropriate for what type of clinical problem and the need for standardization in reporting results. Because of considerable subject-to-subject variability, not only in the cause of the hearing loss but the extent to which there are viable neural elements, as well as the psychological and individual make up of the patients there truly needs to be considerable attention given to recognizing those differences in the description of the results.

Both authors stress the importance of the team of professionals necessary to maximize the potential of the device for the patient. Also both suggest that, as better understanding of neurostimulation and neuroprocessing evolves, more progress with cochlear implants is to be expected.

REFERENCES

J Marquet, S Peeters, M Van Durme

Ballantyne J C, Evans E F, Morrison A 1978 Electrical auditory stimulation in the management of profound hearing loss. Journal of Laryngology and Otology, suppl no 1

Banfai P, Hortmann G, Karczag A, Kubik S, Wustrow F 1984 Results with 8-channel cochlear implants. Advances in Audiology 2: 1–18

Banfai P, Karczag A, Kubik S, Luers P, Surth W, Banfai S 1985 Extracochlear 8 and 6 multichannel cochlear implantation with per- and transcutaneous transmission. Experiences on 129 patients. Melbourne Conference, August

Bosch J, Colomina R 1985 Cochlear implant: comparative study of the mono- and multichannel implantation. In: Myers E (ed) New dimensions in otolaryngology—head and neck surgery, vol 2. Elsevier Science Publishers BV, Amsterdam, p 752–753

Brackman D E 1976 The cochlear implant: basic principles. The Laryngoscope 86: 378–388.

Burian K et al 1984 Clinical experiences with the Vienna cochlear implant. Advances in Audiology 2: 19–29

Bushong J W 1986, Cochlear implants—status. Internal report 3M-Europe

Cazals Y, Aran J-M, Negrevergne M, Portmann M 1984 Activation and inhibition of hearing with electrical stimulation of the ear. Advances in Audiology 2: 30–35

Cazals Y, Celebrier P 1980 Protocole d'evaluation des perceptions auditives et de la parole. Internal report, Paris

Chouard C H, MacLeod P 1976 Implantation of multiple intracochlear electrodes for rehabilitation of total deafness. Preliminary report. Laryngoscope (St Louis) 36: 1745–1751

Chouard C H, Fugain C, Meyer B, Lacombe H, Jegu D 1984 Speech recognition in a deaf subject with a portable multichannel cochlear implant system. Advances in Audiology 2: 36–60

Cochlear implant 1985 Five companies respond to Asha survey. ASHA May: 27–34

Dettmer R 1984 Helping the deaf to hear. Electronics and Power 40: 199–204

Djournd A, Eyries C 1957 Prothese auditive par excitation electrique a distance du nerf sensoriel a l'aide d'un bobinage inclus a demeure. Pressé Medical 65: 1417–1423

Douek E, Fourcin A J, Moore R et al 1983 Clinical aspects of extracochlear electrical stimulation. Annals of the New York Academy of Sciences 18: 332–336

Eddington D K 1982 Multiple channel intracochlear stimulation. In: Brackmann D E (ed) Neurological surgery of the ear and skull base. Raven Press, New York, p 199–205

Eddington D K 1983 Speech recognition in deaf subjects with multichannel intracochlear electrodes. Annals of the New York Academy of Sciences 18: 241–258

Eddington J K, Orth J L 1984 Speech recognition in a deaf subject with a portable multichannel cochlear implant system. Advances in Audiology 2: 61–67

Gantz B J 1985 IOWA cochlear implant comparison project. In: Myers E (ed) New dimensions in otolaryngology—head and neck surgery, vol 2. Elsevier Science Publishers BV, Amsterdam

Gantz B, Tyler R S, Preece J, McCabe B F, Lowder M W, Otto S R 1985 IOWA cochlear implant clinical project: results with two single-channel cochlear implants and one multichannel cochlear implant. Laryngoscope 95: 443–449

Gray R 1985 Cochlear implants. Croom Helm, London & Sydney

Hinojosa R, Blough R R, Mhoon E E 1985 Profound sensorineural deafness. A histopathological study. Abstract Melbourne Conference, August.

Hochmair E S, Hochmair-Desoyer I J 1985 Aspects of sound signal processing using the Vienna intra- and extracochlear implant. In: Schindler R A, Merzenich M M (eds) Cochlear implants. Raven Press, New York, p 101–110

Hortmann 1979 Implex. Implantierbare extracochleare 8-kanal innenohrprothese. Corresponding leaflet.

House W F 1984 3M cochlear implant system. Surgical procedure. November

House W F, Urban J 1973 Long-term results of electrode implantation and electric stimulation of the cochlea in man. Annals of Otology, Rhinology and Laryngology 82: 504–517

Keidel W D, Finkenzeller P 1984 Cochlear implants in clinical use. Advances in Audiology 2: 176

Kriewall T J Why combine multichannel processing with a single electrode? 3M internal report

Lauridsen O, Gunthersen C, Bonding P, Tos M 1983 Experiments with a thinfilm multichannel electrode for cochlear implantation. Acta Otolaryngologica 95: 219–226

MacLeod P, Chouard C-H, Weber J P 1985 French device. In: Schindler R A, Merzenich M M (eds) Cochlear implants. Raven Press, New York, p 110–120

Mecklenburg D J, Brimacombe J A 1985 An overview of the nucleus cochlear implant program. Seminars in Hearing 6 (no 1): 41–51

Merzenich M M 1985 USCF cochlear implant device. In: Schindler R A, Merzenich M M (eds) Cochlear implants. Raven Press, New York, p 121–129

Merzenich M M, Rebscher S J, Loeb G E, Byers C L, Schindler R A 1984 The USCF cochlear implant project. State of development. Advances in Audiology 2: 119–144

Michelson R P 1968 Transactions of the American Laryngology, Rhinology and Otology Society Inc. 23: 626–644

Moore B C J 1984 Electrical stimulation of the auditory nerve in man. Trends in Neurosciences 7 (no 8): 274–277

Moore B C J, Douek E, Fourcin A J et al 1984 Extracochlear electrical stimulation with speech patterns: Experiences of the EPI-group. Advances in Audiology 2: 148–165

Nadol J B 1984 Histological consideration in implant patients. Archives of Otolaryngology 110: 160–163

Patrick J F, Crosby P A, Hirshorn M S et al 1985 Australian multichannel implantable hearing prosthesis. In: Schindler R A, Merzenich M M (eds) Cochlear implants. Raven Press, New York, 93–100

Peeters S, Marquet J, Sansen W et al 1985 Status praesens: cochlear implant UIA-KULeuven-Forelec. Acta Otorhinolaryngology belgica: 39: 763–781

Rosen S, Ball V 1986 Speech perception with the Vienna extracochlear single-channel implant: A comparison of two

approaches to speech coding. British Journal of Audiology
20: 61–83

Sachs M B, Young E D, Miller M I 1983 Speech encoding in
the auditory nerve. Implications for cochlear implants.
Annals of the New York Academy of Sciences 18: 94–113

Simmons F B 1984 BIOEAR Multi-mode cochlear implant
system. Biostim leaflet

Simmons F B 1966 Electrical stimulation of the auditory
nerve in man. Archives of Otolaryngology 84: 2–54

Spillman T, Dillier N 1985 Round window cochlear implant.
In: Schindler R A, Merzenich M M (eds) Cochlear
implants. Raven Press, New York, p 157–166

Tonndorf J 1977 Cochlear prostheses. A state of the art
review. Anals, p 1–20

Van De Heyning P, Marquet J 1985 Diagnosis and prevention
of total deafness in relation to selection criteria of cochlear
implants. Acta Otorhinolaryngologica belgica
39: 678–683

Wever E G, Bray C W 1930 The nature of the acoustic
response: the relation between sound frequency and
frequency of impulses in the auditory nerve. Journal of
Experimental Psychology 13: 378–387

White R L 1985 Stanford cochlear prosthesis system: ten
years of evolution. In: Schindler R A, Merzenich M M
(eds) Cochlear implants. Raven Press, New York,
p 131–142

S D G Stephens

Abberton E, Fourcin A J, Rosen S et al 1985 Speech
perceptual and productive rehabilitation in electrocochlear
stimulation. In: Schindler R A, Merzenich M M (eds)
Cochlear implants. Raven, New York

Berliner K I, Eisenberg L S 1985 Methods and issues in the
cochlear implantation of children: an overview. Ear and
Hearing 6: 6S–13S

Ear and Hearing 1985 The cochlear implant: an auditory
prosthesis for the profoundly deaf child. Ear and Hearing
6: (3) supplement

Fourcin A J, Rosen S M, Moore B C J et al 1979
Experimental electrical stimulation of the cochlea: clinical,
psychophysical, speech-perceptual and histological findings.
British Journal of Audiology 13: 85–107

Goldstein D P, Stephens S D G 1981 Audiological
rehabilitation: Management model 1. Audiology
20: 432–452

Haggard, M P 1986 Straight thinking about cochlear
implants. British Journal of Audiology 20: 5–7.

Haggard M, Gatehouse S, Davis A 1981 The high prevalence
of hearing disorders and its implication for services in the
UK. British Journal of Audiology 15: 241–251

Hochmair E S, Hochmair-Desoyer I J 1985 Aspects of sound
signal processing using the Vienna intra- and extracochlear
implants. In Schindler R A, Merzenich M M (eds) Cochlear
implants. Raven, New York, p 101–110

Kiang N Y-S 1985 Discharge patterns of single fibers in the
cat's auditory nerve. MIT, Cambrige, Mass.

Kirk K I, Hill-Brown C 1985 Speech and language results in
children with a cochlear implant. Ear and Hearing
6: 36S–47S

Martin M C 1986 Total deafness: the need and possibility for
a working definition. British Journal of Audiology
20: 85–88

Rosen S 1984 Patient selection and counselling. Paper
presented at 3Ms symposium on cochlear implantation.
London, 19 November

Rosen S, Fourcin A J 1983 When less is more: further work.
Speech, hearing and language: Work in progress 1: 1–27

Rosen S, Ball V 1986 Speech perception with the Vienna
extracochlear single-channel implant: a comparison of two
approaches to speech coding. British Journal of Audiology
20: 61–83

Simmons F B 1985 Cochlear implants in young children:
some dilemmas. Ear and Hearing 6: 61–63

Spoendlin H 1971 Degeneration behaviour of the cochlear
nerve. Archiv für und experimentelle Ohren-Nasen
-Kehlkopfheilkunde 200: 239–254

Stephens S D G 1982 The role of the state in hearing health
care. British Journal of Audiology 16: 255–263

Thornton A R D 1986 Estimation of the number of patients
who might be suitable for cochlear implant and similar
procedures. British Journal of Audiology (in press)

Tyler R S, Gantz B J, Preece J P et al 1984 Cochlear implant
program at the University of Iowa. Proceedings of the Scott
Reger Conference (ed Glattke T J) University Park Press,
Baltimore

Waters T 1986 Speech therapy with cochlear implant wearers.
British Journal of Audiology 20: 35–43

4

Ménière's disease—an incurable condition?

J.L. Pulec

INTRODUCTION

The majority of patients suffering from Ménière's disease can be cured and almost all can be relieved of their disabling symptoms with treatment currently available. The condition is extremely complex and its successful treatment requires an otologist to have a high degree of specialization and years of experience. Proper management of the patient demands the routine use of sophisticated, high technology diagnostic tests to confirm the presence of endolymphatic hydrops, identify its aetiology and determine the exact state of inner-ear function. When the aetiology and the stage of the disease have been determined, an intelligent choice of treatment can be implemented. The physician's goal should be to cure disease in its early stages before permanent hearing loss, tinnitus or vertigo occur.

DIAGNOSTIC CRITERIA

Signs and symptoms of Ménière's disease include: episodic vertigo with sensorineural hearing loss, tinnitus and pressure in the involved ear. There are two subvarieties of the disorder: 1. cochlear Ménière's disease, 2. vestibular Ménière's disease. Both of these subvarieties will usually progress to the full symptom complex over a period of several months and the pathology is that of endolymphatic hydrops. This produces physical distortion of the structures of the inner ear which affects its function and accounts for the symptoms. Endolymphatic fluid volume changes dynamically moment to moment and can account for the fluctuation in symptoms and findings. Folds in the membranes, with selective involvement of different compartments of the

endolymphatic system, account for the variation and sequence of a patient's symptoms. In addition, actual currents of endolymphatic fluid flowing within the inner ear can abnormally stimulate different parts of the neural end-organ.

Hearing loss is sensorineural, fluctuating and progressive. Early in the course of the disease, deafness is primarily of the low tones. Tinnitus and low-tone hearing loss is produced by the disconnection of the tectorial membrane from the hair cells. Late in the disease when fluctuation decreases, the hearing loss is usually in the high tones. This is presumably caused by gross distortion of Reissner's membrane and cochlear nerve degeneration as shown in the histological examination of tissue obtained at surgery. Tinnitus, pressure and hearing loss often gradually build up before an attack of rotary vertigo, often with nausea and vomiting. Spells of vertigo, characteristically last from 30 minutes to 2–3 hours, after which the patient usually makes a prompt recovery and regains otological function. Nystagmus is common during and after an attack of vertigo. Some patients have constant instability between spells of vertigo, but this is a less common finding. Later in the course of the disease spells of vertigo may occur suddenly without warning and last for only a few minutes.

Cochlear Ménière's disease, or Ménière's disease without vertigo, is characterized solely by fluctuating and progressive sensorineural deafness with all auditory test results typical of Ménière's disease. Many patients notice a fullness in the ear, coincident with a sudden drop in hearing. Some subsequently develop the definitive dizzy spells and the qualifying 'cochlear' is discarded.

Vestibular Ménière's disease, or Ménière's disease without deafness is characterized solely by definitive spells of vertigo. This is more difficult to diagnosis as there are no objective findings between spells. The symptom of pressure in the ears is helpful to differentiate this condition from vestibular neuronitis. Some subsequently develop deafness and the qualifying 'vestibular' is dropped.

In both cochlear and vestibular Ménière's disease electrocochleography is invaluable to confirm the diagnosis. Ménière's disease may affect both ears in 24% of patients.

EXAMINATION

The diagnosis of Ménière's disease is suggested by the clinical history and audiometric findings. However, every patient must be carefully evaluated to confirm the presence of endolymphatic hydrops, establish an aetiology and then carefully be evaluated to rule out acoustic neuromas and other conditions which can mimic the symptoms and findings of Ménière's disease. When the patient is first seen, a complete diagnostic examination should be performed. Every patient should have an audiogram for pure tones and speech, Short increment sensitivity index (SISI) and Bekesy sweep frequency tests. Electronystagmography with both positional and bithermal caloric stimulation and petrous pyramid X-ray including Towne, Caldwell and Stenver Views. Early latency brainstem audiometry should be performed in every case. In most cases in which the possibility of acoustic neuroma is even suggested, good imaging should be performed to confirm the absence of tumour. Each patient should also have a 5-hour glucose tolerance test, a reactive fluorescent antibody absorption (FTA-abs) test for syphilis, and thyroid studies. A lipoprotein phenotype test should be carried out. A careful history of allergies should be taken and, should it be significant, an allergic evaluation may be indicated.

The modern management of the Ménière's patient now includes routine performance of electrocochleography to confirm the presence of endolymphatic hydrops. A characteristic summating potential (SP) is a necessary element in the diagnosis. The physician should be aware that, in early cases, hydrops may be intermittent and that electrocochleography showing positive results during times of hydrops can be normal when the patient is free of symptoms. Although not absolutely necessary to the diagnosis and treatment of Ménière's disease, the use of computerized ocular tracking and sinusoidal harmonic acceleration testing is valuable for the accurate determination of vestibular function and in the sequential follow-up of the patient's condition.

Careful evaluation of these techniques has revealed a specific aetiology in 55% of patients with Ménière's disease. Each of the several differently caused conditions requires a different specific treatment, which is usually successful (Pulec 1972, 1977, Pulec & House 1973).

AETIOLOGY

Allergy

In my experience, the most universally misunderstood and poorly handled aspect of Ménière's disease is that caused by allergy. The problem is compounded when the complex nature of the pathogenesis of Ménière's disease is involved with the complexities of food and inhalant allergy. Allergy by itself, or in combination with other aetiologies, is the cause in more than a quarter of all Ménière's cases. A thorough understanding of the characteristics of this type of Ménière's disease allows us to explain many of the inconsistencies and confusion in the literature. Ménière's disease caused by allergy is the only type which might fit the description that some authors have called 'burned-out Ménière's'. Since allergies can spontaneously cease to be a problem and, especially food allergies, can change after several years, endolymphatic hydrops produced by the allergy will be relieved. This means that, if endolymphatic hydrops and inner-ear symptoms can be controlled, the patient can be ultimately free of all signs and symptoms after several years. If hearing loss is not controlled during the allergic period, the patient will cease to have fluctuation in hearing, but will ultimately have a permanent hearing loss. I have found that intensive antiallergic therapy combined, if necessary, with an endolymphatic subarachnoid shunt operation is useful in preventing permanent sensorineural hearing loss. Endolymphatic subarachnoid shunt surgery is used only when hearing cannot be kept at a normal level with the most intensive antiallergic treatment.

A history of a craving for certain food, seasonal variation in symptoms, or a history of other allergic manifestations such as asthma, postprandial bloating or fatigue, may suggest an allergic aetiology. Investigation of allergic causes is involved, time-consuming and difficult. Cytotoxic and challenge feeding tests, provocative skin food tests, as well as more conventional tests, help identify the offending allergens. I have found scratch skin tests to be the most accurate and cost effective. Tests are made for more than 180 different foods, as well as moulds and inhalants. The physicians must understand the 'rain barrel phenomenon' of allergic response. Relief of aural symptoms can be expected by elimination of the allergens or by desensitization. In contrast to respiratory and many skin reactions, inner-ear allergic reactions show little response to antihistamine. Histamine desensitization and treatment is, however, helpful. Therapy frequently includes intravenous histamine during the acute stages, with chronic use of biweekly intramuscular and twice-daily administration of sublingual histamine.

The condition called autoimmune inner-ear disease is most likely in this category. Some authors question that it is a specific entity (Rubin 1987, personal communication). In almost all cases, a specific antigen will be identified if an adequate examination has been performed. At this time, it would seem that, if the condition of autoimmune inner-ear disease does in fact occur, it is extremely rare.

Adrenal–pituitary insufficiency

Inadequate function of the pituitary and adrenal glands is sometimes associated with allergic manifestations which can cause Méniére's disease, frequently bilaterally. A flat 5-hour glucose tolerance curve suggests this aetiology. Although, in most cases, the condition is clinically treated empirically, thorough diagnostic evaluation is desirable. The ACTH-plasma cortisol stimulation test can be used for both conditions. This test involves the removal of two blood specimens for study, the second 30 minutes after injection of the ACTH or ACTH substitute. A rise of less than 7 μg per 100 ml indicates hypofunction of these glands. The differential diagnosis can be made by a more involved insulin stimulation test to measure growth hormone and lowered adrenocortical reserve. Rarely is low blood pressure present in this group of patients. Treatment involves administration of replacement hormones.

Congenital or acquired syphilis

The pathological disorders caused by syphilis have been shown by Karmody & Schuknecht (1966), to be both endolymphatic hydrops and osteitis of the otic capsule. Collart (1964) showed that live spirochaetes, resistant to all forms of antibiotic therapy, could coexist with their host in late syphilis. The ear symptoms are typical of Ménière's disease and often begin in the fifth decade of life, first in one ear and, after a few years, involving the second ear. Typical low-tone hearing loss with fluctuation, pressure, tinnitus and progressively deteriorating speech discrimination occur. Frequently, hearing loss is sudden and, if not treated promptly, permanent. Caloric vestibular examination frequently indicates bilateral, markedly reduced vestibular responses. When hearing loss is severe and sudden, this condition represents a true medical emergency and treatment is the prompt administration of steroids.

The diagnosis is confirmed by obtaining a reactive fluorescent antibody absorption test (FTA-abs). In over 50% of patients with syphilitic Ménière's disease, their venereal disease research laboratory (VDRL) test or other non-specific test for syphilis will be negative and, for that reason, we have abandoned the use of these other tests and rely wholly upon the FTA-abs test. More than one examination should be done to confirm a positive reaction. This condition can be congenital or acquired and, if it is congenital, there is no method available to eradicate the live circulating spirochaetes. If the condition is acquired, there is a reasonable hope of elimination of the organisms with intensive antibiotic treatment. Diagnostic testing should include an ophthalmologist's examination for interstitial keratitis.

Treatment involves hospitalization and administration of penicillin, 20 million units intravenously daily for 7 days, to remove the risk of overlooking a treatable syphilitic condition. The patient is placed on prednisone, 10 mg q.i.d., with appropriate amounts of an antacid to prevent ulcer formation. The steroid is maintained at this dosage level for 1 month, after which time it is slowly reduced to the lowest level that will maintain hearing. If no improvement in hearing is noted during the month of treatment, the steroid is discontinued and the inevitable permanent loss accepted. It is important that, if the hearing level drops, the patient take more medication immediately until hearing is restored before the dosage level is again gradually reduced to the maintenance level. I have found that steroid administration gives the best results if it is given in small divided doses throughout each day. Patients whose hearing loss cannot be controlled on 20 mg prednisone per day or less should have an endolymphatic subarachnoid shunt operation performed. Following successful surgery, the steroid dosage can often be significantly lowered with satisfactory control. I have followed for as long as 22 years patients whose hearing has been maintained on continued steroid therapy. Unfortunately, a small number will eventually develop a profound hearing loss despite all forms of therapy. When that occurs, steroids are discontinued and a multichannel extracochlear implant is considered (Pulec et al 1985).

Myxoedema

Hypothyroidism is known to produce endolymphatic hydrops and accounts for 2% of cases with Ménière's Disease. The condition is often bilateral and should be detected at initial examination by the routine thyroid function blood test. Thyroid replacement therapy is effective in eliminating the symptoms of Ménière's disease in patients with hypothyroidism. Occasionally, this therapy needs to be combined with antiallergic therapy.

Vascular

In 3% of patients with Ménière's disease, the cause seems to be solely vascular. Symptoms generally occur with obvious other manifestations of vascular disease in association with congestive heart failure, hypertension, diabetes and elevated blood fat. Correction of the primary problems and the use of vasodilators often control symptoms of Ménière's disease.

It is important to differentiate Ménière's disease with endolymphatic hydrops caused by vascular insufficiency from the condition of tinnitus, vertigo or sensorineural hearing loss without endolymphatic hydrops. This subtle, but extremely important, difference is vital to the determination of proper treatment. Studies of 4000 new patients who have come to my office with these complaints have demonstrated that 5% have undiagnosed diabetes and 4.5% have hyperlipodaemia (Pulec & Mendoza 1986). Elevated blood sugar frequently causes significant otological symptoms. Adequate control of blood sugar with diet or medication will result in relief of the otological symptoms within a few days. The return of blood fats to normal will usually result in relief of otological symptoms within three months. These conditions are not Ménière's disease!

Oestrogen insufficiency

Inadequate supply of oestrogen can produce Ménière's disease. No test is currently available to detect the problem. Empirical use of oestrogen replacement prevents the signs and symptoms of Ménière's disease.

Stenosis of the internal auditory canal

Our studies into the aetiology of Ménière's disease have resulted in the identification of a condition called stenosis of the internal auditory canal. This was first noted in the literature by Pulec (1972). The abnormally small internal auditory canal produces compression of its contents with involvement of the ear or the facial nerve. The usual symptoms are progressive hearing loss, instability or tinnitus, but a small number of patients exhibit the signs and symptoms of Ménière's disease with typical fluctuations of hearing, tinnitus, pressure and episodic vertigo. The condition is suggested by the finding of an internal auditory canal measuring 3 mm or less on plain X-ray views and abnormally increased I–V latencies on early auditory evoked response audiometry. It is confirmed by the polytome Pantopaque study, which shows characteristic constriction or non-filling of the canal. Decompression of the internal auditory canal by the use of the middle cranial fossa approach, without disturbing or sectioning any of the nerves, may result in recovery of normal function (Pulec 1972).

Trauma

Physical or acoustic trauma can precede the onset of Ménière's symptoms. The trauma may be a temporal bone fracture or labyrinthine concussion. Exposure to loud noise has been clearly shown to initiate symptoms. The treatment is medical with vasodilator therapy, or surgical by means of the endolymphatic subarachnoid shunt, or a destructive procedure.

Viral

A clear-cut viral aetiology can be demonstrated in only a small number of patients, although it seems evident that the largest group of Ménière's patients classified as idiopathic are caused by a viral injury. Extensive immunological viral investigations suggest that the idiopathic variety is probably of viral aetiology. Absolute proof of this awaits further study. The hypothesis is that a normal ear will sustain a viral infection and injury to the fluid transport or absorption system. This resultant injury is permanent and stable and leads to the development of endolymphatic hydrops, which produces progressive deterioration of the ear. For this condition, no medical treatment is effective in eliminating the hydrops. Surgery is indicated early in the course of the disease to drain the endolymphatic system and eliminate progressive or permanent loss of function. For cases in which effective drainage is unsuccessful, vestibular or vestibular and cochlear nerve section may be required (Pulec 1969).

During the careful follow-up of 120 patients studied over the past 17 years, another variation has been identified. In approximately 3% of the entire group, patients initially develop typical Ménière's disease with fluctuation of hearing, episodic vertigo, tinnitus and pressure; their course, however, is clearly different from the usual situation. Despite all forms of treatment, their symptoms persist for several years with hearing ultimately at the 100 dB level and loss of speech discrimination. The condition is frequently bilateral. At the time of translabyrinthine eighth nerve section, performed for the treatment of unrelenting disabling vertigo, these cases have been found to have severe arachnoiditis involving the VIIth and VIIIth nerves within the internal auditory canal. It would appear that this type of patient sustained, during the original viral infection, not only injury to the fluid transport mechanism, but also a viral arachnoiditis within the internal auditory canal. Initially, the symptoms are primarily those of endolymphatic hydrops, but as the arachnoiditis gradually creates scarring and vascular occlusion within the internal auditory canal, the progressive and persistent symptoms become dominant. At this time, efforts to preserve hearing for such patients have been less than satisfactory. Table 4.1 summarizes the causes of Ménière's disease.

Table 4.1 Causes of Ménière's disease

Primarily medically treatable	
Allergy	14%
Adrenal–pituitary insufficiency	7%
Congenital or acquired syphilis	6%
Hypothyroidism	2%
Vascular	3%
Oestrogen insufficiency	2%
Combination of above	12%
Primarily surgically treatable	
Internal auditory canal stenosis	3%
Physical trauma	3%
Acoustic trauma	2%
Viral	1%
Idiopathic	45%

MEDICAL TREATMENT

In patients for whom a specific aetiology can be determined, such as allergy, hypometabolic state, myxoedema, syphilis, or a small internal auditory canal syndrome, specific therapy should be effective. For those patients in whom no specific aetiology can be determined, medical treatment is only symptomatic and is designed to give temporary relief of symptoms, or allow the ear to function better in a general way. The use of a vasodilator regimen is frequently successful in stopping this severe series of attacks and restoring hearing to a useful level. Unless one is dealing with an allergic or vascular condition which has not been properly diagnosed, the chronic use of vasodilator therapy will seldom be effective. In general, all sedatives will be helpful in reducing acute vertigo. From a practical standpoint, Valium is a good vestibular suppressant. Dramamine, Marezine and Bonine are the most commonly used and are frequently effective when taken 50 mg q.i.d. for the relief of vertigo. Transderm V will often reduce vestibular symptoms, although 25% will have side-effects including the development of a weeping skin lesion from the medication.

Non-specific vasodilator therapy

Patients should be instructed to avoid sodium in their diet. During the acute phases, histamine is given intravenously on 3 consecutive days. This solution contains 2.75 mg of histamine phosphate in 250 ml normal saline. The solution is administered at an initial rate of 20–30 drops per minute, and, if well-tolerated, this dosage may be increased to 50–60 drops per minute after 5 minutes. The time of administration is 90 minutes in the average case. The patient is made aware that mild flushing, headache and increased head noise may develop. Intravenous histamine is commonly given in the physician's office. Following completion of this intravenous series, 0.1 ml of a 1:100 000 dilution of histamine phosphate is administered subcutaneously twice weekly. The patient is instructed to take 2 drops of 1:10 000 histamine phosphate sublingually twice daily. Nicotinic acid tablets, 50 mg, 30–45 minutes before breakfast and before dinner are prescribed. The dose is adjusted by the patient up to 200 mg until a definite flush is obtained. Frequently a flush is obtained by a dose before breakfast greater than that given before dinner. It is important that this drug be administered before meals when the stomach is empty, to ensure rapid absorption and maximum effect. One significant action of nicotic acid may be to reduce atherosclerosis.

In addition, the patient is asked to take Probanthine, 15 mg q.i.d.; Benadryl 50 mg at bedtime and Lipoflavenoid, 2 capsules 3 times daily. There seems to be little question that this form of treatment provides relief of the symptoms of Ménière's disease, although different patients may not respond to each specific medication.

SURGICAL TREATMENT

Patients who have Ménière's disease of a type which requires surgery for treatment should be identified at the initial examination. For such patients, it seems reasonable to use non-specific medical vasodilating treatment for a minimum of 2 months before recommending surgery. Rarely will the delay of 2 months from the onset of symptoms result in a disadvantage of increased long-term hearing loss. On the other hand, by waiting at least 2 months, one has the chance deliberately to repeat specific diagnostic tests and confirm that the diagnosis is accurate. One hopes to avoid surgery for a transitory problem, or a misdiagnosis of perilymph fistula. After deliberate and thoughtful consideration and review of the situation, the physician can recommend surgery and the patient will usually appreciate his efforts at medical treatment and his caution. A possible exception to this rule might be in the patient whose Ménière's disease is in the only hearing ear. For such a patient, risk of delay of surgery might outweigh the benefit (Pulec 1981). The operation of choice is the endolymphatic subarachnoid shunt. I have preferred this procedure because it is not destructive and acts to relieve the endolymphatic hydrops and return the ear to normal hearing and vestibular functions. The risk of hearing loss as a result of the operation is less than 2%. Analysis of long-term results with the shunt operation reveals a successful outcome in 64% of the patients. In order to be considered successful, the hydrops must be relieved, which means that the patient ceases to have fluctuation of hearing, ceases to have vertigo and ceases to have fullness or pressure in the ear. In this context, descriptions of improvement or reduction in the number of attacks seem to be relatively meaningless and indicate that the therapy has not accomplished its goal. The fact that the vestibular system, with its central vestibular efferent suppression effects, can be modified by a host of physical and emotional insults to the body account for many of the inconclusive reports in the literature.

The discussion of the needs for, and merits of, effective endolymphatic drainage will help to support its use. A long-term study of Ménière's disease patients has shown that, with the exception of some whose aetiology is allergic and some whose diagnosis was incorrect, all of the remaining cases will have progressive loss of hearing and vestibular function and unrelenting recurring symptoms indefinitely without specific treatment. The ideal effective therapy results in restoration of normal function without recurrence of symptoms. This can only be accomplished if the therapy is effective. In advanced cases, a shunt operation can produce complete relief of symptoms, although hearing is frequently stabilized at a reduced level. In such cases, the patient will cease to have fullness and pressure in the ear, will have no attacks of vertigo, no instability, tinnitus will be absent, or there will only be a constant high-pitched sound with no episodes of roaring. Speech discrimination will improve and evidence of distortion will subside. Even though such a case may represent the best result obtainable, it is difficult to prove that it has been entirely successful. On the other hand, I have many patients whose symptoms were overt, disabling and present for several months with hearing fluctuating to the 50 dB level and whose vestibular function was grossly reduced, as measured by electronystagmography and sinusoidal harmonic acceleration testing. Following a successful shunt procedure, the patients developed completely normal hearing and vestibular function and have been completely free of all otological symptoms. Such cases are dramatic and support the effectiveness of an adequate shunt. Further evidence of the need for and effectiveness of a shunt is shown in the cases who have had a successful result, but subsequently developed sudden recurrence of symptoms, after being free of their symptoms for months or years. For such patients in whom hydrops is again documented to be present, I have carried out revision of a shunt procedure under local anaesthetic. During surgery, the muscle, which had been placed over the dural opening, is removed. The patient, following this procedure, notices no change in pressure within the ear or hearing function. However, within seconds after the lateral wall of the endolymphatic sac is incised with a knife and endolymph exudes from the endolymphatic sac, the patient will exclaim that the pressure is relieved, or he may hear a gurgling in his ear with relief of pressure, his hearing dramatically improves, both in pure tones and, especially, in speech discrimination. In addition, electrocochleography demonstrates prompt return to normal. In these cases, the shunt tube is generally found to be obstructed within the subarachnoid space. If a subsequent effort provides permanently effective drainage, the patient will again be free of otological symptoms. A third observation to support this view was that of a man whose only hearing ear

had Ménière's disease with a 50 dB hearing loss. A shunt operation was effective in restoring his hearing for 6 weeks followed by sudden recurrence of hearing loss. Revision of the shunt on two subsequent occasions resulted in prompt recovery of hearing for approximately 6 weeks each time, followed by tube obstruction and a drop of hearing. A third revision with a tube placed from the endolymphatic sac into the subarachnoid space of the middle cranial fossa had a similar result. In that patient, an effective shunt could not be maintained because of recurring arachnoiditis about the tube. It seems that an allergic reaction to Silastic shunt tubes occurs in 10% of patients. Use of different materials is sometimes effective in preventing this obstructing reaction. These observations would tend to support the concept that an effective physical shunt and drainage of endolymph is required for success and that simple exposure of the sac or other non-specific trauma to the ear, act only to effect the neural vestibular suppression system.

A number of other shunt-type procedures have been tried, including sacculotomy through the oval window and the otic perotic shunt (Pulec 1968), or modification of it through the round window. I find that these procedures have extremely limited value. They have a high risk of producing a hearing loss from 20% to 100% and frequently result in a slowly progressive and often incomplete deterioration of vestibular function over a period of several months, ultimately requiring VIIIth nerve section.

The use of the middle fossa selective vestibular nerve section, with preservation of the cochlear nerve, has a small but valuable role in the treatment of Ménière's disease. Since the procedure is a destructive one, with a specific result, case selection and goals of treatment must be carefully considered. The procedure is valuable for patients who have stabilized, or otherwise useful, hearing but who are disabled by vertigo. The morbidity is that of a vestibular nerve section, which involves acute vertigo with nausea and vomiting for 3 days followed by reduced instability up to a period of 6 weeks postoperatively. There is a 6% risk of hearing loss with the operation as a result of surgery and vascular involvement of the inner ear. The main reason that it is not generally used, nor desirable for patients with Ménière's disease, is that it in no way affects the cochlear symptoms and pathology. Patients with middle fossa vestibular nerve section continue to have fluctuating and progressive hearing loss with ear pressure and tinnitus (Pulec 1986).

For patients whose symptoms of disabling vertigo persist despite all conservative methods of treatment, and whose hearing is not of concern, or for those patients whose major complaint is cochlear, with pressure, tinnitus and distortion, the best treatment is a translabyrinthine VIIIth nerve section (Pulec 1974). The translabyrinthine technique is the most effective for total ablation of cochlear and vestibular function. It is required when other types of labyrinthectomy have failed and is the surgical treatment of choice in most severe cases. The procedure allows investigation of the internal auditory canal to confirm the absence of tumour and allows section of the cochlear nerve, as well as excision of the vestibular nerve including Scarpa's ganglion, so that there is degeneration to the brainstem and no chance of vestibular or cochlear function. Pressure in the ear resulting from cochlear hydrops in an otherwise destroyed ear does not occur following this procedure unless the cochlear nerve is left intact. Section of the cochlear nerve by this technique offers the best chance for relief of tinnitus. Success is in the 96% range (Pulec et al 1978, Pulec 1964).

Total VIIIth nerve section is also indicated for patients who have severe distortion in an otherwise asymptomatic ear, which makes it difficult for a patient to hear adequately with the normal side. Occasionally, cochlear suppression in the opposite uninvolved ear associated with Ménière's disease is difficult to distinguish from bilateral Ménière's disease. The apparent sensorineural hearing loss can be as great as 25 dB and the true nature of the problem can be suspected when the ear is free of pressure and there are no audiometric findings of recruitment. Translabyrinthine VIIIth nerve section on the involved side will often result in the return to normal of both hearing and vestibular function in the innocent ear. Two patients who had selective vestibular nerve section by the middle cranial fossa approach and had persisting symptoms were found to have complete regrowth of their vestibular nerves, which required excision by the translabyrinthine approach. Even though a 5 mm segment of vestibular nerve is excised, it can apparently regenerate from Scarpa's ganglion to the brainstem by using the intact cochlear nerve as a scaffold. This regrowth had not been observed after translabyrinthine VIIIth nerve section.

CONCLUSION

Is Ménière's disease an incurable condition? Emphatically it is not! The patient and physician must understand that evaluation and treatment of Ménière's disease requires the use of specialized blood tests and audiometry, including pure tones, speech, SISI, Bekesy, brainstem auditory evoked response tests and electrocochleography. Vestibular testing should include, electronystagmography with bithermal caloric tests and ideally, computerized ocular tracking and sinusoidal harmonic acceleration testing. High-quality radiography and imaging facilities are required. The neuro-otologist who undertakes treatment of the patient with Ménière's disease should have a special interest in the condition with thorough training and experience in all details of the condition. Although we cannot yet restore every patient with Ménière's disease to normal, almost all can expect effective relief from disabling symptoms.

Although the title of this chapter is somewhat provocative, a close study of the vast number of publications on the effect of medical and surgical treatment on Ménière's disease casts a legitimate doubt on the objective assessment of the therapeutic effect of management of Ménière's disease. In addition, a frank statement by Jongkees (1980) that 'the existence of a multitude of therapies, with enthusiastic defenders of their efficacy, is the best proof of lack of good therapy' seems to justify the choice of title.

Since the original description by Prosper Ménière of the disease that bears his name, there have been dozens of treatments proposed to cure, control or alleviate Ménière's disease, some in vogue for only a short time, others longer. None has withstood the test of time. Apart from the symptomatic treatment of vertigo, most medical therapies have no logical basis. All treatment is based on some notion of cause, among which are metabolic disorders, sympathetic vasomotor disturbances, endocrine disease, allergies, a-vitaminoses and psychogenic problems. In general, the explanation as to how these conditions affect inner ear physiology are hypothetical and lack supporting data.

The following reflects my experience with patients with Ménière's disease. Most therapies, apart from symptomatic medical therapy and destructive procedures, whether medical or surgical, are most likely quite non-specific in their influence upon the inner ear and the symptoms of the patients.

TERMINOLOGY, DEFINITION AND DIAGNOSIS

In my opinion, Ménière's disease is a clinical and nosological entity based on a disorder of the inner ear. One may assume that endolymphatic hydrops is one of the common histopathological features of Ménière's disease, whereas histopathological evidence of endolymphatic hydrops is not synonymous with this condition. Its characteristic symptoms are recurrent attacks of vertigo, tinnitus and fluctuating hearing loss, sometimes preceded or accompanied by a sensation of fullness in the affected ear. They are caused by a lesion of both the cochlear and vestibular parts of the inner ear and the course of the disease is characterized by periods of remission and exacerbation.

The *diagnosis* is usually based on the patient's history, and audiometric and vestibular tests in many cases only serve to verify an already well-grounded suspicion. In the event of a mono-symptomatic onset of the disease, difficulties may be encountered in establishing the diagnosis, especially if the symptoms at onset are exclusively of the vestibular type. Usually within about one year the symptom triad will be complete in most cases. A final diagnosis of Ménière's disease should not be made until the classic triad of symptoms has fully developed!

In addition, it should be stressed that the presence of a cerebellopontine angle tumour must be excluded in every case.

It has been stated in the literature that *radiographic examination* of the temporal bone is important both in diagnosis and as a prognostic indicator for the outcome of therapy, but evidence has also been presented to the contrary. The general opinion is therefore that information obtained by this examination is of little value, either diagnostically or prognostically.

Testing with *osmotic compounds*, such as administration of glycerol, urea and mannitol, is widely used as a complementary diagnostic tool for Ménière's disease. There is, as yet, no evidence contradicting the opinion that a positive glycerol-test is indicative of Ménière's disease; on the other hand a negative test does not rule out this diagnosis. However, it should be emphasized, that by using the glycerol test for selecting patients for any specific therapy one risks selecting those very patients who will benefit from any form of treatment (Thomsen & Vesterhauge 1979) and therefore significantly bias a cause and effect correlation.

Medical treatment

In a recent survey, Beck (1986) has described the most important methods of medical treatment of Ménière's disease. The multitude of medical therapeutic possibilities are almost without limits. In my opinion, most medical regimes are based on some notion of cause, e.g. metabolic disturbances, sympathetic vasomotor upsets, endocrine diseases, allergies, a-vitaminoses and pyschogenic disorders. To my knowledge, the association of any of these causes with Ménière's disease has not been substantiated. If we look at the supposed relationship between allergy and Ménière's disease, it is evident that in most reports the diagnosis of allergy is based upon case history and allergy testing by the Rinkel-technique of serial dilution titration and Lee's provocative food testing method. Satisfactory studies do not support the validity of these tests (Golbert 1975). The most conclusive report on allergy and Ménière's disease has been published by Stahle et al (1974), who concluded that, if Ménière's disease is caused by a reagin-triggered mechanism, the offending allergen is not to be found in the group of common allergens.

Recently, acupuncture and other natural remedies have been taken 'seriously' in the treatment of Ménière's disease. It is highly probable that this kind of treatment will have a non-specific effect upon symptoms, but this cannot be described as a causal therapy. Acupuncture is an attempt to intervene in autonomic vegetative nervous control of inner ear blood flow, but, as with stellate blockade, there is no experimental evidence that this has any direct influence upon the inner ear.

Results

The most frequently mentioned success rate for any treatment modality lies between 60% and 80%. This is a constant in the survey by Beck (1986), but this 'magic' figure was first mentioned by Torok (1977) in a survey of nearly 1000 papers about medical treatment of Ménière's disease. The same figure appears in each of several double-blind studies, e.g. Thomsen et al (1979), we have performed in our department, and equals the efficacy of placebo. Minor differences in the results have, of course, been reported, e.g. betahistine, but in general this is the exception rather than the rule. The major impact of any treatment modality is entirely non-specific.

Vestibular ablation with aminoglycosides was first suggested by Schuknecht (1956); this method was reactivated by Lange (1968) and by Beck (1986). The aim of local administration of genta-

mycin is the selective destruction of the secretory epithelium within the planum semilunatum of the crista ampullaris and within the stria vascularis, thus reducing the production of endolymph. It is assumed that the secretory epithelium, i.e. the dark cells, are destroyed before the sensory cells of the cochlea-vestibular end-organ. In contrast to this, however, Vosteen & Morgenstern (1986) have concluded that, from an experimental point of view, successful treatment of Ménière's disease with aminoglycosides is not caused by an inhibition of endolymph production. Whatever the mechanism is, the effect upon symptoms are undeniable and local administration of gentamycin is probably a true alternative in 'medical failures' and possibly also as an alternative to surgical intervention. A word of warning has been given by Dix (1986) concerning streptomycin treatment of Ménière's disease. In her experience, patients with Ménière's disease treated by this means have developed imbalance of such severity that they have never walked again, even after prolonged and intensive physiotherapy. However, these patients were treated with systemic aminoglycosides and not by local application.

SURGICAL TREATMENT

The ideal procedure, which had the prime objective of relieving vertigo, is simple and safe and one which could achieve consistent relief of vertigo while preserving hearing. This objective has been elusive. It is a well established clinical observation that any surgical attack on the vestibular membranous labyrinth carries a high risk of injury to the auditory system. Any ablative method that accomplishes less than complete destruction of the vestibular system carries a high risk of continuing or recurring vertigo.

The various procedures described in the literature can be divided into the following four groups: 1. shunt procedures, 2. semidestructive surgery, 3. destructive surgery and 4. vascular surgery.

1. Fistulization of the membranous labyrinth (shunts)

The more commonly used surgical operations aiming at draining the endolymphatic space fall into two groups: a) procedures draining the endo-

Table 4.2 AAOO classification 12 months, 36 months and 84 months after treatment with active surgery or placebo surgery

| | 12 months | | 36 months | | 84 months | |
	Active	Placebo	Active	Placebo	Active	Placebo
Class A	1 (7%)	1 (7%)	3 (23%)	2 (15%)	2 (17%)	5 (39%)
Class B	12 (80%)	6 (40%)	6 (46%)	8 (62%)	3 (25%)	6 (46%)
Class C	0	3 (20%)	0	2 (15%)	4 (33%)	2 (15%)
Class D	2 (13%)	5 (33%)	4 (31%)	1 (8%)	3 (25%)	0
Total	15	15	13	13	12	13

lymphatic sac, and b) endolymph perilymph shunt procedures.

Portmann first described the endolymphatic sac draining procedure in 1927, which was more than 10 years before endolymphatic hydrops was known to occur in Ménière's disease, and nearly 40 years before it was discovered that experimental ablation of the endolymphatic sac causes endolymphatic hydrops (Naito 1959, Kimura & Schuknecht 1965). The concept of draining the sac has some logical basis, but whether it can really be achieved seems doubtful. A number of procedures have been described since Portmann's report and the introduction of the endolymphatic sac–subarachnoid shunt by House (1962) was received with great enthusiasm. The idea of draining the sac into the subarachnoid space, against the pressure of cerebrospinal fluid is incredible, and several surgeons have therefore decided to decompress or drain the endolymphatic sac into the mastoid cavity. Again, there is a lack of solid pathophysiological basis for this modality, because there is no histological evidence that the sac is ever distended in Ménière's disease, and an incision in the sac, including insertion of a drain, would most likely be followed by rapid fibrous healing, rather than a permanent shunt.

Despite the apparent conceptual weaknesses of all the endolymphatic sac drainage procedures, therapeutic success is claimed for 60–80% of patients. However, his reports have not been reproduced by others using the same valve. These rather uniform results make it likely that the effect of sac surgery is not specifically related to the shunt procedure per se, but rather to the non-specific effect of surgery. This opinion is furthermore substantiated by the only existing double-blind study, where the effect of a simple mastoidectomy was compared with the effect of an actual silastic sheet endolymphatic sac-mastoid shunt (Thomsen et al 1981). No significant differences between the groups could be established, and 70% of the patients in both groups could be classified as successes, even after seven years of observation (Table 4.2).

The above study is the only comparison of the efficacy of surgery in Ménière's disease. All other reports on the control of vertigo rest principally on patient testimonials and clinical anecdotes! However, despite these intrinsic weaknesses, the efficacy of the procedures is indisputable. We do not know the actual mechanisms behind the success of the various shunt procedures, and a placebo effect cannot be excluded. It is likely that there is one common denominator, unrelated to the shunt procedure itself, which is effective.

Endolymph-perilymph shunt procedures.

The aim of the endoperilymph shunt is draining of excess endolymph into the perilymphatic space through a surgically created permanent fistula in the membranous labyrinth. This type of operation was introduced by Plester (1967), who approached the saccule through the footplate. Cody (1969) modified the sacculotomy by introducing a fine indwelling 'tack' into the footplate, assuming that the saccule would collapse after puncture. The simplicity of the surgical intervention and the negligible morbidity associated with Cody's tack operation briefly attracted some supporters, but the uncertainty of the results and the high percentage of dead ears forced most surgeons to abandon the technique. In the hands of Cody & McDonald (1983), this operation, however, seems to equal or even surpass most long-term results of endolymphatic sac procedure. Even if the 'tack' operation, from a theoretical point of view, might work there are, however, several problems with this theory: 1. in severe hydrops the dilated saccule appears to be plastered to the walls of the vestibule and probably could not be fistulized into the perilymphatic space, 2. experimental studies have shown that sharp objects implanted through the footplate into the vestibule become ensheathed in a membrane and therefore probably could not function effectively as a puncturing device.

Based on animal experiments, in which a surgical fistulization with fracture disruption of the cochlear duct frequently resulted in permanent fistulas through which endolymph could continuously escape into the perilymphatic space, Schuknecht (1982) introduced the *cochleosacculotomy*.

This surgical modality is intriguing and has some logical basis. However, it is now evident that this operation carries a very high risk of injury to the auditory system. Several authors (Dimitrov & Duckert 1985, Dionne 1985, Montandon et al 1985) have pointed this out, and recently Schuknecht himself (1986) has abandoned the technique in patients with serviceable hearing. It should be mentioned that, during the first 12 months after Schuknecht published his method, 200 3-mm right-angled picks were sold in the United States alone with the purpose of being used for this operation. One can imagine the number of patients now having an unnecessary surgical insult to the auditory system, because the operation is easily performed under local anaesthesia and requires no specific surgical expertise.

2. Semidestructive procedures

Ablation of the vestibular labyrinth

The application of *focused ultrasound* to attenuate the sensitivity of the vestibular function for the relief of vertigo has been in use for several decades. The partial or total ablation of vestibular function, with preservation of hearing by the use of a simple and safe procedure, is an obvious goal for the management of intractable vertigo. Some authors consider the method to be therapeutically useful (Basek 1973, Stahle 1976), resulting in relief of vertigo in about 70% of patients. However, in a recent survey of the literature, together with animal experiments; Peron et al (1983) have concluded

that, in general, the reported pathological changes appear to be nothing more than artifacts of preparations. In animal experiments the temporal bones show no morphological changes which can be attributed to the ultrasound irradiation. It seems doubtful, therefore, if the effects of ultrasound are due to ablation of the vestibular sense organ; it is more likely a non-specific effect of the intervention.

With the intention of locally destroying Reissner's and the basilar membrane, thereby creating a permanent fistula and consequently an endoperilymph shunt, *cryosurgery* has been applied in the treatment of vertigo. However, animal experiments have demonstrated extensive debris within the endolymphatic space around the ampulla in animals killed 2 days after cryosurgical 'destruction' of the lateral ampulla, but in animals allowed to survive for 4 days, the endolymph was clear and the surface of the crista had healed. The fast healing properties of the labyrinthine structures after cryosurgery makes this a fleeting moment in the history of the treatment of vertigo, in spite of the fact that about 70% of the patients were relieved of their symptoms.

Vestibular neurectomy

Selective section of the vestibular nerves in the internal auditory canal, or in the cerebrellopontine angle via the middle or posterior fossa approach, seems to be the method of choice for suppression of vertiginous attacks and preservation of hearing. In the hands of skilled surgeons, vertigo can be relieved in more than 90% of the patients, with little risk (10%) of further hearing loss.

Vertigo induced by unilateral transection of the vestibular portion of the eighth cranial nerve subsides over a 2–3 month period. In elderly patients some unsteadiness, particularly on head movements, may persist over a longer period of time, or even be permanent.

This intervention is correctly considered 'semidestructive', since the sole aim of the operation is destruction of the vestibular afferences. The patient exchanges severe attacks of incapacitating vertigo for complete destruction of a sense organ on the affected side.

The middle fossa vestibular nerve section has been popularized by Fisch (1973) and also recommended by Palva et al (1979) and Glasscock et al (1984).

Other authors (Brackmann 1983, House et al 1984, Silverstein 1981) recommended the retrolabyrinthine approach for vestibular nerve section. This approach offers several advantages over the middle fossa approach; the major advantage is that it offers a wider and easier exposure which does not require temporal lobe retraction. It is applicable to all age groups, in contrast to the middle fossa vestibular nerve section which is limited to patients less than 60 years of age, since increased adherence and friability of the dura increases the morbidity of this procedure in older patients (Plester 1986). The mandatory retraction of the temporal lobe for exposure of the internal auditory meatus can cause injury to the underlying brain.

The change from the middle fossa to the retro-labyrinthine approach is a recent occurrence and a long-term follow-up of the patients operated through this approach will be required to know if the shift is justified.

3. Destructive surgery

Labyrinthectomy is a simple and relatively safe procedure for relieving vertigo in patients with non-aidable hearing, disabling attacks of vertigo and no evidence of disease in the contralateral ear. It is especially indicated for patients who are in poor health carrying an increased surgical risk.

The transcanal labyrinthectomy is a postganglionic section of the vestibular nerve. The distal segment of the nerve does not degenerate and these patients are predisposed to continuing vestibular symptoms even though their definitive attacks are relieved. For this reason most authors prefer a total trans-labyrinthine vestibular neurectomy as being the most certain way of achieving complete ablation of labyrinthine function.

4. Vascular decompression of the vestibular nerve

The question as to whether a vascular loop represents a diagnostic entity causing vestibular and auditory symptoms and thus mimicking Ménière's disease, is still open for debate. Janetta (1975) reports that microvascular decompression of the eighth nerve alleviates symptoms successfully. He states that 'it has been obvious that the nerves of the cerebello-pontine angle are subject to mechanical stresses, especially vascular compression due to arterial elongation'. A statement like this is extremely speculative, and by no means has it been proven to be correct. McCabe & Harker (1983) have demonstrated that in seven patients who underwent vestibular nerve section for intractable vertigo, a vascular loop was found extending far into the internal auditory meatus, pressing upon the superior vestibular nerve. The vestibular nerves were sectioned during surgery and the patients were free of symptoms hereafter; but this does not prove that the arterial loop was the offending factor. When operating on the internal acoustic meatus regularly, I have often found similar conditions, and I consider the presence of an arterial loop inside the internal acoustic meatus as a normal variant.

The existing evidence that vascular abnormalities in the cerebellopontine angle and internal acoustic meatus are causing eighth nerve symptoms are unproven and the basis for vascular decompression is therefore purely speculative.

CONCLUSION

The evaluation of any treatment modality in its ability to alleviate vertigo, or improve hearing, is hampered by the erratic course of the underlying disease process. Discussion of the efficacy of treatments has for many years mainly focused on the control of the vertiginous attack. However, since Torok (1977) demonstrated, from 834 articles, a 60–68% success in controlling vertigo independent of which treatment had been employed, a remarkable change of focus has taken place. It is now more usual to emphasize the ability of a given treatment, be it medical or surgical, to preserve hearing, to stabilize hearing, or even improve hearing.

Up until now there has *not* been published one single report which convincingly proves that a given hearing improvement is the direct result of the intervention, and not merely the result of time and the natural course of the disease. In my opinion, the main issue therefore is still to alleviate the troublesome vertigo and to choose a treatment modality which does not make the hearing worse. In this context, it is interesting to note from the majority of papers presenting results of treatment, that the subjective parameters within the Ménière's symptoms (vertigo, tinnitus and fullness) are improved in the vast majority of cases, while the objective parameter (hearing) is unchanged in the majority of cases. Those cases with deterioration of hearing after treatment occur mainly after surgery.

The number of patients eligible for surgery varies from series to series, probably dependent upon the referral system and the 'aggressivity' of the surgeon. The only indication for surgery in which there is complete agreement is found in a patient whose vertiginous episodes are completely disabling and whose hearing level, by discrimination as well as threshold tests, has dropped almost to the useless level in the affected ear, translabyrinthine labyrinthectomy or translabyrinthine cochleovestibular neurectomy is advisable.

In patients with incapacitating vertigo and serviceable hearing in the diseased ear, and a normal contralateral ear, a selective transection of the vestibular nerve is a rational approach, either via the middle fossa or the retrolabyrinthine route depending upon the individual preference and training of the surgeon. It should, however, be emphasized that this kind of surgery is a major intervention, which should be reserved for the experienced surgeon.

My personal preference is to perform the retrolabyrinthine vestibular nerve section because of a higher morbidity after middle fossa approach.

Most of the surgical treatment modalities contain an inborn risk to hearing in the operated ear. In patients with bilateral disease, and over a period of time this figure will go as high as 40–50%, I would not recommend any form of surgery. This will limit the number of patients eligible for surgery to a few per cent.

Whether to perform surgery on the endolymphatic sac at all, or to use it as a primary procedure before sectioning the vestibular nerve, is a matter of personal philosophy. Many authors continue to perform sac surgery, despite the non-specific nature of the procedure. The argument is that the efficacy is indisputable and no experienced surgeon will reject a low-risk operation that is beneficial to a relatively large number of patients. These remarks may be valid if one always dealt with 'experienced surgeons'. However, not all shunt surgery is performed by such individuals and I tend to agree with Jongkees (1980) that surgery should be avoided for as long as possible while there are safer placebo therapies.

Other otologists have abandoned the sac operation as a primary procedure and go directly to retrolabyrinthine vestibular nerve section. This will cure the vertigo. However, on the way out they put a shunt into the endolymphatic sac, in the pious hope that this will arrest the natural deterioration of the hearing.

In my institution, I believe we can handle the vast majority of patients with Ménière's disease by a combination of symptomatic medical therapy, physical therapy, vestibular rehabilitation, 'psychotherapy', patience in listening to the complaints of the patients and by convincing the patient that he is not suffering from a serious, life-threatening disease.

EPILOGUE

The provocative title of this chapter requires an answer. If 'cure' means removal of some aetiological factor, the answer is: Yes, Ménière's disease is an incurable condition. We do not know the aetiology of Ménière's disease and it is a mistake to interpret the success of therapy in terms of an effect on aetiology. Many otologists have been deluded in their assessment of therapies by the variable nature of the symptomatology (Schuknecht 1981). In terms of symptomatic treatment of the cochlear deficit in Ménière's disease the answer is also: Yes, the hearing problem is an incurable condition. In terms of symptomatic treatment of the vertigo in Ménière's disease the answer is: No, the vertigo can be controlled, either symptomatically by vestibular depressant drugs, or by application of non-specific, possibly placebo, treatment modalities, medical or surgical, or by specific, vestibular ablative procedures, medical or surgical.

A careful reading of the papers by Dr Pulec and Dr Thomsen leaves one with the impression that Ménière's disease is probably 'incurable' by criteria that define *cure* as complete, permanent return to total normality with no recurrences.

The 'dilemma' is introduced by Jack Pulec with the statement: 'The majority of patients suffering from Ménière's disease can be cured'. He then goes on to state that, 'Almost all patients can be relieved of their symptoms by treatments available today'.

Dr Thomsen confronts the dilemma with the statement, 'A close study of the vast number of publications on the effect of medical and surgical treatment . . . casts a legitimate doubt on the objective assessment of the therapeutic effect of management of Ménière's disease.' He quotes the 1980 opinion of Jongkees to the effect that, 'The existence of a multitude of therapies with enthusiastic defenders of their efficacy is the best proof of lack of good therapy', which reminds us that since Prosper Ménière described the disease, dozens of treatments have been proposed to cure, control or alleviate symptoms. 'Apart from the symptomatic treatment of vertigo, most medical definitive therapies have no logical scientific basis.'

Therefore, while both authors are intimately familiar with the problem, they nevertheless present entirely different conclusions to the reader.

Both ably discuss differential diagnosis and do not disagree that the problem is complex. Pulec points out that there are problems in management regardless of aetiology, but, despite this, he is optimistic that in patients 'for whom a specific aetiology can be determined, specific therapy should be effective'. He describes the role of surgery when there is inadequate response to medical therapy and discusses surgical management with reference to endolymphatic drainage, describing shunt techniques, sacculotomy surgery, and otic-periotic procedures, but concludes that these surgical procedures have 'extremely limited value in the occasional patient'. He continues to state that such procedures present a high risk of further hearing loss and discusses the place of middle fossa selective vestibular nerve section with preservation of the cochlear nerve as having a small, but valuable, role in the treatment of Ménière's disease.

Finally, for patients resistant to conservative therapy, he recommends a translabyrinthine eighth nerve section as the most effective approach for total ablation of cochlear and vestibular function. In conclusion, his answer to the theoretical question, 'Is Ménière's disease an incurable condition' is 'emphatically it is not'.

Jens Thomsen seems to approve of the title, particularly the words 'incurable condition'. He concurs with most of the diagnostic recommendations mentioned by Pulec, but mentions the fact that the most frequently mentioned success rate of any medical treatment lies between 60% and 80%, a constant mention by Beck in 1986, which also appeared as a 'magic' figure in Torok's classic 1977 study of almost 100 papers of medical treatment of Ménière's disease. The same figure appeared in the various double-blind studies reported by Thomsen et al in 1979. These approaches, in Thomsen's words, 'equal the efficacy of placebo' and he concludes that the 'impact of any treatment modality is entirely non-specific'.

With reference to surgical treatment, his opinion is that the prime objective of surgery is relief of vertigo with preservation of hearing and the success of this objective has been elusive. He points out that 'any surgical attack on the vestibular membranous labyrinth carries a high risk of injury to the auditory system' and 'any ablative method that accomplished this with less than complete destruction of the vestibular system carries a high risk of continuing or recurring vertigo'.

The four major surgical approaches are: 1. shunt procedures, 2. semidestructive surgery, 3. destructive surgery and 4. vascular surgery.

Regarding shunt procedures, the idea of *draining the sac into the subarachnoid space against the pressure of cerebrospinal fluid is incredible!* He feels that there is a lack of solid pathophysiological evidence for this modality because there is no evidence, as far as he is concerned, that the sac is ever distended in Ménière's disease and that an incision in the sac, including the insertion of a drain, would most likely be followed by rapid fibrous healing, rather than maintenance of a permanent shunt. He states that we do not know the actual mechanisms behind the 'successes' of the various shunt procedures and therefore considers it is unlikely that there is one common denominator, *unrelated to the shunt procedure itself*, which is effective. He discusses the 'tack' operation, ultrasound and cryosurgery with varying results.

Vestibular neurectomy by selection section of the vestibular nerve 'seems to be the method of choice for suppression of vertiginous attacks and preservation of hearing'. It appears that, in the hands of skilled surgeons, vertigo can be relieved in more than 90% of patients, with little risk (10%) of further hearing loss. It is correctly considered to be 'semidestructive', since the sole aim of the operation is destruction of the vestibular afferent nerve. The patient exchanges severe attacks of incapacitating vertigo for complete destruction of a sense organ on the affected side.

Fisch, in 1973, popularized the middle fossa vestibular nerve section and other authors (Brackmann 1983, House et al 1984, Silverstein 1981) recommended the retrolabyrinthine approach for vestibular nerve section, an approach which offers several advantages over the middle fossa approach, the major one being that it offers a wider and easier exposure which does not require temporal lobe retraction, and it is applicable to all age groups.

The change from the middle fossa to the retrolabyrinthine approach is recent and a long-term follow-up of the patient operated through this approach will be required to evaluate the procedure.

Destructive surgery through labyrinthectomy is a relatively simple and safe procedure for relieving vertigo in patients with non-aidable hearing and for patients with disabling attacks of vertigo, where there is absolutely no evidence of disease in the contralateral ear. It is especially indicated for patients who are in poor general health.

The issue of vascular decompression of the vestibular nerve has been discussed with reference to the question as to whether a vascular loop can cause vestibular and auditory symptoms mimicking Ménière's disease.

In the conclusion to his paper, Thomsen starts with this statement, 'The evaluation of any treatment modality in its ability to alleviate vertigo, or improve hearing is hampered by the erratic course of the underlying disease process', while 'Discussions of the efficacy of treatments has for many years been mainly focused on the control of the vertiginous

attack . . . a remarkable change of focus has taken place. It is now more usual to emphasize the ability of a given treatment, be it medical or surgical, to preserve hearing, to stabilize hearing, or even improve hearing'.

Thomsen states that, 'up until now there has not been published one single report which convincingly proves that a given hearing improvement is the direct result of the intervention, and not merely the result of time and the natural course of the disease'. In his opinion, therefore, the main issue is alleviation of troublesome vertigo and the choice of treatment modality is one which does not make the hearing worse. He points out, in this context that in the majority of papers presenting results of treatment the subjective parameters of Ménière's symptoms, namely vertigo, tinnitus and fullness, are improved in the vast majority, while the objective parameter, hearing, is unchanged in the majority of cases.

The author states that, in his institution, the vast majority of patients with Ménière's disease can be managed effectively by a combination of systematic medical therapy, physical therapy, vestibular rehabilitation, psychotherapy, listening to complaints and convincing the patient that they are not suffering from a serious life-threatening disease.

He concludes that the provocative title of this chapter requires an answer. His position is that 'cure' means removal of some aetiological factor. Ménière's disease is an incurable condition since we do not know the precise aetiology.

Since the two major symptomatic problems are 1. *dizziness* and 2. *hearing loss* (with or without 3. tinnitus), results of treatment modalities must deal with all three presenting symptoms.

Both authors present differing yet valuable points of view. Obviously, there is a wide range of patient responses to symptoms, depending on many factors relating to general health, age and personality differences.

My experience, and that of my colleagues, has been that conservative measures, including careful study of previously undetected otological disease, attention to general health and allergy and the use of various antivertigo drugs can relieve or 'cure' vertigo in many patients. However, in spite of such management, a very small number of patients continue to have significant unpleasant and even disabling attacks. For such patients surgery should probably be considered.

In terms of systematic treatment of the cochlear defects in Ménière's disease, the hearing problem is an incurable condition. In terms of symptomatic treatment of vertigo, symptoms can be controlled.

'Is Ménière's disease an incurable disease?.' Today it is still 'incurable', if defined as complete and permanent, but it *is* 'relievable' in a majority of patients.

REFERENCES

J L Pulec

Collart P 1964 Persistence of treponema pallidum in late syphilis in rabbits and human, nothwithstanding treatment. Proceedings of the forum on syphilis and other treponematosis. Public Health Service Publication no. 997 United States Government Printing Office, Washington, DC, p 285–294

Karmody C S, Schuknecht J F 1966 Deafness is congenital syphilis. Archives of Otolaryngology 83: 18

Pulec J L 1968 The otic-perotic shunt. Symposium on Ménière's disease. Otolaryngology Clinics of North America October 643–648

Pulec J L 1969 The surgical treatment of vertigo. Laryngoscope 79: 1783–1822

Pulec J L 1972 Ménière's disease: results of 2½ year study of etiology, natural history and results of treatment. Laryngoscope 82: 1703–1715

Pulec J L 1972 Idiopathic hemifacial spasm: pathogenesis and surgical treatment. Annals of Otology, Rhinology and Laryngology 81: 664–676

Pulec J L 1973 Ménière's disease: etiology, natural history and results of treatment. Otolaryngology Clinics of North America 6, no 1: 25–39

Pulec J L 1981 Endolymphatic subarachnoid shunt for Ménière's disease in the only hearing ear. Laryngoscope 91, no 5: 771–783

Pulec J L 1984 Tinnitus: surgical therapy. American Journal of Otology 5, no 6: 27–38

Pulec J L 1974 Labyrinthectomy: indications, technique and results. Laryngoscope 84, 9: 1552–2573

Pulec J L, Hodell S F, Anthony P F 1980 Tinnitus: diagnosis and treatment. Annals of Oto-Rhino-Laryngology 87, no 6: 821–833

Pulec J L, House W F 1973 Ménière's disease study: three-year progress report. Equilibrium Research 3: 1

J Thomsen

Arenberg I K 1982 The fine point of valve implant surgery for hydrops: an update. American Journal of Otology 3: 359

Basek M 1973 Ultrasound for Ménière's disease. Archives of Otolaryngology 97: 133

Beck C 1986 Medical treatment. In: Pfaltz C R (ed) Controversial aspects of Ménière's disease. Georg Thieme Verlag, Stuttgart, p 88

Brackmann D E 1983 Ménière's disease: surgical treatment. In: W J Oosterveld (ed) Ménière's disease: a comprehensive appraisal. John Wiley & Sons Ltd, New York, p 91

Cody D T R 1969 The tack operation for endolymphatic hydrops. Laryngoscope 79: 1737

Cody D T R, McDonald T J 1983 Tack operation for idiopathic endolymphatic hydrops: an update. Laryngoscope 93: 1416

Dimitrov E A, Duckert L G 1985 Morphologic changes in the guinea pig cochlea following cochleostomy—a preliminary scanning electron microscopic study. Otolaryngology and Head and Neck Surgery 93: 408

Dionne J 1985 Cochleosacculotomy. The Journal of Otolaryngology 14: 1

Dix M R 1986 Physical therapy and rehabilitation. Biochemical aspects of inner ear pathophysiology. In: C R Pfaltz (ed) Controversial aspects of Ménière's disease. Georg Thieme Verlag, Stuttgart, p 113

Fisch U 1973 Excision of Scarpas ganglion. Archives of Otolaryngology 97: 147

Glasscock M E et al 1984 Current status of surgery for Ménière's disease. Otolaryngology and Head and Neck Surgery 92: 67

Golbert T M 1975 A review of controversial diagnostic and therapeutic techniques employed in allergy. Journal of Allergy and Clinical Immunology 56: 170

House W F 1962 Subarachnoid shunt for drainage of endolymphatic hydrops. Laryngoscope 72: 713

House J W, Hitselberger W E, McElveen J et al 1984 Retrolabyrinthine section of the verstibular nerve. Otolaryngology and Head and Neck Surgery 92: 212

Janetta P J 1975 Neurovascular cross-compression in patients with hyperactive dysfunction symptoms of the eighth cranial nerve. Surgical Forum: 26: 467

Jongkees L B W 1980 Some remarks on Ménière's disease. ORL Journal for Oto-Rhino-Laryngology and Its Related Specialities 42: 1

Kimura R, Schuknecht H F 1965 Membranous hydrops in the inner ear of guinea pig after obliteration of the endolymphatic sac. Practica-Oto-Rhino-Laryngologica 27: 343

Lange G 1968 Isolierte Medicamentöse Ausschaltung eines Gleichwichtorganes beim Morbus Ménière mit Streptomycin-Ozothin. Archiv für klinische und experimentelle Ohren-Nasen-Kehlkopfheilkunde 191: 545

McCabe B F, Harker L A 1983 Vascular loop as a cause of vertigo. Annals of Otology, Rhinology and Laryngology 92: 542

Montandon P B, Hausler R J, Kimura R S 1985 Treatment of endolymphatic hydrops with cochleosacculotomy. Clinical results and experimental findings. Otolaryngology and Head and Neck Surgery 93: 615

Naito T 1959 Clinical and pathological studies on Ménière's disease. 60th Annual Meeting 22 Oto-Rhino Laryngological Societies of Japan

Palva T, Ylikoski J, Paavolainen M et al 1979 Vestibular neurectomy and saccus decompression surgery in Ménière's disease. Act Oto-Laryngologica 88: 74

Peron D L, Kitamura K, Carniol P J et al 1983 Clinical and experimental results with focused ultrasound. Laryngoscope 93: 1217

Plester D 1967 Surgical treatment of Ménière's disease. Proceedings of the Royal Society of Medicine 60: 4

Plester D 1986 Surgery of Ménière's disease. In: C R Pfaltz

(ed) Controversial aspects of Ménière's disease. Georg Thieme Verlag, Stuttgart, p 104

Portmann G 1927 Saccus endolymphaticus and operation for draining same for relief of vertigo. Journal of Laryngology and Otology 42: 809

Schuknecht H F 1956 Ablation therapy for relief of Ménière's disease. Laryngoscope 66: 859

Schuknecht H F 1981 Rationale of surgical procedures for Ménière's disease. In: Vosteen K H, Schuknecht H F, Pfaltz C R et al (eds) Ménière's disease. Georg Thieme Verlag, Stuttgart, p 236

Schuknecht H F 1982 Cochleosacculotomy for Ménière's disease: theory, technique and results. Laryngoscope 92: 853

Silverstein H 1981 Surgery for vertigo (you don't have to live with it). Journal of Otolaryngology 10: 343

Stahle J 1976 Ultrasound treatment of Ménière's disease. Long-term follow-up of 356 advanced cases. Acto Otolaryngologica 81: 120

Stahle J, Deuschl H, Johansson S G O 1974 Ménière's disease and allergy. Equilibrium Research 4: 22

Thomsen J, Bech P, Prytz S et al 1979 Ménière's disease: Lithium threatment. Demonstration of placebo effect in a double blind, cross-over trial. Clinical Otolaryngology 4: 119

Thomsen J, Bretlau P, Tos M et al 1981 Placebo effect in surgery for Ménière's disease. Archives of Otolaryngology 107: 271

Torok N 1977 Old and new in Ménière's disease. Laryngoscope 87: 1870

Vosteen K H, Morgenstern C 1986 Biochemical aspects of inner ear pathophysiology. In: C R Pfaltz (ed) Controversial aspects of Ménière's disease. Georg Thieme Verlag, Stuttgart, p 16.

5

The need for skull-base surgery in glomus tumours

D.E. Brackmann

Since first described in 1945 by Rosenwasser, therapy of glomus tumours of the temporal bone has been controversial. Some have advocated no treatment because these tumours may be very slow growing and produce minimal symptoms, others have advocated surgical removal, while others have recommended X-ray therapy as the primary treatment modality. It is difficult to evaluate the efficacy of the various forms of therapy since the clinical course and growth rate of these tumours is variable. Patients who have survived over 40 years without treatment have been reported (Bickerstaff & Howe 1953, Steinberg & Holz 1965). That all tumours are not clinically benign is shown by the studies of Brown (1985), Spector et al (1976) and Rosenwasser (1973), who found mortality rates ranging from 5% to 13% with glomus jugulare tumours.

In general, I favour surgical treatment of glomus tumours of the temporal bone. In this chapter I will outline the surgical therapy which I employ and then discuss this treatment in comparison to radiotherapy.

EVALUATION OF GLOMUS TUMOUR PATIENTS

Great strides have been made in recent years in the evaluation of patients with glomus tumours. New techniques have allowed accurate assessment of size and involvement of temporal bone and skull base with glomus tumours. These new techniques allow preoperative planning and assessment of the risk of surgery. Following are the tests routinely used in the evaluation of patients with glomus tumours of the temporal bone.

Routine hearing test. Routine air, bone, and speech hearing tests are performed to assess the degree of both conductive and sensorineural hearing impairments.

Polytomography. This technique was once our mainstay for the assessment of the degree of involvement of the temporal bone by glomus tumours. It has now been replaced by computerized cranial tomography and is no longer used routinely in assessment.

Computerized cranial tomography. Thin section (1.5 mm thickness) computerized cranial tomography using the bone algorithm has become the standard method of assessment of glomus tumours of the temporal bone. Tumours confined to the middle ear and mastoid are delineated from those tumours which involve the jugular bulb. Extensive lesions, which extend onto or medial to the internal carotid artery and those which extend transdurally, are also defined by this technique. In many cases CCT is the only examination that is necessary for planning of treatment. As will be described shortly, involvement of the jugular bulb is the major consideration in preoperative planning. Rarely is it necessary to perform retrograde jugular venography.

Arteriography. Four-vessel angiography is used when computerized cranial tomography has demonstrated a large glomus tumour. There are several justifications for this examination, the first being to assess the involvement of the internal carotid artery. This is necessary to assess the advisability of surgery and, if surgery is undertaken, planning for management of involvement of the carotid artery.

With four-vessel angiography one can also assess the blood supply to the tumour, particularly studying the vessels arising from the internal carotid artery or from the vertebral artery in tumours that extend intracranially. Finally, at the time of angiography, embolization is frequently employed. Embolization may be used as preoperative adjunctive therapy, as the primary treatment modality, or as a combination.

CLASSIFICATION OF GLOMUS TUMOURS

Several schemes for classification of glomus tumours of the temporal bone have been proposed. At the Otologic Medical Group we use a classification developed by Antonio De la Cruz. This is a clinical surgical classification, the extent of the tumour being described by the involvement of structures of the temporal bone and skull base. A series of operations is used which correspond with the extent of the tumour.

Tympanic tumour

This is a tumour which has arisen from the glomus tympanicum body of the promontory alongside Jacobsen's nerve, being confined entirely to the mesotympanum. All of its borders can be seen with routine otoscopy. In tumours of this type no other studies are necessary for one knows that this small tumour could not arise from the jugular bulb or it would extend beyond the inferior margins of the tympanic annulus. One consideration in this, or any other vascular tumour of the middle ear, is to rule out an aberrant carotid artery or a dehiscent jugular bulb. The aberrant internal carotid artery lies anteriorly and is paler in colour than the glomus tumour. The jugular bulb lies posteriorly and is dark blue in colour. If there is any question about the existence of either of these lesions, computerized cranial tomography must be carried out.

Tympanomastoid tumour

This tumour arises from the glomus body on the promontory, but has enlarged so that it extends beyond the tympanic annulus either inferiorly or posteriorly. Once a tumour has reached this size, there is no way clinically to delineate its true extent. Any patient with a tumour that extends beyond the tympanic annulus must have thorough radiographic evaluation. Studies will show this tumour not to involve the jugular bulb. It may extend into the mastoid and retrofacial air cells, but the jugular bulb itself is not involved.

Jugular bulb tumour

This tumour arises from the glomus body on the dome of the jugular bulb. It then extends into the middle ear to a variable degree and also into the jugular bulb. By definition, it is limited to involvement of the middle ear, mastoid and the jugular bulb. It does not extend onto the carotid artery nor medially into the skull base, or intracranially.

Carotid artery involvement

This tumour has arisen from the jugular bulb, but has extended beyond its confines and is contacting the carotid artery. Smaller tumours of this type may only contact the internal carotid artery at the skull base. Larger tumours may extend far medially and involve not only the ascending, but also the horizontal portion of the internal carotid artery and petrous apex.

Transdural tumours

Transdural tumours arise from the jugular bulb and extend not only onto the internal carotid artery, but also through the jugular foramen intracranially.

SURGICAL APPROACHES TO GLOMUS TUMOURS OF THE TEMPORAL BONE

A series of operations are used for removal of glomus tumours of the temporal bone (Sheehy & Brackmann 1984). The extent of the surgery is determined by the preoperative evaluation and classification of the tumour.

Transcanal approach

The transcanal approach is used for small glomus tympanicum tumours limited to the mesotympanum. Surgery is performed under local anaesthesia with preparation as for a stapes operation. The tympanomeatal flap is elevated, the inferior incision extending so that the inferior aspect of the tympanic membrane can be elevated. The tumour is identified on the promontory, but one must always consider the possibility of an aberrant internal carotid artery in these cases.

The blood supply to the glomus tympanicum tumour is the inferior tympanic branch of the ascending pharyngeal artery. This vessel may either be coagulated bipolarly, or a small piece of Surgicel may be used to occlude the bony canaliculus from which it arises. The tumour is then removed with a cup forceps. There is often brisk bleeding from the distal end of the artery anterior to the stapes near the cochleariform process. It is difficult to control this artery directly, but if left alone it will usually clot readily. It is important not to use monopolar cautery on the promontory as this may produce damage to the inner ear. Additional small pledgets of Surgicel may be placed over the promontory and, when haemostasis is secure, the tempanomeatal flap is replaced and the ear canal packed.

Mastoid approach

This approach is used for glomus tumours of the tympanomastoid variety. The tumour may extensively involve the middle ear and mastoid, but it has arisen from the glomus tympanicum body and does not involve the jugular bulb.

The incision is made 1.5 cm posterior to the postauricular sulcus, a simple mastoidectomy is completed and the facial recess is opened. The surgeon extends the facial recess opening inferiorly by severing the chorda tympani nerve and following the fibrous annulus of the tympanic membrane as a landmark. This is referred to as the extended facial recess approach and allows complete exposure of the middle ear and the hypotympanum.

After exposure, Surgicel packs are used to tamponade the main arterial supply in the hypotympanum and the tumour is removed with cup forceps. The tumour can be stripped from the ossicles if necessary.

Glomus tympanicum tumours often spread into the regrofacial air cells. A cutting burr is used to remove the air cells inferior to the labyrinth beneath the facial nerve, thereby leaving the facial nerve suspended within a thin layer of bone. This allows the surgeon access to the entire hypotympanum. A small curette is used to remove bits of tumour from crevices in the hypotympanum. The dome of the jugular bulb can be inspected to be certain that it is free of tumour.

If the ossicles are involved by tumour, they may be removed and ossicular reconstruction accom-plished from the posterior tympanotomy. Some tumours extend through the tympanic membrane and tympanoplasty and ossicular reconstruction may be accomplished in the routine manner.

In some cases there is extensive destruction of the canal wall by large glomus tympanicum tumours. In these cases it may be better to utilize a canal wall down technique combined with tympanoplasty and mastoid obliteration following complete tumour removal.

Mastoid and neck approach

This approach is used for small glomus jugulare tumours. By definition, these involve the jugular bulb but do not extend onto, or medial to, the internal carotid artery, nor into the neck or posterior fossa. The approach for removal of these tumours is to first complete the dissection described above. The next step is to amputate the mastoid tip, drilling laterally, both anteriorly and posteriorly, thus freeing the entire mastoid tip. The incision is then carried into the neck along the anterior border of the sternocleidomastoid muscle, which is freed from the mastoid tip and retracted posteriorly. The internal jugular vein is identified and freed from surrounding tissues and 2-0 silk sutures are placed around it. The vein is then followed over the transverse process of the first cervical vertebra into the base of the skull. The 11th cranial nerve is identified (usually lying on top of the vein) and preserved.

This approach is used for limited tumours that do not extend into the neck or skull base and it is usually possible to preserve the 9th, 10th and 11th cranial nerves. The main reason for the neck exposure is to ligate the jugular vein.

Exposure of the sigmoid sinus and jugular bulb is then completed with diamond burrs. The limited tumours do not involve the medial wall of the jugular foramen and the proximal sigmoid sinus is controlled with extraluminal packing of Surgicel. The jugular vein is then tied in the neck and the sigmoid sinus is opened just distal to the proximal packing; Surgicel is advanced into the jugular bulb to control bleeding from the inferior petrosal sinus. Care is taken not to pack this area too firmly or a weakness of the 9th, 10th and 11th cranial nerves might result. The dome of the jugular bulb is then excised along with the tumour. If the tympanic membrane or ossicles are involved, these may be reconstructed as described above. If intact, the tympanic membrane and ossicular chain is preserved, as is the posterior canal wall. Unless there is preoperative involvement of the 9th, 10th and 11th cranial nerves, it is not necessary to sacrifice them in removal of this limited tumour.

Infratemporal fossa approach

The development of the infratemporal fossa approach by Fisch (1982) has been a significant advance in our ability to remove large tumours. This approach is used for large glomus tumours that extend to the carotid artery, into the neck, skull base, or intracranially. This approach has allowed adequate exposure and control of vital structures so that tumours which previously were considered non-resectable can now be totally removed with safety and limited morbidity.

The dissection described above under the mastoid and neck approach is first accomplished. After the facial recess is open, the incudostapedial joint disarticulated and the external auditory canal is transected at the level of the bony cartilaginous junction. The skin of the meatus is everted and closed with 5–0 nylon sutures. The periosteum of the postauricular area is sutured behind the opening in the meatus to reinforce closure. The skin of the external auditory canal is removed along with the tympanic membrane, malleus and incus. The bony external auditory canal is then removed. Following this, the facial nerve is freed of bone from the geniculate ganglion through the stylomastoid foramen. Fisch originally described exposure of the facial nerve through the stylomastoid foramen into the parotid with permanent anterior transposition of the facial nerve. In my experience, this always produced a temporary facial paresis and sometimes a minor permanent residual facial weakness. I have modified this approach as follows.

Rather than exposing the facial nerve into the parotid, I elevate the entire tail of the parotid along with the periosteum of the stylomastoid foramen and nerve. The facial nerve is then carefully freed from the fallopian canal with sharp dissection. There are multiple fibrous connections which are sharply incised in the descending portion of the nerve. In the tympanic portion of the nerve there are no adhesions and this section elevates readily. The entire tail of the parotid with contained facial nerve is then elevated lateral to the mandibular ramus. A large silk suture is placed through the periosteum of the stylomastoid foramen and attached to the soft tissue in the area of the root of the zygoma. This elevates the facial nerve and prevents it being stretched when retractors are placed. After the facial nerve and parotid are elevated, I place a large Perkin's retractor beneath the angle of the mandible and retract the entire mandible forward. I have not had to resect the mandibular condyle, even in large tumours that extend into the infratemporal fossa extensively.

Transposition of the facial nerve allows exposure of the skull base in the area of the jugular foramen and carotid artery. The common carotid artery is identified and the external carotid artery ligated. The internal carotid artery is followed through the skull base into its intratemporal course. The 9th, 10th and 11th cranial nerves are identified in the neck and followed into the jugular foramen. The 12th cranial nerve is also identified and followed to its foramen.

The sigmoid sinus is doubly ligated with silk sutures and the tumour is then freed from the carotid artery anteriorly. Bleeding caroticotympanic vessels are controlled with bipolar cautery. If the tumour is adherent to the internal carotid artery, it is best to leave a portion of it on the artery at this point and remove the bulk of the tumour. The tumour is freed superiorly, posteriorly and then medially and a total removal of the tumour is thus accomplished.

If there is intracranial extension of the tumour, a decision must be made at this point whether to attempt a total removal of the tumour. We base this decision upon the amount of blood loss and if limited to less than 3000 ml, we proceed with removal of the intracranial extension of the tumour. If there has been greater blood loss, one may encounter problems with bleeding despite the replenishment of the known clotting factors with fresh frozen plasma and platelet packs. In such a case we prefer a two-stage procedure, with removal of the intracranial portion of the tumour approximately 6 months after primary surgery.

Removal of the intracranial portion of the tumour is often easier than removal within the temporal bone. By the time one is ready for removal of the intracranial extension, the blood supply has often been controlled.

If tumour has been left along the internal carotid artery, this is now removed. Closure is accomplished by obliterating the mastoid defect with strips of abdominal fat. If the cerebrospinal fluid space has been entered, continuous lumbar drainage is used for approximately five days until the wound is sealed.

There are considerable risks and complications to this extensive surgery. Large tumours, particularly those that extend transdurally, often intimately involve the 9th, 10th, 11th and 12th cranial nerves. The approach itself produces a permanent conductive hearing impairment because of removal of tympanic membrane and ossicles and blind sac closure of the external auditory canal. With management of the facial nerve and the method described, approximately 50% of patients will have no facial weakness at any time. I have only had 2 patients out of 25 who have had a significant permanent facial weakness. Both of these patients had preoperative X-ray therapy as a curative measure, but then had recurrence of tumour.

The internal carotid artery is at risk in extensive tumours which involve its wall. Usually it is possible to remove the tumour from the artery and preserve it. The problem that I most commonly encounter is producing a defect in the internal carotid artery at the origin of the caroticotympanic branch, which is often hypertrophied. I have been able to repair these small defects in the internal carotid artery and none of the patients has had a stroke.

Cerebrospinal fluid leak and infection is an occasional problem. Continuous lumbar drainage has avoided the problem of persistent c.s.f. leak and appropriate antibiotics have quickly cleared the few cases of infection that have occurred.

I do not routinely perform a tracheostomy or gastrostomy on patients in whom we have had to sacrifice the 9th, 10th, or 11th cranial nerves. Most patients can manage their secretions adequately. Teflon injection of the vocal cord is done in patients with permanent loss of vagus nerve function. Nasogastric feeding tubes are used early in the postoperative course and, if patients are not able to maintain adequate nutrition by mouth, a percutaneous gastrostomy is performed as a temporary measure. All patients have eventually been able to maintain adequate nutrition by the oral route and none has had a problem with persistent aspiration. There have been no deaths in my series.

X-RAY THERAPY OF GLOMUS TUMOURS

Besides surgery the most commonly used modality for therapy of glomus tumours is irradiation. Fifteen years ago we performed a study of the effect of X-ray therapy on glomus tumours (Brackmann et al 1972). Seven patients who had received irradiation for glomus jugulare tumours subsequently were operated on by members of the Otologic Medical Group. We compared the pre-irradiation biopsy specimen with the biopsy taken following various doses of X-ray therapy. The effect of irradiation that was apparent in these cases was on the blood vessels and fibrous elements of the tumour rather than on the tumour cells themselves. We found that the effect of 2000–3000 R was similar to the effect of 4000–6000 R. Following this study we developed a protocol which uses relatively small doses of external irradiation in the 2000–3000 R range for patients who have non-resectable tumours, for the elderly, or those in poor health. The palliation afforded by this small dose of irradiation appears to be equal to that obtained with the larger dose with much less morbidity.

EMBOLIZATION

Embolization is a relatively new modality for treatment of glomus tumours. In large tumours we now routinely utilize embolization with gelfoam 24 hours preoperatively. We have found this to reduce blood loss and facilitate total tumour removal. On occasions, in very large tumours where there is some question as to whether total removal can be accomplished, polyvinyl alcohol sponge is used for embolization. This fulfils the same purpose as gelfoam for promotion of haemostasis, but has the additional benefit of permanent embolization of the vessels in case total removal cannot be accomplished.

DISCUSSION

From the above description of techniques available for treatment of glomus tumours, one can see that smaller tumours can be removed with a minimum of morbidity and there is little argument that this is the preferred method of management of glomus tympanicum tumours and smaller jugulare tumours. Where the debate arises is in the treatment of larger tumours where surgery may produce morbidity with regards to hearing, facial nerve function, function of the 9th, 10th, 11th and 12th cranial nerves and risks to the carotid artery. It is interesting to review the radiotherapy literature which discusses the radiosensitivity of glomus jugulare tumours and at the same time describes radioresistance of the histologically identical carotid body tumour (Brackmann et al 1972). This misconception arose years ago when surgical techniques in the temporal bone were undeveloped and attempts at removal of glomus tumours of the temporal bone were often disastrous. From our study of the effect of X-ray therapy on glomus tumours, it is apparent that the glomus tumour cell itself is not radiosensitive. What responds to external X-ray treatment is the blood supply to the tumour. A radiation vasculitis is produced and this does result in shrinkage of the tumour and slowed growth. It does not, however, cure a glomus tumour.

I agree that, in elderly patients or in those in poor health, X-ray therapy is a reasonable method of controlling a tumour. On the other hand, I believe that total excision is the preferred treatment in younger patients. Newer microsurgical techniques, particularly the infratemporal fossa approach, now allow total exposure of even large tumours and total removal with safety. Rehabilitative measures can be instituted, which provide good quality of life when total tumour removal requires sacrifice of the involved cranial nerves.

One might argue that X-ray therapy might first be used to ascertain the biological behaviour of the tumour and its response to X-ray, with reservation of surgery for those cases which do not respond well or exhibit aggressive growth. I have considered that argument and believe it reasonable in some cases. This would be in older patients where the expected 8–10 years of palliation corresponds with their normal life expectancy. On the other hand, in younger patients I do not think this is ideal, because if surgery is later necessary, it does increase the morbidity of extensive surgical procedures. The only patients in whom I have encountered problems with wound healing or persistent facial paresis have been in patients who have received preoperative X-ray therapy. I, thus, agree with Brown (1985) and Spector et al (1976), who prefer surgery as the primary modality for glomus tumour treatment. X-ray therapy is reserved for those patients who have incomplete removal and show signs of recurrent tumour growth or for the elderly or those in poor health.

CONCLUSION

After a review of the literature, as well as my personal experience in the management of glomus tumours, I agree with Rosenwasser (1973) who stated, 'Long-term follow-up of my cases of glomus jugulare tumours (30 years) and wide experience with cases referred to me have convinced me that surgery, when feasible, is the method of choice in treatment of this lesion.'

Glomus jugulare tumours are rare, with an incidence of 0.012% of all head and neck tumours. As a result, very few surgeons will see a sufficient number of patients to enable them accurately to assess the merits of the different treatment modalities and they are therefore dependent on the evaluation of the comparatively few large series published in the world literature.

This also presents difficulties because of the following facts:

1. The natural history of these untreated tumours is very long with a slow rate of growth.

2. As a result, the length of follow-up after treatment must be adequate, probably to the order of 10–15 years at least, if results are to be at all meaningful.

3. Accurate, pretreatment classification with regard to the size of the tumour is difficult, with no uniformity between various authors.

4. Assessment of the effect of treatment is not easy as comparison of results is made more difficult by the variation among authors concerning the criteria for a 'cure', as distinct from clinical control.

Before discussing the various possible treatments a brief comment on histology and clinical behaviour is required as it has significant bearing on the problem.

HISTOLOGY

Glomus jugulare tumours are merely one type of chemodectoma involving the head and neck. They are composed of groups of epithelioid cells (of two types) closely applied to the endothelium of capillaries in richly vascular connective tissue. Frequently, there is a 'feeder vessel' from the external carotid artery, or one of its branches, with numerous venules draining into the internal jugular vein, or inferior petrosal sinus.

CLINICAL FEATURES

These tumours are very slow growing, but by virtue of their anatomical location have the potential to cause serious symptoms, even though their activity is biologically low. Infiltration occurs into bone, but nerves are frequently compressed and displaced rather than invaded.

TREATMENT

The various treatments possible are as follows:
1. Surgery
2. Radiotherapy
3. Surgery with either pre- or postoperative radiotherapy (combined treatment)
4. Embolization with, or without, surgery
5. No treatment

1. Surgery

Jenkins and Fisch (1981)

Jenkins and Fisch (1981) reported a series of 16 patients in whom total extirpation was accomplished in all cases. From a technical point of view, they stressed the necessity of freeing the internal carotid artery early on in the procedure. Complications consisted of a CSF leak in 4 patients, dysphagia in 3 and facial paralysis in all the patients, although eventually 75–80% obtained a good return of function. To minimize the dysphagia caused by damage to the 10th cranial nerve, a cricopharyngeal myotomy is done routinely. The authors classify tumours into four types, ranging from involvement of the middle ear only, up to varying degrees of intracranial extension.

Comment. This article is of limited value as no follow-up is mentioned. Operation details concentrate on the management of the internal carotid artery, with the authors maintaining that it is possible to remove tumour and adventitia without residual neurological sequelae.

Jackson et al (1982)

Jackson et al state that amongst the various options possible, curative therapy can only be achieved when surgery (with or without irradiation) is used, radiotherapy being only palliative. They stress the necessity of determining preoperatively the relationship of the tumour to the internal carotid artery and state that 'large tumours can be expected to involve the artery and thus sharp dissection is required'. With regard to complications, the authors point out that injury to cranial nerves 9 to 12 is all too common and patients may well require temporary nasogastric tube feeding and a tracheostomy.

Their series involved 40 cases between 1970 and 1982 with a follow-up ranging from 2 months to 12 years.

Total tumour removal was achieved in 83%, with complications including a 'dead ear' (7%), CSF leak (22%), damage to 9th to 12th cranial nerves (50%) with aspiration pneumonia not infrequent and death occurring in 7% of the cases (1 patient succumbing from occlusion of the carotid artery).

Comment. This is a good article drawing attention to the considerable degree of morbidity following surgery. The follow-up time is too short to draw any definite conclusions and no mention is made as to the feasibility of completely removing a large tumour adjacent to the internal carotid artery without fear of damage to it.

Brown (1985)

Brown reviewed a very large series of 231 patients over a period of 10 years. The smaller tumours were treated by surgery, moderate-sized ones by surgery with pre- or postoperative radiotherapy and the very large lesions by radiotherapy alone.

The results obtained on 75 patients treated mainly by surgery alone were 66 alive and free of disease.

It is worth mentioning the fate of the 42 cases with large tumours, 19 being treated by radiotherapy and surgery, 19 by radiotherapy alone and 4 having no treatment at all.

Fifteen were alive and free of tumour, another 12 alive but with residual disease and 12 had died.

Comment. The length of follow-up in this series is insufficient, particularly as the author says that 'the tumour is benign and slow growing in most cases, so that patients can survive without treatment, even with CNS involvement of 20 years'.

No criteria are given as to how freedom from tumour is determined and there is no mention of complications, morbidity or the problem of proximity of the tumour to the internal carotid artery.

2. Radiotherapy

Sharma et al (1984)

Sharma et al present the largest recorded series in the literature of 60 patients treated at St Bartholomew's Hospital, London between 1942 and 1982.

The average duration of follow-up was 13 years with a dose of 4–5000 cGy used in nearly every case.

Sufficient radiotherapy details and follow-up information are available to assess the results in only 42 patients, but with an overall success rate of 82.5%. In this connection the authors suggest that if, following radiotherapy, symptoms remain static or improved and the tumour regresses and remains inactive over many years, it would be reasonable to regard this as a 'cure'.

Comment. This is an excellent article with a large number of patients and a more than adequate follow-up period. However, no mention is made of side-effects, or possible complications of treatment.

Cummings et al (1984)

Cummings et al reviewed 45 patients treated between 1958 and 1978 with a median follow-up of 10 years, and a smaller dose of 3500 cGy (9 patients had had incomplete pretreatment surgery). The majority obtained symptomatic relief with, in particular, tinnitus and hearing improved. Pain was completely abolished, but cranial nerve abnormalities were unchanged, or only particularly relieved.

Three patients did not respond to radiotherapy and subsequently underwent surgery (at 1, 7 and 16 years later), and 2 patients had a further course of irradiation.

There were no deaths or serious complications, with chronic otitis externa occurring in only a small percentage of patients. Otherwise no permanent deterioration of any symptom or objective findings was noted.

Comment. This was another well documented and interesting article. The authors point out that the mechanism by which radiation reduces the symptoms caused by these tumours is still unclear, and there seems very little in the way of histological change following DXR. Gross angiographic appearance may not change significantly, even when masses previously detectable on clinical examination have regressed, and bone defects generally persist.

In the above report there was no difference in the degree or duration of response to DXR following clinical diagnosis, limited biopsy, or incomplete resection and others have also reported no apparent benefit from 'surgical debulking'.

Regrowth of glomus tumours appears to be as likely after high irradiation doses as after low doses, with the authors suggesting the latter protocol enabling a further course of treatment to be given if recurrences develop. They consider that a persistent, but stable, tumour mass is not evidence of radiation failure.

Kim et al (1980)

Kim et al have the longest recorded follow-up of 5–30 years in 30 patients treated between 1932 and 1978. They state that almost all patients obtained complete or significant relief of presenting symptoms, with some showing partial or complete improvement in cranial nerve deficits.

The authors consider that tumour is controlled (88% in their series) if there is no progression of cranial nerve lesions, increase in size of visible tumour, or progression of radiographic findings.

Comment. This is an important article by virtue of the long follow-up evaluation. The authors consider that there is no demonstrable increase in tumour control at doses greater than 4000 cGy. Cases of brain necrosis have occurred from doses higher than 5000 cGy, especially when given in shorter time intervals.

Maruyama et al (1971)

Maruyama et al, using angiography as a method of assessing the effect of radiotherapy were surprised to find that, despite the excellent clinical response, there was not a corresponding change in the vascular mass. They suggest that part of the results of radiotherapy is an injury to small blood vessels below that of angiographic visibility.

Gibbin and Henk (1978)

Gibbin and Henk describe a small series of 14 patients in South Wales followed up for 20 years (mean time 8.7 years). Twelve patients were alive and well and free from clinical evidence of active tumour. The other 2 died from unrelated causes.

Comment. A short article exemplifying the importance of considering survival and freedom from symptoms rather than radio (or surgical) curability.

3. Combined treatment

Spector et al (1976)

Spector et al compared the various therapeutic modalities in 65 patients with a follow-up of 2–27 years, average 9.1 years. The various 'success rates' (a satisfactory therapeutic response) were reported on as surgery 78%, radiotherapy 70% and combined treatment 60%. However, in the latter group there were only 10 patients, the radiotherapy being used either pre-or postoperatively in equal numbers.

Comment. The article is loaded in favour of surgery, but makes the point that primary radiotherapy may make subsequent surgery easier. However, the authors' data on postirradiation specimens showed 'no significant response of the chief cells to radiation and a persistence of tumour vasculature'. They maintain that the inherent tendency of glomus jugulare tumours to slow growth is a more important determinant than its actual response to irradiation.

Gardner et al (1981)

Gardner et al treated 19 cases of glomus jugulare tumours, 10 by combined therapy (8 with preoperative irradiation and 2 following surgery). The follow-up time, however, was short, with a maximum of 8 years.

The interest in the article lies in the comparison of the pathological findings in 6 patients who had preoperative DXR and 6 treated by surgery alone.

In the irradiated group histology showed tumour still present in 5 out of the 6 cases. There were changes in the endothelium of the blood vessels which also contained thrombi. Occasional necrotic tumour due to infarction was noted, but fibrosis was the same in the two groups. It should be noted, however, that only 4–6 weeks elapsed between the radiotherapy and surgery.

Comment. These are two excellent articles by the above authors, this particular one quoting infrequent histological findings. The authors conclude that perhaps it will be demonstrated at some future date which modality can be expected to provide the highest cure rate, the lowest mortality and morbidity and the best functional results, along with the least expenditure of the patient's time and resources.

Reddy et al (1983)

Reddy et al treated 17 patients with primary surgery with 10/15 (70%) incidence of recurrence. Radiation therapy was then used and, at follow-up ranging from 2 to 22 years, all patients were living with disease controlled.

Comment. The authors feel that DXR, either as a primary modality or as adjuvant therapy, has an important role in the management of glomus jugulare tumours. They reckoned that the above study shows that the incompletely excised and recurrent lesions often respond extremely well to radiotherapy.

4. Embolization

References in the literature to this technique are few.

Ruggiero et al (1976) make the point that embolization can be repeated and Gryskiewicz et al (1984) reported a case where histology showed large tumour vessels occluded by gelfoam.

Shick et al (1979) described a patient in whom a postembolization arteriogram indicated 90% occlusion of tumour vascularity with, at subsequent surgery, lack of arterial bleeding and considerable tumour necrosis.

Comment. Various articles would suggest that embolization's main value is as a preoperative measure to reduce tumour vascularity. An experienced radiologist is essential, with the inherent risk of the internal carotid artery being affected.

5. No treatment

Mention should be made that observation alone may be fully justified, for example in the elderly patient. There are a number of well documented cases of tumours remaining 'static' and inactive for many years, with no worsening of symptoms. The author himself has two such cases followed up for 8 and 10 years respectively with the clinical situation unchanged.

CONCLUSION

The problem of assessing the effectiveness of the various forms of treatment in this condition is made difficult by the natural history of the disease, i.e. the tumour is biologically relatively benign (analagous to the acoustic neuroma) and very slow growing, with, in some patients, significant periods when it remains completely static. A very long follow up, possibly 15–20 years is therefore necessary to make any evaluation worthwhile.

At the outset, a difference has to be made between a true tumour cure and symptomatic clinical control.

There is no doubt that in terms of complete cure (total eradication of the disease), surgery is the only answer. It is, however, a very long and protracted operation, most authors quote 8–10 hours, ideally both an otological and neurosurgeon are required, with the tumour often being removed piecemeal and not intact. There are potentially serious complications, especially with the larger lesions, e.g. a CSF leak, and the procedure is attended by significant postoperative morbidity from damage to 7th, 9th and 10th cranial nerves. Even in those cases where there are no neurological symptoms beforehand, some damage to the nerves would seem inevitable by virtue of the proximity of the tumour to the jugular foramen. Varying degrees of facial weakness are universal, as mobilization of the 7th nerve is an integral part of the surgical exposure.

With large tumours radical removal runs the risk of damage to the internal carotid artery with evidence to suggest that, even if it is not injured at the time of surgery, the adventitia over the artery may necrose several weeks later (even the most ardent of surgeons agree that tumours extending to the foramen magnum are inoperable).

With regard to radiotherapy, all authorities agree that it does not eliminate the tumour, but is palliative in effect. It is important, therefore, when assessing results to consider survival and freedom from symptoms rather than radiocurability. However, there is overwhelming evidence that radiotherapy, whatever its effect (? vascular ? fibrosis ? tumour kill), slows down the progress of the disease and relieves symptoms. In certain instances nerve palsies improve, carefully planned treatment will often maintain ear function, there is minimal morbidity and many of the surgical complications are removed. It should be noted that when a dosage of 4000 cGy is applied, a further course of treatment is possible several years later.

Embolization is used in the main as an adjunct to surgery by reducing vascularity preoperatively. In certain rare instances it may have some value in relieving symptoms in large unresectable tumours that have not responded to radiotherapy. It is obligatory that this technique is only carried out by a very experienced neuroradiologist.

When trying to make a balanced, overall view of the correct management of this difficult condition (and the place of base of skull surgery), a fundamental question has to be asked as to whether radical excision is necessary, as distinct from long-term palliation by radiotherapy. Obviously, the age of the patient, size of the tumour, etc., will be important factors. In the older age group with a large tumour, it may be felt that surgery is unjustified, whereas in the younger patient with a small lesion an operation is deemed a practical possibility.

However, a good case can be made out for initially treating glomus jugulare tumours by radiotherapy (4000 cGy), with a meticulous long-term follow-up when further radiotherapy or surgery is perfectly possible if recurrences occur.

In the event of primary surgery being advised all patients should be clearly informed about the incidence of facial nerve weakness, dysphagia, voice change, etc.

Whatever treatment plan is arrived at it is suggested that these rare tumours should be dealt with in a few special centres where radiotherapy, neurosurgical and neuroradiological facilities are available. It is only by concentrating the patients in such hospitals that sufficient experience will be obtained to arrive at a sensible judgement.

Until recently, the inability of surgeons to remove successfully extensive glomus tumours strongly favoured the use of radiation therapy. With the introduction and development of skull base surgery, the situation has changed and there is now a body of opinion which supports the view that the majority of these tumours are resectable. Nevertheless, because of the high degree of skill and technical resources which are necessary and the inherent risks of the most serious morbidity which are involved, a controversy exists. This controversy, in which ethical considerations are paramount, is increasingly assuming importance and requires for its solution the accumulation and analysis of data and experience. The rate of development of our knowledge and, thus, our arrival at a sound judgement, is hampered by factors such as the slow growth rate of the tumour and improvements in radiotherapeutic therapies, which have rendered much of what was previously reported no longer appropriate.

Dr Lund and Dr Brackmann have presented their case for radiotherapy and for radical surgery in a most capable and comprehensive way. The title proposed to these authors absolves them from all but limited reference to the treatment of glomus tympanicum. Although considerable skills are necessary for total excision of tumours arising from glomus bodies in the mesotympanum and which often invade the retrotympanic air cells, there is general agreement that surgical treatment in these cases is both necessary and appropriate. Among those surgeons adequately trained and fully competent in temporal bone surgery, the necessary expertise can be expected to be available. Therefore, the debate between Dr Lund and Dr Brackmann is focussed on the treatment of tumours arising from and involving the jugular bulb, often with extensive and life-threatening extensions throughout the anatomically crowded petrous bone, and even intracranially—the glomus jugulare.

In putting the case for radiotherapy, Dr Lund makes several important points:

1. The natural history of glomus tumours renders the evaluation of results for all therapies unreliable unless patients are followed-up for a minimal period of 15 years.

2. There is a need to differentiate between tumour cure and symptomatic control.

3. While surgical treatment is the only means of curing the disease, the price may be extremely high in terms of immediate and delayed sequelae. The duration of the operation, the need for substantial blood replacement and the unavoidability of piecemeal removal present serious intraoperative hazards. Although the tumour does not infiltrate associated cranial nerves, these, by virtue of their proximity to the anterior margin of the jugular foramen, are usually in jeopardy. As a consequence, nasogastric tube feeding and tracheostomy may be necessary for prolonged periods postoperatively. Facial paresis, although often largely recoverable, is virtually unavoidable and, when there is tumour involvement of the internal carotid artery, serious central nervous system catastrophes or death may ensue.

4. Although there is no certainty on the mechanism whereby radiation affects the tumour, there is general agreement amongst authors on its palliative effect. The point is made that survival and freedom from symptoms are more relevant than radiocurability. If carefully planned, using a dose no greater than 4000 cGy, which permits subsequent repetition of treatment if the initial response is inadequate, preoperative hearing levels are maintained and morbidity is relatively moderate. Radiotherapy decelerates tumour growth and, in many cases, enables attempts at surgical excision to be avoided. Thus, a period of tumour control greater than the life expectancy of many patients can be anticipated. In addition, subsequent surgery is not precluded for tumours whose aggression exceeds the capability of radiation.

5. Embolization has been shown to be of benefit, not only as a preliminary to surgery, but also as a definitive method of treatment for the frail and elderly, provided it is performed only by those highly skilled in the technique.

6. In view of what is known about the benefits of radiation, with relatively minor morbid effects, in contrast to the sequelae of surgery, the question is asked as to whether long-term palliation by radiation is not preferable to radical excision. The argument in favour of radiotherapy for patients in the older age group with large tumours is strongly presented. There may be a case for surgical treatment in young fit patients with smaller tumours, provided they are fully informed of and understand the possibility of

permanent facial weakness, dysphagia and voice changes.

7. Finally, it is pleaded that, whichever treatment is accepted, this should be provided only at a few specialized centres where all requisite facilities are available and where there is a concentration of experience and expertise.

In advocating surgical treatment for glomus jugulare, Dr Brackmann most clearly details his methods of preoperative evaluation and operative management. In order to justify his preference, Dr Brackmann has clearly rationalized his methods of evaluation and underlines the enormous value of recently introduced investigative techniques—notable by its absence from his protocol was retrograde venography, which provides information about tumour extension within the internal jugular vein and bulb and levels of catechol amine secretion. The classification described facilitates planning the surgical procedure in relation to the extent of the tumour.

The surgical approaches as determined by the preoperative findings are clearly and succinctly described with useful practical innovative advice on methods of haemorrhage control and facial nerve transposition. Control of bleeding from the internal carotid artery is also usefully discussed. With the procedures described, tracheostomy and gastrostomy are not routinely required and sequelae have been effectively managed in all the author's patients without mortality.

In justifying his preference for surgical treatment, Dr Brackmann emphasizes the following:

1. The effect of radiotherapy was observed in his own research to be on the blood vessels and fibrous elements of the tumour rather than the tumour cells themselves and that relatively small doses were effective in this respect. A dose of 2000–3000 cGy is recommended for non-resectable tumours and for elderly or frail patients. With such relatively small doses, palliation is equal to that achieved with a larger dose with much less morbidity.

2. Embolization 24 hours preoperatively reduces total blood loss and is used routinely.

3. Although radiation retards tumour growth it does not cure a glomus tumour.

4. Putting aside the case of elderly patients, Dr Brackmann believes that total excision is the treatment of choice, even for large tumours. He justifies this view on the basis of the advantages provided by new microsurgical techniques and the capacity of rehabilitative measures to minimize the effects of sequelae. He believes that a policy consisting of initial radiotherapy to assess the biological behaviour of the tumour and its response to radiation, with subsequeht excision of those tumours which do not respond satisfactorily, is inadvisable because of surgical complications due to irradiation.

5. Although it is undoubtedly an unintentional omission, no information is provided about the protocol for postoperative evaluation.

COMMENT

Although Dr Brackmann's arguments are certainly persuasive, they lack support from long-term follow-up and this must surely weaken his case. By contrast, the advocates of radiotherapy can point to extensive periods of tumour control. The balance is further affected by the relative scarcity of skills appropriate to skull base surgery, even among developed nations. By comparison, oncology centres capable of providing skilled radiotherapy are relatively numerous, certainly throughout Europe, North America and Australasia, which are the principal areas in which the diagnosis of glomus jugulare is likely to be made before the tumour becomes inoperable. In terms of therapeutic input, it can be argued that in the case of radiotherapy, this is much more objective. The dose can be measured accurately and the extent of its effects controlled with precision. By contrast, the ability of the surgeon to cure the disease is undoubtedly variable and events, which are unforeseen and frequently incorrectable, can occur intraoperatively. Although several excellent reports on skull base surgery have been published during the last decade, their value in terms of this controversy is limited by the relatively small number of patients involved and their relatively brief follow-up times.

In choosing between the opinions expressed by Dr Lund and Dr Brackmann, the most relevant factor is the relative ability of each therapy to provide freedom from, or limitation of, symptoms, together with the long-term effects each exerts on the quality of the patients' lives.

On the basis of the information provided by these two authors and that available from a variety of published reports, the following conclusions appear to be inescapable to this reviewer:

1. In general, radiotherapy has much more to offer the majority of patients suffering from glomus jugulare than excision.

2. Radiotherapy is the only appropriate available method for inoperable tumours and for elderly or infirm patients.

3. For young healthy individuals, surgical excision may be justified only if the operation is performed by those few surgeons who possess Dr Brackmann's undoubted and unusually developed technical skills.

4. In examining the case presented by both sides in this controversy, I conclude that the evidence presented by Dr Lund carries most weight and that, for the majority of patients with glomus jugulare, radiotherapy is the treatment of choice. It is axiomatic that this be administered only by those with considerable experience and also that, thereafter, there be regular observation of the tumour by sophisticated investigative methods, utilizing the combined expertise of both surgeon and radiotherapist.

REFERENCES

D E Brackman

Bickerstaff E R, Howell J S 1953 The neurological importance of tumours of the glomus jugulare. Brain 76: 576–593

Brackmann D E, House W F, Terry R, Scanlan R L 1972 Glomus jugulare tumors: effect of irradiation. Trans AAOO 76: 1423–1431

Brown J S 1985 Glomus jugulare tumors revisited: A ten-year statistical follow-up of 231 cases. Laryngoscope 95: 284–288

Fisch V 1982 Infratemporal fossa approach for glomus tumors of the temporal bone. Annals of Otology, Rhinology and Laryngology 91: 474

Rosenwasser H 1973 Long-term results of therapy of glomus jugulare tumors. Archives of Otolaryngology 97: 49–54

Sheehy J L, Brackmann D E 1984 Technique of mastoidectomy. In: English G M (ed) Otolaryngology. Harper & Rowe, Philadelphia, PA, ch 21

Spector G J, Fierstein J, Ogura J H 1976 A comparison of therapeutic modalities of glomus tumors in the temporal bone. Laryngoscope 86: 690–696

Steinberg N, Holz W G 1965 Glomus jugularis tumors. Archives of Otolaryngology 82: 387–394

W S Lund

Brown J S 1985 Glomus jugulare tumors revisited: a ten-year statistical follow-up of 231 cases. Laryngoscope 95: 284–288

Cummings B J, Beale F A, Garrett P O et al 1984 The treatment of glomus tumors in the temporal bone by megavoltage radiation. Cancer 53: 2635–2640

Gardener G, Cooke E W, Robertson J T, Turnbull M L, Palmer R E 1981 Glomus jugulare tumors—combined treatment. Part II. The Journal of Laryngology and Otology 95: 567–580

Gibbin K P, Henk J M 1978 Glomus jugulare tumors in South Wales—a twenty year review. Clinical Otolaryngology and Allied Sciences 29: 607–609

Gryskiewicz J M, Atwell D, Pois A, Mackinon S M 1984 Inoperative arterial embolisation followed by excision of large chemodectoma. Wisconsin Medical Journal 83: 21–25

Jackson C G, Glasscock M E, Nissan A J, Schwaber M K 1982 Glomus tumor surgery: the approach, results and problems. The Otolaryngologic Clinics of North America 15: 4 897–916

Jenkins H A, Fisch U 1981 Glomus tumors of the temporal region. Technique of surgical resection. Archives of Otolaryngology 107: 209–214

Kim J, Elkon D, Lim M L, Constable W C 1980 International Journal of Radiation, Oncology, Biology, Physics 6: 7 815–818

Maruyama Y, Gold H A, Kieffer S A 1971 Radioactive cobalt treatment of glomus jugulare tumors. Clinical angiographic investigation. Acta Radiologica Therapy, Physics, Biology 10: 239–247

Reddy E K, Mansfield C M, Hartman G V 1983 Chemodectoma of glomus jugulare. Cancer 52: 337–340

Ruggiero G, Grillo B A, Santoro G 1976 Two cases of glomus tumor treated by unusual embolisation. Neuroradiology 11: 265–269

Schick P M, Hieshima G B, White R A et al 1980 Arterial catheter embolisation followed by surgery for large chemodectoma. Surgery 87: 4 459–464

Sharma P D, Johnson A P, Whitton A C 1984 Radiotherapy for jugulo-tympanic paragangliomas (glomus jugulare tumours). The Journal of Laryngology and Otology 98: 621–629

Spector G S, Fierstein J, Ogura J H 1976 A comparison of therapeutic modalities of glomus tumors in the temporal bone. The Laryngoscope 86 (i): 690–696

6

Problems of conservation surgery in middle ear disease

W.M.S. Ironside

During the past 40 years, development of micro-surgical techniques and their application to patients suffering from deafness has led to benefits for the patient undreamed of by surgeons starting practice at the beginning of the period. Replacement of fenestration by stapes mobilization, followed by full-plate stapedectomy—the latest procedure with preservation of chorda, stapedius tendon and a small hole in the footplate—give the otosclerotic patient a better than 96% chance of a good long-term hearing result.

However, such progression to a more limited procedure has not been seen in the treatment of chronic otitis media.

TUBOTYMPANIC DISEASE

Whilst antibiotics control very effectively acute infections of the middle ear, with resulting decline in the need for mastoidectomy, the patient with a central perforation is still common. The management of the resulting symptoms of deafness and recurrent discharge seems to vary. It would appear that some of these patients are unnecessarily subjected to mastoidectomy, for this operation is advocated in some centres when there is no irreversible pathology of the middle ear or mastoid (Jackler & Schindler 1984).

It is well to recall earlier times when Banham (1947) reported the results of conservative treatment of chronic otitis media in 200 consecutive cases in Royal Air Force personnel. The treatment consisted of daily mopping, suction, removal of any small polyps through the perforation under local anaesthetic and insufflation of one of three powders, boracic with 1% iodine, boracic sulphapyridine with 1% iodine, and boracic and sulphathiazole. During this period any pathology of the nose, sinuses or nasopharynx was also treated.

Without the advantages of the wide range of antibiotics now available, 93.2% of the patients with a central perforation gained a dry ear and another 3.7% had only a small amount of residual mucus in the ear.

Today, even better results should be obtained, making exploration of the mastoid rarely necessary before closing the perforation by myringoplasty through a permeatal approach, usually found to be adequate even when, occasionally, a convex anterior wall has to be drilled to expose the anterior margin of the drum. Initially, skin was recommended for grafting these perforations (Wullstain 1952), but later, other autogeneic material was advocated, such as periostium, vein (Clos-Domenech 1959, Shea 1960). Eventually fascia became the most widely used graft (Ortegren 1959), giving a closure rate better than 90%.

Over the years there have been discussions as to whether the underlay or overlay techniques held an advantage, but it would seem that, if adequate control of haemorrhage is achieved, and thus good visualization and a dry bed, mastery of either technique gives equally good results.

Occasionally, when the annulus has been destroyed by infection or sacrificed during surgery, an allogeneic tympanic membrane (Marquet 1966) can be used in order to obviate the disappointing results which occur when fascia is used under these circumstances. The allogeneic graft can be used to advantage when the maleus handle is absent, making reconstruction between the tympanic membrane, attached malleus and residual ossicles.

In children there remains some doubt as to whether myringoplasty should be undertaken, as the results

105

tend to be less impressive due to poor eustachian function, which may persist even after adenoidectomy, or clearance of infection in the nose and sinuses.

Even though Strong (1972) pointed out that there is a change in the eustachian tube at the age of 8 years, it has been shown that there is no significant difference in the results obtained with myringoplasty before or after this age (Buchwack & Birck 1980).

The majority of surgeons advocate delaying closure of a perforation until after the age of 15 years, coincident with the decline in lymph tissue throughout the body.

However, if a bilateral perforation exists, resulting in an educational and social handicap, then surgery is surely indicated no matter that the rate of success is less.

The choice of ear under these circumstances is usually the more deaf one, but this is dependent on a period of observation over weeks to make sure that the ear is free of infection and to attempt to determine function of the eustachian tube (Sheehy 1981).

CHRONIC TYMPANOMASTOID DISEASE

When chronic otitis media is associated with a perforation in the attic, marginal posterosuperiorly, or both, it is usually an indication of a disease process that extends beyond the middle ear and it is suspected that cholesteatoma may be present. In these circumstances mastoidectomy is usually recommended. This decision is independent of X-ray examination, many surgeons accepting that this is of little benefit in diagnosis or modifying management. Tomography may show some detail, including erosion of bone, but does not alter treatment. Probably the most helpful steps in ascertaining diagnosis is regular microscopic examination over a long period, if necessary under general anaesthetic with the use of suction. These, combined with the use of local and systemic antibiotics, reduce bacterial infection and discharge facilitating choice of surgery (McGuckin 1958).

In his paper, Banham showed that, with the simple measures then available, 83% of ears with attic perforations became dry and, of those with a marginal perforation, 49% achieved a dry state with 7.6% left with only a minor discharge.

After this period of observation, some ears will show no evidence of cholesteatoma and can be treated by simple myringoplasty, thus reducing the number of unnecessary mastoidectomies undertaken on ears that contain no irreversible changes. In some mastoidectomy series the incidence of patients without cholesteatoma has been over 40%.

Whilst it is hard to accept Korner's theory that cholesteatoma is a tumour, from common experience it is known that all matrix must be removed and, furthermore, the bone underlying the matrix should be drilled, as one would remove a tumour with a margin of apparently healthy tissue. If there is the slightest suspicion that this has been unsuccessful, as for instance in the sinus tympani or over a fistula, then these areas must not be cut off from the meatus by surviving bone, soft tissue or grafting unless a second operation is planned.

It follows, from the variety of ways in which the problem of cholesteatoma is tackled, that there is not one correct or widely accepted method. This is hardly surprising when one considers the vagaries of cholesteatoma, the circumstances under which the surgery is performed and the variation in experience and aptitude of the surgeon.

There is a considerable difference in the extent of this process when first seen by the surgeon. Some surgeons find only a small bead of cholesteatoma readily eradicated and would suggest that the large open cavity and the more complicated postauricular combined approach techniques are rarely necessary. Others see this pathology only when it is extensive and has already destroyed the contents and boundaries of the mastoid and frequently presents as an intracranial complication—for them the open cavity method seems to be the only solution.

The latter group of surgeons may well be practising in areas where the number of ENT surgeons is extremely low, where much of the mastoid surgery is still performed by general surgeons and where the distances to be travelled to see a specialist may be counted in hundreds of kilometres. This is a totally different experience from that of the surgeon in a large hospital, supported by screening programmes, in the middle of a city containing a relatively stable population, patients who can be easily contacted and persuaded to attend for regular examinations.

There are four surgical techniques which have an accepted place in the treatment of cholesteatoma:

1. Cortical mastoidectomy
2. Attico antrostomy
3. End of postaural mastoidectomy
   a. Open cavity
   b. Obliterated
   c. Delayed reconstruction
4. Combined approach tympanoplasty, (CAT)

There are variations of these four basic operations, such as modifications of the incisions used and the way in which the operation site is closed.

1. Cortical mastoidectomy

The most conservative of operations, using either an endaural or postauricular approach, this has little place in the management of cholesteatoma, although occasionally it is possible to remove the matrix without having to carry out a posterior tympanotomy or take down the posterior meatal wall.

2. Attico antrostomy

Through an attico antrostomy, it is possible to deliver a cholesteatoma into the meatus, but once the lateral wall of the attic has been drilled away and, possibly, an extension has been made posteriorly, there is a commitment to an open cavity with or without obliteration. However, when correctly applied, the patient is left with a small shallow cavity which does not accumulate epithelial debris and necessitates minimal attention; the patient can wear a hearing-aid with insert and can swim with little fear of infection.

3a. Mastoidectomy with open cavity

This is the most widely accepted operation, whether by an endaural or postaural incision, for the treatment of cholesteatoma. It should be emphasized that the modern operation, carried out with drill and microscope, bears little relation to the procedure performed more than 40 years ago and reported in the 1960s by the protagonists of the combined operation.

Whereas, in the past, possibly as many as 35% or more had a discharge following surgery, it would now be disappointing to see more than 12% and, in some of these, the discharge would amount to no more than occasional episodes. This has been achieved by attempting to eliminate those factors which may cause residual discharge.

Residual cholesteatoma

This may occur in any part of the mastoid or middle ear originally affected by cholesteatoma; the most common sites are in the mesotympanum, the region of the sinus tympani and oval window and in the epitympanum, particularly anteriorly. The necessity of dissecting carefully in these regions, of opening up the attic by removing the outer wall and making the tegmen turn smoothly into the anterior wall of the middle ear, has been appreciated. However, there will still be some 5% of patients (personal series) with a postoperative cholesteatoma.

Eustachian tube

An open eustachian tube with perforation of the tympanic membrane from sacrifice of the remainder of the drum in the radical operation, led to recurrent infections of the middle ear cleft, but this is now avoided by an adequate myringoplasty at the time of primary surgery.

Active cells

The problem of the actively secreting cells with connection to the cavity has largely been eliminated by drilling, grafting and cauterization on an outpatient basis.

Poor drainage

The need to undertake a meatoplasty, lower the facial ridge almost to the nerve obliterating the tip, has been accepted as essential to provide adequate drainage. The majority of surgeons pack the cavity at the end of the operation, not only to control bleeding, but to prevent septa forming and thus avoid pocketing.

With the application of new techniques and re-learning old lessons, discharge from the mastoid cavity has become a minor problem.

3b. Mastoidectomy with obliteration of cavity

Since the first report by Zaufal (1890) of the fashioning of a mastoid cavity, postoperative discharge had been accepted as a significant and troublesome complication. In an attempt to stop this discharge, flaps were fashioned to turn soft tissue into the cavity and reduce its size. In the 1950s the Rambo (1957) muscle flap, which also obliterated part of the middle ear, had some acceptance, but within 15 years evidence of further cholesteatoma and other complications led to its abandonment. Beales in 1969 collected the records of 880 patients who had been subjected to obliterative myoplasties with a short follow-up. This report included Thornburn's experience with the technique. He had subjected 198 patients to this type of obliterative surgery, the complications were not inconsiderable, 12% discharged and 5.5% developed cholesteatoma, including one that did not have cholesteatoma at primary surgery. Particularly disturbing was the development of infections and cholesteatoma deep to the obliterating flap. As the complication rate was so high, with a relatively short follow-up, he abandoned this procedure.

The Palva (1963) flap is similar, being a musculoperiostal flap, but hinged anteriorly and used to obliterate cavity either on its own or augmented with gelatine sponge, free muscle grafts or bone patty. Where this obliterative procedure differs from the Rambo operation is that the posterior bony canal wall is reduced by varying amounts; that is to say, the basic operation is not a classical radical or modified mastoidectomy and the flap does not enter the middle ear. Like the Rambo flap, there is the tendency for the flap to shrink with the passage of time and there is risk that infections and cholesteatoma develop deep to the flap, delaying presentation until further complications develop.

Another similarity is the incidence of postoperative cholesteaoma, 5.4% obtained by Ojala & Palva (1982) compared with Thornburn's rate of 5.5%. One can understand the acceptance of the Palva operation before the Rambo procedure was condemned, because of the popularity of combined approach tympanoplasty which most surgeons find gives poor results.

3c. Delayed reconstruction

This is a planned two-stage procedure, during the second stage of which the cavity is closed off by restoring the posterior meatal wall and reconstructing the middle ear. The cavity must be stabilized and there must be no evidence of cholesteatoma—this can be considered after 12 months. The wall can be rebuilt by autogeneic bone from mastoid, or allogeneic bone from iliac crest supported by cancellous allogeneic bone. By rebuilding, the patient is relieved of the care of a cavity and also a more complete reconstruction of the middle ear mechanism is possible, either with fascia and allogeneic ossicles or a tympanic membrane ossicular chain block. There is no justification for reconstruction at the time of the primary surgery.

4. Combined approach tympanoplasty

The final method of managing cholesteatoma is by the combined approach or intact wall technique advocated by Jansen (1958), who claims that in nearly all cases it is impossible to gain an adequate view through the meatus, the lateral approach to the epitympanum and posterior tympanotomy, to clear all matrix in middle ear and mastoid. However, there are some 2% of patients who have an extremely oblique or narrow external auditory canal and another 17%, according to a personal series, in which the dura is very low and the sinus far forward making visualization impossible.

Early results reported by the enthusiasts suggested that incidence of postoperative cholesteatoma was only 7%, but long-term follow-up showed that this was nearer 35%. Cody (1977) and Abramson (1977) predicted that only 36% of patients would be free of disease at the end of 5 years. With an appreciation of these long-term results, a second operation at 1 or 2 years was considered necessary to check for postoperative cholesteatoma and a more cautious application of this surgery led most surgeons to reduce the numbers performed. In the author's experience this now amounts to no more than 4% of all operations for cholesteatoma.

Bearing in mind the advantages and disadvantages of the different operations that are available, the surgeon has to consider other factors which may influence the choice of method to treat cholesteatoma.

Age

Although it is desirable in the child to undertake a CAT, the chances of sucess are slim as the cholesteatoma tends to be diffuse, extending occasionally from mastoid tip to the eustachian tube and the possibility of complete eradication of the matrix is reduced (Abramson 1977, Cody 1977). In the older patient the lesion tends to be more confined, but is it really justified in a 60-year-old, who is not active in sports and who does not enjoy swimming, to subject him or her to a closed method which will necessitate a further operation in 1 or 2 years time to have a 'second look'? If, at this time, cholesteatoma has developed then that ear will obviously require to be opened again. Unfortunately, these recurrent or residual cholesteatomas tend to occur in those sites which were, at the time of the original surgery, difficult to approach and so the incidence of secondary postoperative disease is high. It is easy to understand why some patients have been reported as having had no less than nine operations!

With experience, it has been the author's policy that, if a recurrence has developed, to convert the ear to an open cavity. Even then 56% of CAT patients had 2 operations, 24% had 3, 7% had 4 and 1 had 5. Few of these patients had expressed a desire for further surgery in order to close the cavity 2 or more years after the ear has become stable.

Both ears affected

When both ears are affected by cholesteatoma an attempt should be made to treat these ears by a canal-preserving or obliterative technique, even if this entails a second operation on each side.

It can be assumed that, even with the best possible hearing results, the patient will eventually require a hearing aid, or, as occurs occasionally, an instrument will be required immediately. In these circumstances the normal meatus gives a better response.

Work on activities

Obviously, every patient hoped for the best possible hearing after surgery to eliminate the disease process. There are some—service and police personnel—whose livelihood depends on their hearing and must, because of their active lives, have trouble-free ears. They would accept the need for exploratory surgery in a year or two and, if necessary, further surgery to improve hearing in order to pursue their careers. A closed technique should be attempted.

Eustachian tube dysfunction

Unfortunately, there are no accurate repeatable methods of determining the function of the eustachian tube preoperatively and it is only during surgery or postoperatively that dysfunction is detected. This is treated by a transtympanic ventilation tube and, according to Sheehy (1981), is required in 4% of operations for cholesteatoma.

Matrix that cannot be dissected

If the matrix is found dipping into the sinus tympani, it cannot be followed during an intact wall operation and blind scraping is inadequate to deal with such persistent and insidious pathology. Even if the posterior wall is taken down, it is not possible to be sure of seeing the whole of this region and it should not be grafted.

When matrix is adherent over a fistula, there is no justification for leaving it behind an intact wall for, if it does not reform macroscpic cholesteatoma in a year, it may later. Similarly, obliterative flaps should not cover the remaining matrix and a graft placed in an open cavity should have a hole cut to lie around the area. A similar situation arises when matrix cannot be dissected from dura, or when an intracranial complication develops; the affected area should not be cut off from the meatus.

CONCLUSION

In the management of chronic otitis media, after assessment and any conservative treatment, a decision is made where the patient requires a simple myringoplasty or mastoidectomy. If the latter, there is a number of options open to the surgeon depending on the extent of the pathology, skill and experience of the operator and the possibility of long-term follow-up. While pursuing the primary reason for undertaking surgery, complete eradication of irreversible pathology, as much healthy tissue as possible should be preserved in order to facilitate restoration of function.

Chronic middle ear disease manifests itself in a variety of forms. Some of these conditions can be treated successfully by fairly standard procedures, while others present considerable difficulties in terms of complete eradication of the disease. This applies especially to squamous epithelium ingrowth or cholesteatoma formation and it is also in this area that surgical policies differ most markedly. I will discuss some of the problems associated with certain procedures and also outline the techniques that, in my own experience, lead to stable results, using single-stage surgery.

TYMPANIC MEMBRANE

Reconstruction of the pars tensa of the tympanic membrane can confidently be achieved using fascial underlay after creation of meatal skin-tympanic membrane remnant swing door flaps (Palva et al 1969). The upper flap should be dissected loose from the malleus handle and the fascia placed to lie lateral to the handle. Anteriorly, the fascial graft should be medial to the tympanic membrane remnant. The flaps are turned back on to the fascia, fixing it to the malleus handle. An underlay graft does not lateralize, if placed in this fashion. Use of fibrin glue is optional, but may prove helpful on some occasions.

The problem that one should be aware of in conservative approach is that squamous epithelium may line the entire medial part of the pars tensa and even continue into the middle ear, possibly without apparent cholesteatoma as the keratin is still migrating. If the membrane remnant is exceptionally thick, it may contain ingrowing extensions of squamous epithelium in its subepithelial layers (Palva et al 1982). The only safe way of handling this problem is to excise all remaining membrane at the annular level and to roll up the meatal skin sleeve laterally for 0.5–1 cm in 3–4 strips.

Total reconstruction of the tympanic membrane—in the above situation Shrapnell's membrane must also be excised, or rolled up—this can be done with a large piece of wet fascia placed on top of the malleus handle, annular bone and epitympanum. However,

since the fascia is not premoulded, inexperienced surgeons find this difficult and, postoperatively, these ears often show marked graft lateralization and anterior blunting. Here, tympanic membrane homografts are preferable to fascia (Marquet 1976). My only objection to homografts is the tedious work needed for their preparation. Unless this work can be done by assistants, I prefer to use the commercially available moulded calf jugular vein xenograft (Neotymp) (Sanna et al 1985). It conforms to the shape of the tympanic membrane, is equipped with a meatal sleeve and can be fixed firmly in place with fibrin glue, apparently accepted without any adverse reaction. The meatal skin strips, turned down again on the meatal sleeve of the graft, provide a squamous epithelium surface for the graft.

A similar problem is sometimes encountered even in perforations which show both ingrowth of squamous epithelium and a huge tympanosclerotic plaque, forming the medial layer of the tympanic membrane. The only solution is total removal of the ingrowing epithelium of the plaque, which leaves a tympanic membrane rim only at the annulus. In this situation, a preformed xenograft with meatal sleeve provides an easy means for rapid reconstruction.

OSSICULAR CHAIN

Undoubtedly, the most conservative method—preservation of the patient's own ossicular chain if intact and mobile—gives optimum sound conduction. In disease involving the mastoid with no squamous epithelium ingrowth in the middle ear, the best results are obtained by simple mastoidectomy and tympanic membrane reconstruction. This is the one real indication for intact canal wall surgery, as the facial recess approach is sufficient for checking the intactness of the incus long process and stapes. One must drill out a sufficient amount of bone in the zygomatic area to expose adequately the head of the malleus. The mucosal folds, which occasionally cause compartmentalization in the form of non-ventilating pockets around the incus, malleus, tensor tendon and eustachian tube orifice, are severed.

Fixed chain

In an ear with a stiff ossicular chain, one must first make sure that the footplate is mobile. when this is the case, one should not attempt to break the malleus loose, wrap the head in silastic, or drill the bone around the head. Even if it seems conservative, it carries unnecessary risks of damage to the inner ear and invariably fixation recurs. If the incus becomes mobile after cutting the malleus head, the latter can be interposed between the long process and malleus handle, or, if the handle lies too far to the front, between the long process of the incus and tympanic membrane. Should the incus also be fixed, I cut its long process with a delicate malleus head nipper, or with the argon laser, and reconstruct the ossicular chain from the lenticular process (Palva 1983a). A stapes initially fixed, either by otosclerosis or by severe tympanosclerosis, should be handled conservatively and surgery staged. Stapedectomy is performed later when the tympanic membrane, has completely healed, no signs of infection are present and the middle ear is well ventilated.

Destroyed incus

If the stapes superstructure is intact, reconstruction from the head of the stapes generally present few problems. I use the time-proven conservative techniques, either with homograft incudi or, if not available, the patient's own cortical bone. One step that is often neglected is to check the length of the prosthesis properly. This is especially important if it must reach the tympanic membrane as there is no malleus handle to act as an anchor. A columella that is too short will be pulled out from the stapes and no hearing gain obtained. Use of fibrin glue is again optional, but can often be useful. However, the principle to bear in mind is to make the reconstruction so stable that it will not slip, regardless of whether the glue is used or not. In my opinion, there is no need for artificial prostheses in this situation, as non-reactive material can always be used effectively.

Destroyed stapes

In the majority of ears in which ossicular reconstruction must be made from the footplate, the malleus handle is still present. Again, I prefer to use an autograft incus, the lenticular process of which will be placed on the footplate. This gives sufficient height for the columella. A U-shaped trough is then made with a small diamond drill on the short process to fit the malleus handle. The prosthesis must be shaped carefully to avoid contact with the canal and it is usually wise to interpose a small piece of silastic as a safeguard against osseous union. If the tensor tympani tendon can be kept intact, it will be easier to place the incus process under the malleus handle. A drop of fibrin glue at both ends of the columella is of definite benefit.

A difficult situation arises when the prosthesis must be placed at a very oblique angle to reach the footplate, because of an overhanging facial nerve. Normal positioning might cause pressure on the facial nerve with possible paralysis. My solution in those ears in which the malleus handle is also missing is to use an obtuse-angled L-shaped bone columella, the thin, short leg of which will make contact with the footplate. The long leg will rest on the promontory on top of a small piece of lyophilized dura to prevent bony union. The freely mobile footplate leg of the prosthesis affords good stapes movements, provided that the arch of the L-shaped prosthesis has been made sufficiently high to allow creation of a normal sized tympanic cavity.

Substitution of the stapes with various artificial materials has been suggested by many surgeons. Autologous material needs shaping and adjusting during surgery and some time may be gained by using prefabricated prostheses. Years ago I used stainless steel-wire prostheses with favourable short-term results, but abandoned the method because eventually some 25% of the prostheses became visible through the drum as a result of adhesive changes in the middle ear. This is also true of hard polyethylene, which will be extruded in many cases, although the material per se is tolerated without obvious foreign-body reaction. Porous polyethylene is widely used, as it is easy to shape and adjust. It is quite clear, however, that it causes a marked foreign body reaction (Palva & Makinen 1983), which amounts to non-acceptance at this site and my advice is against its use.

Ceramic prostheses represent the latest development in this field. They seem to be well tolerated by the ear and, to date, no foreign body reaction has been reported. We have used these prostheses in 40 ears and the few revisions that we have carried out indicate good acceptance. However, this prosthesis also needs reshaping and drilling and I have found it to be a good alternative only in narrow window niches in which a bony prosthesis would inevitably be fixed. On the other hand, it should be remembered that one has to extract the footplate and make a direct columellization from the perichondrium, or fascia-covered window to the tympanic membrane. The ceramic prosthesis may work its way into the vestibule if the prosthesis is not an adequate length.

SURGERY FOR CHOLESTEATOMA EARS.

It is part of our policy to obtain X-ray films of the mastoid of every patient who is to undergo surgery for chronic ear disease. This helps us to evaluate the duration of the disease, as a non-pneumatized or sclerotic mastoid indicates disease in childhood. On the other hand, good pneumatization, with no cloudiness of the air cells, generally indicates disease confined to the vicinity of the middle ear.

Tympanic cholesteatoma

The commonest condition indicative of future problems is squamous epithelium ingrowth from the margin of a pars tensa perforation. In ears where X-ray examination has shown air-containing cells in the mastoid, a long endaural incision is made and the posterior meatal skin sleeve lifted up to provide unhindered visibility. If necessary, the anterior bony overhang is drilled away, care being taken to spare the ear canal skin. The middle ear cavity is opened up by the swing door technique and squamous epithelium and cholesteatoma can be removed. Drilling may be necessary in the area of the pyramidal process to obtain an unimpeded view of the oval and round window niches and access to the tympanic sinus. With good indications this radical, but still conservative, procedure is rewarding, although it may take time to remove all squamous epithelium.

The tympanum is the site where I find the best use for the argon laser, because it can be employed to evaporate mucosa in all areas of the tympanum, i.e. footplate, stapes crura, round window area and with the aid of a small mirror, the sinus tympani. If both stapes crura are enclosed in squamous epithelium, there is no place for conservatism and the crura are cut with the laser. This will not disturb the footplate and reconstruction can be made with a properly shaped ossicular homograft. In my view, the introduction of the argon laser in middle ear surgery is one of the greatest technical advancements made in the last 20 years.

Attic cholesteatoma

X-ray examination gives some indication of the size of the cholesteaoma sac. If the air cells are intact, one can confidently expect to employ a conservative approach using an endaural incision as described above. The removal of annular bone should be more extensive than in otosclerosis surgery and one proceeds directly to exposure of the long process and body of the incus and neck of malleus. In my experience, only 1% of attic cholesteatomata are so superficial that one can peel the squamous epithelium off all areas, including the entire Shrapnell's membrane, without disturbing the ossicular chain. One must make certain that epitympanic and fibrous folds are severed and the space to the anterior epitympanum and eustachian tube orifice opened up to guarantee future aeration. There is no doubt that the argon laser is a better and safer instrument for penetrating these crevices than any knife or needle. I have found that a small piece of split-thickness lyophilized dura placed on the neck of the malleus and under the fascia and meatal skin surface effectively restores the contour of the attic space. Its stiffness prevents problems of medial shift that might occur with soft fascia alone. With an intact chain, hearing will be superior to that obtained by any ossicular reconstruction. Generally, however, the cholesteatoma envelopes the incus body and malleus head, and conservation with preservation of the ossicular chain is no longer possible. The head of the malleus and also the long process of the incus must be cut, or the whole incus removed, if the cholesteatoma involves its lenticular process (Palva 1983a). The ear canal must be enlarged in the postero-superior area and the attic space opened with a drill so that the exposure of the anterior epitympanum is unrestricted. Once the incus and the malleus head and neck have been removed, drilling carries no risk of damage to the inner ear. The bony defect in the annular region is repaired with suitably tailored pieces of lyophilized dura, fixed in place with fibrin glue. At reconstruction the fascial graft must be placed so that its anterior edge is flush with the protympanum and the fascia inserted under the cut handle of the malleus which abuts against the fascia from a lateral direction. Narrow ear canals are enlarged by drilling, and by ample conchal cartilage resection to obtain a wide meatus.

The ear with limited attic disease also shows cloudiness of the mastoid cells; postauricular mastoidectomy should be performed and all cells harbouring cholesterol granulomatous disease removed. One should never leave a cloudy air-cell system unexplored. If drilling through cortex to antrum reveals no pathological changes, nothing further need be done in the mastoid.

Intact canal wall

The possibility of using the intact canal wall procedure is controversial if the cholesteatoma involves the mastoid. The advocates of the intact canal-wall technique claim that they can handle any kind of cholesteatoma through a facial recess approach and still keep the canal wall intact. However, the intact canal wall will prevent the operator from seeing the posterior area of the oval window and tympanic sinus. The angle of the facial recess approach also makes visualization of these areas impossible. The most practicable solution is to remove a good deal of the medial part of the bony canal wall by endaural attic surgery, improve the view of the posterior tympanum and keep a sizeable part of the lateral part of the canal wall intact. This is what many intact canal-wall advocates admit they are doing (Jansen 1982). The annular ridge for fascial (reconstructed tympanic membrane) attachment is lost, but can, of course, be repaired with lyophilized dura or cartilage. The recurrence rate is high due to hidden residual squamous cell rests, or due to retraction pockets through the attic or the open facial recess (Palva 1983c).

Another hazardous feature of the intact canal-wall method is the attempt to create a large mastoid air space connected to the tympanum. This inevitably results in development of a retraction pocket in 30–35% of cases, as eustachian tube function is likely to be deficient in at least one-third of chronically infected ears with extensive tympanic cleft and mastoid cholesteatoma. In these patients adhesive changes gradually develop in the middle ear and reformation of cholesteatoma, due to open auditus or facial recess retraction, inevitably occurs in the next 3–10 years. At revision surgery I have found that many such ears show a fistula in the horizontal canal and under the cholesteatoma matrix the bone covering the facial nerve has been destroyed.

Canal wall down and obliteration

This is my own routine procedure in ears where the cholesteatoma extends to the mastoid. The open approach provides a direct view of the epitympanum, facial recess, both labyrinthine windows, hypotympanum and eustachian tube. Exposure of the sinus tympani is also better than with any other approach. Systematic study of tympanic biopsies has established that clinical diagnosis of squamous epithelium in cholesteatoma ears receiving open surgery fails in as many as 15% of cases (Palva 1983). Thus, adequate excision cannot be accomplished through restricted approach and requires as wide an exposure as possible of the mucosa adjoining the cholesteatoma. The canal wall down procedure gives by far the best chance of complete eradication of cholesteatomatous epithelium.

Obliteration of the mastoid bowl can be made with the patient's own healthy tissues, i.e. cortical bone pate, mastoid bone chips and a meatally based musculoperiosteal flap (Palva 1982). If bone pate is mixed with fibrin glue 2 minutes before application, it can be used both to fill the antrum and epitympanic space and form a new sufficiently high annulus for lateral attachment of the tympanic membrane graft. Additional bone chips and an adequate flap will fill even large cavities. I must again emphasize that a narrow external meatus should be enlarged during the early steps of surgery by a wide meatoplasty, with ample resection of conchal cartilage. This is important to create a self-cleaning ear canal and facilitates future inspection of the medial part of the canal.

Labyrinth fistula

If one elects to leave cholesteatoma membrane covering the fistula in place, it will be necessary to leave at least a small operation cavity. With a closed procedure, a second operation must be carried out in 6 months to clean the fistular area. At primary surgery, the fistula can be covered temporarily, for instance with a free graft of crushed temporal muscle. Open cavities may be subject to infection with some risk of involvement of the inner ear and the patient must be seen at least once a year for the rest of his life. During the fenestration era in otosclerosis surgery, some of the cavities created in entirely normal mastoids caused considerable problems postoperatively. For these reasons I have abandoned conservative methods and remove cholesteatoma epithelium from a fistula at the primary operation (Palva 1983b).

The presence of a fistula should always be suspected in cholesteatomatous ears and the, dome of the horizontal canal approached with respect. It is not advisable to use instrumental palpation of the dome to ascertain whether the bone is intact. This may result in disruption of the membrane, which sometimes is very thin, the instrument entering the perilymph space, infecting it, or damaging the membranous labyrinth. The cholesteatoma membrane and granulations are removed by microscissors to make the fistular area clearly visible.

At this stage the fistula is left undisturbed but covered with ampicillin-soaked gelatine sponge pledgets. One should return to the fistula only after completing removal of diseased tissue, when the ear is ready for reconstruction.

During the final removal of the cholesteatoma membrane covering the fistula, the membrane is dissected from all sides towards the edges of the fistula by using large round knife-elevators. A thin sucker needle with low power is held at 4–5 mm from the fistula towards the vertical canal; it is kept in this position as the membrane is gently pushed off with the elevator-knife. Its round end must be larger than the fistular lumen so that there is no possibility of the instrument slipping into the canal. The loose membrane is picked out with cupped microforceps. Forceps may also be used primarily to extract the membrane gently from the fistula.

The next step is to remove any particulate matter with wet antibiotic-containing gelatin sponge pledgets. The sponge must be thoroughly wet, because a non-soaked gelatin sponge will absorb a large amount of perilymph, resulting in unnecessary postoperative vertigo. If the edges of the fistula look thin and rough, they can be smoothed with instruments used for fenestration surgery. Movements must always be directed away from the fistula lumen, on the right margin to the right and vice versa. When one is certain that the fistula is clean, a periosteum graft is placed over the opening and adjusted, the side which originally faced the bone lying against the fistula.

If fibrin glue is available, a few drops are applied to the periosteum and surrounding bone. While the glue is still sticky, some bone pate and small bone chips are added. This promotes effective bone formation on top of the fistula. The use of fibrin glue is optional and bone pate and chips can be applied without it. Subsequent steps include obliteration of the mastoid segment with more bone pate, bone chips and, finally, the musculoperiosteal flap. Ossicular reconstruction and tympanic membrane repair are made in the usual fashion. Provided that there has been no loss of perilymph, patients experience no, or only slight vertigo, which last for 1–2 days and there is no inner ear damage.

It may be appropriate in this context to add some remarks on accidental opening of one of the semicircular canals. Should this mishap occur, a wet, ampicillin-soaked gelatin sponge pledget is immediately placed over the opening. A periosteum graft is then taken and pressed on top of the defect. If fibrin glue is available, it is used to fix the graft securely in place. If there is no glue, wet gelatine sponge sheets are pressed on to the periosteum, care being taken not to dislodge them as surgery is completed. Opening a canal in chronic ear surgery is not a catastrophe, but it must be immediately recognized and handled properly.

Open, discharging cavities

When energetic conservative treatment fails to make an operated ear dry, it indicates irreversible pathological changes in the soft tissue lining of the cavity and also infection of adjacent bone, which may contain many unopened air cells with osteitis. In some cases, undue conservatism may lead to complications such as development of fistula, labyrinthitis, facial paralysis or intracranial infection. It should clearly be understood that open discharging cavities always carry definite risks. Revision and reconstruction should follow all the principles described above in connection with canal wall down surgery.

CONCLUSION

The basic principle in surgery for chronic middle ear disease is to apply the procedure to the individual needs of the patient and not to have only one technique to fit all patients. Many ears can be cured by conservative limited surgery, which is ideal for recovery of function. Squamous epithelium medial to the outer layer of the tympanic membrane must, however, be removed meticulously, and the structures that are sacrificed to accomplish this recon-structed. It should also be realized that, in time, adhesions will invariably develop in one-third of ears with a seriously diseased tympanic cleft. All precautions against the development of postoperative retraction pockets should therefore be taken at the primary operation in order to spare the patient revision surgery. Only in ears where, for fear of causing inner ear complications, squamous epithelium may have been purposely left in place at primary surgery, should a second exploration be performed as a staged routine procedure.

INTRODUCTION

Despite the enormous progress made since the first publications of Moritz, Wullstein & Zollner (1952) in the field of reconstructive surgery of chronic middle ear disease, there is still a non-ending discussion concerning the advantages and disadvantages of certain operative procedures advocated by several groups of experienced otologists. Some of them claim that their method should be accepted as a standard procedure, others prefer to modify their technique again and again, publishing merely their first and favourable results and rarely presenting a critical analysis of their failures. In this situation, the resident in training and the inexperienced practising ear surgeons become bewildered and feel insecure, realizing that there is no standard operation taking into account, in each case, the problem of pathology and its functional consequences. They try to explain their failures primarily by a lack of technical skill and ignore the fact that lack of pathophysiological understanding of the problems with which they are confronted during surgery is far more important. The papers of both Ironside and Palva reflect this dilemma, which is due to the abundance of surgical techniques and the shortage of clear-cut criteria which allow the surgeon to choose the 'right operation'. I should like to present a pathophysiological and clinical concept of middle ear surgery:

Long-term results of reconstructive surgery of the middle ear depend as much on the technical skill of the surgeon as on his knowledge of middle ear pathology. He should keep in mind that there exist two entirely different types of chronic otitis media, each of which necessitate a different surgical approach:

1. CHRONIC SUPPURATIVE OTITIS MEDIA AND MASTOIDITIS (Schuknecht 1974)

This middle ear disease is characterized by a central perforation of the tympanic membrane and intermittent, or constant, purulent discharge associated with irreversible pathological changes in the middle ear, eustachian tube and the pneumatized compartments of the temporal bone. The mucous membrane

is hyperplastic, caused by oedema, submucosal fibrosis and infiltration with inflammatory cells. Formation of polyps, mucosal ulceration and granulation tissue are not infrequent pathological changes. It may even be associated with rarifying osteitis of the ossicles, the otic capsule and the mastoid bone (Schuknecht 1974).

I agree only to a certain degree with Ironside's statement that antibiotics effectively control acute infections of the middle ear with resulting decline in the need for mastoidectomy. In my own material of 150 cases of mastoiditis, observed and treated between 1978 and 1983 (Pfaltz & Griesemer 1984), 30% of the patients showed practically normal otoscopic findings and 55% of our adult patients suffered from a chronic, granulomatous mastoiditis, discovered only at surgery. Both in children and adults the rate of complications (facial palsy, labyrinthine fistula, meningitis) is still rather high (10%). We disagree that better results in tympanoplasty will be obtained by rarely exploring the mastoid before closing the perforation. Chronic infection of the middle ear inevitably spreads into the mastoid space, despite adequate antibiotic treatment. It becomes a highly treacherous condition and will sooner or later cause complications during the postoperative course following simple myringoplasty, without control of the pneumatized compartments of the mastoid.

For these reasons we advocate in all cases of chronic suppurative otitis media a *cortical mastoidectomy*, with complete eradication of cholesterol granulomatas and inflammatory tissue within the pneumatic cells of the temporal bone, enlargement of the connecting passages between the antrum and the attic and the removal of polyps within the tympanic cavity, aiming at the primary goal of restoring unimpaired drainage and ventilation. Tympanoplasty, i.e. closure of the tympanic perforation and reconstruction of the ossicular chain, should always include surgical revision of the mastoid cavity, performed at one stage.

Even in the presence of a dry perforation, tympanoplasty should include an inspection of the oval window niche and the attic. A simple myringoplasty should only be carried out in cases with a central perforation and a negative history of aural discharge for many years, including a normal audiogram.

2. THE SECOND TYPE OF CHRONIC OTITIS MEDIA IS CHOLESTEATOMA

Ironside's rather pessimistic statement that '. . . it follows that there is not one correct or widely accepted method from the variety of ways in which the problem of cholesteatoma is tackled' can only be accepted with great reserve and not without a critical comment.

The area of sophisticated reconstructive surgery of the middle ear has demanded an intense search into the basic mechanisms of cholesteatoma. Cholesteatoma, or keratoma as it has been termed by Schuknecht (1974), is simply an

> . . . accumulation of exfoliated keratin in the middle ear, or the adjacent pneumatized areas of the temporal bone, arising from keratinizing squamous epithelium— the matrix—that has invaded these areas from the deep meatal and tympanic epidermal layer. Basal cells in the stratum germinativum of the meatal skin adjoining the postero-superior margin of the drum show a special growth potential, which is the point of departure of cholesteatoma formation. The principle tissue reaction responsible for the spread of cholesteatoma is the surrounding inflammatory granulation tissue within the subepithelial layer of the mucoperiosteum of the middle ear, i.e. the perimatrix.
>
> (Friedmann, 1977)

Pathogenesis of cholesteatoma

This may be summarized as follows: the first step in the development of inflammatory middle ear disease begins with respiratory pathology. This is usually a combination of adenoidal hypertrophy and repeated nasopharyngeal infections. An appropriate medical and surgical treatment (adenoidectomy, paracenteses with insertion of a ventilation tube) may be successful in the majority of the cases. Not infrequently, however, immunological disorders, as well as allergy, also play a prominent role and may result in a chronic seromucous otitis media. The ultimate results of these processes are reduced ventilation of the middle ear cavities, as well as deficient pneumatization of the temporal bone. Purely mechanical phenomena resulting in ventilation and drainage problems are the first to occur. But, with time, the inflammatory component becomes more and more important. This combined process—impairment of ventilation and chronic hyperplastic, non-bacterial inflammation of the middle ear mucosa—results in a permanent retraction of the pars tensa, later in a localized or total collapse of the tympanic membrane. Thus, a retraction pocket is formed, representing a prospective or potential cholesteatoma. This may become an active tensa cholesteatoma as soon as the self-cleaning mechanism within the retraction pocket is impaired; because epidermal migration is disturbed, keratin then collects serving as an ideal medium for bacterial growth, particularly for Gram negative organisms, such as pyocyaneus and *Proteus mirabilis*. Thus, the infectious inflammatory process is started and cholesteatoma is born (Litton, 1977).

If acute inflammation is present from the outset, a tympanic membrane perforation may occur early. As long as the annulus fibrosus remains intact, the perforation is centrally located. If the inflammatory process becomes invasive, both the fibrous and osseous tympanic annulus will be destroyed (rarifying osteitis) and the perforation becomes marginal. This is the starting point of a marginal migration of squamous epithelium from the meatus into the tympanic cavity, resulting in the formation of *tensa cholesteatoma*.

Attic or flaccida cholesteatoma

Attic cholesteatoma is characterized by retraction and invagination of Shrapnell's membrane into the attic, due to recurrent otitis media in infancy. This invagination of Shrapnell's membrane into the epitympanic space (attic retraction) and, at the same time, active epithelial immigration are the primary causes of attic cholesteatoma (Nager 1977). With time, this invaginated epidermic sac accumulates keratin and epithelial debris, which is an ideal medium for the growth of Gram negative proteolytic bacteria. This secondary infection, in return, is stimulating proliferation of the matrix, formation of osteoclasts, as well as the release of proteolytic enzymes (collagenase), thus initiating the bone resorption process which is typical for cholesteatoma.

Surgery

Surgical procedures have to be adapted to the type and extension of cholesteatoma, bearing in mind that eradication of the disease (matrix and perimatrix) is of primary importance and restoration of function only secondary. Skill and experience of the operator, as mentioned by Ironside, are necessarily important prerequisites to a successful surgical intervention. However, without a profound knowledge and understanding of middle ear pathology, failures will become inevitable. Palva emphasizes that '. . . the basic principle in surgery for chronic middle ear disease is to apply the procedure to the individual needs of the patient and not to have only one technique to fit all patients'. This statement is valid on the assumption that the surgeon is respecting certain principles which are based on his precise judgement of the surgical situation and its underlying pathology. If one of these factors is disregarded he will be tempted to modify his technique too frequently, because he becomes insecure and attributes his failures to the use of an established method. Based on the results of a long-term follow-up study, carried out in a series of 500 patients operated for chronic otitis media (Pfaltz et al 1982), we have adopted the following surgical strategy:

Attic cholesteatoma

1. Attic cholesteatoma without erosion of the lateral attic wall and without extension into the antrum (restricted lesion):

Antroatticotomy, with preservation of the posterior canal wall and the annulus tympanicus osseus, posterior tympanotomy, followed by tympanoplasty.

2. Attic cholesteatoma with erosion of the lateral wall but without extension into the mastoid process:

Removal of the lateral attic and postero-superior canal wall, immediate reconstruction with autologous cartilage and perichondrium, followed by tympanoplasty.

3. Attic cholesteatoma with extension into the sclerotic mastoid process, the tympanic sinus and the facial recess:

Modified radical mastoidectomy with partial removal of the posterior canal wall and exposure of tympanic sinus and facial recess, followed by an immediate reconstruction of the partially removed canal wall, but only if the intact cholesteatoma sac can be completely removed; otherwise an *open cavity* technique is carried out. In either case a tympanoplasty is performed.

Extensive cholesteatoma

Extensive cholesteatoma with spread into the pneumatized temporal bone, and/or paralabyrinthine space, middle fossa, posterior fossa, tympanic segment of the facial nerve:

Modified radical mastoidectomy with total removal of the posterior wall, without reconstruction, formation of an *open cavity*. Reconstruction of the tympanic membrane and the ossicular chain (autologous bone or cartilage, or ceramic prosthesis).

Tensa cholesteatoma

Tensa cholesteatoma develops on the basis of a chronic tubotympanic disease and is, therefore, associated with manifestation of decreased tympanic pressure. It arises usually in the postero-superior quadrant of the drum, originating from a deep retraction pocket which has lost its natural self-cleansing mechanism. Keratin collects in this pocket and the debris becomes infected.

Surgical management depends on the site and extension of the lesion:

1. Tensa cholesteatoma, postero-superior localization, limited to the oval window niche, attic and antrum:

Antroatticotomy, with removal of the postero-superior portion of the canal wall and immediate reconstruction with perichondrium and autologous cartilage, followed by tympanoplasty with perichondrium and/or temporalis fascia.

2. Extensive tensa cholesteatoma, with invasion of the mastoid cavity, tympanis sinus and facial recess, demands:

Modified radical mastoidectomy with complete removal of the posterior canal wall, open cavity, followed by tympanoplasty.

Results

We have followed this strategy for about 15 years and the results of our long-term follow-up study may be summarized as follows:

Residual cholesteatoma occurred in 8% of our cases, recurrent cholesteatoma in 1%, the average interval between surgery and the diagnosis of the complication varied between 3 and 10 years.

An analysis of our postoperative audiometric follow-up showed that the type of the middle ear lesion and the type of tympanoplasty are determining factors with respect to the attained functional results. If the ossicular chain was intact, no failures could be observed. If there was only a small defect of the ossicular chain, which coul dbe bridged either by a cartilage graft or by transposition of the incus, in all groups of middle ear pathology the success rate was equally good. In cases with extensive defects of the ossicular chain functional results were both unfavourable for chronic otitis media cases with and without cholesteatoma.

The problem of the retraction pocket needs more detailed discussion. As mentioned above, a retraction pocket may be regarded as a prospective, i.e. potential tensa cholesteatoma. In the current literature on chronic otitis media, there is little agreement as to whether this type of lesion should be operated on or allowed to heal by long-term ventilation of the middle ear. Eliachar & Joachims (1982) emphasize that localized atelectatic retraction pockets signal impending irreversible complications. Re-establishment of adequate middle ear ventilation is, in the view of these authors, the key in every attempt to arrest and reverse this pathology. They present the results of a study on 177 advanced cases in which they were able to demonstrate the reversibility of a seemingly irreversible pathology in the middle ear, achieved by application of long-term silicon ventilating tube.

In our opinion, this type of management should always be tried in children before a more invasive type of ear surgery is performed. In adults, however, tympanoplasty is indicated if the following conditions are present.

1. The self-cleansing mechanism of the retraction pocket seems to be impaired (intermittent discharge).

2. There is a considerable conductive hearing loss.

3. The pocket is formed by an atrophic membrane, floating back and forth with respiration, thus causing annoying noises or even painful sensations.

Portmann (1982) has based his indications for surgical treatment of retraction pockets on the following criteria: anatomical structure of the mastoid (reduced pneumatization), functional state, extension of the local lesion and the general condi-

tion of the patient. He summarizes that there is no method of choice for the management of retraction pockets and that the selection of a particular surgical technique for each particular case will always be a compromise. Sade (1982) emphasizes that it is often not easy to distinguish between a large retraction pocket with an intact self-cleansing mechanism and an active tensa cholesteatoma originating from a deep pocket. He recommends treating shallow retraction pockets with conservative methods (regular microscopic control with suction of the debris). Deep retraction pockets are removed by an endaural or retroauricular approach, if necessary with eradication of an infected 'dead space' in the region of the sinus tympani. His follow-up study of 308 atelectatic ears with retraction pockets showed that most of them did not progress, some of them even regressed. These findings account for the favourable prognosis of the conservatively treated and operated retraction pockets.

According to our own experience (long-term follow-up of more than 6 years) radical removal of a retraction pocket and reconstruction of the tympanic membrane demands the use of solid, resistant autologous grafting material, particularly in cases presenting a partially destroyed (either spontaneously, or by surgery) annulus tympanicus osseus. Both fascia and perichondrium do not have a structure which allows resistance to the retraction forces arising again postoperatively. Within a short time there will form first a shallow and later a deep retraction pocket. From experience we know that autologous grafts like perichondrium and fascia are still the best material to be used for reconstruction of the tympanic membrane, because they are biologically resistant and the take rate is high. If we need grafting material with more solid physical properties resisting retraction, as in the case of a retraction pocket repair, we use thin cartilage foils (taken from the tragus) which reinforce the tympanic graft without impairing its vibration properties. The same method is used for the repair of defects in the postero-superior canal wall, following antroatticotomy, and by this technique postoperative retraction pockets have become a rare complication in our series of cases operated by an antroatticotomy. Human fibrin glue is an excellent technical aid to keep the grafts in place, whereas polymerizing plastic adhesives like histoacryl may cause a chronic inflammation behind an intact graft, resulting in the formation of recurrent cholesteatoma even more than 2 years after the first operation. Histological examinations have shown a foreign-body tissue reaction around the acrylic beads imbedded in the subepithelial layer; at the same time there was papillary proliferation of the stratum germinativum, inducing invasive growth of the squamous epithelium covering the reconstructed postero-superior part of the reconstructed lateral attic and posterior canal wall.

Also, our own experiences with xenografts (lyophilized dura, pericard—Pfaltz & Griesemer 1985), which are recommended by Palva, were disappointing in the long run. Although there was a very high immediate take rate (98%), a short period of healing and no antigenicity, 3 years postoperatively long-term controls showed, in about a third of cases, the appearance of a central necrosis in the reconstructed area, resulting in a dry perforation of the neotympanum.

CONCLUSION

As mentioned above, the primary goal the surgeon is aiming at is eradication of the disease, the secondary goal improvement of hearing. Whereas there is some agreement with respect to the advantages and disadvantages of the various ossiculaoplasty methods and the real chances of an overall hearing improvement, there still is some argument concerning the quickest and safest way to achieve a dry, i.e. healthy, middle ear without the risk of recurrence. Both Ironside's and Palva's paper reflect their concern for this crucial problem. Should a closed or a combined approach tympanoplasty technique be used, as advocated by Marquet, Jansen & Sheehy (1982), or should an open cavity be developed, as emphasized by Smyth et al (1982)? From the conclusions drawn at the end of the second cholesteatoma conference (Paparella 1982), it may be considered that there is a definite trend to return to open cavity procedures, that CAT is a useful tool, but not for every case, and that it is unnecessary to recommend two or more planned procedures when one careful operation will provide a safe ear with suitable hearing in most cases. Moreover, we should not teach residents to perform CAT procedures because serious complications, which are totally avoidable, may occur. Together with Portmann, Paparella stresses that the ear surgeon should be flexible and select various methods to adapt to the patient's particular ear pathology and functional problems. A strategy, which I highly recommend!

REFERENCES

W M S Ironside

Abramson M 1977 Results of conservative surgery for middle ear cholesteatoma. Larynoscopy 87: 1281–1286

Banham T M 1947 The conservative treatment of chronic suppurative otitis in adults. In: Contributions to aviation otology. Hedley Bros, London, p 84–103

Beales P H 1969 Complications following obliterative mastoid operations. Archives of Otolaryngology 89: 222–225

Buchwach K A, Birk H G 1980 Serous otitis media and type 1 tympanoplasties in children. A retrospective review. Annals of Otology, Rhinology and Laryngology (suppl 68) 89: 324–325

Claros-Domenebh A 1959 100 Tympanoplasties practised with the aid of the use of free periosteal membrane graft. Revue de Laryngologie, Otology, Rhinologie (Bordeaux) 80: 817–921

Cody D T R, Taylor W F 1977 Mastoidectomy for acquired cholesteatoma—long-term results, In: Cholesteatoma, 1st international conference. Aescalapius Publishing Co, Birmingham, Al, p 337–373

Jackler R K, Schindler B A 1984 Role of mastoid in tympanic membrane reconstruction. Laryngoscope 94 (4): 495–500

Jansen C 1958 Uber radikaloperation und tympanoplastik. Sitz ber fortbild arztik. Obv.

Korner O 1964 Cited in: Portmann G, Portmann M,

Claverie G (eds) The surgery of deafness. Progress Press, Malta

McGuckin F 1958 Recent advances in tympanoplastic surgery. Journal of Laryngology and Otology 72: 535–548

Marquet J 1966 Reconstructive microsurgery of the eardrum by means of a tympanic membrane homograft. Acta Otolaryngologica 62: 459–464

Ojala K, Palva A 1982 Late results of obliterative cholesteatoma surgery. Archives of Otolaryngology 108: 1–3

Ortegren U 1959 Tromhinne plastik. Für handlingar i Svensk otolaryngologisk fürening. Archives of Otolaryngology, suppl 244

Palva T 1962 Reconstruction of ear canal in surgery of chronic ear. Archives of Otolaryngology 75: 329–336

Rambo J H T 1957 A new operation to restore hearing in conductive deafness of chronic suppurative origin. Archives of Otolaryngology 66: 525–532

Shea J J Jnr 1960 Vein graft of ear drum perforations. Journal of Laryngology 74: 358–362

Sheehy J L 1981 Testing eustachian tube function. Annals of Otology, Rhinology and Laryngology 90: 562–566

Strong M S 1972 The eustachian tube: basic considerations. Otolaryngology Clinics of North America 5: 19–27

Wullstein H 1952 Functionelle operationen in millelohr mit

hilfe des frelen spaltlappen transplantates. Archiv für Ohren
-Nasen-und-Kehlkopfheikunde 161: 442–435

Zaufal E 1890 Technik der trepanation des process mastoid.
Nach kusterchen. grundsatzen. Archiv Ohrenh. 30: 291

T Palva

Jansen C 1983 The combined approach for tympanoplasty.
Journal of Laryngology and Otology (suppl 8): 97: 90–91

Marquet J 1976 Ten years of experience in tympanoplasty
using homologous implants. Journal of Laryngology
and Otology 90: 897–905

Palva T 1982 Obliteration of the mastoid cavity and
reconstruction of the canal wall. In: Gibb A G, Smith M F
(eds) Otology. Butterworth, London, p 19–29.
(Butterworths International Medical Reviews:
Otolaryngology 1)

Palva T 1983a Preservation of the lenticular process of the
incus in surgery for chronic ear disease. Laryngoscope
93: 1362–1363

Palva T 1983b Treatment of ears with labyrinth fistula.
Laryngoscope 93: 1617–1619

Palva T 1983c Why does middle ear cholesteatoma recur?
Archives of Otolaryngology 109: 513–518

Palva T 1985 Chronic otitis media—obliterative techniques.
In: Marquet J F E (ed) Surgery and pathology of middle
ear. (Proceedings of the international conference on the
postoperative evaluation in middle ear surgery. Medical
Media International, Brussel, p 45–51 (Ars Medici,
Congress Series No 6)

Palva T, Mäkinen J 1983 Histopathological observations on
polyethylene-type materials in chronic ear surgery. Acta
Otolaryngology (Stockholm) 95: 139–146

Palva T, Palva A, Kärjä J 1969 Myringoplasty. Annals of
Otology, Rhinology and Laryngology 78: 1074–1080

Palva T, Karma P, Mäkinen J 1982 The invasion theory. In
Sadé J (ed) Cholesteatoma and mastoid surgery.
Proceedings of the second international conference on
cholesteatoma and mastoid surgery. Kugler, Amsterdam,
p 249–264

Sanna M, Zini C, Gamoletti R 1985 Xenogenic material
for tympanic membrane reconstruction. In: Marquet J F E
(ed) Surgery and pathology of middle ear. Proceedings of
the international conference on the postoperative evaluation
in middle ear surgery. Medical Media International,
Brussels, p 108–113 (Ars Medici, Congress Series No. 6)

C R Pfaltz

Eliachar I, H Z Joachims 1982 Arrest of cholesteatoma
formation by long-term ventilation of the middle ear;
Proceedings of the 2nd international conference on
cholesteatoma and mastoid surgery: Kugler, Amsterdam,
p 605–610

Friedmann, I 1977 The pathology of epidermoid
cholesteatoma; Proceedings of the international conference
cholesteatoma. Aesculapius, Birmingham (Al), p 10–22

Goodhill V 1982 Alternative approaches to CAT.
Proceedings of the 2nd international conference on
cholesteatoma and mastoid surgery. Kugler, Amsterdam,
p 527–532

Jansen C 1982 Combined approach tympanoplasty in

cholesteatoma surgery. Proceedings of the 2nd international
conference on cholesteatoma and mastoid surgery. Kugler,
Amsterdam, p 455–459

Litton W B 1977 Epidermal migration patterns in the ear
and possible relationship to cholesteatoma genesis.
Proceedings of the 1st international conference on
cholesteatoma. Aesculapius, Birmingham (Al), p 90–92

Marquet J 1982 Cholesteatoma—eradication of disease.
Proceedings of the 2nd international conference on
cholesteatoma and mastoid surgery. Kugler, Amsterdam,
p 475–78

Moritz W 1952 Plastische Eingriffe am Mittelohr.
Zeitschrift für Laryngologie und Rhinologie 31: 338–344

Nager G T 1977 Cholesteatoma of the middle ear—
pathogenesis and surgical indication. Proceedings of the
1st international conference on cholesteatoma. Aesculapius,
Birmingham (Al), p 193–203

Palva T, Ojala K 1982 Late results of obliteration
surgery in cholesteatoma. Proceedings of the 2nd
international conference on cholesteatoma and mastoid
surgery. Kugler, Amsterdam, p 495–496

Paparella M M 1982 Epilogue of the cholesteatoma and
mastoid surgery conference. Proceedings of the 2nd
international conference on cholesteatoma and mastoid
surgery. Kugler, Amsterdam, p 613–618

Pfaltz C R, Pfaltz R, Finkenzeller P 1982 Short and long-term
results in ossiculoplasty in cholesteatomatous ears.
Proceedings of the 2nd international conference on
cholesteatoma and mastoid surgery. Kugler, Amsterdam,
p 559–566

Pfaltz C R, Griesemer C 1984 Complications of acute middle
ear infections. Annals of Otology, Rhinology and
Laryngology 93 (suppl 112): 133–136

Pfaltz, C R, Griesemer C 1985 Pericard—a new biomaterial
for tympanoplasty. American Journal of Otology
6: 266–268

Portmann M 1982 Definition of success and failure in
cholesteatoma and mastoid surgery. Kugler, Amsterdam,
p 431–432

Sade J 1982 Treatment of retraction pockets and
cholesteatoma and mastoid surgery. Kugler, Amsterdam,
p 511–525

Schuknecht H F 1974 Keratoma (cholesteatoma), In:
Pathology of the ear. Harvard University Press, p 225–228

Sheehy J L, Robinson J V 1982 Revision tympanoplasty—
residual and recurrent cholesteatoma. Proceedings of the
2nd international conference on cholesteatoma and mastoid
surgery. Kugler, Amsterdam, p 443–448

Smyth G D L, Hassard T H 1982 What do we find at the
revision of mastoid surgery? Proceedings of the 2nd
international conference on cholesteatoma and mastoid
surgery. Kugler, Amsterdam, p 439–441

Wullstein H 1952 Funktionelle Operationen im Mittelohr.
Archiv für Ohren-Nasen-Kehlkopfheilkunde 161: 422–438

Yanagahira N 1982 Surgical treatment of cholesteatoma.
Proceedings of the 2nd international conference on
cholesteatoma and mastoid surgery. Kugler, Amsterdam,
p 483–490

Zoellner F 1954 Die Schalleitungsplastiken. Acta
Otolaryngologica 44: 370–384

7

Are we agreed as to the management of idiopathic facial palsy?

I. Munro

INTRODUCTION

The answer is 'no' for there is still controversy as regards both aetiology and treatment. Jongkees (1951) has pointed out that idiopathic facial palsy (Bell's palsy) is not the disease described by Sir Charles Bell in 1829. He did describe the sensory function of the trigeminal nerve and the motor function of the facial nerve. He did not describe the disease that now bears his name.

Until recently, Bell's palsy was accepted as an acute mononeuritic peripheral facial palsy of unknown aetiology. Kedar Adour, in his paper, 'The medical management of Bell's palsy', read at the VIth international workshop on otomicrosurgery and based on his experience of over 2000 cases, states that he has proven without doubt, with May in Pittsburgh, Djupesland in Norway, Korcyzn in Israel, and McGovern in West Virginia, that Bell's palsy is primarily a sensory craniopolyganglionitis in which the facial nerve is involved and is an innocent bystander in an inflammatory demyelinization. He also proposed that Bell's palsy be used as a general classification for all cases of peripheral facial paralysis and the term 'Antoni's palsy' be used in honour of the man who, in 1919, first described acute infectious polyneuritis cerebralis acusticofacialis, correctly interpreting the disease as a localized neuritis of the cranial and spinal ganglia.

My own interest in Bell's palsy, or Antoni's palsy, was stimulated in 1956, suffering a complete Bell's palsy myself.

I had treated some patients, by this time, with prednisolone and thought it had some effect, although Taverner (1954), having made the initial controlled clinical study, had concluded that the drug was not beneficial. Thomas (1955) believed it did have some effect. I took 120 mg of prednisolone in the first 24 hours, 100 mg in the second and third. Recovery started to take place on the ninth day and by the twelfth day was complete. I took the prednisolone for a further week in diminishing doses (Campbell 1954).

The dilemma was obvious—should one give all patients prednisolone immediately they were seen—both complete and incomplete cases, which would mean that a large number of cases would be given prednisolone who did not require it—or should one do nerve excitability tests and only give it to the patients who showed signs of degeneration? A decision was made to use prednisolone only in those cases who showed degeneration, but this was abandoned because signs of degeneration in some cases did not begin until after the seventh day and I could not convince myself that prednisolone was of value started so late after the onset of paralysis. I also decided not to give prednisolone to any patient under the age of 16 years, to pregnant women, or to patients whose medical condition contraindicated its use. At the beginning, we also excluded patients with hypertension.

The following results are not a scientific evaluation of prednisolone, or ACTH, but an appraisal of the results obtained in a retrospective study of 200 consecutive patients with Bell's palsy seen in the late 1950s and 1960s, which included recurrent cases of which there were 16, making a total of 216 cases. Of these, 60% were female, 40% male. There was no increase or decrease according to seasonal incidence. In 110 cases the right side was affected, in 106 the left side.

Frequent nerve excitability tests were carried out

in the first 3 weeks and those patients who showed evidence of degeneration were followed up for a year or more.

The age groups were as follows:

0–9: 13	40–49: 31
10–19: 35	50–59: 20
20–29: 42	60–69: 17
30–39: 31	70–79: 11

The results of patients who develop Bell's palsy under-30 years of age present a very different picture from the over-30 age group.

The under-30 age group, which comprised 101 cases, including recurrent ones, showed that: 87% recovered completely, 10% showed minimal degeneration, 3% showed moderate degeneration.

In the age group under 10, 13 children, including 1 little boy who had a recurrence on the other side of his face, making 14 cases in all, had a complete recovery. Only 1 case received prednisolone, although the policy was not to give steroids to patients under 16 years of age.

In the age group 20–29, there were 46 cases. Of these, 34 recovered completely, 9 showed minimal degeneration, 3 showed moderate degeneration.

Prednisolone was given to 5 of the cases out of the 12 who developed degeneration. Three cases who were started on prednisolone on the second, fourth and fifth day, had minimal degeneration and the other 2 cases developed moderate degeneration, having been started on prednisolone on the seventh and fourteenth day. These results make one believe that the earlier in the course of the disease prednisolone is given, the better.

In the under-30 age group, 25 cases were given prednisolone and 12 cases ACTH—a total of 37. Four cases given prednisolone developed minimal degeneration and 2 cases moderate degeneration. All 12 cases given ACTH recovered completely.

Included in this age group were 11 cases of recurrence. Five recurred on the same side and 6 on the opposite side. Four of the 11 cases showed minimal degeneration.

The 30 and over age group, which comprised 115 cases, including the recurrent ones, present a very different picture:

56% recovered completely
17% showed minimal degeneration
24% showed moderate degeneration
3% showed severe degeneration.

In this group 51 cases were given prednisolone and 13 cases were given ACTH (a total of 64 cases) of which:

41 recovered completely
13 showed minimal degeneration
10 showed moderate degeneration.

Of the remaining 51 cases who were not given prednisolone or ACTH:

23 recovered completely
9 showed minimal degeneration
15 showed moderate degeneration
4 showed severe degeneration.

These results again suggest the value of prednisolone or ACTH in limiting degeneration.

There were 5 recurrences in the over 30 age-group; 2 on the same side and 3 on the opposite side. In the much larger series of Adour's, there was no statistical difference in the two sides. Two of the 5 cases of recurrence showed minimal degeneration, and 1 showed moderate degeneration. Taken in conjunction with the 11 cases in the under-30 age-group, there is a greater liability in recurrent cases to show degeneration. In the 12 cases treated with ACTH:

7 recovered completely
5 showed minimal degeneration
1 showed moderate degeneration (this case, a female with hypertension, was given ACTH on the fourteenth day).

The total number of cases, 25 in all, treated with ACTH showed the following results:

20 recovered completely
5 showed minimal degeneration
1 showed moderate degeneration.

This small group of cases would support Deryck Tavener's view that ACTH diminishes the degree of denervation in Bell's palsy cases. In this small series, the patients attended the hospital for their injections under controlled conditions.

It is interesting that Ekstrand (1980) has advised treatment with ACTH instead of surgical management. I consider that the results, which have been described as recovered completely, minimal degeneration, moderate degeneration and severe degeneration, would compare closely with Erik Peiterson's table (Peiterson 1985, Table 7.1).

An opinion on the management of Bell's palsy necessitates some knowledge of the aetiology and diagnosis.

Table 7.1 Evaluation of ACTH in Bell's palsy

Grade	Palsy	Contracture	Ass. movements
0	No	No	No
I	Slight	Just visible	No
II	Moderate	Clearly visible	Yes
III	Severe	Disfiguring	Yes
IV	Complete	No	No

AETIOLOGY OF BELL'S PALSY

In October 1950, in a paper entitled, 'The treatment of facial paralysis' published in the *Proceedings of the Royal Society of Medicine*, Josephine Collier, in discussing Bell's palsy, stated that more than one pathological process may produce spontaneous facial paralysis. Since cases tend to appear in groups, or small epidemics and are sometimes associated with herpetic eruptions, not only of geniculate ganglion origin, but with involvement of other ganglia, it may be asked whether most cases are of viral origin. Occurrence in children of cases indistinguishable from Bell's palsy during epidemics of anterior poliomyelitis have been observed.

In support of the virus theory, six cases in one week convinced me of the 'cluster effect' and, also, a colleague had three cases of Bell's palsy in the same ward at the Maternity Hospital in Glasgow at the same time. In the late 1950s and early 1960s, I arranged for virology studies to be done and these revealed high titres to Herpes simplex in several cases. The result (in a letter from Virology Department to Mr Munro, dated 27.9.63) impressed me so much that it is printed in full below. It left no doubt in my mind that Bell's palsy could be associated with a primary infection by Herpes simplex:—

Dear Mr Munro,
Re: J.H.—facial paralysis:

I thought I would comment further on the report which was sent to you yesterday about the above patient. It was impossible to find an end point for the antibody titration within the normal limits of the tests with herpes simplex antigen. The record of such a high level of antibody must, I think, indicate that the patient is currently suffering from an infection with this virus and, if you could exclude facial herpes around the lips, then I think we have produced a diagnosis for you this time.

The person who suffers from recurrent herpes simplex on the lips, usually has a high antibody titre,

somewhere in the region between 32 to 128. It would obviously be worthwhile in this instance collecting a further specimen in a few weeks time, when the facial paralysis is healing, so that we might observe what is happening to the antibody. It is curious that this case has coincided with the appearance of a few others in Glasgow with enormous titres of herpes simplex antibody and I thought it worthwhile drawing your attention also to this fact, in case there is a minor epidemic of Herpes infection in general, picking out the facial nerve in a few instances, on the go at the minute.

Yours sincerely,
Dr R. G. Sommerville.

I am able to confirm that the patient had no facial herpes around the lips.

Interest now focuses on the Herpesviruses, or, at any rate, four of the five which commonly infect humans:
1. Herpes simplex virus—type 1
2. Varicella zoster virus
3. Cytomegalovirus
4. Epstein–Barr virus

1. Herpes simplex virus has been mentioned.

2. Varicella zoster virus. Clinical, immunological and virological findings have demonstrated that one virus (VZV) causes both varicella and herpes zoster. The epidemiology of the primary infection, varicella, is distinct from that of herpes zoster. Varicella is seen world-wide, occurs in seasonal epidemics and is a generalized erythematous disease, usually of childhood. Herpes zoster is a sporadic endemic disease. It generally occurs years after varicella and is the result of VZV reactivation within latently infected individuals. The clinical picture suggests that VZV latently affects dorsal root ganglion cells which are the focus of reactivation in herpes zoster (Bacon 1985).

The Ramsey Hunt syndrome is a lower motor neurone facial paralysis, ear pain, a varicelliform rash of the external auditory canal or pinna, and is assumed to be caused by the VZ virus.

The herpex simplex virus may produce disseminated lesions resembling varicella and may also produce segmentally focal lesions that resemble herpes zoster (Weller 1983). Further known herpes zoster reactivation occurs without the pathognomonic vesicles (zoster since herpete) (Ogino et al 1985).

In 1507 patients evaluated consecutively for facial

palsy, 185 (12%) of cases were attributed to herpes zoster (Robillard et al 1985). In the cases diagnosed as Bell's palsy, 4% proved to have herpes zoster. Diagnosis was based on acute and convalescent serum titres for varicella zoster virus or on the characteristic clinical presentation of the Ramsey Hunt syndrome. It also confirmed what had previously been accepted, that herpes zoster facial palsy was found to be more severe and have a less favourable recovery.

3. *Cytomegalovirus.* I.W.S. Mair, Department of Otorhinolaryngology, University of Tromso, Norway (Mair 1985) reported a series of 88 consecutive APFP cases in which significant CMV antibody levels were found in 64 (73%) and in only 3 of 94 (3.2%) controls. The epidemiology of CMV (Bacon 1985) is difficult to describe for at least two reasons. Firstly, no clear syndrome has been associated with primary infection, and secondly, isolation of CMV from an individual could indicate a recent primary infection, reactivation of a latent infection, or infection with an exogenous strain of CMV.

After a primary infection, an individual becomes persistently infected but it is unclear whether CMV is maintained in a latent (non-replicating) form or whether there is slow production of small amounts of virus by infected tissues. CMV may persist in epithelial cells of the renal tubules, the parotid gland, the cervix and possibly also in polymorphonuclear leucocytes. The interaction between CMV and humans resembles a chronic infection by a commensal virus which poses medical problems only in unusual circumstances when CMV acts as an opportunistic pathogen.

There is comparatively strong evidence for the aetiologic role of CMV in the Guillain–Barré syndrome (Bale 1984). The clinical course of Bell's palsy and the possibility of its recurrence are themselves similar in many respects to GBS (Abramsky et al 1975). Also, the same lymphocyte sensitization to the same purely neuritogenic basic protein P_1L, isolated from human peripheral nerve myelin, possibly indicates that Bell's palsy may represent a variant of GBS. In most cases it is a mononeuritic variant but occasionally it is possible that systemic polyneuropathy develops where only one facial nerve exhibits paralysis and the other side, or even other peripheral nerves, are involved sub-clinically, as has been proved by electrophysiological examination.

4. *Epstein–Barr virus* (Bacon 1985) is a ubiquitous virus in all populations and is transmitted horizontally in saliva. Primary infection occurs early in life in children living in developing countries. It is almost invariably subclinical and, by the age of 3 years, 99% of the children have been infected with EBV. In developed countries, infection is often delayed until late childhood or early adult life because of improved living conditions and standards of hygiene. Between 75% and 80% of the population in developed countries are seropositive for EBV. Primary infection results in specific immunity and persistence of EBV in the host, both of which are maintained for life. EBV has adopted two distinct strategies to persist throughout the life of the individual. The first involves a latent infection in some B-lymphocytes. Secondly, EBV also persists within the oropharynx, where a low level of infection is maintained.

Significant titre changes have been reported against EBV antigens in acute peripheral facial palsy patients, both with and without clinical symptoms of mononucleosis. Grose et al (1975) judged 3 out of 16 patients to be definitely associated with EBV and 2 others gave suggestive evidence.

Further support for the viral theory comes from the report by Bruce Proctor et al (1976). The patient was a man with an early case of Bell's palsy who suffered cardiac arrest during induction of anaesthetic for a decompression of the facial nerve and died three days later. The findings were of acute inflammation and demyelinization without evidence of vascular occlusion. Changes were evident throughout the entire course of the facial nerve from the internal auditory meatus to the stylomastoid foramen.

Kedar Adour (1981) believes that the herpes simplex virus, which is a DNA virus, is specific for sensory nerves once it enters the system and subsides to latency in the sensoriganglion nucleus. When it reactivates, the virus replicates in the nerve cell before migrating either up or down the axon and eventually breaks out of the neural compartment. When leaving the neural compartment, the virus picks up a coat of lipoprotein from the cell membrane and sets up a secondary autoimmune 'allergic reaction', or demyelinization.

Edstrom et al (1985) supports the view that Bell's

palsy is frequently associated with cranial neuropathy or brain-stem impairment, as judged by otoneurological, general neurological and neuro-ophthalmological examination. The fraction of the classic form of Bell's palsy, the true mononeuropathy of the facial neuron, seems to decrease along with refinements of the diagnostic procedures used. Their results have shown that Bell's palsy is frequently associated with different CNS disorders including central auditory pathways, the trigeminal nerve system, the ophthalmological system and degeneration of CNS myelin. He concludes that Bell's palsy is frequently associated with a cranial neuropathy with secondary manifestation of the extrapontine part of the facial nerve.

The diagnosis of Bell's palsy (cranial polyneuritis, cranial polyneuropathy, Antoni's palsy) is a facial paralysis of peripheral origin and of acute onset with no evidence of systemic disease (Deryck Taverner). Adour would add concomitant sensory cranial polyneuritis. The symptoms and signs are: 1. epiphora, 2. retroauricular pain, 3. taste disturbance, 4. hyperacusis, 5. numbness of the face, 6. decreased tears.

The physical findings include hypoaesthesia of cranial nerves V, IX, and cervical 2. Djupesland (1977) in Norway was the first to demonstrate hypoaesthesia of the 2nd cranial nerve. Motor paralysis of branches of the Xth cranial nerve are seen as unilateral shift of the palate or shortening of one vocal cord with rotation of the posterior larynx to the affected side. On experience based on over 2000 cases, Adour (1980) states that the superior laryngeal nerve is paralysed 10 times more frequently than the facial nerve and there is no bony canal to account for a 'compression palsy'. He also states that physical examination almost always reveals inflammation of the fungiform papillae of the tongue since the geniculate ganglion is the primary source of infection.

Topographic diagnosis is first of all to determine the anatomic site of the lesion and also the physiological extent of the nerve involvement. It is founded on the anatomy of the facial nerve and the site of the lesion is determined by:

1. Lacrimal flow (subjective and Schirmer's test)
2. Stapedial reflex (impedance audiometry)
3. Taste (qualitative—sweet, sour, acid and bitter)
4. Salivation—comparison of salivary flow by catheterizing Wharton's ducts.

The information gained from these tests should tell us:

1. Whether the entire motor portion of the facial nerve as it leaves the stylomastoid foramen, is involved (paralysis of all ipsilateral facial muscles).

2. Whether the lesion of the facial nerve is lateral to the geniculate ganglion, which should be the information gained in 1. plus,

   a. Impaired salivary secretion.

   b. Impaired taste in the anterior two thirds of the tongue.

   c. The stapedius muscle may be paralysed resulting in loss of the stapedial reflex.

Noise intolerance (hyperacusis) on the affected side is not related exclusively to paralysis of the stapedius muscle. It can occur with a normal stapedial reflex. Adour believes that it probably represents loss of inhibition to the cochlea and Edstrom, that lacrimal testing, salivatory testing and test of taste, as far as topographic value is concerned, are doubtful since each of them represent a specific function originating from its respective nucleus in the brain stem. This means that an injury of the facial nerve at the CNS level must not necessarily involve lacrimation, salivation or chorda tympani function. Partial destruction of the facial nucleus may even preserve the function of the stapedius reflex since the nerve fibre function units of the facial nerve correspond to their respective nuclear regions in the central nervous system.

3. Lesions of the facial nerve at, or medial to, the geniculate ganglion produce all the deficits described in 1. and 2. and impaired lacrimation on the side of the lesion is a consequence of destruction of the preganglionic parasympathetic fibres, leading to the sphenopalatine ganglion.

The results of these tests show discrepancy. For example, a marked decrease in lacrimation with a normal stapedial reflex. The validity and reliability of topographic tests is doubtful. Electric diagnostic testing helps to determine the physiological extent of nerve damage and predict prognosis. Most electrical tests are comparative, using the normal side as the control for the abnormal side. In cases of incomplete paralysis, repeat examination days later is necessary to obtain accurate results. The tests commonly used are minimal and maximal nerve excitability tests, electromyography (EMG) and evoked electromyography. This test is variously labelled as electroneuronography, electroneurography and neuromyography. In this test, instead of estimating by visual inspection the effect of nerve stimulus, the muscle action potential is recorded. The interval between the nerve stimulation and the start of the muscle potential—the facial nerve latency—can be measured accurately and is an acceptable indication of nerve function.

Interpretation of electrical tests.   In the surgical management of facial paralysis, electrodiagnosis is used for selection of cases. In the non-surgical management of facial paralysis, it is used to predict prognosis. Each test has limitations and all tests show abnormality days to weeks after degeneration. Serial nerve excitability tests are necessary and useful only in the early weeks of Bell's palsy. If testing indicates equal muscle response on both sides of the face, the patient can be expected to have complete return of facial function within 3–6 weeks, without complications of faulty nerve degeneration. If denervation has progressed from minimal to severe degeneration in 7–10 days, a greater and earlier return of volitional muscle motion can be expected than in patients with progression from normal to severe degeneration in 3–4 days.

TREATMENT

Prednisolone

The treatment of Bell's palsy is the same today for my patients as it was 30 years ago—prednisolone. Taverner et al (1971) and Adour et al (1972) felt that prednisolone was the treatment of choice. Lewis & Cochrane (1986) in their paper on systemic steroids in chronic severe asthma, pointed out that prednisone in itself is inactive and requires conversion by hepatic hydroxylation to its active form of prednisolone, but the rate of hydroxylation is affected by liver disease and shows individual variation. The dosage I used in 1956 was 60 mg per day for 3 days and 40 mg a day for 2 days, then 30 mg a day for 2 days, 20 mg a day for 2 days, 10 mg a day for 2 days and 5 mg a day for 2 days. This was far below the dose I had taken, so it was with great interest that I noted that Eberhard Stennert (1982) (University of Goettingen) gave a dose of 200–

250 mg a day of prednisolone by an infusion technique. Despite the high dosage, atrophy of the renal cortex was not expected because of the short term of therapy. In addition, for improved microcirculation with the aim of increased perfusion of the peripheral nerve with oxygen, he used low molecular dextran in combination with Pentoxifylline.

Closed head injuries have been treated with small, large and mega doses of steroids. Bracken and associates (1984), in a large clinical series, clearly demonstrated lack of any effect of high dosage (1000 mg of methyl-prednisolone daily for 10 days) compared with normal dosage (100 mg of methyl-prednisolone for 10 days) steroid treatment. The incidence of gastrointestinal haemorrhage and fluid electrolyte changes were greater in patients treated with high doses.

ACTH

Deryck Taverner, at the 2nd British Academic Conference, read a paper on the management of facial palsy in which he recommended using repeated injections of adrenocorticotrophic hormone (ACTH gel). In 77 consecutive cases of Bell's palsy, he reported an incidence of 16% denervation, which compared favourably with the 40% of denervation he had always found previously. At that meeting, the surgical decompressionists had their full team out—Cawthorn, Sullivan and Jongkees. Professor Miller and Deryck Taverner represented the non-surgical approach. Comment from Professor Miller: 'an operation, although feasible, may not necessarily be indicated'. Deryck Taverner commented, 'there is now strong evidence that early treatment with ACTH significantly diminishes the incidence of denervation and therefore of permanent sequelae. Properly applied, these methods should relegate the treatment of idiopathic facial palsy by the scientifically untested manoeuvre of surgical decompression to the realms of history'.

These are strong words, but I believe, in the stage of our present knowledge, are true. In the discussion that followed I related my own history and how I had been treating cases with prednisolone since the late 1950s, considering it the treatment of choice if given early, preferably in the first three days. I also considered that age, hypertension and severe pain were bad prognostic signs.

Surgical decompression

Depression was based on the vascular ischaemic theory (Hilgar 1949, McGovern 1968), which postulates dysfunction of blood vessels producing vasoconstriction on exposure to cold or other stimuli. Ischaemia and thrombosis lead to swelling and compression of the nerve within its rigid and bony canal— the vascular entrapment phenomenon. Later, the oedema was attributed to viral inflammatory swelling or to an abnormal immunological response.

Wolferman (1974), in his critical evaluation, shows the rationality of decompression can be challenged.

Anson and his co-workers (Anson et al 1963, 1970, 1973) have demonstrated that the facial nerve occupies only a small portion of the lumen of the fallopian canal, leaving a vast space for expansion.

Jongkees (1972) believed that compression is caused by the fibres of the sheath and, as soon as the sheath is incised, the nerve bulges out. The significance of bulging is questionable, as all nerves bulge when their sheaths are split. Sade et al (1966) believe that bulging of the nerve does not indicate any pathology. The theory of sheath constriction can also be challenged in view of electromicroscopic investigations by Harkin & Skinner (1970). They found that, in generating nerves, the sheath is highly cellular and any constricting or unyielding property of either the myelin or the Schwann sheath is difficult to imagine.

Devriese (1972) investigated the effects of decompression on the normal facial nerve in cats and found the nerve was damaged in 7 out of the 12.

Adour states that facial nerve palsy does recur even though a technically complete decompression has been performed. He also has knowledge of five documented cases of acute facial paralysis who have had no recovery of facial function. All five of these cases received facial nerve decompression, which indicates that further damage was done to the nerve by surgery.

Olson et al (1973) published the first series of auditory complications associated with facial nerve decompression.

The histology report of Bruce Proctor shows that the nerve is involved throughout its whole length. The questioning of topographic diagnosis, which is no longer assumed to be 100% accurate and which negates the belief that the nerve impulse is blocked out at a specific site of involvement, challenges the rationality of decompression.

The appearance of oedema of the nerve at operation has been described by many surgeons who have had experience of facial nerve decompression: Ballance & Duel (1932), Cawthorne (1946), Kettel (1947), Sullivan & Smith (1950), Fisch & Esslen (1972). The existence of oedema is not supported by Josephine Collier who, on decompressing the nerve for Bell's palsy, found a normal nerve, at other times an attenuated nerve compressed by fibrous tissue at the stylomastoid foramen, or with dense scar tissue extending over the various lengths of the vertical course. The success or failure of the operation had little relation to the operative findings or treatment, suggesting that, in the cases in which there was no return of movement, the lesion was central to the middle ear.

The existence of oedema of the facial nerve has also been questioned by Sunderland (1946), Sade (1972), Diamond & Frew (1979). Adour & Diamond (1982) point out that the operation has been abandoned in Great Britain. In 1971, Adour & Swanson (1971) concluded that surgery performed on the basis of electic tests was not beneficial to recovery.

Adour and Diamond have shown in each decade, as the time in which to perform surgical intervention has decreased, the anatomic extent of decompression has increased to the entire length of the nerve. Brockman (1974) and Fisch (1977) returned to decompressing segments of the nerve. The timing of surgical intervention after the onset of the paralysis has undergone wide fluctuation from two months to nine months and back again to two months, then two weeks, and finally to within a few days. Peter Bumm et al (1982) decompress only patients with complete degeneration and state that the time factor after the onset of paralysis is irrelevant. Ugo Fisch, where electroneuronography study shows that 90% of facial nerve fibres have undergone degeneration within two weeks from onset of the palsy, decompresses the meatus and labyrinthine segments through a middle cranial fossa approach.

CONCLUSION

Bell's palsy would appear to be acute cranial polyneuritis which can present as a mononeuritis. The aetiology may be herpes simplex reactivation caused by different factors, such as draughts, other viruses or pregnancy. Prednisolone seems to be helpful in limiting the degree of degeneration and is widely used throughout the world. It should be given as soon as possible after the onset of palsy, certainly within three days. Possibly larger doses should be used than are being used at present. At hospital level, patients' progress can be monitored with the stapedial reflex—which is accurate in 80% of cases and electrodiagnosis. The evidence against decompression appears now to be overwhelming, but one must accept that there is still a percentage of patients who develop degeneration with contracture, synkinesia and facial spasm, and sometimes gustatory tears (crocodile tears), for which we have no answer.

Does the future lie in antiviral drugs or even in producing a vaccine against the herpesviruses? Adour, who now has experience of managing over 2000 cases, is at present carrying out a double-blind study: 1. the patients get prednisone, 2. the patients get prednisone plus acyclovir (personal communications).

I also understand from Adour that, in a multi-centre investigation in the USA a controlled study of decompression as performed by Ugo Fisch (1982) and based on electroneuronography studies is at present being carried out.

The results of these studies are awaited with great interest and hope for the approximately 15% of cases who still develop moderate to severe permanent degeneration.

When discussing any aspect of idiopathic facial nerve palsy (Bell's palsy) we must first be sure of the diagnosis. Although the diagnosis is eventually one of exclusion, we can make a provisional diagnosis based on Taverner's (1965) criteria:

1. Paralysis of all the muscles of expression on one half of the face, but not necessarily complete.

2. Sudden onset.

3. Absence of any symptom or sign of disease of the central nervous system.

4. Absence of any symptom or sign of disease of the ear or posterior fossa.

However, Adour has found that the majority of his cases of Bell's palsy had involvement of other cranial nerves, especially the trigeminal and glossopharyngeal. He said (Adour 1978), 'Bell's palsy was an acute, benign, cranial polyneuritis (probably caused by reactivation of the herpes simplex virus) and that the dysfunction of motor cranial nerves (V, VII, X) may represent inflammation and demyelination rather than ischemic compression.' However, Bento et al (1985) from Sao Paulo examined this point in 107 consecutive cases very carefully and concluded:

1. We didn't find a significant difference between the control group and the 107 patients tested.

2. The idiopathic facial palsy was an isolated pathology in the great majority of cases.

3. If there occurs some other involvement of cranial nerves, it was subclinical.

To reach a diagnosis of Bell's palsy it is therefore necessary to take a careful history—the exact date of onset of the palsy and whether it was of slow or sudden onset. The patient is questioned regarding the presence of aural pain or discharge, taste alterations, dryness of the affected eye, hearing loss or vertigo. Whether or not any trauma to the head or ear has occurred recently is an important part of the history. Careful examination of the patient's face is made to assess the palsy and every attempt made to see if there is any voluntary movement. A careful examination of the head and neck, especially the parotid, and a full neurological examination are necessary. Special attention is given to the ear on the affected side looking for any sign of local disease, e.g. carcinoma of the external auditory meatus, cholesteatoma, etc. A careful look for blebs or blisters in the canal and on the soft palate is especially necessary in order to exclude Ramsay Hunt syndrome. Some investigations are necessary, such as a full blood count, sedimentation rate and serological tests such as a fluorescent treponemal antibodies test. If there is any suspicion of diabetes, such as obesity or family history, a glucose tolerance test is necessary. It is debatable whether a fasting glucose test is worthwhile. It is the practice of the author to order a computerized tomogram of the petrous temporal bones in all cases of idiopathic facial nerve palsy. Dr Bruce Doust of the Department of Radiology, St Vincent's Hospital, Sydney, Australia has described the procedure:

> The examination should be performed on a high resolution CT scanner. Prior to the study, the patient should be instructed to remain motionless throughout the examination so that the axial slices can be used to produce off-axis reformated images if necessary. Axial slices 1.5 mm thick, at 1.5 mm intervals, should be taken throughout the petrous temporal bone and reconstructed using an algorithm designed to optimize spatial resolution. The resulting images should be displayed with a window of 4000.

Again, in some cases, it may be necessary to investigate the function of the labyrinth (e.g. where there is a complaint of vertigo, or nystagmus has been seen), but it is not necessary in all cases.

The question arises as to whether prognostic electrical tests should be carried out immediately. The author believes it is highly advantageous to have the chosen electrical tests carried out at the primary visit to establish base levels. No specific electrical test is so superior that it is used to the exclusion of all others. The tests of motor nerve function available are:

1. Minimal nerve excitability test (NET)

2. Maximal stimulation test (MST)

3. Electroneuronography (ENOG)

4. Electromyography (EMG)

Whatever test or tests are used, they should be regarded as a guide and used in conjunction with clinical examination and judgement. It is important to remember that the most slight or fleeting voluntary movement is the best indicator of a good prognosis. The electrical tests are only indicated when there is complete or total paralysis of all the muscles of expression. Also available are tests of efferent parasympathetic fibres to the lacrimal and submandibular gland, e.g. lacrimation studies, salivary flow, and pH levels.

The minimum nerve excitability test (NET) was devised by Jongkees (1969, 1977) and further described by Cawthorne (1965), Hilger (1964) and May (1977). The test is a comparison of the electrical conductive capacity of the paralysed facial nerve as against the normal side. The test can be performed with any electrical stimulator in which the strength of the current and its direction can be varied. The author has used the Medelec type FS1 as described by Cawthorne (1965) and Cawthorne et al (1963, 1969). This is a small battery-operated stimulator giving a square wave impulse of 1 millisecond duration at a constant voltage. The strength of the current can be varied from 1 to 10 milliamps and is similar to the one described by Hilger (1964).

It is important to remember that you are comparing the muscle response to electrical stimulation on the normal side to the paralysed side. Therefore, you must be sure that the muscle response on the normal side is truly normal. There may be a congenital neuromuscular disorder or some acquired disorder on the 'normal side'. There may have been a previous Bell's palsy, injury to the nerve or muscles, myasthenia gravis, or other facial myopathies.

The patient is seated and reassured that no pain or discomfort arises from the test. The skin is prepared for the application of electrodes in the usual manner with alcohol and gentle rubbing. The reference electrode in Hilger's (1964) description is placed in the groove between the mastoid and mandible. In Cawthorne and colleagues (1965, 1963, 1969) description, the indifferent electrode is attached to the skin of the upper arm by means of a saline-soaked pad and held there by means of a perforated rubber belt. The stimulating electrode, anode, is placed about 2–3 centimetres anterior to the posterior border of the ramus of the mandible. Jongkees (1969, 1977) felt there should be as small a distance as possible between the cathode and the anode. May (1977) (and Cawthorne et al) felt that this was not important. The stimulation begins on the normal side and the stimulus is increased. The minimum amount of current required to give rise to a just perceptible muscle flicker is determined. This varies between 1 milliamp to 4 milliamps, about 1.5 milliamps is commonly seen. The stimu-

lating electrode is then placed in the same position on the paralysed side and, again, the current required to give rise to some perceptible muscle flicker is determined. A difference in current of 2 milliamps to 3.5 milliamps is considered to be significant.

The test has considerable test–retest variability, so it should be repeated several times to be sure of the observations. The test should be repeated every other day—if the excitability remains the same, confidence in an early recovery is justified. A rapid rise in the difference in excitability between the normal and the paralysed side is thought to indicate that myelin degeneration is taking place.

The maximum stimulation test (MST) is Landau's modification of the Jongkee's test, using maximum rather than minimal stimulation. The same battery-powered apparatus is used. The patient is told that the application of the current is designed to give rise to maximum stimulation and may give rise to some discomfort. For some patients, the discomfort is extreme.

The current output is increased on the non-paralysed side to the maximum amount that can be tolerated by the patient without extreme discomfort. The amount of muscle contraction is observed carefully. Then the probe is placed on the paralysed side and the same current that produced the maximum contraction on the non-paralysed side is turned on. The amount of contraction produced is observed. The contraction produced could be described as the same (normal), reduced, or greatly reduced. A significant result is present if the amount of contraction produced is greatly reduced or absent altogether.

May's studies (May et al 1971) on 37 patients with Bell's palsy using the MST are considered to be extremely valuable. He examined all of his patients within 10 days of the onset of the Bell's palsy and assessed them again at 6 months. He concluded that if the MST results on the non-paralysed and the paralysed side were equal, there was a 92% chance of complete recovery. If the results of the MST were greatly reduced or absent, there was only a 14% chance of complete recovery.

The author now only uses the MST test. It is valuable and can be carried out in the office quickly and repeated every second day, and the results carefully documented. The MST in the author's opinion is more reliable because it is not subject to test-retest variability. Different observers on the same day can obtain the same results invariably. The MST is a subjective test, while the next test to be described has the valuable advantage of being objective.

Electroneuronography (ENOG) has many names. In the USA, it is commonly known as evoked electromyography or EEMG.

In this test, the facial nerve is stimulated and the resultant combined action potential (CAP) is detected in the nasolabial crease and recorded. The CAP is the summation potential produced by the simultaneous firing of many motore units. The CAP recorded is assumed to be typical of the response that would be found as a result of stimulation of any of the major branches of the facial nerve.

The skin of the face is prepared for electrode placement in the usual way. The patient is seated and reassured that the test is not painful, nor will they feel any discomfort. The ground electrode is placed in the depression between the mastoid and the mandible. The reference and recording electrodes are placed alongside the nasal alae. The stimulating electrode is placed about 2 centimetres in a horizontal line anterior to the ground electrode.

The skin resistance is important—the preparation of the skin must be thorough to reduce the resistance to less than 10 000 ohms. The author, uses a Medelec Sensor as a stimulus generator. According to Hughes and his associates (1983) the following protocol has reduced test-retest variability. Firstly, the stimulus intensity should be increased until the pain threshold is reached, and then reduced. Secondly, it should be ascertained if this stimulus intensity is causing contraction of the muscles. If there is muscle contraction, the stimulus must be reduced until this is absent. 'The ideal stimulus intensity is one that avoids discomfort and trigeminal nerve artifact, but attains maximal response. This ideal stimulus intensity is not possible in every patient' (Hughes 1985). As is usual in all electrical tests of the facial nerve, there is considerable test-retest variability and several test procedures must be carried out. The CAP is measured from peak to peak. The CAP is compared—the paralysed to the non-paralysed—and the result is documented as a percentage. This percentage comparison is said to represent the number of non-degenerated fibres present. Experimental evidence confirms this 1:1 ratio between the ENOG finding and actual nerve fibre loss. Fisch (1981) has written about ENOG as a prognostic test and an indicator for surgical decompression. He states that a better than 90% CAP predicts a satisfactory outcome for the Bell's palsy: 'as long as 10% of the facial nerve fibres remain conductive for electrically evoked nerve impulses, a sufficient number of endoneural tubes remain intact and ensures proper regeneration of the degenerated nerve fibres'. When there is less than 10% fibres active it indicates the need for surgical decompression. He reviewed a small number of cases (7 patients) in which these strict criteria were observed and reported that surgical decompression had improved the chance of satisfactory facial function.

Electromyography (EMG) is a traditional test that still has usefulness. In a patient with complete paralysis, EMG will give the following results:

1. Normal motor unit response to attempted voluntary contraction of the muscle group being tested.

2. Fibrillation potentials, i.e. no motor unit potential when voluntary contraction is attempted, but a continuous state of involuntary contractions with a variable amplitude between 10 and 200 mV. These fibrillation potentials indicate that the nerve supply to the muscle being tested has undergone degeneration.

3. Recovery potentials. These are the so-called nascent motor units that are irregular, small in amplitude and polyphasic (four phases usually). These nascent units are seen in the early stages of nerve regeneration and hence are a valuable sign.

EMG is not a valuable test in the prognosis of early complete paralysis, because fibrillation potentials (indicating nerve degeneration) do *not* appear until about 14–21 days after the beginning of nerve degeneration.

Although there is evidence (May et al 1976) that salivary flow studies may be good indicators of likely degeneration, the test has never become popular and the author has no personal experience. Recently, Rosen and his associates (1985) from Emek Hospital, Israel, in an article entitled 'Submandibular salivary gland scan', concluded: 'as one can see from the results the validity of the test shown here is no better than other time-honoured tests. With our test we did not get any breakthrough in the prognostic tests of facial palsy. But if you believe in the salivary collecting test, then we suggest that you try our method'.

The only real question to be decided, when considering the question of medical management, is whether or not to use steroids. There have been many trials but Stankiewiez (1983) concluded that most had faulty study design and methodology. Ardour (1972) started a most ambitious and well designed study, but unfortunately aborted the study when he felt that steroid administration was so superior that he could not withhold this treatment from his control group. May's study (May 1976), four years later, was again well designed, but the number of patients in the study (51 patients) is thought to be too small. May concluded that steroid administration conferred no significant benefit to patients with Bell's palsy.

Why is it that no universally accepted study has been carried out that will definitely solve the question of whether steroid administration is beneficial in Bell's palsy? Many modern investigators feel the dosage of steroid in these early studies was far too small for any meaningful results to emerge.

The author's opinion is that steroid administration is necessary. The only question to be decided is the dosage schedule. Two schedules are popular:

1. Low dosage schedule: 60 mg to 5 mg in a daily dose, tapering over twelve days.

2. High dosage schedule: 250 mg (per day for 4 days) and then tapering off by 25 mg per day for 10 days. The author favours schedule (2.). The usual absolute contraindications to steroid therapy do, of course, apply: e.g. pregnancy, peptic ulceration, psychiatric disturbance, diabetes or hypertension. With the careful advice and management of a consultant physician, some of the above contraindications may be overcome.

The most controversial question has been the value or not of surgical decompression. The opponents of surgery in the management of Bell's palsy state that not only is if of unproven value, but that it is based on an old and outmoded notion of the pathology of Bell's palsy. That is, that the paralysis is due to ischaemia based on oedema—causing more ischaemia. Decompression (i.e. removing the constricting bony confines) was thought to break this vicious cycle. The proponents of surgical decompression must now rely on carefully controlled and documented prospective studies to prove their case. Fisch (1982) has carried out such a study and concluded that decompression of the geniculate

ganglion and labyrnthine segment of the facial nerve was worthwhile in carefully selected cases.

The question is, where should one decompress and what cases justify the operation? The question of where decompression should be carried out is one that has fuelled the fire of opponents of surgical management of facial palsy. At first, those surgeons who advocated surgery advised that only the lowermost portion of the descending (mastoid) segment should be decompressed. Gradually, the amount of decompression extended up to the cochleariformus process.

Careful evaluation of the patient's palsy (Schirmer's test) may show a very small percentage of patients that would justify surgery on the tympanic and mastoid portions only, but in those patients who can justifiably be put forward as candidates for surgery, the decompression should take place in the region of the geniculate ganglion and the labyrinthine segment of the nerve. Although it can be shown that the geniculate ganglion can be reached by this mastoid approach (dislocating the incus and later replacing it) the proximal portion of the labyrinthine segment of the facial nerve can rarely be safely seen from this approach (Goin 1982). The labyrinthine segment of the facial nerve slopes rapidly downwards as well as medially from the geniculate ganglion, that is why the proximal half of the labyrinthine segment is especially difficult to visualize from the mastoid approach.

Therefore, the author stongly feels that if a decompression of the ganglion region is going to be attempted, the middle fossa approach should be the approach of choice. Naturally, this operation requires special training and neurosurgical co-operation and, sometimes, neurosurgical consultation, especially in a middle-aged or elderly patient. Another consideration is the incidence of sensorineural deafness (at least 5%) that occurs in middle fossa decompression. The patients who may be candidates for decompression need a detailed audiological work-up. The basal coil of the cochlea and the facial nerve are most intimately associated in the labyrinthine segment, and, indeed in some cases, the bony division may be lacking.

To summarize, decompression of the geniculate ganglion and the labyrinthine segment of the facial nerve, in a middle cranial fossa approach, is indicated only if the following criteria are met, and it must be stressed that this is an extremely uncommon situation.

1. There is complete paralysis of all the facial muscles on one side.

2. By careful exclusion, it is certain that the paralysis is indeed idiopathic (Bell's palsy).

3. An adequate course of steroids (schedule 2.) has been given.

4. MST is absent or *greatly* reduced.

5. ENOG shows that less than 10% of fibres are active.

6. No fibrillation potentials are obtained on EMG, and there is a complete absence of action potentials on attempted voluntary movement.

7. Speech discrimination on the normal (non-paralysed) side is adequate.

AETIOLOGY

The aetiology of idiopathic facial nerve palsy is still uncertain. For this reason it is to be expected that its management is controversial. A possible relationship between Bell's palsy and a reactivated herpes simplex virus (HSV) infection has been considered by both authors. However, other viral agents such as varicellazoster virus (Leeming 1976), Epstein–Barr virus (Proctor et al 1976) and cytomegalovirus (Mair 1985) have also been associated with Bell's palsy. Furthermore, there is recent evidence that the tick-borne spirochaetes causing Lyme disease and Bannwarth's syndrome have been aetiologically related to Bell's palsy (Steere et al 1983). Figure 7.1 illustrates possible neuropathological pathways in this disease. Whatever the causation agent, it is reasonable to assume that there are several different pathogenetic mechanisms resulting in facial palsy. In this respect, it must also be considered that recent findings of polyneuropathy (Rosenhall et al 1983, Hanner et al 1986, Edström et al—in press, Hanner et al—submitted for publication) suggest CNS impairment and also may demonstrate secondary changes in the peripheral part of the facial nerve (Aldskogius 1974). This means that the cited criteria of Taverner, concerning absence of CNS features in Bell's palsy, can be abandoned. In fact, similarities have previously been discussed between Bell's palsy and multiple sclerosis regarding age of onset, relapses and recoveries (Hedner et al 1980), signs of migration, evidence of demyelination, axonal degeneration of the optic nerve (Hanner et al—submitted for publication) and auditory brain stem

abnormalities (Rosenhall et al 1983, Edström et al—in press). Furthermore, Bell's palsy is 15 times more frequent in patients with multiple sclerosis than in a normal population (Hedner et al 1980). This suggests that Bell's palsy occasionally may be part of a more widespread neuropathy.

CLINICAL INVESTIGATION

We agree with Tonkin that it is necessary to take a careful history and to perform a clinical examination in order to distinguish trauma, tumours and ear infections from Bell's palsy. Furthermore, an accurate clinical examination is usually sufficient to predict a satisfactory prognosis of the facial palsy. It is well recognized that the following factors are associated with an unfavourable prognosis: 1. elderly patients (> 60 years), 2. slow onset (> 3 days), 3. postauricular pain, 4. complete paralysis, 5. diabetes, 6. herpes zoster, 7. failing remission within 3 weeks after onset of disease.

In this respect, electrical tests may provide additional prognostic information. However, it is probable that the physician's own experience of different tests play the most important role to obtain reliable predictive information. This also concerns lacrimation tests, salivatory tests and tests of taste which have been demonstrated to be beneficial in predicting the outcome of the facial palsy. It seems quite clear that the value of these tests is dependent upon the particular experience of each doctor. While the prognosis in many cases may be fairly well established, the topographical significance of these non-motor tests is doubtful, since each of them represents a specific function originating from its respective nucleus in the brain stem (Edström et al 1985). This means that injury of the facial nerve at the CNS level need not necessarily involve lacrimation, salivation or chorda tympany function. A partial destruction of the facial nucleus may even preserve the function of the stapedium reflex, since the nerve fibre function units of the facial nerve correspond to their respective nuclear regions in the CNS.

Dr. Tonkin suggests computerized tomography (CT) of the petrous temporal bone in all cases of idiopathic facial nerve palsy. We cannot understand

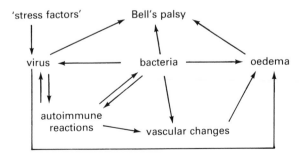

Fig. 7.1 Neuropathological dynamics in Bell's Palsy.

the reason for this investigation in every single case. From our point of view we order a CT of the brain stem and cerebral tissues as well as the temporal bone in cases of persistent complete facial paralysis for more than 2 months, primarily in order to eliminate the possibility of malignancy. In addition, when using CT with contrast enhancement in a consecutive series of 13 patients with acute facial palsy, Edström and Hanner (unpublished) found a plaque localized adjacent to the lateral ventricle on the right side in 1 patient in the acute stage of the disease. The facial palsy was on the contralateral side! Obviously, there was no anatomical connection between the plaque and the facial tracts. The patient was re-examined 3 months later and this alteration, as well as the facial palsy had disappeared. Such tomographic findings have previously been demonstrated in the acute stage of multiple sclerosis (Weinstein et al 1978). Recently, cortical alterations have been demonstrated in another study by using nuclear magnetic resonance (Thomander et al, personal communication).

TREATMENT

Both authors advocate steroid administration. However, it must be emphasized that objections can be raised against steroids since no study has yet demonstrated definite differences with respect to recovery. This is partly due to the high spontaneous recovery rate of > 75% and also due to difficulties in obtaining objective measurements of the recovery progress. Although different opinions exist about the value of steroids, adverse side-effects are extremely rare with short-term therapy. We delay steroid administration in patients with Bell's palsy until better scientific evidence is available.

A possible relationship between HSV and Bell's palsy has recently become of particular interest since specific therapy is now available. If HSV is aetiologically involved in some cases of Bell's palsy, there is experimental support for the view that the site of the lesion producing the facial nerve dysfunction should be located in the CNS rather than in the extrapontine part of the facial nerve (Townsend & Baringer 1978). This means that antiviral treatment probably needs to be administered in high doses compared to HSV-induced skin eruptions. A possible HSV aetiology cannot be ruled out, since virus replication might well have ceased at the time of onset of the facial palsy. This means that, even if antiviral therapy is started immediately after development of the facial palsy, it may already be too late.

During the last few years, increased interest has been focused on *Borrelia spirochaetosis* associated with a variety of neuropathological disorders. At the ENT department in Göteborg, Dr Hanner has demonstrated significant serum titres in 33% of patients with Bell's palsy. Age-matched healthy individuals showed no antibodies against *Borrelia*. These findings may encourage a new view of the management of some patients with Bell's palsy. An investigation is in progress in Göteborg for the evaluation of intravenous administration of Bensyl penicillin.

Both Drs Monroe and Tonkin have restrained opinions about the clinical benefits of surgical intervention in Bell's palsy. Decompression was early regarded as a therapeutic means directed against the frequently recognized oedema in the intratemporal part of the nerve. Subsequently, surgical decompression frequently included the middle fossa with obvious risks, even in experienced hands. Our experience of surgical decompression has decreased in Sweden during the last decade. Nevertheless, wherever the primary injury may be located it must not be forgotten that surgical decompression of the facial nerve in Bell's palsy may improve peripheral nerve conduction.

REFERENCES

I Munro

Abramsky O, Webb C, Teitelbaum D Arnon 1975 Journal of the Neurological Sciences 26

Adour K K 1981 Proceedings of 6th Shambaugh International Workshop and 3rd Shea Fluctuant Hearing Loss Symposium. Strobe Publications

Adour K, Diamond C 1982 Otolaryngology: Head & Neck Surgery 90

Adour K K, Swanson P J 1971 Transactions of the American Academy of Opthalmology and Otolaryngology 75 Transactions of The American Academy of Opthalmology and Otolaryngology 77

Adour K K, Wingerd J 1972 New England Journal of Medicine 287: 1268

Adour K K, Schneider G D, Hilsinger R L, Jun., 1980 Otolaryngology and Head and Neck Surgery 88: 418–424

Anson B J, Harper D G, Werpeka R C 1963 Annals of Otology, Rhinology and Laryngology 72
Anson B J, Donaldson J A, Werpeka R C et al 1970 Annals of Otology, Rhinology and Laryngology 79
Anson B J, Donaldson J A, Werpeka R C 1973 Archives of Otolaryngology 97
Bacon T 1985 Hospital Update 2, no 8
Bale J 1984 Archives of Neurology 41
Ballance, Duel 1932 Archives of Otolaryngology 15
Bracken & associates 1984 Journal of The American Medical Association 251, no 1: 45–82
Brockman S J 1974 Laryngoscope 84
Bumm P, Hirschberger H, Thumfart W, Wigand M 1982 In: Graham M D, House W F Raven Press, New York
Campbell E D R 1954 British Medical Journal 17: 215
Cawthorne T 1946 Laryngoscope 56
Collier J 1951 Proceedings of The Royal Society of Medicine 44
Devriese P P 1972 Archives of Otolaryngology 95
Diamond C, Frew I 1979 Oxford University Press, p 142
Djupesland G, Degre M, Stein R, Skrede S (eds) 1977 Archives of Otolaryngology 103: 641
Edstrom S, Aldskogius H, Hanner P, Rosenhall U 1985 In: Myers E (ed) New dimensions in otorhinolaryngology—head and neck surgery, vol 1. Elsevier Science Publishers
Ekstrand T 1980 Bell's palsy: Prognosis and treatment: A study of the accuracy of some prognostic indicators and evaluation of treatment with adrenocorticotrophic hormone. Thesis: Umea, Sweden
Fisch U 1977 Proceedings of the Shambaugh 5th international workshop on middle ear microsurgery and fluctuant hearing loss, Huntsville, Ala Strode Publishers Inc
Fisch U 1982 In: Graham M D, House W F (eds). Raven Press, New York
Fisch U, Esslen E 1972 Archives of Otolaryngology 95
Groves J, Scott Brown W G, Ballantyne J, Groves J (eds) 1965 Diseases of the ear, nose and throat, vol 2. Butterworth & Co, 2nd edn
Grose C, Henle W, Henle G et al 1975 New England Journal of Medicine 202
Harkin J C, Skinner M S 1970 Experimental and electron microscopic studies of nerve regeneration. Annals of Otology, Rhinology and Laryngology 79: 218–226
Hilgar J A 1949 Laryngoscope 59
Jongkees L B W 1951 Journal of Neurology
Jongkees L B W 1972 On peripheral facial nerve paralysis Archives of Otolaryngology 95, 317–323
Kettel K 1947 Archives of Otolaryngology 46
Lewis D, Cochrane G M 1986 British Medical Journal 292: 1289–1346
McGovern F H 1968 Laryngoscope 78
Mair I W S 1985 In: Myers E (ed) New dimensions in otorhinolaryngology—head and neck surgery, vol 1. Elsevier Science Publishers, BV
Ogino S, Okada M, Tamaki H, Matsunaga T, Takahashin 1986 Early diagnosis of 'zoster sine herpete'. In: Portmann M (ed) Proceedings of the 5th international symposium on the facial nerve, Sept 3–6. Bordeaux. Masson, New York
Olson N R, Goin D W, Nicholas R D et al 1973
Peiterson E 1985 In: Myers E (ed) New dimensions in otorhinolaryngology-head and neck surgery, vol 1. Elsevier Science Publishers, BV
Proctor B, Corgil D A, Proud G 1976 Transactions of The American Academy of Opthalmology and Otolaryngology 82: 70–80
Robillard R B, Hilsinger R L, Adour K K 1985 Herpes zoster facial paralysis: presented in part at the annual meeting of the American Academy of Otolaryngology–Head and Neck Surgery. Atlanta, Georgia, October 19–24
Sade J 1972 Archives of Otolaryngology 95
Sade J, Levy E, Chaco J 1966 Archives of Otolaryngology 82
Stennert E 1982 In: Graham M D, House W F (eds) Raven Press, New York
Sullivan J A, Smith J B 1950 Annals of Otology, Rhinology and Laryngology 59
Sunderland S 1946 Brain 69
Taverner D 1954 Lancet ii: 1052
Taverner D, Cohen S B, Hutchinson B C 1971 British Medical Journal 4: 80
Thomas M H 1955 Neurology 5: 882
Weller T H 1983 Varicella and Herpes zoster. New England Journal of Mecicine
Wolferman A 1974 The present status of therapy of Bell's paralysis—a critical evaluation. Annals of Otology, Rhinology and Laryngology, May–June

J P Tonkin

Adour K K 1972 Prednisone treatment for idiopathic facial paralysis. National English Journal of Medicine 287: 1268–1272
Adour K K et al 1978 The true nature of Bell's palsy: analysis of one thousand consecutive patients. Laryngoscope 88: 787–801
Bento R F et al 1985 Cranial nerve alterations during Bell's palsy. In: Myers E (ed) New dimension in otorhinolaryngology, head & neck surgery, vol 2. Elsevier Science Publishers BV, Amsterdam p 266–267
Cawthorne T 1965 Geniculate ganglion facial palsy. Archives of Otolaryngology 81: 502
Cawthorne T 1969 Gowers Memorial Lecture: Intratemporal facial nerve surgery. Archives of Otolaryngology 90: 794
Cawthorne R, Wilson T 1963 Indications for intratemporal facial nerve surgery. Archives of Otolaryngology 78: 429
Fisch U 1981 Surgery for Bell's palsy. Archives of Otolaryngology 107: 1–11
Fisch U 1982 Results of surgery vs conservative treatment in Bell's palsy and herpes zosta oticus. In: Graham M D, House W F (eds) Disorders of the facial nerve. Raven Press, New York, 273–278
Goin D W 1982 Proximal intratemporal facial nerve in Bell's palsy surgery—a study correlating anatomical and surgical findings. Laryngoscope 92: 263–271
Hilger J A 1964 New instrument. TransAmerican Academy of Ophthalmology & Otolaryngology 14: 510–520
Hughes G B 1985 Textbook of clinical otology. Thieme-Stratton, New York, p 235
Hughes G B et al 1983 Analysis of test-retest variability in facial electroneuronography. Otolaryngology, Head & Neck Surgery 91: 290–293
Jongkees L B W 1969 Tests for facial nerve function. Archives of Otolaryngology 89: 153–156
Jongkees L B W 1977 Nerve excitability test. In: Fisch U (ed) Facial nerve surgery. Aesculapius, Birmingham, Al, p 83–86

May M 1976 The use of steroids in Bell's palsy: a prospective controlled study. Laryngoscope 86: 1111–1122

May M 1977 Maximal excitability test. In: Fisch U (ed) Facial nerve surgery. Aesculapius, Birmingham, Al, p 87–91

May M et al 1971 The prognostic accuracy of the maximal stimulation compared with that of the nerve excitability test in Bell's palsy, Laryngoscope 81: 931–938

May M et al 1976 Natural history of Bell's palsy: the salivary flow test and other prognostic indicators. Laryngoscope 86: 704–712

Rosen G et al 1985 Submandibular salivary gland scan: A prognostic indicator of Bell's palsy—a preliminary report, In: Myers (ed) E New dimensions of otorhinolaryngology, head & neck surgery, vol. 2. Elsevier Science Publishers BV, Amsterdam, p 274–276

Stankiewicz J A 1983 Steroids and idiopathic facial paralysis. Otolaryngology, Head & Neck Surgery 91: 672–677

Taverner D 1965 Treatment of facial palsy. Archives of Otolaryngology 81: 489

H Diamant, S Edström

Aldskogius H 1974 Indirect and direct Wallerian degeneration in the intramedullary root fibres of the hypoglossal nerve. Advances in Anatomy, Embryology and Cell Biology 50: fasc 1

Edström S, Aldskogius H, Hanner P and Rosenhall U Facial nerve pathology in Bell's palsy. In: Myers E (ed) New dimensions in otorhinolaryngology—head and neck surgery, vol. 1 Excerpta Medica, Elsevier Science Publishers, Amsterdam, p 100–103

Edström S, Hanner P, Karlsson B, Andersen O, Rosenhall U and Vahlne A Elevated levels of myelin basic protein in CSF in relation to auditory brainstem responses in Bell's palsy. Acta Otolaryngologica (Stockholm)

Hanner P, Badr C, Rosenhall U and Edström S 1986 Trigeminal dysfunction in patients with Bell's palsy. Acta Otolaryngologica (Stockholm) 101: 224–230

Hanner P, Andersen O, Frisén L, Rosenhall U, Edström S (submitted for publication) Clinical observations of CNS affections in patients with Bell's palsy.

Hedner M-L, Andersen O, Edström S et al. Perifer facialispares vid MS. Sv. Otolaryngol Fören Förhandl 1

Leeming R D 1976 Varicella-zoster virus and facial palsy. Journal of Laryngology and Otology 90: 365–371

Mair J W S 1985 Ethiology and pathogenesis of the peripheral facial palsy. In: Myers E N (ed) New dimensions in otorhinolaryngology, head and neck surgery, vol 1. Excerpta Medica, Amsterdam, p 82–85

Proctor B et al 1976 The pathology of Bell's palsy. TransAmerican Academy of Ophthalmology and Otolaryngology 82: 70–80

Rosenhall U, Edström S, Hanner P, Badr G, Vahlne A 1983 Auditory brainstem response abnormalities in patients with Bell's palsy. Otolaryngology, Head and Neck Surgery 91: 412–416

Steere A C, Grodzicki R L, Kornblatt A N et al 1983 The spirochetal etiology of Lyme disease. New England Journal of Medicine 308: 733–740

Townsend J J, Baringer J R 1978 Central nervous system susceptibility to herpes simplex infection. Journal of Neuropathology and Experimental Neurology 37: 255–262

Weinstein M, Lederman R, Rothner D et al 1978. Interval computed tomography in multiple sclerosis. Radiology 129: 689–694

8

Medical or surgical treatment of sudden deafness?

B.F. McCabe

The entity known as 'sudden deafness' is that sensori-neural deafness which occurs in one ear over minutes to hours, is severe to profound in degree and without obvious cause on history or physical examination. Patients commonly report it presents upon awakening. It has been the subject of medical reports for many decades. One would hazard that, if a search of the ancient literature were to be carried out, it would be found back to the time of the classic Latin and Greek physicians, or earlier. Over these hundreds of years many different treatments for sudden deafness have been proposed as efficacious, but always within limited degree and with small numbers of subjects.

Treatment has been almost entirely medical. We have gone through many phases of medical regimens depending upon the aetiological vogue at the time: vascular (haemorrhage, stroke, vasospasm, 'blood-sludging'), neural (viral, demyelinating), endorgan (endolymphatic hydrops, suppurative and viral labyrinthitis of pars inferior, endocochlear membrane rupture, window membrane rupture with perilymph fistula) and systemic (diabetes mellitis, cancer, leukaemia). Undoubtedly, most of these can still be accepted as actual causes of sudden deafness, but in many we have no way of delineating the cause by examination and testing. Specific cause then cannot be followed by specific therapy; this is the case in the vast majority of patients with sudden deafness.

The sum total is then that treatment of sudden deafness is a matter of the state-of-the-art. The therapist is dependent upon soft clues in diagnosis as to selection of therapy. Indeed, the clues may be so soft or non-existent that some (or most) otologists offer no therapy at all! It is hard to fault these since that may be the most logical scientific course: no action, since there is in this case no clearly indicated intervention. However, state-of-the-art in otology suggests that there are some sudden deafness cases that do seem to have enough evidence, either on history, physical examination or testing, to indicate a *feasible* course of action. I use the word feasible because the evidence for a certain action is not yet established. Let us examine some possibilities of diagnosis and the soft clues to them that might lead to treatment for that particular patient.

Perilymph fistula

This can (and did, in our series, Selzer & McCabe 1986) cause mild to profound sudden deafness. The most surprising aspects in this series of over 100 fistulas were that they may exist with hearing loss and no dizziness, or the reverse, that there is a high relative incidence in children, decades can elapse between onset and treatable correction, and that there is a high rate of statistically significant hearing improvement (49%) irrespective of the duration of loss. It is difficult to identify the patient with a sudden moderate to profound hearing loss for a tympanotomy. The panoply of symptoms of patients with perilymph fistula is large: sudden (sometimes fluctuating) deafness, spells of brief vertigo, motion intolerance, motion sickness, episodic ataxia, chronic fatigue secondary to constant control of balance and a feeling of desperation that they are getting no help or even understanding from the series of doctors they have seen. Signs of importance are a progressive unilateral (adults) or bilateral (children) sensorineural deafness, and a positive fistula test objectively (conjugate deviation of the eyes), or subjectively (no eye deviation but a definite sensation of motion geared to the pressure pulse).

We believe from our experience there is no valid diagnostic test or symptom pattern to indicate clearly exploratory tympanotomy. It is a matter of clinical judgment. We urge that at least two of the 'markers' described above be present before tympanotomy is advised. Admonitions, vis-a-vis recognizing the leak, best graft materials, etc., are presented in the *Laryngoscope* paper and need not be repeated here.

Skull base trauma

This, of course, is not sudden deafness as defined above, but is included for the sake of completeness in discussion of treatment of acute massive hearing loss. There should be no controversy here over the majority of cases, at least in the first two categories.

1. Transverse temporal bone fracture

This produces a profound and permanent sensorineural deafness through fracture across the inner ear or internal auditory canal. The only problem is recognizing the lesion, which should not be difficult if the patient is responsive. There is no treatment to restore hearing. Fortunately this constitutes only 15% of temporal bone fractures.

2. Longitudinal (75%) fracture

This fracture traverses the external canal, tegmen tympani and eustachian tube roof. In the process it produces a sudden conductive deafness through ossicular injury, in order of frequency, incudal displacment and crural fracture.

3. Transverse – longitudinal and interwindow fractures

The remaining 10% of temporal bone fractures causing major hearing loss are combined transverse and longitudinal fractures and the rarest pure form of fracture, the inter-window fracture. The latter is diagnosable only at postmortem and is not worthy of clinical discussion.

4. Direct injury

The final form of skull base trauma causing significant sensorineural deafness is direct injury to the outer ear, canal, or tympanic membrane. It is this which causes sudden conductive deafness with or without vertigo and nystagmus. The proper course of action is delayed treatment if there is no vertigo. Let healing take place. However, if vertigo is present, it constitutes an otological emergency. In this case the sun must not set on an exploratory tympanotomy, the patient's general condition permitting. The stapes is prolapsed into the vestibule and must be extracted. This can always be done under local anaesthesia in the adult. The vertigo and nystagmus can be titrated to zero by intravenous diazepam in 2.5 mg increments as needed, as determined by manipulation of the prolapsed stapes. After the ossicle is removed, the oval window should be sealed by a connective tissue graft and reossicularization be done, if there is adequate inner ear reserve.

Idiopathic sudden deafness

This is the most common cause of this disorder, comprising the largest group of sudden deafness patients. There is no clue to aetiology. This is the group we define as having a severe to profound sudden loss, *not* moderate to mild. It is the group in which we seldom see any return and which were treated (if at all) with steroids, anticoagulants, aspirin, carbogen, intravenous histamine, etc. There have been several reports out of Japan of some quite remarkable recoveries of hearing by daily infusions of radiocontrast iodinated compounds of the type used for pyelograms. We have tried this with some success, but a prospective clinical study needs to be carried out with appropriate controls. It will require a number of years before statistical significance can be reached (if, indeed, at all), but it is a study that needs to be done.

Endolymphatic hydrops (cochlear Meniere's disease)

This aetiology is clearly the most common cause of sudden non-conductive hearing loss. It can take many forms audiometrically, most commonly mild to moderate in degree at onset, and in the low to mid-frequencies. It least frequently involves the high frequencies. The 'markers' that identify it as hydrops, as opposed to all the other causes of sudden deafness, are the presence of recruitment (and hyperrecruitment), fluctuation of the loss and eventual involvement of the pars superior as well as the pars inferior of the labyrinth. Cochlear microphonic recording (Aran, Morrison) may also be very helpful in the distinction.

Drug ototoxicity

This requires but little comment because it is dose-related and any good doctor takes a careful drug history. One might only need to be reminded of the synergistic effects of two mildly ototoxic drugs, and of one ototoxic drug and damaging levels of noise.

Dialysis deafness

It is commonly heard in verbal comments and repeated anecdotally in the literature that patients with renal failure undergoing dialysis may incur sensorineural deafness. However, it is known that renal failure alone is associated with sensorineural deafness and, also, that most patients with renal failure have treatment with known ototoxic antibiotics. In a literature search going back to 1964 (about the time when significant numbers of patients were being dialysed), we could find only seven patient reports where the deafness was severe to profound, sudden and clearly related in time to a dialysis event, and the picture not clouded by ongoing ototoxic antibiotic therapy.

Thus, dialysis deafness may be an entity, but it appears to be rather rare judging by the literature. Since there is no known way of treating dialysis deafness and no one would cease dialysis for the sake of hearing, it is mentioned here only for the sake of completeness.

Autoimmune inner ear disease

We now have more than 60 patients with this diagnosis which we have treated and followed closely over a long enough post-treatment period to assess results. The variations in onset of the deafness from our first report (McCabe 1979), consisting of 17 patients, have become apparent. In that group, the deafness was relatively slowly progressive, over a period of months rather than hours, days or years. We now have a distinct group of patients who can be classified in the category of sudden deafness.

Case 1. L.D.F. is a 49-year-old man who received a diagnosis of Ménière's disease in the right ear at age 15. He had fluctuating hearing loss, high pitched tinnitus and recurrent spells of incapacitating vertigo. At age 29 he received an operation across the middle ear which he was told would destroy all residual hearing

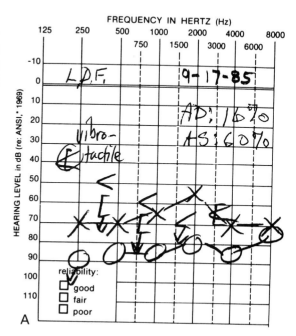

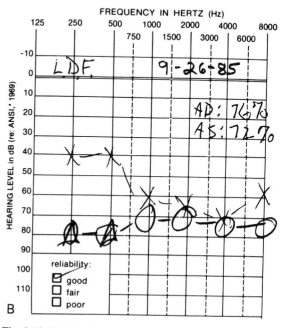

Fig. 8.1A The hearing of patient L.D.F. prior to treatment. **B** Response to nine days of treatment.

but stop the spells. He had no further spells and no useful hearing in that ear. Six weeks before being referred, the patient had a severe loss of hearing in his left ear over a 24-hour period of non-fluctuating nature. He had a vague feeling of fluctuating pressure in his left ear and a low pitched tinnitus. He was hospitalized by his referring physician for intravenous medication including diuretics, antihistamines and cortisone. After a 10-day course of treatment his hearing improved significantly, but after discharge his hearing resumed its prior level over a 1-week period.

The patient was admitted for treatment. An immune screen was normal, except for a significantly elevated sedimentation rate and a rheumatoid factor which was three times normal. The patient received oral dexamethasone 16 mg/day and daily infusions of 2.5 mg/kg of cyclophosphamide. He received twice-weekly white blood cell counts. At the time of discharge on the 14th day of treatment speech reception threshold on the right had improved 15 decibels and the discrimination improved from 16% to 76%, and on the left the SRT improved 20 decibels and the discrimination 12% (Fig 8.1). The patient received a second course of infusions by his referring physician and the dexamethasone was continued for a further two months. Hearing has been further improved and maintained off treatment.

Of note is that the patient did not have Ménière's disease, in the usual sense of the term, in his right ear with onset 20 years prior, but autoimmune inner ear disease. It is apparent that this disorder may take a clinical picture highly suggestive of Ménière's disease. Also of note is that for many years this patient's disease was unilateral and also that the hearing loss in each ear was rapidly progressive, as in the sudden deafness syndrome.

Case 2. M.G.I. is a 60-year-old woman whose only health problem prior to her hearing loss was occasional relapsing polychronditis. Eight months before being seen by one of my colleagues she awoke in the morning with severe vertigo and unilateral hearing loss. She was admitted to a local hospital and treated symptomatically while the vertigo subsided over a 6-day period, leaving her with significant motion intolerance which she still had. Audiometry at that time showed no hearing in the right ear and normal hearing in the left.

Admission audiometry demonstrated a 50 dB SRT on the left, her only hearing ear, and 34% discrimination. She was entered into our sudden deafness protocol (Renagrafin and Rheomacrodex), but her hearing continued to fall. Ten days later the SRT was at 60 DB and the discrimination was 18% (Fig. 8.2A). Her motion intolerance was increasing. At this time the situation was reassessed. An immune screen was obtained and she was found to have an elevated sedimentation rate and an antinuclear antibody eight times normal. On the basis of the relapsing polychronditis, which at different times involved the extremities,

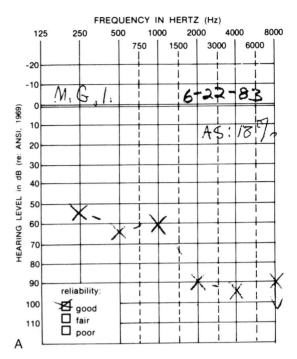

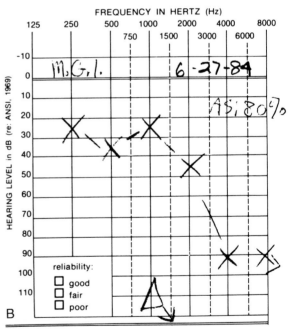

Fig. 8.2A The hearing of patient M.G.I. prior to treatment. The hearing in the right ear had been lost eight months prior in what was probably the sudden deafness syndrome. **B** Three months after treatment the hearing level in the left ear was 25 dB with 80% discrimination. Over the next two years the hearing fluctuated mildly but three days before readmission began to deteriorate rapidly. **C** The hearing upon readmission. After treatment, hearing was restored.

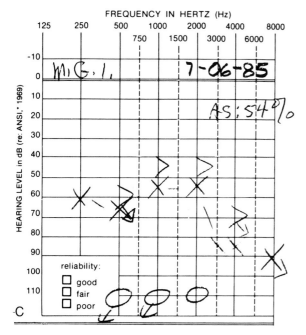

-C

Over the next 2 years the patient had mild fluctuation of hearing but 3 days before being readmitted noticed a rapid deterioration. At the time of readmission her SRT was 50 dB and discrimination 54% (Fig. 8.2C). She was re-treated in exactly the same way and, at the end of the 3-month treatment period, her SRT was 20 dB and discrimination 84%. It has been stable over the past 12 months.

This is one of the very few patients to have had a relapse. The fact that the patient has a polyimmunopathy suggests the relapse is on this basis.

It is apparent that the otolaryngologist who diagnoses and treats sudden deafness must be aware of this entity as a cause, for it responds to no other treatment save immunosuppression.

SUMMARY

There are many causes of sudden deafness. It no longer suffices that a patient with the documented complaint of a quite recent and significant sensorineural hearing loss be categorically compartmentalized, each to receive the same treatment, whatever it might be, according to the vogue of the time or the whim of a particular otolaryngologist. Second and third opinions should rule, for the good of the patient whose diagnosis is not crystal clear. Finally, at least some cases of sudden deafness are reversible on appropriate treatment. Perhaps quite a few!

back, auricle, nose and eye and which on each occasion responded promptly to cortisone, and the time course and character of her hearing loss in the left ear, the patient was considered to have a polyimmunopathy. She was started on cyclophosphamide 2 mg/kg intravenously and dexamethasone 12 mg/day. She received a second course of infusions at her home hospital. Three months after treatment was stopped her hearing was stable at 25 dB SRT and 80% discrimination (Fig. 8.2B).

Over the past 10–20 years there has been considerable controversy regarding the medical and surgical management of sudden hearing loss (SHL). This controversy has existed and will continue for some years to come for a variety of reasons. One problem has been the lack of any universally accepted definition of the terms, 'sudden hearing loss' or 'sudden deafness'. Wilson et al (1980) defined SHL as not less than a 30 decibel sensorineural hearing loss in three contiguous frequencies occurring within a 3-day time limit. Mattox & Simmons (1977) consider the hearing loss as sudden if it occurred within 12 hours or less. Other authors have been less specific with both the rapidity and severity of the hearing loss. A second factor in fuelling the controversy about the management of SHL is the relative infrequency with which it occurs. A busy otologist may see only a dozen cases or so a year. In addition, many of these cases have markedly different causes so that comparisons of treatments and prognoses are difficult.

It is important to remember that sudden hearing loss is a symptom rather than a diagnosis. As with most symptoms in medicine, categorizing SHL relies on the patient's subjective assessment of its severity and timing. Since patients can be vague about the duration of symptoms, it is difficult to be rigid in our definition of 'sudden hearing loss'. It seems, however, that Wilson's definition of sudden sensorineural hearing loss is a reasonable starting point.

Patient evaluation

Prior to discussing treatment it would be helpful to discuss the usual evaluation for patients with SHL, bearing in mind that special tests may be necessary when the history justifies it. First, an in-depth history is obtained from the patient, reviewing not only the presenting problem, but also reviewing the past medical history in an effort to find some underlying cause for the disorder. A thorough physical examination is performed. We routinely obtain a complete blood count, urinalysis, serum chemistry panel (electrolytes, lipids, cholesterol, kidney function) and serological tests for syphilis (fluorescent treponemal antigen test, serological test for syphilis).

A sedimentation rate is also obtained, because of evidence by Mattox & Simmons (1977) that an elevated sedimentation rate (over 30 mm/h) is associated with a poor prognosis. Our initial audiological evaluation includes speech and pure-tone audiometry, acoustic impedance audiometry with acoustic reflex testing and auditory brain stem response (ABR) tests. We usually obtain a computerized tomography scan (CT) or a magnetic resonance imaging (MRI) study, unless the auditory brain stem response test is unequivocably normal. An electronystagmogram (ENG) is routinely obtained, even if there are no vestibular complaints. We look specifically for ipsilateral canal paresis as being a significantly abnormal finding. If clinically indicated, an ENG fistula test is performed, as reported by Daspit et al (1980). In this technique, a pneumatic otoscope or impedance audiometer is used to generate a sustained negative and then positive pressure for 15 seconds while an ENG records any nystagmus. Daspit reported five out of six patients with proven fistulas had a direction-fixed nystagmus, usually (four out of five) toward the affected ear. It has not been our experience, however, that the fistula test is of great help in deciding whether or not to explore the patient for a perilymph fistula. As has been reported by Harris (1980), fistula tests are positive in only half of the patients with surgically proven fistulas.

The role of temporal bone polytomography has not been well defined. Shea & Emmett (1980) have reported finding large cochlear aqueducts in 16 of 34 patients with proven perilymph fistulas. Schuknecht et al (1973) reviewed seven temporal bones of patients with sudden hearing loss and found that two of these had enlarged cochlear aqueducts. It has been postulated that this enlargement in the cochlear aqueduct may be responsible for labyrinthine membrane rupture, resulting from a rapid increase in cerebrospinal fluid pressure. Despite these two studies, we do not perform polytomography routinely because this information would rarely determine the management of the patient. In addition, there is the expense and irradiation risks.

Mattox & Simmons (1977) have performed a thought-provoking and interesting analysis of sudden hearing loss patients by having their pure-tone audiograms performed at 100 Hz intervals to detect patients with very narrow frequency band hearing loss. Although the practising otolaryngologist may not have the ability to perform this type of analysis, it is innovative techniques like this that may eventually clarify our understanding of SHL.

Specific causes and management

The differential diagnosis of SHL is quite long and more obscure cases are being found every year. A large number of viruses have been implicated. Mumps, measles, rubella, herpes zoster, Epstein–Barr, hepatitis, Coxsackie, influenza, parainfluenza and adenoviruses have all been mentioned in the literature over the past 10 years as possible causes of SHL. We believe that these patients are best managed with high-dose steroids such as dexamenthazone, 4 mg four times a day orally for 10 days and then tapered over another 10 days. There have also been scattered reports in the literature demonstrating the effectiveness of Acyclovir (Meyers et al 1982, Wade et al 1982) as an antiviral drug most specifically against the herpesvirus family. This drug may prove very helpful in the future, but its efficacy in SHL is lacking.

Bacterial meningitis has long been known to cause both unilateral or bilateral deafness. When this occurs, total deafness usually results within 24 hours after the onset of meningitis (Vienny 1985). This phenomenon makes it imperative that we diagnose and treat meningitis as a true medical emergency.

Multiple sclerosis has been recognized as a cause for sudden deafness for many years. These patients have neurological symptoms and signs that vary considerably in severity, timing and location, such that the aetiology of their problems may remain obscure for years. They can have one of a variety of audiometric patterns, but most frequently have poor word discrimination. A hallmark of this disease is abnormal and, at times, bizarre waveforms seen during auditory brain stem response testing. Neurology consultation is imperative if the diagnosis is being considered.

There are now several well recognized autoimmune related causes of sudden deafness. Certainly, the patient with neurosyphilis can have a Ménière's-like syndrome and present with rapidly progressing sensorineural hearing loss. We treat these patients, with the co-operation of our infectious disease colleagues, with both systemic penicillin and high-dose steroids. Initially, they appear to respond to this treatment, but will frequently have a relapse if the steroids are withdrawn. At that point, the patient must help decide whether he/she will withstand the side effects of long-term steroid usage or risk further hearing deterioration. In addition to syphilis, both systemic lupus erythematosus (SLE) and Cogan's syndrome are two of the more commonly recognized autoimmune causes for sudden deafness. As reported by McCabe (1979), there also appears to be a group of patients with idiopathic autoimmune SHL. These patients are treated with high-dose steroids (dexamethazone 4 mg *po qid* initially and tapered over three weeks) and, at times, remarkable results can be seen. McCabe is presently studying the use of Cytoxan in these patients (Personal communication, 1986). Preliminary results are encouraging.

There are a large number of vascular-related causes of sudden deafness. Thromboembolic disease, such as cryoglobulinaemia, sickle cell anaemia crisis and certain rare coagulopathies all have been reported to cause sudden deafness. Although it is difficult to prove these aetiologies, it is reasonable to presume that they exist. Studies by Suga & Snow (1969) on the vascular supply to the cochlea reveal that with 30 minutes of anoxic injury to the cochlea there is irreversible cochlear neuronal death. Given the prevalence of vascular disease in our society and the experimental data on cochlear blood supply, it seems reasonably certain that many patients, especially those with vertebral artery or intracranial vascular disease, have had SHL because of anoxic damage. In those patients where thromboembolism is hypothesized, therapeutic anticoagulation with intravenous heparin/oral coumadin is used. In less severe cases a milder anticoagulation can be achieved using dipyridamole (Persantine) or aspirin. There have been reports by Haug et al (1976) advising a stellate ganglion block to perform a sympathectomy to enhance the blood supply to the cochlea. In reviewing the literature, there appears to be some question as to whether autonomic nervous system control exists over cochlear blood flow. Animal studies have shown that the sympathetic nervous system does not have a significant role in regulation of cochlear blood flow (Suga & Snow 1969). In our opinion, further research is needed to document the efficacy of this technique.

It is occasionally mentioned that Ménière's patients can present with sudden deafness. In our experience, this is quite rare. The deafness that is associated with Ménière's disease often occurs slowly over a period of many years. These patients are best treated with a salt-restricted diet, diuretics and vestibular suppressants.

There is a large list of medications that can result in deafness. In our present experience the most common of these are cisplatin and aminoglycosides. Most often these drugs cause a mild to moderate bilateral sensorineural hearing loss. Other than the prompt discontinuation of these medications, there appears to be no other reliable treatment to restore the hearing. Prompt identification of this side effect appears to be the best treatment at present.

Patients with acoustic nerve tumours can definitely present with sudden deafness. In the series by Shaia & Sheehy (1976), which is the largest series on SHL ever reported, they found 10 cases of acoustic neuromas out of 1220 cases of sudden deafness. In a review of the senior author's (Pensak et al 1985) series of 506 acoustic nerve tumours, we found that approximately 15% presented with sudden hearing loss as their main complaint.

In addition to all of the causes mentioned above, there are countless other specific aetiologies for SHL. Jaffe (1973), for instance, has reported that there have been over 100 aetiologies for SHL reported in the literature. Despite the large differential diagnosis discussed above, we are able to define an exact cause of the deafness in no more than 25% of the patients. In Shaia & Sheehy's report (1976) they established a firm diagnosis in only 15% of the cases. Clearly, there is a large group of patients who have idiopathic sensorineural hearing loss. There have been literally several dozen different treatments for these patients over the past 20 years; most of them have had a marginally positive effect on the patient's outcome.

IDIOPATHIC SUDDEN DEAFNESS – MEDICAL MANAGEMENT

At the present time our treatment regimen for sudden deafness includes systemic steroids, carbogen and also placing the patient at bed rest with sedation, if necessary. In reviewing the literature, there appears to be good scientific evidence that both systemic steroids and carbogen treatment will benefit sudden deafness patients. In the study by Wilson et al (1980) and in a second study by Moskowitz et al 1984, prospective randomized trials of systemic steroids were more effective than placebo in improving SHL recovery. Wilson's study revealed that 78% of patients treated with high-dose systemic steroids had complete recovery of hearing, whereas only 38% of those patients treated by placebo recovered. In his study, which was performed at two different hospitals, two dose regimens with similar potency were used. One group of patients was treated with a two-week tapering dose of dexamethazone starting with 4.5 mg orally twice daily. At the second study centre the patients were treated with a two-week tapering course of methylprednisolone starting with 16 mg orally twice daily. Wilson et al found that those patients with mild hearing loss nearly universally recovered, regardless of the treatment. Those patients who had a profound hearing loss (greater than 90 dB sensorineural hearing levels at all frequencies) had no response to the steroids. In those patients with the moderate to severe hearing loss, between 40 dB and 90 dB, the best steroid response was obtained. In Moskowitz's study, dexamethazone 0.75 mg orally four times a day tapered over two weeks was used. They found that 89% of those patients treated with steroids had greater than 50% hearing improvement. Conversely, only 44% of those patients treated with placebo had a similar improvement. In summary, it would appear from these two well-performed studies that systemic steroids have a role in the treatment of idiopathic sudden hearing loss.

Our second mode of treatment is carbogen inhalations. Patients receive this treatment for approximately 20 minutes every hour to every other hour, while they are awake. We have experienced no significant adverse side effects from this treatment in hundreds of cases and occasionally a patient will note an improvement in hearing immediately after the treatment. In addition to our clinical observations, there are several rather elegant studies which have been performed during the past 10 years by Fisch (1983). Fisch has shown, in both an animal model and also in clinical cases, that carbogen is beneficial in SHL. He has found that the peri-lymphatic oxygenation in sudden hearing loss patients is approximately 30% of what it is in normal hearing patients. Experimentally, he has found that carbogen increases perilymphatic oxygenation approximately 200% in these patients. In his randomized controlled prospective study he found no significant difference in the audiograms of patients treated with five days of carbogen when compared to five days of dextran and Papaverine. When the audiograms of these patients were compared after one year, however, there was a statistically significant improvement in those patients treated with carbogen. Although his results were by no means overwhelming, there seems to be experimental evidence that would suggest that its use is beneficial, and there are no reports of serious adverse effects with its use.

Other patient care issues include psychological support and rehabilitation with hearing aids. SHL can be devastating to the patient's socioeconomic and emotional life. We try to reassure them that the incidence of bilateral SHL ranges between 1% and 10% (Shaia & Sheehy 1976). If the hearing does not return, we promptly start counselling on the use of CROS or BICROS hearing aids.

There are many other treatments that have been used in the past for sensorineural hearing loss. Many have been discontinued, whereas others are still in use at different centres throughout the United States.

In 1974 Morimitsu et al reported on the effectiveness of diatrisoate meglumine (Urograffin) in the treatment of sudden hearing loss. These patients received 10 cc of Urograffin daily intravenously for one to two weeks until maximum recovery was obtained. Hearing recovery occurred in 54% of the patients treated with Urograffin whereas only 19% of those treated with vasodilators recovered. Several studies have also been published by Shea & Emmett (1980) documenting the effectiveness of this treatment. It has been hypothesized that the Urograffin acts as a molecular plug in a leaky stria vascularis to allow the sodium potassium pump to be reactivated. This is an attractive theory and the results are somewhat encouraging. We have no personal experience with its use.

Meyerhoff & Paparella (1980) have advised using a treatment protocol including heparin, dextran, adrenocorticotrophic hormone (ACTH), sedation and stool softeners. We have, at times, used heparin on patients who have known thromboembolic or vascular disease, but do not feel it is warranted in every patient. We have had extensive experience in the past with the use of intravenous dextran, both in patients with sudden hearing loss and with severe vertigo, but do not feel it has any dramatic effect and rarely use it now. In addition, dextran can cause significant side effects, including electrolyte abnormalities and also a rare severe allergic reaction. In 1980, Wilson & Nadol reported on an anaphylactic-related death due to the use of dextran. We also have not used the hormone ACTH because it seems quicker, easier and less expensive to give the patient high-dose systemic steroids such as dexamethazone.

Vasodilators have also been used in many centres throughout the country and we have used them extensively in the past. This vasodilator effect can be achieved using nicotinic acid, 50 mg orally 30 minutes before breakfast and before the evening meal, or up to four times per day. We have also used intravenous histamine (histamine 2.75 mg in 250 cc of normal saline, infused over a $1\frac{1}{2}$-hour period), as well as sublingual histamine (histamine 1:10 000 solution) four times a day. Papaverine has also been used by many otologists, including us, during the past 10–15 years. Unfortunately, there appears to be very little experimental evidence to support the use of any of these vasodilators. Suga & Snow (1969) have found that vasodilators actually decrease the cochlear blood flow, possibly by a vascular steal phenomenon. Mattox & Simmons (1977) have reported that histamine may actually have a negative effect on recovery of hearing when compared with no treatment at all. Fisch (1983) has also found that the perilymphatic oxygenation can actually decrease in response to histamine. In view of these studies and our own personal impression of their lack of efficacy, we are reluctant to use these medications in the future.

When analysing the results of any of these medications, it is important to put their effectiveness into perspective by comparing them to the classic study by Mattox & Simmons (1977) in which they determined the natural course of patients with sudden hearing loss. They found that 65% of patients had a complete recovery of hearing spontaneously. They calculated the pure-tone averages between 500, 1000 and 2000 Hz for SHL patients. In the overall group, the patients had a 67 dB pure-tone average when first diagnosed with sudden hearing loss and on the average had a recovery to 35 dB pure-tone average with no treatment whatsoever. In their study, they found that several factors determined the prognosis in the patients. An upward sloping audiogram (preservation of low frequency hearing) was almost universally associated with recovery. For example, those patients who had retention of hearing at one frequency, 8000 cps, had a 78% incidence of good or complete recovery. Conversely, absence of hearing at 8 kHz reduced the prognosis to only 29%. A poor prognosis has also been associated with a sedimentation rate in excess of 30 mm/h, a downward sloping audiogram pattern, poor word discrimination and also severe vertigo associated with a downward sloping audiogram. It was their conclusion that the most important factor in the patient's recovery appears to be the actual nature of the injury as reflected by the audiogram and not any therapeutic manoeuvre by the physician. In view of these findings, it seems unjustified to endorse enthusiastically the use of any medication, including those we use ourselves (steroids, carbogen). If we are aiding SHL patients with these drugs, we appear to be doing so marginally.

SURGICAL TREATMENT OF SUDDEN DEAFNESS

Exploratory tympanotomy in adults

If the medical treatments of sudden deafness appear controversial, the surgical treatment is no less so. There is support in the literature for operating on these patients nearly at any time; immediately (Shea 1980, Pullen et al 1979), after a 5-day waiting period (Harris & Goodhill 1977), after a 10–14 day period (Mattox & Simmons 1977), or never (Bly 1984). Simmons and Mattox's study has shown that those patients with an upward slowing audiogram have a good or complete recovery without surgery 92% of the time. They advise performing an exploratory tympanotomy to repair a perilymph fistula only after a waiting period of 10–14 days to see if spontaneous recovery will occur. They advise a more urgent exploration if the patient has progressive hearing loss during this waiting period. It is their impression that repairing perilymph fistulas is quite effective in eliminating the vestibular symptoms, but is minimally effective in stabilizing or improving hearing. They felt that only 2 of 19 patients that they operated on improved more than would have been expected if no operation had been performed and spontaneous healing was allowed to occur.

Pullen et al (1979) advises immediate exploration for all patients having traumatic sudden hearing loss, unless they have a high frequency loss pattern on their pure-tone audiogram. He feels that patients with high frequency losses, as noted by Simmons, have a universally poor prognosis and that the exploratory tympanotomy may in fact be detrimental to the recovery process. Fisch advises exploring these patients with sudden hearing loss after one week if they are not better. Shea (1980) advises a more urgent exploration, basically as soon as the diagnosis is suspected. Since the results of surgical closure of perilymph fistulas are fair in stabilizing or improving the hearing and possibly no better than the natural healing process itself, we advise a conservative approach to management of these patients. We believe that, even in those patients with significant trauma, a 10–14 day waiting period to see if spontaneous improvement will occur seems reasonable. The only time earlier exploration is advised is when vertigo is severe or the hearing is progressively deteriorating.

There are several other issues to address when considering surgical treatment of SHL. These include exploratory tympanotomy surgery for suspected perilymph fistula in children, the technique of the exploration and also the material that is used to plug the perilymph fistula.

Exploratory tympanotomy in children

Grundfast & Bluestone (1978) have advised performing exploratory tympanotomy in children who have unexplained vertigo/dysequilibrium or sudden/fluctuating sensorineural hearing loss. In addition, those patients who have unexplained recurrent meningitis should be explored to see if a congenital cerebrospinal fluid-middle ear communication exists. It seems important to stress that these children with sensorineural hearing loss must have a progressive loss with no other possible aetiology before a surgical procedure is advised. Also, the vestibular symptoms must be significant in severity and there must be some evidence by history, audiogram,

ENG, ABR or CT scan that the aetiology is a labyrinthine dysfunction rather than a central nervous system disorder.

Exploratory tympanotomy—technique

We prefer the technique be done under local anaesthesia with adequate sedation. For children, teenagers, or anxious adults the procedure can be performed under general anaesthesia. Our technique is as follows: the ear is sterilely prepped and draped. The ear canal, with special attention to the vascular strip, is injected with 2% xylocaine with 1:10 000 adrenaline (epinephrine) to achieve adequate anaesthesia and promote haemostasis with the adrenaline-induced vasoconstriction. An angled canal knife is used to incise a tympanomeatal flap several millimetres lateral to the tympanic annulus. A No. 2 House knife is used to elevate the canal skin down to the level of the annulus. Using a No. 1 or No. 2 House knife, the annulus is raised out of the bony sulcus and the middle ear entered. Special care is taken to control all bleeding on the tympanomeatal flap prior to entering the middle ear. This is most easily achieved by packing the ear canal with Gelfoam soaked in 1:1000 adrenaline after the flap has been raised down to the level of the annulus. The Gelfoam soaked in epinephrine is left in place for 5 minutes, timed by the clock. After entering the middle ear the oval window and round window niches are carefully observed for several minutes to see if perilymph leakage occurs. If no leakage is obvious, several manoeuvres are performed to try to enhance cerebrospinal fluid pressure in an effort to make a perilymph leak more obvious. These methods include positioning the patient in reverse Trendelenburg, compressing the jugular veins on both sides of the neck and having the patient perform a Valsalva manoeuvre. There are often some small mucosal adhesions in the oval window niche that can be stripped away carefully using a small right angle pick. The round window niche is carefully observed for a fistula, especially around the periphery of the round window membrane where the leaks commonly occur. Special attention is paid to the anterior portion of the oval window near the area of the annulus where the leaks most often occur. Both niches must be carefully observed for several minutes to confirm the absence of a perilymph leak. Regardless of whether a leak is observed, both the oval window and round window niches are then stripped of surrounding mucosa and a small piece of fat or areolar tissue is packed into each niche.

We advise against using Gelfoam to plug a suspected perilymph leak because of the incidence of fistulas noted when it is used in stapedectomy. Many other authors, however, advise the use of a connective tissue plug, such as a vein or fascia graft. Singleton et al (1978) performed surgical repair of perilymph fistulas in 19 patients. In 9, there was no return of hearing, or continued vertigo and, as a result, these patients were re-explored. He found that 6 of the 7 patients repaired with fat had a persistent perilymph fistula, whereas only 2 of 8 patients repaired with perichondrium had a recurrent fistula. A more recent study by Seltzer & McCabe (1986) also found that recurrent fistulae occurred more commonly after use of a fat graft. It seems quite reasonable to use fascia in preference to ear lobe fat, especially considering these two studies.

We have reviewed our own experience with exploratory tympanotomy for the repair of perilymph fistulas. We have been quite conservative in exploring patients because of the rather modest results for hearing preservation that have been reported in the literature by many authors. In approximately 15 years of practice by the senior author (MEG) (Glasscock et al 1986), only 36 patients have been explored and only 25% of these had unquestionable evidence of a fistula. The fistula repair has been generally successful in eliminating the patient's vestibular symptoms, but has been mediocre in returning the patient's hearing to the previous level.

SUMMARY

We evaluate the patient with sudden hearing loss in a rigorous and systematic fashion. The history is the key in making the diagnosis, especially if there is a history of direct or barometric trauma. A thorough physical and neurotological exam is performed. A battery of testing is performed, including pure tone and speech audiometry, impedance tympanometry, ABR, ENG and, at times, a CT scan. Routine laboratory studies, including a complete blood count, serum chemistry analysis, sedimentation rate, and serum syphilis tests are also routinely performed.

Using the above technique we have been able to identify an underlying cause in the sudden deafness patients approximately 25% of the time. The remaining 75% are treated as idiopathic sudden hearing loss patients. We have selected a treatment plan that is based on what we feel are currently the most reliable and sensible modes of therapy. We use carbogen inhalations, systemic steroids, bed rest and then closely monitor the hearing loss and vestibular complaints. Many of these patients respond rather quickly and are able to be discharged in less than one week of hospitalization. In a small minority of the patients the hearing loss will progress in severity, or vestibular symptoms will persist after 10 days of observation. In these patients we do advise a middle ear exploration in search of a perilymph fistula. We believe that repairing these fistulas is successful in stopping their vestibular symptoms and at times will stabilize or improve their hearing.

Unfortunately, the aetiology of sudden hearing loss eludes us in most patients. The treatments, both medical and surgical, appear to have only a modest beneficial effect on the patient. As a result, we will continue to treat these patients in a conservative fashion. We advise against the exploration of all patients with sudden or progressive sensorineural hearing loss. We continue to support and encourage the continued research both in animals and in humans, as this is where the answers are to be found.

A.W. Morrison

When a disease is understood there is little argument about its therapy or, if there be no therapy, about symptomatic palliation. The trouble with 'sudden deafness' is that it is not a disease but a manifestation of one of any number of diseases. Frequently the cause cannot be ascertained. The sceptic delights in this situation and can, with a measure of logic, discard all therapies and recommend neither investigation nor treatment. This is not a helpful approach.

The reader need hardly be told that the two preceding monographs on sudden deafness, though having a few common denominators, are very different in content and in approach, reflecting the interests and expertise of the writers. The Glasscock paper takes a much broader view of the subject; the McCabe paper concentrates on a few aspects.

Points of agreement

Included amongst the common denominators is the paucity of any reference to non-American literature on this vast subject. Not that a review of world bibliography is required, indeed it would make dull reading, but rather that horizons might have been widened. This criticism is not directed in any personal way towards the authors, but is intended as a comment upon an American attitude to much otological writing which, no doubt, seems quite natural in the United States, yet is an obvious omission when viewed from elsewhere. There are, of course, outstanding exceptions to this generalization!

Both papers agree that the cause of sudden deafness is seldom found (75% not found, Glasscock; the vast majority, McCabe). This has not been the experience at the Royal National Throat, Nose and Ear Hospital, nor at The London Hospital where, over the years, the aetiology has been ascertained in about 75% of cases (Morrison & Booth 1970, Morrison 1975, 1976, 1978).

Neither paper examines the postmortem pathological changes in idiopathic sudden sensorineural deafness, which must surely have a bearing on investigation and treatment. Schuknecht has described these repeatedly from 1962 (Schuknecht et al 1962) to the most recent publication in 1986 (Schuknecht & Donovan 1986), which also reviewed

the literature. In most of the temporal bones the pathology was end-organ and similar to the changes seen after viral labyrinthitis, especially post-mumps and post-rubella. A minority of cases demonstrated primary neuronal loss, which could also be viral in origin. Of particular note was the absence of any evidence of vascular pathology and certainly no evidence of any membrane ruptures or perilymph fistulae.

The search for a cause

Glasscock and his colleagues give a good account of many of the causes of sudden sensorineural deafness and of the investigations required to unmask them. They rightly emphasize the importance of excluding space-occupying lesions of the internal auditory canal and cerebellopontine angle. Most large series of such cases, including our own from The London Hospital, indicate that about 15% present with sudden deafness. Emphasis is placed on excluding syphilis. Whereas the viruses which are recognized as causing sudden sensorineural hearing loss are enumerated, neither of the papers mentions the viral immunological studies which, if performed, would confirm the clinical disease and which, at times, would indicate the subclinical infection which had been responsible. Nor does either paper mention psychogenic or non-organic sudden deafness, not common but definite entities.

The major point of disagreement between the two papers is the frequency of endolymphatic hydrops as a cause of sudden deafness. In Nashville it is quite rare; in Iowa it is the most common cause of sudden non-conductive hearing loss. The London experience places it at 1 in 10 cases (Morrison 1978) and a more recent analysis would probably increase this frequency. McCabe correctly points to transtympanic electro-cochleography as a means of confirming this diagnosis. The enhanced negative summating potential in response to high-intensity acoustic stimulation is characteristic. Dehydration studies (Morrison et al 1980), hydration tests (Brookes et al 1982) and otoadmittance changes in ears affected by endolymphatic hydrops may also provide diagnostic clues (O'Connor et al 1983).

Glasscock et al, while denying the frequency of

cochlear hydrops, quote the Mattox and Simmons paper of 1977 and the much greater likelihood of spontaneous fluctuation to a better hearing level in those patients with a low tone rather than a high tone sensorineural loss. This much quoted paper claims that 65% of patients make a complete spontaneous recovery, a Californian feat which patients in the south of England are unable to equal (Morrison 1975)!

Perhaps the most difficult group to identify are those with a vascular aetiology, since cardiovascular disease is such a common pathology in most populations. A posterior inferior cerebellar infarct, sudden unilateral inner ear symptoms and signs in a patient with recurrent episodes of transient ischaemia, inner ear haemorrhage in leukaemia, sludging episodes in sickle-cell disease, or polycythaemia, or macroglobulinaemia and possibly vertebrobasilar migraine. These are all conditions which should be recognizable. It is faulty to label a sudden unilateral sensorineural deafness as vascular with no other evidence than perhaps hypertension and some evidence of arteriosclerosis.

There are two further aspects of investigation which merit mention. Neither paper places emphasis on localization of the lesion, i.e. whether sensory, neural or a combination of both, yet this has some bearing on further tests and on treatment. The difficult decision about when to start treatment and its relationship to the outcome of therapy is also important. Valuable treatment time can be wasted by prolonged and delaying investigations. Sudden deafness *is* an otological emergency.

Definitions

There is another area of apparent disagreement between the two papers. In Nashville, a sudden hearing loss of as little as 35 dB in three contiguous frequencies is accepted for inclusion, whereas in Iowa sudden deafness signifies severe to profound loss, not moderate to mild. One suspects that, in practice, there would be little difficulty about this definition. Both papers agree that the rapidity of onset is the qualifying criterion. After all, in cerebral cortical 'deafness' or psychogenic hearing loss, the pure tone threshold is meaningless, yet the patient may have a sudden presentation.

The term idiopathic is and will continue to be acceptable, although the more thorough the investigation the smaller the group will become.

Membrane ruptures and perilymph fistulae

This is without doubt the most controversial and worrying aspect of this subject, as acknowledged by Glasscock et al. They tend to sit on the fence, whereas McCabe has little doubt about this entity.

One would not argue with much of the paper by Seltzer & McCabe (1986), which details the findings in 91 patients with perilymph fistulae, some of whom presented with sudden deafness. Oval window fistulae after stapedectomy, middle ear tympanoplastic surgery, head injuries which might fracture or dislocate the footplate, or in children with certain congenital anomalies of the inner ear who usually present with recurrent meningitis; these are all well recognized otological conditions which merit exploratory tympanotomy. It is even possible that sudden severe middle ear pressure changes could subluxate the stapes footplate. The quarrel is with round window fistula and the quite remarkable number and gathering pace of publications on the subject, recently culminating in the respectability of a Leading Article in the British Medical Journal (O'Donoghue & Colman 1986).

Round window fistula may occur after chronic ear surgery, which has involved removal of disease from the round window niche; it may follow the insertion of intracochlear electrodes, and has been seen after acid burns have destroyed the primary and secondary tympanic membranes; it has followed singular neurectomy and the membrane may be ruptured after severe head injuries which have fractured the otic capsule and destroyed the ear. But does it occur spontaneously, or after relatively minor pressure changes? To visualize the round window membrane, it is necessary to drill the promontory quite widely and almost up to the oval window niche. If this is done expertly, round window fistulae *will not* be seen. The membrane is small and tough. The literature reports indicate that this exposure is never, or almost never, done. Holes are described in the mucous membrane folds, an error which many have been guilty of; mostly however, as in the Iowa experience (Seltzer and McCabe), *the niche is viewed over 5 minutes and a suggestion of moisture or an alteration in the light reflex after* jugular compression or head-down tilt is considered evidence of a leak. Little attention is given to the consequence of local anaesthetic and/or vasoconstrictor solutions injected or applied during the tympanotomy. Some of this fluid usually gets into the middle ear where it can collect in rudimentary cells and mucosal folds.

Goodhill and his colleagues (Goodhill et al 1973) certainly started a vogue. In 1976 Morrison wrote:

When Victor Goodhill introduced to use the entity of spontaneous rupture of the round window as a treatable cause of sudden sensorineural deafness, he unleashed a great potential of surgical energy. For the otologist the concept of a simple operation to cure or partially reverse hearing loss is so attractive that it carries the risk of replacing adequate investigation by exploratory tympanotomy. There seems no reason in 1986 to change this view.

The other hypothetical rupture involves parts of the membranous labyrinth. Simmons (1978) followed his admixture of endolymph and perilymph hypothesis with a double membrane break (Simmons 1979), where a rupture of one of the labyrinthine windows resulted in secondary pressure tears of the membranous labyrinth. Pure-tone audiograms at 100 Hz increments in three patients showed a number of notches, the theory being that these corresponded to areas of rupture in the cochlear duct. Schuknecht (1986) has demolished these ideas! Nevertheless the concept of membranous labyrinthine rupture causing sudden total or subtotal hearing loss cannot be dismissed. It may be one explanation for the catastrophe which is sometimes seen in deep sea divers, while basilar membrane tears in syphilitic ears have a similar consequence.

Autoimmune disease

Both papers raise the subject of autoimmune inner ear disease. Since McCabe's 1979 paper there has been gathering interest in this subject. There is no doubt that some patients with a recognized autoimmune disease, especially with pathological vasculitis, can suffer sudden hearing loss, usually bilateral, often fluctuant and normally progressive with or without vertiginous symptoms. The intralabyrinthine neo-osteogenesis of Cogan's disease would be compatible with the vascular changes. Sometimes these inner ear changes are associated with abnormal circulating immune complexes (Brookes 1985), and even Ménière's disease may have an autoimmune basis (Xenellis et al 1986).

McCabe also mentions dialysis deafness and the difficulty of excluding ototoxic drugs as the cause of the sudden deafness. Most otologists who work in hospitals with renal dialysis units have encountered these problems and they are possibly not as rare as the literature suggests. One wonders about the possibilty of an abnormal immunological response to the membranes in the dialysing equipment as a cause.

At all events, there are probably several different syndromes, including hypersensitivity reactions, which may cause sudden or fluctuant inner ear symptoms. They require elucidation.

Treatment

If we exclude surgery for the traumatic or postsurgical causes of sudden deafness, there remains steroids and vasodilators.

Both papers and most (but not all) otologists are agreed that high-dose steroids, say dexamethasone 4 mg *qds*, carry the best prospect of reversing the sudden hearing loss in recognized viral disease, in syphilis, in idiopathic cases, some of the immunological disorders and even in acoustic neuroma. The contraindications to steroid therapy have to be considered. The time factor is important; steroids started later than two weeks after onset carry a poor prognosis compared with the good prospects if therapy is started within a week (Morrison & Booth 1970, Morrison 1975, 1976, 1978).

The evidence that vasodilator therapy is beneficial is controversial. Apart from a number of vasodilator drugs, carbogen inhalations and intravenous urograffin act as vasodilators. Glasscock and his colleagues have reviewed these therapies. There is one aspect of vasodilator therapy which is seldom mentioned; if given to a patient with peripheral vascular disease then the vasodilation would affect the more normal blood vessels and further embarrass the blood supply to the affected area.

REFERENCES

B F McCabe
McCabe B F 1979 Autoimmune sensorineural hearing loss. Annals of Otology, Rhinology and Laryngology 88: 585–589

Selzer S, MaCabe B F 1986 Perilymph fistula – Iowa experience. Laryngoscope 96: 37–49

M E Glasscock, K X McKennan, S C Levine
Bly F 1984 Sudden hearing loss: eight years experience and suggested prognostic table. Laryngoscope 94: 647–661

Daspit C P, Churchill D, Linthicum F H 1980 Diagnosis of perilymph fistula using ENG and impedance. Laryngoscope 90: 217–223

Fisch U 1983 Management of sudden deafness. Otolaryngology, Head and Neck Surgery 91: 3–8

Glasscock M E, McKennan K X, Levine S C 1986 Perilymph fistulae—spontaneous and traumatic. Personal review

Grundfast K M, Bluestone C D 1978 Sudden or fluctuating hearing loss and vertigo in children due to perilymph leak. Annals of Otology, Rhinology and Laryngology 87: 761–771

Harris I, Goodhill V 1977 Oval and round window fistula repair. In: Proceedings of the fifth Shambaugh international workshop on middle ear microsurgery and fluctuant hearing loss. Strode Publishers, Huntsville, Alabama, p 452–457

Harris I 1980 Detection and therapy of perilymph fistulas. In: Proceedings of the sixth Shambaugh international workshop on otomicrosurgery and third Shea fluctuant hearing loss symposium. Strode Publishers, Huntsville, Alabama, p 153

Haug O, Draper W L, Haug S A 1976 Stellate ganglian blocks for idiopathic sensorineural hearing loss: a review of 76 cases. Archives of Otolaryngology 102: 5–8

Jaffe B F 1973 Clinical studies in sudden deafness. Advances in Otorhinolaryngology 20: 221–228

Mattox D E, Simmons F B 1977 Natural history of sudden sensorineural hearing loss. Annals of Otology, Rhinology and Laryngology 86: 463–480

McCabe B F 1979 Autoimmune sensorineural hearing loss. Annals of Otology, Rhinology, Laryngology 88: 585–589

Meyerhoff W L, Paparella M M 1980 Medical therapy for sudden deafness. In: Snow J B (ed) Controversy in otolaryngology. W B Saunders, Philadelphia, Pennsylvania, p 3–11

Meyers J D, Wade J C, Mitchell C D et al 1982 Multicenter collaborative trial of intravenous acyclovir in treatment of mucocutaneous herpes simplex virus infection in the immunocompromised host. American Journal of Medicine 73 (1A): 229–235

Morimitsu T, Hirashima N, Yasuda K 1974 Sudden deafness treated successfully with amidotrizoate. Otologia Fukuoka 20: 599–604

Moskowitz D, Lee K J, Smith H W 1984 Steroid use in idiopathic sudden sensorineural hearing loss. Laryngoscope 94: 664–666

Nadol J B, Wilson W R 1980 Treatment of sudden hearing loss is illogical. In: Snow J B (ed) Controversy in otolaryngology. W B Saunders, Philadelphia, Pennsylvania, p 23–32

Pensak M L, Glasscock M E, Josey F A, Jackson C G, Gulya A J 1985 Sudden hearing loss and cerebellopontine angle tumors. Laryngoscope 95: 1188–1193

Pullen F W, Fosenburg G J, Cabeza C H 1979 Sudden hearing loss in divers and fliers. Laryngoscope 89: 1373–1377

Schuknecht H F, Kimura R S, Naufal P M 1973 The pathology of sudden deafness. Acta Otolaryngologica 76: 75–97

Seltzer S, McCabe B 1986 Perilymph fistula: the Iowa experience. Laryngoscope 94: 37–49

Shaia F T, Sheehy J L 1976 Sudden sensorineural hearing impairment: a report of 1220 cases. Laryngoscope 86: 389–398

Shea J 1980 Panel: sudden hearing loss management. In: Proceedings of the sixth Shambaugh international workshop an otomicrosurgery and third Shea fluctuant hearing loss symposium. Strode Publishers, Huntsville, Alabama, p 153

Shea J, Emmett J R 1980 Hypaque treatment of sudden hearing loss. In: Proceedings of the sixth Shambaugh international workshop on otomicrosurgery and third Shea fluctuant hearing loss symposium. Strode Publishers, Huntsville, Alabama, p 153

Singleton G T, Post K N, Karlan M S, Bock D G 1978 Perilymph fistulas diagnostic criteria and therapy. Annals of Otology, Rhinology and Laryngology 87: 761–771

Suga F, Snow J B 1969 Cochlear blood flow in response to some vasodilating drugs and some other agents. Laryngoscope 79: 1956–1979

Vienny H 1985 Early diagnosis and evolution of deafness in childhood bacterial meningitis: a study using brainstem auditory evoked potentials. Pediatrics 73(5): 579–586

Wade J C, Newton R, McLaren C, Flournoy N, Keeney R E, Meyers J D 1982 Intravenous acyclovir in treatment of mucocutaneous herpes simplex virus infection after marrow transplantations: a double-blind trial. Annals of Internal Medicine 96(3): 265–269

Wilson W R, Byl F M, Laird N 1980 The efficacy of steroids in the treatment of idiopathic sudden hearing loss. Archives of Otolaryngology 106: 772–776

A W Morrison
Brookes G B 1985 Immune complex-associated deafness: preliminary communication. Journal of the Royal Society of Medicine 78: 47–55

Brookes G B, Hodge R A, Booth J B, Morrison A W 1982 The immediate effects of acetazolamide in Meniere's disease. Journal of Laryngology and Otology 96: 57–72

Goodhill V, Harris I, Brockman S et al 1973 Sudden deafness and labyrinthine window ruptures. Annals of Otology, Rhinology and Laryngology 82: 2–12

Mattox D E, Simmons F B 1977 Natural history of sudden sensorineural hearing loss. Annals of Otology, Rhinology and Laryngology 86: 463–480

McCabe B F 1979 Autoimmune sensorineural hearing loss. Annals of Otology, Rhinology and Laryngology 88: 585–589

Morrison A W 1975 Sudden deafness. Management of sensorineural deafness. Butterworths, London, p 175–216

Morrison A W 1976 Sudden sensorineural deafness: outline of management. Proceedings of the Royal Society of Medicine 69: 572–574

Morrison A W 1977 Acute deafness. British Journal of Hospital Medicine 11: 237–249

Morrison A W, Booth J B 1970 Sudden deafness: an otological emergency. British Journal of Hospital Medicine 4: 287–298

Morrison A W, Moffat D A, O'Connor A F 1980 Clinical usefulness of electrocochleography in Meniere's disease: An analysis of dehydrating agents. Otolaryngologic Clinics of North America 13: 703–721

O'Connor A F, Morrison A W, Shea J J 1983 Glycerol induced changes of acoustic conductance in Meniere's disease. American Journal of Otology 41: 200–201

O'Donoghue G M, Colman B H 1986 The leaking labyrinth. British Medical Journal 293: 220–221

Schuknecht H F, Benitez J, Beekhuis J, Icarashi M, Singleton C, Ruedi L 1962 The pathology of sudden deafness. Laryngoscope 72: 1142–1157

Schuknecht H F, Donovan E D 1986 The pathology of idiopathic sudden sensorineural hearing loss. Archives of Otolaryngology 243: 1–15

Seltzer S, McCabe B F 1986 Perilymph fistula: the Iowa experience. Laryngoscope 94: 37–49

Simmons F B 1978 Fluid dynamics in sudden sensorineural hearing loss. Otolaryngologic Clinics of North America 1: 55–61

Simmons F B 1979 The double membrane break syndrome in sudden hearing loss. Laryngoscope 89: 59–66

Xenellis J, Morrison A W, McClowsky D, Festenstein H 1986 HLA Antigens in the pathogenesis of Meniere's disease. Journal of Laryngology and Otology 100: 21–24

9

The early diagnosis of the deaf newborn

W.P.R. Gibson

A recent study of early childhood hearing loss showed that 50% of children with a hearing loss of 50 dB or worse had passed their third birthday before the hearing loss was confirmed (Martin et al 1981). Simmons (1978) estimated that the national age average in the USA for the detection of hearing loss in children was 2.7 years (Simmons 1978).

It is widely accepted, though difficult to prove, that the earlier a hearing loss is detected and remedial steps are taken, the better the child's chance of achieving language, speech and education.

The present level of achievement of a severely or profoundly deaf child is a matter of concern. Few of these children achieve normal language. Countries such as Australia have moved to a system of total communication, which allows signing in an attempt to improve language even though many children given this opportunity will converse only by signing and lose the opportunity of joining the hearing world. Such deaf children average a reading age equivalent only to an 8-year-old and few can achieve even modest educational goals. Most profoundly deaf children will chose to spend their lives within the protective confines of a deaf community, marrying only a similarly afflicted person, and rarely venture into the hearing community.

There is hope. There is now, at long last, a realization that conventional hearing aids are not the only technical assistance available. New devices, such as vibrotactile devices, frequency transposing hearing aids and the cochlear implant, offer glimmers of hope. Much has to be done to prove the effectiveness of these devices, but soon it can be hoped they will be available to help the deaf child.

The task is to identify the deaf child as soon as possible to institute effective help. Ideally, all children with severe or profound hearing loss should be identified soon after their birth. This author will argue the need for an 'at risk register' and careful behavioural testing of all suspected babies, which should be supplemented by electrophysiological tests in many instances.

THE 'AT RISK REGISTER'

The World Health Organization have suggested that there is a minimum incidence of childhood deafness of 2 per 1000 live births (WHO 1966). In Australia, the incidence was estimated at 2.605 per 1000 live births for the years 1944–1980 (Upfold & Ispey 1982).

An 'at risk register' identifies groups which are likely to contain born deaf children. Galambos & Dupesland (1980) identified the following factors: preterm low birth weight (>1000 g), Apgar score of $>5/6$ at 1 minute, postnatal blood pH >7.25, ototoxic drugs, brain haemorrhage, deep coma, respiratory distress syndromes requiring more than 11 days on a ventilator, congenital cardiac and facial malformations and possibly status epilepticus and trisomy 18. Downs & Silver (1972) produced a much simpler ABCDS of risk factors: A—affected family regardless of the claimed cause, B—serum bilirubin levels over 20 mg/100 ml, C—congenital rubella, D—defects of the ears, nose or throat at birth, S—small at birth (>1500 g). Use of such an 'at risk register' identifies 60–70% of those born deaf (Downs & Northern 1984), but also places approximately 1 child in every 40 births into the 'at risk register'.

The argument now becomes is an 'at risk register' cost effective if, to identify 60–70% of 2.6 children per 1000 live births (i.e. 1.56–1.82 children), 25 children have to be assessed? How many of the children would have been detected anyhow due to parental worries etc.? At present, Australia does not maintain an 'at risk register', following these criticisms and others outlined by Rosen & Austin (1979).

In 1986, the US Department of Health, Education and Welfare estimated an annual cost of 1.75 million dollars in staff salaries, etc., to test behaviourally all children on their 'at risk register'. It has also been estimated that if the 1.3 million deaf persons in the USA had been diagnosed at birth and provided with proper language input, it would save 360 million dollars per year.

The author argues that 'at risk' factors should be considered again in view of the technological developments of the past decade. There should be a reappraisal of past standards. With the advent of electrophysiological tests, the aim should be to establish a certain diagnosis within a few days of birth.

DETECTION OF DEAFNESS IN NEONATES

The following suggestions are proposed: All neonates should be considered according to the criteria suggested by Downs & Silver (1972). If an 'at risk' factor exists, then the parents and medical staff are informed so an assessment of possible hearing loss can be undertaken.

Behavioural testing

At birth the normal hearing baby should be aroused during light sleep by a female voice at 70–100 dB SPL. The nursing staff can easily be trained to undertake this task and their opinion should be sought. It should be remembered that such simple screening will only detect severe or profound hearing loss. Alternatively, a trained audiologist can conduct the tests, but unlike the nurses such a person can usually only test the baby once and the babies sleep state may not be ideal. There is no statistical evidence to show which method is the most accurate.

If the baby is thought to be hearing then no further testing is undertaken unless the parents become worried. At age 7–9 months, ideally further behavioural tests should be undertaken as a baby's responses become more clear at this age, with head turning towards the direction of a sound, and more minor degrees of hearing loss can be detected.

If the neonate is suspected of not hearing, further tests are indicated. It is also worthwhile to have an expert examine the child's ears medically.

The auditory response cradle

The auditory response cradle (ARC) (Bennett 1979) provides a semiautomated multiresponse screening procedure which can identify neonates with severe or profound hearing loss. It is a simple to use device which can be used by nursing staff after a brief training period. Each child takes about 15 minutes to test.

The full description of the device can be read in an article by Shepard (1983). In brief, the baby is placed into a special cot. A microprocessor stores and analyses information on five types of activity: body movement, head turn, startle (backward head movement) and two types of changes in respiration. A sound with a frequency range of 2.6–4.3 kHz at 85 dB SPL is presented via plastic tubes and ear inserts.

The test procedure comprises a variable number of sound and blank or control trials. Each recording includes three 5-second periods: prestimulus, perstimulus and poststimulus. During the prestimulus period the base motor activity and breathing patterns are continuously monitored and the test only proceeds if the baby is in a passive state. The baby's activity is monitored throughout the stimulus period and in the poststimulus period. The five types of activity during these periods are compared and the microprocessor decides whether or not a positive response occurred. A complete test can consist of between 2 and 10 trial blocks (each block being four trial elements—two sound and two control). After the first two trial blocks, the machine compares the number of positive responses to sound and to control periods and, if the number of responses to sound exceeds the number of responses to silent control period exceeds the preset decision criteria, a green light (pass) is illuminated. If the number of responses to sound and control periods is not significantly different, the machine continues and presents up to 10 blocks in total. If the baby still has not scored a significant number of more positive responses to sound than to control periods, the red light (fail) is illuminated.

The auditory response cradle has been suggested as a test for neonates in special care units, because the incidence of hearing impairment is much higher there than in unselected neonates. McFarland et al (1980) reported an incidence in the special care units of 1 in 60 against 1 in 1000 for the general population of births.

Bennet & Wade (1980) report a false alarm in 5.3% of 150 normal neonates. Davis (1984), however, reports that the incidence of false alarms on testing special care babies is higher, although he does not specify by how much. The tester has therefore to expect at least 1 baby in 20 will need further testing (usually by brainstem audiometry).

Davis (1984) has calculated that there is a risk that there will be a failure to detect a significant hearing loss in about 1 child in 10 000. Although this seems adequate, he explains that this would mean that 1 out of 10 severely deaf neonates could pass undetected. There are probably methods of increasing the sensitivity of the test, but unfortunately this will also increase the number of false alarms.

In conclusion, the auditory response cradle is a very worthwhile tool for detecting hearing loss in neonates, but it has some limitations which should be realized. Further testing of the neonates at 7–9 months is still needed.

Electrophysiological tests

A number of different electrophysiological tests have been evaluated over the past 20 years, including the cortical responses (Appleby 1964) and the postauricular myogenic responses (Ashcroft et al 1975), but there is no question that the best electrophysiological measure of neonatal hearing at present is provided by the brainstem auditory responses (BAEP).

The brainstem auditory evoked potentials (BAEP)

These potentials were first reported by Sohmer and Feinmesser in 1967 and were further evaluated by Jewitt and Williston in 1971. Since then the BAEP have become the backbone of the auditory evoked potentials.

The BAEP are a series of potentials (Fig. 9.1) and the origin of each wave can be closely linked as follows:

Wave I   (NI)   The first order cochlear fibres
Wave II   (NII)   The cochlear nuclei
Wave III   (NIII) The superior olivary nuclei
Wave IV   (NIV)   The nuclei of the lateral lemnisci
Wave V   (NV)   The inferior colliculus
Wave VI   (NVI)   Also from the inferior colliculus
(Wave VII when seen is probably myogenic in origin)

Premature babies provide potentials with smaller amplitude and longer intervals between each wave. As the infant ages, the interwave intervals decrease. The adult waveform of the BAEP is obtained after the first 6 months of life. (The author allows a delay of 0.2 ms of the NI-NV interval for the first 2 years.)

In most neonates the NI is as large, or even larger, in amplitude than the NV. Either can be used to estimate the threshold. Usually it takes 2000 responses at a rate of 15–33/second to provide a

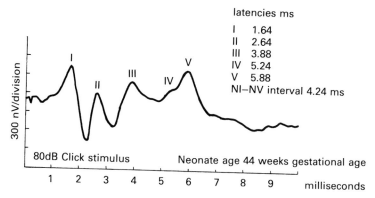

latencies ms

I   1.64
II   2.64
III 3.88
IV   5.24
V   5.88
NI–NV interval 4.24 ms

300 nV/division

80dB Click stimulus   Neonate age 44 weeks gestational age

1   2   3   4   5   6   7   8   9   milliseconds

Fig 9.1 The brainstem auditory evoked potentials (BAEP) from a neonate.

recognizable averaged potential (60–113 seconds per trial). The response is quite obvious at 50 dB SL, but may require more averaging and some experienced judgement within 30 dB of the threshold.

The test is unaffected by sedation or even general anaesthesia; but most neonates can be tested during natural sleep after feeds.

The test is extremely reliable and the author has not encountered any false positive or false negatives in distinguishing normal hearing from severe or profound hearing loss in over 10 years of personal experience of testing approximately 100 babies and older children per year. Exact estimation of hearing thresholds is another matter: the BAEP are best at estimating threshold of frequencies above 2 kHz. Various authors (e.g. Davis & Hirsh 1976) have used a slow brainstem response at approximately 10 milliseconds to estimate thresholds at 500 Hz but the author has not been impressed by the accuracy of the results he has obtained. Residual islands of low frequency hearing are difficult to detect using BAEP.

Thus the BAEP could easily be used as a screening test for severe or profound hearing loss in neonates. Most hospitals already possess the necessary equipment, which is no longer expensive by today's standards. Two trials, each at 80 dB HL and 50 dB HL, could be completed using a binaural stimulus within 8 minutes with a further 5 minutes sufficient for preparing the neonate for testing.

The advantage of the BAEP is that they provide neuro-otological diagnostic data in addition to acting as a means of estimating hearing. For example, the author has seen three babies with hydrocephalus; each has been behaviourally severely deaf and yet the electrocochleogram and NI of the BAEP were normal (Fig. 9.2).

Test procedure

Neonates can be tested during natural sleep after feeds. Indeed it is usually possible to test babies in this manner until they are about 6 months old; after this time it is usually necessary to use a sedative such as chloral hydrate. After the age of 2 years, simple sedatives may not suffice and often general anaesthesia is needed to get reliable recordings.

The neonates are lain in a cot. It is wise to have the ears inspected for wax before testing, or for the presence of serous otitis media. Surface electrodes are attached to the vertex (active), skin over the mastoid processes (references) and to the forehead (earth). The sound stimuli may be delivered binaurally for screening purposes or to each ear separately if monaural information is sought. However, masking the opposite ear can be a problem as it tends to disturb the babies. Most clinicians are content to know that a neonate has binaural hearing with a loss no greater than 30 dB HL; further testing for a possible monaural hearing loss can be undertaken when the child is much older without any serious compromise to the child's educational hopes.

The stimuli are presented at 80 dB HL and, if clear BAEP are obtained, the stimulus levels can be reduced by 20 dB on each trial until either a threshold is obtained, or until a hearing level of 30 dB HL has been demonstrated.

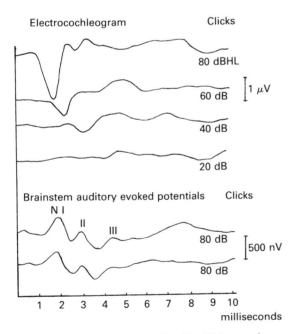

Fig 9.2 A child with hydrocephalus. The NI is normal, showing normal cochlear function, but the NIII, NIV and NV is grossly abnormal, showing severe dysfunction of the brainstem auditory pathways.

Electrocochleography

This test is rarely needed for neonates. The electro-cochleogram (ECochG) is a recording of the eighth nerve action potential from an active electrode placed near the basal turn of the cochlea. It provides a very large response which can be traced to a threshold very quickly and the reliability of the test is superb. The author has used the test in a few special instances when neonates have either failed to give reproducible responses, or have had multiple handicaps which have made a general anaesthetic essential, or when it has been necessary to inspect the ears under general anaesthetic.

FINAL CONCLUSIONS

New electrophysiological tests, in particular the brainstem auditory evoked potentials, have re-opened the debate concerning the need to establish an 'at risk register' for neonates that may have a severe or profound hearing loss. The neonates should be tested initially by behavioural methods and any which are suspected of a hearing loss, or who give doubtful responses, should undergo further testing. Such testing should be conducted either by using the auditory response cradle, or, preferably, by using BAEP.

DETECTION AND DIAGNOSIS

The process of early detection of hearing loss is virtually inseparable from the concept of screening. Screening is carried out in nearly all health districts and authorities in the UK and there is general agreement on the basic details of the test, with considerable variation in practice. It is based on the behavioural response of the normally developing child aged 7–10 months, the optimum age being about 8 months. At this stage in development the child can sit well, with good control of his head, he is less preoccupied visually and will turn his head and eyes to look directly at the source of the sound stimulus. It is necessary to ensure that the sound is presented in such a way that the child is given every opportunity to respond to the stimulus, whilst excluding visual and other cues. The response is not the motor component of a reflex analogous to the startle or auropalpebral reflexes, but is a learned response demonstrating that the child has achieved the fusion of events taking place in the separate sensory spaces of sight and hearing. It is therefore susceptible to all the experiences of the child up to that time and is more difficult to evaluate than is generally realized. Yet it is assumed that health visitors, doctors, or even teachers can carry out this screening procedure with perhaps no more preparation than a morning of lectures and the practical experience of testing one or two children under supervision.

The results are much as one might imagine. In a survey of nearly 3000 8-year-old children born in the EEC countries (CEC 1979), the diagnosis of hearing loss was achieved in just under 10% of them by the first birthday. In order to be included in the study, the child had a minimum loss averaging 50 dB; such is the distribution of deafness that half the children had severe to profound losses, averaging 85 dB or more. Despite the adoption of a national screening programme, the results for the UK were scarcely more impressive: just over 10% were diagnosed by 12 months. Recent scrutiny of the age at diagnosis in children attending the Nuffield Hearing and Speech Centre in London (Martin 1985, Unpublished data) shows that there has been no significant improvement in early diagnosis since

the European study was published in 1979. Individual centres can, with sufficient determination, achieve a much improved rate of detection.

A screening test which identifies 1 in 10 of the children is falling woefully short of the 95% level of detection, which is a reasonable requirement of screening procedures, and indicates a very low level of efficiency. The position is worse than this. Some of the children with severe hearing losses are not diagnosed till months or years later, because their hearing has been passed as normal. In other, much younger children in whom parents, relatives or others suspect the child might be deaf, the diagnosis is delayed until the 8-month hearing screening test (8MHST) because it is thought that hearing cannot be tested until that time.

The tragedy of the deaf child is that for many years it has been possible to identify the presence of congenital hearing loss in the neonatal period. The pioneering work of Marion Downs (Downs & Sterritt 1967) was an attempt to achieve this by using a team of trained observers to identify behavioural responses following the administration of sound stimuli. As is often the way, progress was dependent on advances in other fields. In order to overcome the considerable difficulties the neonate poses to the human observer, the procedure was made more objective by using instrumentation. The Crib-o-gram, introduced by Simmons & Russ (1974), incorporates a motion-sensitive transducer over which the baby is placed. Serial recordings of spontaneous activity are made, and of any change consequent upon the presentation of a loud sound-stimulus. The procedure is repeated a number of times automatically during a 24-hour period. The procedure was refined in a number of important respects by Bennett (1979); he increased the number of behaviours recorded to include head, neck and respiratory activity. Alternating periods of control and stimulus-related activity are compared and the number of trials is adjusted depending on the number of anomalous responses. A reliable test result can be obtained in a few minutes. In a prospective follow-up study of 6000 newborn infants by Bhattacharya et al (1984), 8.1% gave equivocal results; on retesting, this number dropped to 1.7%. Of this latter group, all of whom were subjected to brainstem evoked response audiometry, there were 9 children with significant bilateral hearing loss.

The work of Sohmer and Feinmesser (1967), amongst those studying evoked auditory potentials (of which more detail is provided in the contribution by Gibson) provided the basis for a non-invasive, reliable technique for the identification of hearing loss in almost any age of subject. The procedure would be the nearest approximation to the ideal screening test were it not for the constraints imposed by application of electrodes, the bulk of the equipment and the overall time required to complete the test. Royston et al (1984) have developed a miniaturized, portable and relatively inexpensive unit for administering the BSER which removes one major problem; it should be possible to overcome the problems of electrode design and the test protocol, adapting it for a screening procedure, which, perhaps, in the software design carries on automatically to a threshold measurement if there is no response within the limits set for normality in the paridigm.

The fundamental value of the BSER technique is that it provides a virtually direct measure of threshold hearing function. The 8MHST requires the administration of stimuli at, or as near as possible to the auditory threshold of the normally hearing child. Functionally, it can be looked upon as coming into the same category of test, but the complexity of the neural pathways and the involvement of learning in order to obtain an identifiable response makes it a very different test neuropsychologically. The disadvantages of the Crib-o-gram, auditory response cradle and tests such as the postauricular myogenic response (Flood et al 1982) and other sonomotor test procedures is that the intensity of the presenting stimulus must be far above normal threshold, not less than the 75–80 dB level, in order to elicit a detectable response. Nor is the BSER without considerable drawbacks of its own. It is not foolproof and, in inexperienced hands, can give seriously misleading results. Even when administered by highly trained individuals, the test gives a relatively crude measure of auditory threshold. It is disappointing that 20 years after the introduction of these short latency electrophysiological techniques, we have no adequate measure of threshold in the 1–2 kHz range, nor in the 250 Hz region. In the normal development of voice and speech

perception in the very young child, it is these regions of the auditory spectrum which are the most important. The need for accurate clinical testing techniques, modified to meet inescapable developmental criteria, are no less important today despite, or perhaps because of, the auditory evoked response.

This brief review of the current status of early detection of hearing loss reveals not one but several dilemmas which need to be considered and, where possible, resolved. The first audiology clinic to be established as part of a local health authority child service was in Leicester in 1952 (Humphreys 1960). The screening procedures, based on the pioneer work of the Ewings (1944) in their development of hearing tests in children, have remained essentially unaltered since then. A great many deaf infants have been diagnosed and the appropriate forms of management instituted much earlier than would ever have been thought possible. But we have seen that the detection rate of severe congenital hearing loss remains nearer the 10% rather than the 95% level at which we must aim. This is a field which is more noted for earnest hopes in diagnosis and communicative ability than for their realization in the majority of deaf children.

The EEC study (CEC 1979) showed that 30% of children had been suspected of having a hearing loss in the first year of life, so that if the suspicion of parents and others coming in contact with the child had been acted on expeditiously, the detection rate would have been of the order of three times greater than was actually achieved. One's personal view is that there needs to be a major revision in the approach to hearing screening. Ideally, we should be in a position where the level of health education, knowledge of child development available to parents and specific training for the providers of primary health care would result in detection of poor auditory response long before the 8MHST becomes necessary. In order to facilitate this, McKormick (1983) and Scanlon (1986, unpublished data) have introduced brief guideline questionnaires which are effective in alerting parents and care providers to the possibility of hearing loss at an early stage.

But we are immediately confronted by another dilemma. Even supposing that all congenitally deaf and other children acquiring severe hearing losses in the first few months of life were diagnosed by 8-months-old, would this materially affect the outcome in terms of the quality of spoken language? The results of the EEC study give no evidence to support this long-held view. There is an intuitive appeal in the view that early diagnosis leads to good speech, but there was no positive correlation between the intelligibility of speech and the youngness of the child when the diagnosis was made. Many factors are involved in the development of speech in the deaf child, some of which will be considered in the next section. The question which needs to be considered here is, is early diagnosis early enough? In other words, can we persist in the assumption that to diagnose a child as being deaf at 8–10 months is sufficiently early to overcome all the problems of not having heard the sounds of speech during these vitally important first few months?

It is still widely believed that the child with severe hearing impairment babbles normally until approaching his first birthday. Defining babble as the repetition of the same consonant-vowel combination for two, three or more times in a string, personal observation finds no support whatever for this assumption. In the vocal development of the normally hearing child, the stage before the incorporation of consonant-like sound is the one in which control of the prosodic features of pitch contours, volume and rhythm which comprise the speech carrier wave is largely achieved. This stage is well in evidence by 10–12 weeks (Martin 1981), serving as a constant reminder of the use to which the very young child is putting his developing auditory and vocal skills. The child with a sensorineural hearing loss fails to achieve this vital, earlier stage, let alone the subsequent stage of babbling. If this complex neurological process is not to be distorted, and possibly affected irreparably in some children, one cannot avoid the conclusion that the diagnosis, and the provision of amplification, should be achieved by 6–8 weeks.

Where does this leave the 8MHST? The view expressed here is that it has an unacceptably low level of efficiency, taking the results for the UK as a whole. The detection rate for congenital deafness being significantly worse than if the parents' concern had been used as the alerting factor. The procedure cannot be looked at in isolation: it is not the test procedure itself which is at fault in this respect, but the organizational and clinical framework within which it is placed. Screening is first carried out at 8 months or thereabouts; there may then be one, two or several repeats if the results are equivocal. The child, by now often well past his first birthday, is then referred to one or more medical doctors, perhaps a community paediatrician, the general practitioner, an otolaryngologist, or to a non-medically qualified audiological scientist, technician or teacher of the deaf. At each stage of referral, delays mount up and the parents become increasingly frustrated and despairing. If the procedure is to continue in use, it can only do so effectively when all the intermediate stages are eliminated. The ideal chain is the briefest possible: from failed test, repeated no more than once, to a clinician who is both competent as the secondary level screener and who is also proficient in arriving at the correct diagnosis of type, pattern and extent of hearing loss. It will be appreciated that the 8MHST, if it is to be carried out efficiently, is demanding in terms of manpower, training, facilities and time—all expensive components. Paradoxically, the procedure becomes progressively more expensive in the demands it makes on manpower resources and clinic facilities as equivocation persists and an accurate diagnosis is delayed. The logic of the situation is simple: either the child has a hearing loss, or normal hearing, and there is no longer any technical reason why the hearing loss cannot be identified.

A more cogent reason for replacing the 8MHST than its inefficiency and cost is that it is almost certainly achieving the diagnosis several months too late, even when the sequence of screening-referral–diagnosis–management is completed as expeditiously as one could hope. Fortunately, we have arrived at that point in time when these considerable dilemmas, of excessively low detection rate and of lateness in diagnosis, can both be resolved. In considering the optimum approach to very early diagnosis it is necessary to have constantly in mind the size of the problem. If all newborn children are to have their hearing screened, the screening procedure must be specific, sensitive, non-invasive and capable of being administered quickly and easily. Furthermore, it must be acceptable to the parents and make as little demand as possible on limited resources of trained staff and finance.

The most suitable candidate in many respects

would be the BSER but it is not realistic to suppose that it could become the primary screening procedure without further, considerable development, particularly at the commercial level. It has an important screening role where numbers are relatively small, especially if there is an increased risk of hearing loss, as in those infants who have been nursed in intensive care units. At the present time the most effective and economical approach would appear to be the initial use of the auditory response cradle. A trained nurse, working in close co-operation with the maternity unit nursery, can achieve a through-put of about 2500 newborn infants a year (Tucker 1986, personal communication). Once again it is essential not to think of the screening test in isolation, but to consider the requirements as a whole. Electrophysiological testing must be readily available for all those infants who fail the second cradle test and there must be an experienced team to whom referral can immediately be made for clinical assessment, initiation of management and careful follow-up.

DEVELOPMENT OF COMMUNICATION

The prevailing model on which the management of the hearing-impaired child is based, may be schematized thus:

'If a child cannot hear he will not learn to talk.'

'Give him hearing aids and he will learn to talk.'

This is true for numbers of children, some of whom, despite severe and occasionally profound loss, learn to talk in complex sentences, naturally and fluently, with minimal articulatory defects. Their achievement is remarkable! It is also unusual and until 8 or 9 deaf children in every 10 develop this facility in the use of spoken language the system is failing them. The quality of speech in the 8-year-old children in the EEC study showed that it was not possible for virtually half of them to be understood by those outside their immediate family circle; in 27% the children's speech was grossly defective or unintelligible to members of their own families. In Conrad's (1979) study of all children leaving the special schools for the deaf in England and Wales, the results were much the same. Using a similar five-

point scale of evaluation, he found that no less than 2 out of every 3 children were difficult to understand or unintelligible to strangers. The more recent survey carried out by Markides (1983) confirms the depressing overall picture. He asked the teachers to evaluate the intelligibility of their pupils' speech: of the 2429 children in partial hearing units attached to mainstream schools, 32% came into the categories of 'rather difficult to follow' to 'unintelligible or no speech'. There were 2743 in schools for the deaf, and the comparable figure for them was no less than 58%.

In none of these major studies was any attempt made to evaluate the level of language development. Had it been, the full extent of their communicative deficits would have been laid bare. It is a commonplace in clinical experience to find that many children in the 10–11 year range are unable to put more than an expanded subject-verb-object sentence together in speech. This level of syntactical development is reached in the majority of normally hearing children by their third birthday. The next, more advanced sentence structure, representing stage 5 in the developmental syntax of Crystal, Fletcher and Garman (Crystal et al 1978) may never be adequately mastered. Yet the ability to combine the elements of simpler sentences into utterances with a variety of dependent clauses, incorporating such words as 'and', 'because', 'if . . . then' and so on, marks the gateway to mature language, readily achieved by the typical 4-year-old. There can be no doubt that some of the worst disorders of speech and language, which one sees in clinical practice, affecting otherwise normal children, arise from the effects of hearing loss in the young child.

Why are the results so poor? We are faced by a massive dilemma. What is the nature of the problem? Is it so fundamemtal as to be insuperable, something which we are obliged to accept and do the best we can, whilst knowing that 1 in every 2 severely deaf school-leavers will never achieve the speech skills of the 3- or 4-year-old? Is it one problem, or is it compounded of many—late diagnosis, inadequate hearing aid design and provision, poor teaching of speech mechanics and of the basic structures of language? If we are honest—and if there is to be any progress, it is essential for these children and their families that we are—we would have to acknowledge deficiencies in each of these fields.

But the full depth of the problem has not yet been plumbed.

If we return to the theoretical schema, which might be termed the 'audiological model' of management, there is no recognition of all the many features of normal infant development which have been disrupted by the lack of hearing. Detailed observation of the vocal behaviours of normal infants during the first 18 months of life from birth (Martin 1981) shows that the newborn is modifying his vocalizations from the first or second day. There can be little doubt that he has an innate, specific sensitivity to the human voice. Support for this conclusion comes from the work of Condon & Sanders (1974) who described the 'interactional synchrony' which takes place in the form of various bodily movements occurring in time with the mother's speech. This sensitivity allows a remarkably intense, close-knit process of interaction between the very young child and those around him, with all the implications this holds for bonding. It has other implications: from the time of birth the infant is hearing the human voice and modifying his own innate propensity to vocalize. He first learns to control the basic features of the voice, varying pitch, volume, stress and rhythm, and by 3–4 months the carrier wave for speech is developing well. This demonstrates the integrity of another crucial neurological function, the auditomotor process by which 'sounds-heard' are transformed into motor activity in the various parts of the speech apparatus, resulting in 'sounds-said'. The process is related to, but distinct from, language as such: that it can be an isolated behaviour is clear to all familiar with the parrot and other talking birds, where it is a constant source of amused incredulity. This fundamental process is taken for granted, it has to be; but one sees normally hearing children who demonstrate normal speech perception, but who show severe delay in developing through all the various stages of voice and speech acquisition. A few such children remain truly mute.

The prosodic features of intonation, stress and rhythm, with their high energy, low frequency and slow temporal patterns are salient for the infant in the early weeks and months, and he soon learns to imitate them. Differentiation of acoustically more complex, shorter duration sounds takes place and differing vowel-like sounds and certain voiced consonants such as 'b', 'm' and 'd' begin to appear in the repetitive patterns of babble. All this is normally achieved well before eight months of age. In comparison the deaf child may never gain fluent control of the speech carrier wave and his voice shows poor variation of pitch, with numerous incorrect intonation contours, the rhythm is jerky and laboured and the stress patterns exaggerated and abnormal. Despite this, the emphasis in management is on the production of words: the child is being made to control the articulators of speech before the voice, and the carrier wave for speech, have developed. Intelligibility suffers drastically because it is the prosodic features which convey so much in this respect.

The plea was made above for earlier diagnosis and it was argued that the congenitally deaf child should be provided with amplification by the age of 8 weeks. An added cautionary note, ensuring the greatest respect for the complex neurology of the young developing child, requires that no child be provided with a hearing aid before the age of 6 months or so unless the deafness has been confirmed by electrophysiological investigation. It is not appropriate here to discuss the practical details of exactly how such a young child, vulnerable in so many vitally important respects, should be managed. One can only say that it throws a heavy burden of responsibility on all who undertake this work and I see no alternative to concentrating the supervision of management in the first 8–10 months of life in special centres where the staff have received the requisite developmental training.

One of the major contributions to solving the dilemma of management is to alter the framework of reference and to put the child and his mother at the centre, rather than his deafness. This is not to discard the audiological model of management, but to see that it is, and always has been, inadequate. It is a component of a more comprehensive approach, based on detailed knowledge of child development, interactive behaviour and communication, which might best be labelled the 'developmental communication model'.

What are the benefits of very early diagnosis? Two major deficits of present regimes of management will be overcome. The infant's family will know that he is deaf and, intuitively, with suitable guidance from the management team, will be able to make adaptive changes in their patterns of interaction with him. The other concerns his ability to perceive the prosodic features of his parents' and siblings' voices. Unless he is quite exceptionally deaf, there is a high probability that he will hear sufficiently, with amplification, to develop the basic features of the speech carrier wave and to monitor his own vocal output.

Does this mean that the cordon of dilemma surrounding the deaf child, and impeding so severely his communicative development, will be overcome? Regretfully, no. Experience with a dozen or more deaf children, diagnosed at between 4 and 16 weeks, confirms definite gains in the two major parameters outlined above. But the problem of adequate speech perception, and so of accurate articulation in the child's own speech, remains. The auditory differentiation of vowels and especially the brief duration, low energy (and numerous high frequency) consonants is beyond the scope of the central neural processing mechanisms, given such degraded signals from the inner ear in many children. It is almost certainly the nature of the damage inflicted on the lower reaches of the auditory pathways which determines which children will speak well, despite severe audiometric loss, and those who have little or no speech perception. Diagnostic tools which permit measurement of auditory perception, such as the speech pattern approach of Hazan & Fourcin (1985) and other discrimination tests, are desperately needed in work with the hearing impaired as a routine part of the investigatory armamentarium.

One way of circumventing the speech perception dilemma will lie in improving the technology of the hearing aid. Whilst amplification of the incoming speech signal is sufficient for many hearing impaired, it is manifestly inadequate for many more, despite the refinements of frequency response, volume compression and so on. The deaf child, and numerous deafened adults, require a prosthesis which will process the signal in various ways, so that, for instance, transient, high frequency sounds are rendered more salient, or the contrast between nearby frequency bands is sharpened and becomes discriminable. An essential requirement for the child learning to talk is that the sounds, injected into his auditory nervous pathways through such devices, remain within the possibility of limitation so that his speech is as near normal as possible.

There are other ways by which the problems centering on defective speech perception may be circumvented. In the profoundly deaf it may, in due course, be necessary to consider the place for cochlear implants. It is important to remember that a number of children with hearing losses off the lower edge of an audiogram chart will show remarkable gains with powerful ear level hearing aids, and the audiometric threshold cannot of itself ever be the criterion on which the decision is based. One's own view is conservative, considering it an essential obligation of the proponent to demonstrate a reasonably high probability of speech perception which will lead to the (near-)normal development of spoken language. Unless this is forthcoming, it is advisable for parents and their professional advisers to await further developments in the field. A sorry victim of the interest in cochlear implant surgery is the non-auditory approach to speech perception. It is an unceasing source of amazement to discover how many profoundly deaf young people become adept in music and dance. There is little doubt that vibro-tactile devices, converting acoustic into vibratory energy, have been seriously neglected, and deserve to be actively pursued.

A further approach needs to be considered, especially in view of the widespread opposition to its use. The problem for the child, especially if he is diagnosed late, say during the second year of life or later, is his severe deficit in communication. The only effective approach open to him is by facial expression, manipulative behaviour, pushing, pulling and pointing. The appalling emotional effects on the child and the extent of his frustration are frequently a serious source of anxiety within the family and, not infrequently, lead to overt psychiatric disturbance in later childhood and adolescence (Denmark 1973). The use of manual communication as an adjunct to speech can result in remarkable benefits for the child and his family. Its introduction has a twofold benefit: it facilitates communication so that parents and child can, at long last, have some mutuality of understanding, and it makes visually concrete the parts of speech which go to make up a spoken utterance, however brief. In this way it provides a framework for language learning and, despite widely held views to the contrary, is invariably discarded if no longer of value. The child who persists in using signing is the child who needs to, for his spoken language is inadequate to his needs.

J.A.M. Martin and W.P.R. Gibson have each produced a thoughtful, comprehensive account of the problem of the early diagnosis in very young children and it is very agreeable to me, as adjudicator, to state that I am in general agreement with most of the major points that each has made in his review. Naturally, given the inherently idiosyncratic disposition of most professionals, I hope that any criticisms that I offer will not be considered as carping or pettifogging, as they are solely intended to round out the discussion of the whole problem.

In contributing chapters on a particular topic to a book dealing with dilemmas in otolaryngology it might be expected that the authors would specify such dilemmas as identified in their particular subject. In this case Martin, in the course of an extensive and erudite account of the problems of early diagnosis in congenital hearing loss, mentions the subject of dilemma five times.

However, it is only by studying the context carefully that the dilemma or dilemmas can be clearly identified. Gibson on the other hand does not specify any dilemma or dilemmas at all! A dilemma is generally defined as 'being the state of affairs where one is forced to choose between two alternatives, or two courses of action, each of which involves considerable inherent disadvantages.'

In considering Martin's extensive review of the problem, it emerges that his reference, to 'another dilemma' and 'a massive dilemma' are one and the same, namely the question whether or not striving for earlier diagnosis of infant deafness than is now generally achieved would lead to better results in respect of acquisition of speech, language and education. Gibson, without specifically mentioning this dilemma, alludes to it briefly but clearly. In my opinion this is the first major dilemma associated with this subject. The other major dilemma in this context is the long-standing controversy of oralism versus manualism. The controversy has been formally debated for more than a century and opinions, particularly between opposing groups of educationalists, have become strongly entrenched. It is, of course, a classical two-horned dilemma where either option can involve considerable disadvantages as well as advantages, but, as both authors point out, a refreshing spirit of compromise is visible today

whereby both techniques can often be usefully combined to the advantage of the profoundly deaf child. This is likely to be more productive than the rigid 'either . . . or' position so often adopted in the past. Gibson, in this context, refers to the method of total communication now widely adopted in Australia and in many other countries, where oralism is combined with signing. Martin, reviewing this problem, quotes Denmark and a strong plea is made for manual communication in the case of disturbed profoundly deaf children and adolescents.

The two authors, and no doubt the majority of clinicians who deal with hearing-impaired children, are, by preference, oralists in the sense they would *prefer* the hearing-impaired child to be taught in such a way that his residual hearing is used to promote understandable speech and language. Both authors point out very clearly that this laudable object is often not achieved, leading to failure and frustration. It would seem to me that the introduction of signing before the child has become discouraged by failure to achieve adequate progress by purely oral methods is a sensible idea. It means that the teachers would have to decide, after a reasonable trial with oral methods, which children are likely to progress adequately under this regime, which children would be helped by a combined method and whether profoundly deaf children, who are not progressing at all, should perhaps change over to a manual system entirely.

Both authors, and Martin in particular, draw attention to the shortcomings of behavioural screening tests of hearing, based on the observation by the tester of the child's reaction to voice and various other test sounds and culminating in the tests carried out when the child has attained the age of 6 months. This is referred to by Martin as the 8-month hearing screening test (8MHST) as described in EEC report, or the 7–9 month screening test referred to by Gibson. By the age of 6 months a child can generally sit unsupported on the mother's knee, has satisfactory head control and is able to respond by turning towards sounds presented to right of left ear, visual clues being carefully eliminated. Under good testing conditions with experienced testers the result of such an assessment is quite good, but in general use over the whole child population the results are depressingly poor. Martin discusses the shortcomings of screening tests in considerable detail and both authors list the lamentably poor results achieved in various countries where such screening is widely carried out and both come to the conclusion that, in addition to more and better training for those engaged in screening in the community, two particular technological advances of recent years should be more widely employed to screen for hearing impairment in the neonatal period. These are the auditory response cradle, which should be the first line of attack, with the brainstem electric response test used to check those who fail the cradle test. If such a scheme were followed, it should be possible to detect the presence of significant hearing impairment in virtually all neonates. Both authors refer to the savings in money and resources if these two techniques were widely deployed, because expensive screening testing in the community would become less necessary. I am by no means convinced that this is so, as confirmation of the presence of adequate hearing by behavioural testing in the 7–9 month period would still be necessary in my opinion, even if the cradle or BSER results indicated adequate hearing in the neonatal period. It is not unknown for sensorineural hearing loss to develop in early infancy, or for minor S–N loss to progress, despite clear evidence of hearing in the neonatal period. Some savings would be possible as earlier informal tests of hearing in the community could probably be omitted if the auditory cradle, backed by BSER, were to be generally used for neonatal assessments. Thus, there seems to be little likelihood of appreciable savings in resources to offset the costs of introducing these technological innovations and this may be seen as yet another unwelcome dilemma.

Gibson argues cogently for the establishment of an 'at risk' register for neonates liable to congenital hearing impairment. The main objection to 'at risk' registers is that many of them are not sufficiently discriminatory and that too many children are caught in the net. There may be some virtue in such a register for congenital hearing loss if one is proposing to proceed directly to brainstem testing. He quotes Galambos' and Djupesland's list of neonatal disorders and children with these particular conditions would constitute the bulk of neonates receiving treatment in special care baby units. He

also refers to Marian Downs and Silver's simpler criteria which consists of five factors referred to as ABCDS. Such a scheme would include 1 neonate in 40 (or of all births), but in this group 60–70% could be expected to have a significant degree of congenital sensorineural hearing loss. But, settling on a specific group of at-risk neonates, say 3% or so of all births, there would be every prospect of identifying those with hearing problems by proceeding immediately to BSER a few days after birth. On the other hand, the entire newborn population, but not the high-risk group mentioned above, could more reasonably be tested by means of the auditory response cradle and only those who failed this test would be rechecked by BSER testing. This would seem the way to proceed if scarce high-technology resources are to be most economically employed. A behavioural follow up should be carried out on *all* children in the 7–9 month age group to detect that small number who may have either developed sensorineural hearing loss, or in whom a minor and undetected sensorineural loss may have progressed until it constituted a significant disability for which urgent audiological management and specialized educational measures would be necessary. The behavioural hearing testing at 7–9 months would also provide a valuable second filter in which to trap those infants with impaired hearing who may have slipped through the technological diagnostic net due to technical or procedural shortcomings.

Although both authors either suggest or imply that the technological innovations of the auditory response cradle and auditory brainstem testing method would yield much in the way of savings of scarce reserves and funds, I personally think that such savings would be less than the two authors anticipate, because it is impracticable to abandon the 7–9 months hearing screening tests on all infants, except for those already confidently diagnosed as having a significant hearing loss and who are receiving appropriate management. The whole hearing screening service in the community could no doubt be streamlined and made much more efficient. This should lead to steadily improving results as far as the promotion of speech and language is concerned in these severely handicapped children.

While the two authors have given an excellent review of the current status of the methods of early diagnosis of hearing loss in the very young, and have dealt implicitly with the two major dilemmas one encounters in this field of medicine and audiology, they have neglected to specify them unequivocally.

These two dilemmas are:

1. Very early diagnosis is difficult to achieve clinically especially in the neonatal period, and, while early diagnosis should lead to better results as far as acquisition of speech, language and education is concerned, the outlook for a severely deaf infant in this respect does not seem to have improved as a result of earlier diagnosis.

Fortunately, the one horn of this dilemma, the difficulty of really early diagnosis, has been severely crumpled by improved clinical awareness and technological innovations to the point where confident diagnosis of significant hearing impairment in all cases is now within our grasp. The other horn of the dilemma is the realization that, despite diagnostic improvements, the management of the severely hearing-impaired infant is still a difficult and sometimes unrewarding task. This horn, too, may be blunted and finally eliminated as a danger to the child's development if the improvements in hearing aid design, teaching methods, the importance of the speech carrier wave and even cochlear implants or vibrotactile devices (in the case of the profoundly deaf) are steadfastly applied to the problem, or discarded in favour of others if found to be ineffective. One would expect progress in coping with each aspect of the problem to be a slow piecemeal affair. If slow, it should nevertheless lead to a steady improvement in results if the efforts are sustained and a sudden acceleration in the rate of progress should encourage those whose difficult job it is to help these unfortunate infants. Not to capitalize on the possibilities raised by the fact that diagnosis, even in the neonatal period, is now feasible, is unexceptably nihilist. In spite of the practical difficulties our efforts must be concentrated on improving the capability of these infants to achieve worthwhile communication ability.

I do not necessarily believe that the present state of the art means that hearing aids have much practical benefit before the age of 6 months, although I am sure that many colleagues would say otherwise. Up to the age of 6 months the child cannot even sit unaided and is, in effect, his mother's captive. She has a golden opportunity at this stage of speaking to the child at a short distance—a few inches—which

goes some way to overcoming the effect of the hearing deficit. If the mother talks to the child as often as possible in a firm, clear voice, sings to him with her mouth close to his ear while jogging him on her knee to the rhythm of her singing, she will do much to develop the child's awareness of the important carrier wave of the human voice which carries vital prosodic information about human speech. The problem with fitting aids at the age of 2, 3 or 4 months is the practical difficulty of making really well-fitting ear-moulds. If this difficulty can be overcome then, of course, aids could be very valuable for the infant. If satisfactory ear-moulds cannot be supplied at this early age, and usually this is the case, then one might consider the method advocated by some French audiologists whereby the child is 'bathed in sound'—*baignade sonore*—by placing a small loud speaker in the crib so that the infant in those early weeks of life is constantly exposed to his mother's voice and to the common environmental sounds of the home.

By the age of 6 months I think that aids should be fitted, as in a few short weeks or months the child will become increasingly mobile. It is essential to have the use of hearing aids firmly established before he becomes more mobile and increasingly intolerant of any form of restraint. Failure to introduce adequate amplification in this period will mean that he will increasingly feel the effects of deprivation of early learning of the nature of sound, including his own vocalization, as Martin clearly points out.

2. The second great dilemma is the controversy of oralism versus manual communication. The one horn of this dilemma is that, while the child taught by the oral method will, hopefully, develop adequate speech and language so that he can converse with members of the hearing world and receive a satisfactory education, some children fail dismally to achieve this goal, leading to frustration, dismay, depression and sometimes antisocial and destructive behaviour. The other horn of the dilemma is that, while severely hearing impaired, or even totally deaf children can indeed communicate using manual signs and thereby receive a satisfactory education, they do this at the expense of hearing and speech and can therefore communicate only with their teachers and their classmates. This means that such children may learn more, but communicate less

than a hearing-impaired child who learns to lip-read and to speak successfully. Inability to understand speech and to use it to communicate, not just with their teachers or close family, but with the generality of normally hearing persons, leads those so handicapped to lead an increasingly isolated life, which is not a desirable outcome of years of painstaking teaching.

Finally, I would like to discuss just one practical aspect of brainstem testing, which both authors have rightly described as being the most reliable arbiter of hearing impairment in very young infants. Gibson gives a very clear account of the technique as used in newborn infants and this shows that he has a very good practical insight into the method based on personal experience. The obvious advantages of this method are that this particular series of responses is readily recorded from young infants either awake, or, better still, in natural sleep. If necessary, sedation or even general anaesthesia can be employed without suppressing the responses and, in the young infant as opposed to older subjects, the NI wave (which is identical to the compound auditory nerve action potential of the electrocochleogram) is readily recorded from surface electrodes in young infants. Feinmesser & Sohmer in 1967 described this test as a form of non-invasive cochleography. The clearly recordable responses of the brainstem test give information concerning acuity of hearing as well as auditory function at the periphery and in the neural pathways up to the collicular level. It may also be informative in cases of CNS anomalies or immaturity. Martin, who refers to the imminent commercial availability of a small portable battery-driven brainstem recorder deplores the fact that frequency information is restricted as the brainstem response provides auditory information only from 2 kHz and above. Low frequency information below 2 kHz is almost entirely lacking, despite the best efforts of researchers to rectify this shortcoming. He says that the test therefore gives no information about the important low frequency prosodic features of the continuously varying, low frequency carrier wave of speech, the fundamental speech frequency. I think that this shortcoming is more apparent than real in practical terms, because, if it is impossible to construct an audiogram by the brainstem method by testing with a number of important frequencies, one has to be content to use a wide-band click which contains all frequencies, knowing that only those of 2 kHz and above give recordable responses. What is obtained is a mean decibel level of the response across the frequencies of 2 kHz and above. It is well known that congenital sensorineural hearing loss causes either a flat loss, or more commonly, one which slopes steadily downwards over the higher frequencies. If there is evidence of high frequency hearing as a result of the brainstem test, one can infer that the low frequency hearing is either similar to high frequency hearing acuity where there is a flat loss, or better than the high frequency hearing where there is a sloping high tone loss. The only case where this assumption is misleading would be in the excessively rare cases where the hearing loss profile slopes *upwards* from low to high frequencies, a situation seen in early hydrops in adults, but almost unknown in hearing impaired infants.

In conclusion, I would like to report that, apart from a few minor criticisms, I am in close general agreement with the views expressed in these two highly informative papers.

REFERENCES

W P R Gibson

Appleby S V 1964 The slow vertex maximal sound evoked response in infants. Acta Otolaryngologica suppl 206: 146–152

Ashcroft P B, Humphries K N, Douek E E 1975 New developments in the use of the crossed acoustic response as a screening test in children. Paper read at the second British conference in audiology

Bennett M 1979 Trials with the auditory response cradle: I. British Journal of Audiology 13: 125–134

Bennett M, Wade K 1980 Automated newborn screening using the auditory response cradle: II. British Journal of Audiology 14: 1–6

Davis A 1984 Detecting hearing-impairment in neonates—the statistical decision criteria for the auditory response cradle. British Journal of Audiology 18: 163–168

Davis H, Hirsh S K 1976 The audiometric utility of brain-stem responses to low-frequency sounds. Audiology 15: 181–195

Downs M P, Northern J L 1984 Hearing in children, 3rd edn. Williams & Wilkinson, Baltimore

Downs M P, Silver H K 1972 The ABCDs to HEAR, Clinical Paediatrics 2: 563–565

Galambos R, Dupseland P 1980 The auditory brainstem response evaluates risk factors for hearing loss in the newborn Paediatric Research 14: 159–163

Jewitt D L, Williston J S 1971 Auditory-evoked far fields averaged from the scalp of humans. Brain 94: 681–696

McFarland W, Simmons W, Jones F 1980 An automated hearing screening technique for newborns. Journal of Speech and Hearing Disorders 45: 495

Martin J A M, Bentzen O, Colley J R T et al 1981 Childhood deafness in the European community. Scandinavian Audiology 10: 165–172

Rosen J K, Austin A M 1979 The high risk register for neonates at risk of deafness: limitations of presently recommended procedures. Australian Journal of Audiology 2: 67–71

Shepard N 1983 Newborn hearing screening using the Linco-Bennett auditory response cradle: a pilot study. Ear and Hearing 4: 109–115

Simmons F B 1978 Identification of hearing loss in infants and young children. Otolaryngology Clinics of North America 11: 19–26

Sohmer H, Fiennmesser M 1967 Cochlear action potentials recorded from the external ear in man. Annals of Otology, Rhinology and Laryngology 76: 427–435

Upfold L J 1979 21 birth years—a look at early intervention in Australia. Australian Journal of Audiology 1: 41–44

Upfold L J, Isepy J 1982 Childhood deafness in Australia: incidence and maternal rubella 1949–1980. Medical Journal of Australia ii: 323–326

J A W Martin

Bennett M J 1979 Trials with the auditory response cradle; 1. Neonatal responses to auditory stimuli. British Journal of Audiology 13: 125–134

Bhattacharya J, Bennett M J, Tucker S M 1984 Long-term follow-up of newborns tested with the auditory response cradle. Archives of Disease in Childhood 59: 504–511

CEC (Commission of the European Community) 1979 Childhood deafness in the European community. No EUR. 6413. CEC, Luxembourg

Condon W S, Sander L W 1974 Neonate movement is synchronised with adult speech: interactional participation and language acquisition. Science 183: 99

Conrad R 1979 The deaf school child; language and cognitive function. Harper and Row, London

Crystal D, Fletcher O, Garman M 1978 The grammatical analysis of language disability. Arnold, London

Denmark J 1973 The education of deaf children. Hearing (Sept): 1–12

Downs M P, Sterritt G M 1967 A guide to newborn and infant hearing screening programs. Archives of Otolaryngology 85: 15–22

Ewing I R, Ewing A W G 1944 The ascertainment of deafness in infancy and early childhood. Journal of Laryngology and Otology 59: 309–314

Flood L M, Fraser J G, Conway M J, Stewart A 1982 Assessment of hearing in infancy using the post-auricular myogenic response. British Journal of Audiology 16: 211–214

Hazan V, Fourcin A J 1985 Microprocessor-controlled speech pattern audiometry: preliminary results. Audiology 24: 325–335

Humphreys E B B 1960 The ascertainment of deafness in maternity and child welfare centres. In: Ewing A W G (ed) The modern educational treatment of deafness. University Press, Manchester

McCormick B 1983 Hearing screening by health visitors: a critical appraisal of the distraction test. Health Visitor 56: 449–451

Markides A 1983 The speech of hearing-impaired children. University Press, Manchester

Martin J A M 1981 Voice, Speech and language in the child: Development and Disorder. Springer Verlag, New York

Royston R E, Beagley H A, Vickery J C 1984 A portable brainstem evoked response audiometer. In: Computer-aided biomedical imaging and graphics physiological measurement and Control. Proceedings of the Biological Engineering Society, July

Simmons F B, Russ F N 1974 Automated newborn screening. The Crib-o-gram. Archives of Otolaryngology 100: 1–7

Sohmer H, Feinmesser M 1967 Cochlear action potentials recorded from the external ear in man. Annals of Otology 76: 427–435

10

Are ventilation tubes essential in the management of secretory otitis media?

G.A. Gates

INTRODUCTION

Background

Otitis media is the most common condition of childhood treated by a physician. Estimates of incidence suggest that 75–86% of children have at least one bout of otitis media and that 40% of children experience three or more episodes. The prevalence of acute otitis media (AOM) is highest in 1–3-year-old children and peaks again in the 4–6-year-old group, presumably because of the increased exposure to upper respiratory infections in school classrooms. In an elegant longitudinal study of a day-care population, Henderson et al (1982) showed the strong correlation of AOM to acute viral upper respiratory infections, thus leaving little doubt as to the role of nasal infection in the pathogenesis of otitis media.

The duration of a given episode of AOM is quite variable. Teele et al (1980) noted persistent middle ear effusion (MEE) in 40% of children one month after their first case of acute otitis media, at two months in 20%, and for three or more months in 10%. By convention, an effusion that persists for more than one month is labelled as chronic. Terms often used to name the condition of chronic effusion in the middle ear are chronic otitis media with effusion, persistent otitis media with effusion, and chronic secretory otitis media. The interchangeability of these terms is generally accepted, although some attach particular meaning to each.

Even though the causal relationship of chronic effusion that persists after documented acute infection is obvious, a substantial problem exists regarding the classification of asymptomatic (i.e. painless) middle ear effusion, which is, by definition, of unknown duration. Logically, asymptomatic MEE might be the sequel to an unrecognized episode of AOM, or it could be a separate disorder. From the otolaryngic literature of the past has remained the tacit presumption that asymptomatic chronic middle ear effusion may be the result of factors other than AOM. This conceptualization of persistent effusion is reflected in the frequently used term, secretory otitis media (SOM). Secretory otitis is held to be an abnormal condition of the middle ear mucosa, characterized by mucosal and goblet cell hyperplasia, due primarily to poor eustachian tube function; it is sometimes perceived as a precursor rather than a sequel of AOM.

It is important to recognize that a single episode of inflammation in the middle ear cleft may have both an acute and a chronic phase, each being but one side of the same coin, that is otitis media. To separate and place the chronic stage into a different pathological category is to force a conceptual razor onto our understanding of the disorder. To be sure, much of what we know about otitis media is conjectural (even though based on considerable data) so that the many unresolved dilemmas about treatment may be viewed in more than one light. However, because it is essential to have a consistent view of the pathophysiology of any condition in order to have a logical treatment plan, I feel that any consideration of the chronic stage of otitis media that does not include its acute side as well does a disservice to our understanding of the subject.

While the foregoing rhetoric may seem a bit tedious, it has direct relevance to the discussion at hand. Physicians, logically, apply treatment concepts according to their understanding of the pathophysiology of the disorder. For example, if a condition is perceived as a pathological collection of fluid resulting from a necrotizing infection, i.e. an abscess, the obvious therapeutic principle is to drain the fluid. But an accumulation of infected fluid interspersed within the tissue would be conceived of as a cellulitic process and would be treated medically, not surgically. Similarly, if otitis media is thought of as being the result of outlet obstruction, relief of obstruction is the logical treatment principle. If it is understood to be the result of inlet incompetence, an entirely different approach would be required. Unfortunately, our concepts of the pathogenesis of chronic otitis media with effusion are not uniform and, correspondingly, neither is our treatment.

Definitions

1. Acute otitis media (AOM) is a middle ear effusion accompanied by signs of inflammation such as redness of the tympanic membrane, fever, irritability, or pain. AOM in the infant, as opposed to the older child, has a substantially different clinical presentation: the older child may have no fever and little pain, but redness and middle ear effusion will be present. Younger children with a mild infection may be asymptomatic, that is to say, without pain.

2. Chronic otitis media with effusion (COME) is a middle ear effusion that has been present for more than 30 days. Although the physical nature of the effusion may vary from serous to purulent to mucoid across patients and from the same ear at different times, the underlying pathological disorder is the same. I consider the terms secretory otitis media and chronic otitis media with effusion to be generically equivalent. To be precise, however, one should be able to document the duration of effusion when using COME as a diganosis.

3. Middle ear effusion (MEE) refers to an accumulation of liquid in the middle ear cleft regardless of its presumed aetiology. This term is convenient to use when discussing effusions whose temporal course is unknown. Because it is not possible to distinguish the aetiology of an effusion on the basis of its physical characteristics (i.e. serous, mucoid, purulent), I lump all types of chronic effusion into a single category.

4. Secretory otitis media (SOM) describes an hyperplastic condition of the middle ear mucosa that produces continuing middle ear effusion. Implicit in the use of this term is the possibility that the effusion may be non-infectious in nature. SOM is often used as a synonym for asymptomatic (i.e. painless) middle ear effusion of any aetiology.

Pathophysiology

1. AOM results from bacteria entering the middle ear and inducing an inflammatory response. The principal route of entry is retrograde from the nasopharynx via the eustachian tube. Three factors appear to enhance bacterial reflux into the middle ear: bacterial colonization of the nasopharynx, incompetence of the protective function of the eustachian tube and a pressure differential between the middle ear and the nasopharynx.

That AOM follows an upper respiratory infection is well documented clinically (Henderson et al 1982) and experimentally (Giebink et al 1976). Viral rhinitis causes a loss of mucosal integrity, which, in turn, permits bacterial adherence and growth in the nose and nasopharynx. In addition, swelling of the adenoid pad and nasal mucosa alters the normal aerodynamics of the upper respiratory airway. The bacteria in the nasopharynx are similar to those cultured from the middle ear effusion, namely S. pneumoniae and H. influenzae.

The eustachian tube has three functions: protection of the middle ear, equalization of pressure between the nose and middle ear and clearance of middle ear secretions. In children, where the tube is short, horizontal and composed of relatively flaccid cartilage, the protective function of the tube is impaired and retrograde reflux of nasopharyngeal secretions occurs (Bluestone et al 1972). Clearance is primarily the result of the ciliary action of the tubal mucosa. It is presumed that ciliary function of the middle ear and eustachian tube is impaired during an AOM to the same extent as the nasal mucosa is during an acute upper respiratory infection. If this is indeed the case, we may assume that fluid forming during AOM accumulates in the middle ear primarily because of ciliary paralysis and, further, that clearance of fluid should follow recovery of ciliary function.

Pressure equalization is the third function of the eustachian tube. 'Popping' of the ears during rapid ascent or descent (as in an elevator or airplane) is a common experience. It is mediated by opening of the eustachian tube, permitting the pressure of the gas in the middle ear to equilibrate with the atmospheric pressure. The opening is passive when the middle ear pressure exceeds atmospheric, generally by 100 mmH$_2$O, but must be active when the middle ear pressure is negative. Should the middle ear pressure reach -300 mmH$_2$O or less, the tube may be functionally locked and equilibration through muscular effort to open the tube may be impossible.

The third factor in the genesis of AOM—pressure differential—appears to require both a negative pressure in the middle ear and positive pressure in the nasopharynx to drive infected material up the eustachian tube. Obstruction of the nose secondary to the viral rhinitis results in the equivalent of the Toynbee manoeuvre with every swallow. The Toynbee manoeuvre, designed to ventilate the middle ear, is done by swallowing with the nostrils pinched shut. Since most upper respiratory infections result in nasal obstruction, swallowing during a URI results in increased nasopharyngeal pressure which will open the tube and tend to 'push' secretions earward. Negative pressure in the middle ear may assist in the process by 'pulling' any material in the eustachian tube into the middle ear.

2. Chronic otitis media with effusion: current concepts of the pathogenesis of COME fall into two broad categories: (i) that it is a chronological sequel to acute otitis media, and (ii) that it represents a chronically altered state of the middle ear due to multiple causes, of which eustachian tube dysfunction is the chief. There is evidence to support both concepts which I will summarize in a superficial and reductionist manner, with apologies to those whose diligent efforts have expanded our knowledge of them.

The work of the Greater Boston Collaborative Otitis Media Study Group (Teele et al 1980) gives firm credence to the fact that persistent effusion is a common sequel of AOM and, as any pediatrician knows, is a major problem in the management of this disease. Further support comes from the work of many investigators who, like Liu et al (1976), have demonstrated pathogenic bacteria in the fluid obtained from the middle ears of children with COME. Stengerup & Tos (1985) repeatedly examined a cohort of 360 children and found a significantly higher incidence of abnormal tympanograms in those who had had an acute episode of infection in the preceding three months. It is likely that eusta-

chian tube obstruction and retained secretion in these cases is the result of the acute infection rather than the cause of it. Thus, we may conclude that COME is a sequel of AOM and should be classified as a stage in the pathological spectrum of that disorder. However, we do not know if this concept applies to all cases of asymptomatic MEE in children.

The theory that COME is a primary disorder which predisposes to AOM is supported by the careful and diligent work of Sade et al (1979) and Tos (1974), who have demonstrated that hypersecretory state of the middle ear mucosa exists in patients with SOM. This is attributed to multiple causes, infection included, but the primary pathogenic mechanism is classically ascribed to eustachian tube dysfunction. Such dysfunction, which results in underaeration of the middle ear and negative middle ear pressure, leads to goblet cell hyperplasia and hypersecretion. Hypoxia and hypercapnia of the mucosa, allergy and immune complex formation are also thought to play a role in the genesis of SOM.

The therapeutic implications of these differing concepts is profound. In the first case, antimicrobial therapy would seem to be the primary treatment strategy; in the second, surgical drainage, ventilation and pressure equalization. Our state of knowledge is not yet to the point that the issue can be resolved with great degree of certainty but, as the evidence pointed out below will suggest, it is likely that both treatment concepts have usefulness.

If one accepts the idea that the majority of cases of COME have their beginning in acute infection of the middle ear and that postinflammatory alterations in the middle ear mucosa and eustachian tube lead to persistence of effusion and that obstruction of the eustachian tube is secondary to the infection, rather than the cause of it, we then have a conceptual framework from which to proceed to the task at hand, namely, how best to treat COME.

Consequences of COME

Before discussing therapy, however, it is prudent to examine the natural history of the disorder in order to identify the principal consequences of COME that we wish to avoid. These may be divided into infectious, educational and anatomical sequelae.

1. *Infectious.* It is clear that children with COME are at high risk for recurrent acute exacerbations of their chronic middle ear disorder. Indeed, in our studies in progress (Gates et al 1985a) episodes of AOM are common even in older children who have been treated for typical asymptomatic chronic middle ear effusion. Therefore, prevention of acute infection must remain part of the therapy of COME.

2. *Educational.* It is common knowledge that severe hearing loss creates a severe educational impairment, but it is widely debated whether mild and intermittent hearing loss, such as that due to otitis media, is also educationally handicapping. And, if so, whether its effects are permanent or susceptible to remediation. Klein et al (1984) provided considerable insight into this problem when they demonstrated more retardation of educational achievement in children with frequent otitis media in families of middle versus lower socioeconomic class. Hubbard et al (1985) demonstrated substantial decrements in auditory and articulatory performance in children with cleft palates not treated routinely with tympanostomy tubes.

The educational issue is too complex to treat in any greater detail here. Further, because of problems with accuracy of test measures and difficulties in experimental design, it is likely that a study definitive enough to resolve the issue firmly may never be done. Therefore, one must make a personal judgement on this issue and act accordingly. It is my belief that hearing loss secondary to middle ear effusion imposes a definite risk of limiting the development of cognitive, speech, language and auditory comprehension functions of the child and that correction of that hearing loss is the principal objective of therapy.

3. *Anatomical.* End-stage otitis media is characterized by severe retraction of the tympanic membrane (often with atelectasis and obliteration of the middle ear space), ossicular necrosis, tympanosclerosis and cholesteatoma formation. It is likely that these pathological sequelae are all related, ultimately, to poor ventilatory function of the eustachian tube. Until and unless subsequent research proves this assumption untenable, prevention should be attempted by measures to increase the aeration of the middle ear (see below).

Finally, the natural history of COME should be discussed. It is clear that this is a disease of childhood and that growth brings about changes, presumably in the anatomy and function of the eustachian tube as well as in the immune system, that inhibit the further occurrence of otitis media. Cooper et al (1975) examined the point-prevalence of abnormal otoscopy/tympanometry in school-aged children and found that 20% of kindergarten first-grade children had an abnormal examination, whereas in the fifth grade it was 5%. Tos et al (1982) in their careful, repeated surveys have also noted decreasing prevalence of abnormal middle ears with age. If one considers that inflammation and effusion in the middle ear cleft are symptoms of an underlying diathesis consisting of unknown amounts of eustachian tube dysfunction, immaturity of the immune system, genetic predisposition and environmental factors, it is certain that we can only treat the symptoms and attempt to prevent irreversible sequelae while waiting for development to correct the underlying diathesis.

TREATMENT

Goals

The goals of treatment of chronic otitis media with effusion are prevention of: 1. recurrent acute infection, 2. educational handicaps and 3. anatomical sequelae. Treatment should be carried out until the underlying anatomicophysiological diathesis is resolved.

General measures to prevent acute infection include limiting exposure, insofar as practical, to upper respiratory infection, treating nasal allergy, and decreasing tobacco smoke in the home. Children with frequent acute infections benefit from medical prophylaxis (Perrin et al 1974). Failing this, Gebhardt (1981) showed the value of prophylactic intubation of the middle ear in younger children with recurrent acute otitis media.

Prevention of educational handicaps requires the attention of parents, teachers and physicians alike. Parental awareness will bring about a proper home communication environment with care being taken to facilitate face-to-face conversations and careful enunciation of speech during the times when MEE is present. Preferential seating in the classroom and modification of teachers' communication habits are advisable in this regard. Finally, for children with truly persistent MEE, drainage and aeration of the middle ear via ventilation tubes is advisable.

Children whose middle ears are developing anatomical sequelae should be considered candidates for the full spectrum of medical and surgical treatment (as discussed below) to assist in proper aeration of the middle ears.

Treatment choices.

1. *Non-operative therapy.* Healy (1984) randomly assigned 200 children with asymptomatic MEE to treatment with placebo, or the combination of trimethoprim-sulfa, and evaluated the outcome otoscopically. He found resolution of the MEE at 4 weeks in 58% of the treated group and in 6% of the control group. Gates et al (1986a) administered a 10-day course of erythromycin ethyl succinate plus sulfimethoxizole to 1054 children with asymptomatic MEE and found clearance rates of 64% by 60 days. Thus, there is good evidence that a course of an antimicrobial agent is useful in the treatment of MEE.

Other measures designed to clear the middle ear, such as Politzerization, self-use of the Toynbee manoeuvre and eustachian tube catheterization with retrograde insufflation, do not appear to affect appreciably the ultimate course of chronic otitis media with effusion. One reason may be that the gas that is introduced into the middle ear is quickly absorbed.

For children with persistent effusion who have failed all forms of therapy, use of a hearing aid is encouraged to assist them in critical learning situations such as the classroom, tutoring and special events where even a mild conductive hearing loss might be detrimental.

2. *Myringotomy.* Simple drainage of the tympanum via a myringotomy incision has been shown to be of value in acute otitis media (Roddey et al 1966) and has been used in special cases of recurring effusion in the absence of inflammation. Unfortunately, as a first-line therapy for COME it has little value. Gates et al (1985b) and Mandel et al (1984), in randomized clinical trials, have demonstrated that simple drainage of the middle ear has a limited and short effect. In situations where the procedure can be carried out with local anaesthesia, repeated myringotomy may be a useful technique. However, the majority of young patients would not accept this form of treatment without general anesthesia and, in that instance, the procedure is not effective enough to warrant, in my opinion, the extra risk and expense.

3. *Tympanostomy tubes.* Variously known as grommets, PE tubes, pressure equalizing tubes and ventilation tubes, these tiny cannulae, which are manufactured in a variety of sizes and shapes, have become the most widely used medical devices since their introduction in 1954 (Armstrong 1954); Paradise (1977) estimated that over 2 million were inserted in 1976 in the United States alone. That evidence alone is testimony to their perceived usefulness.

Currently available are additional data indicating their efficacy. In 1980 my colleagues and I began a randomized clinical trial designed to assess the efficacy of tympanostomy tubes and adenoidectomy in the treatment of chronic otitis media with effusion. Although the two-year follow-up period is not complete, we have analysed the outcome of those treated with myringotomy versus tympanostomy tubes (Gates et al 1985a). It is clear that in all measures used to assess outcome, children treated by tubes fared substantially and significantly better than

Table 10.1 Comparison of outcome measures between children treated with myringotomy (MX) or tympanostomy tubes (TT)

	MX (N = 84)	TT (N = 78)	P
Recurrent effusion	75 (89%)	58 (75%)	0.0001
Time to first recurrence	53 d	223 d	0.0001
Medical retreatments	1.82 ± 0.11+	1.2 ± 0.12+	0.0001
Surgical retreatments	0.5 ± 0.08+	0.22 ± 0.05+	0.0001
(number)	31	15	
Time with effusion	23	15 weeks	0.0001
Time with abnormal hearing	16	11 weeks	0.001

+ (mean ± s.e.)

those without (Table 10.1). The average time to recurrence of middle ear effusion was 53 days in the myringotomy group and 223 days in the tympanostomy tube group. This difference corresponds closely to the average duration of intubation (170 days).

4. *Adenoidectomy*. Though not strictly part of the charge of this chapter's assignment, the effect of adenoidectomy must be addressed since the issue of the efficacy of tympanostomy tubes is relative to other options and cannot be discussed in isolation. Long held to be a key factor in the development of otitis media and in poor eustachian tube function, the clinical importance of the adenoid has been downplayed by several studies (Roydhouse 1980, Fiellau-Nikolajsen et al 1984) showing that adenoidectomy has little effect upon the outcome of COME. If one examines closely the design of the studies and reviews them in the light of new evidence, it is clear that the question of efficacy of adenoidectomy must be reopened.

Maw and colleagues (1984) tested the efficacy of adenoidectomy in an interesting manner. They randomized children with bilateral MEE (based on otoscopy and tympanometry) to receive adenoidectomy, tonsilloadenoidectomy, or no adenoid surgery. A tube was inserted into one ear and clearance of the effusion from the opposite, untreated ear was the main outcome variable. Clearance rates were substantially and significantly higher (64% v 16%) in the adenoid-removed group compared to the adenoid-unremoved group. In a later report (Maw 1985), the effect of adenoidectomy was correlated with adenoid size; the larger the adenoids, the greater the impact of removing them.

Adenoidectomy has three possible benefits in the management of chronic otitis media. First is relief of nasal and nasopharyngeal obstruction, second is removal of a source for pathogenic bacteria and third is its effect upon eustachian tube function.

That an enlarged adenoid interferes with nasal respiration and, along with nasal oedema, contributes to reflux of secretions into the eustachian tube is well known. However, most patients do not have high-grade nasopharyngeal obstruction and, therefore, the upper limit of adenoid size that contributes to otitis media is not known. We measure the size of the adenoid on a lateral radiograph of the neopharynx. If it fills two-thirds of the airway we recommend removal.

The crypts of the adenoid, like those of the faucial tonsil, provide a favourable physical environment for harbouring bacteria which cause infection following an upper respiratory infection. Removal of the adenoid creates a smooth nasopharyngeal lining which, presumably, decreases the adherence of pathogenic bacteria and consequently should lower the incidence of otitis media.

Whether adenoidectomy has a direct effect upon eustachian tube function is not well understood. The studies of Bluestone et al (1975) suggest that it does not and, in some cases, eustachian tube reflux may increase after adenoidectomy. Our own data on the efficacy of adenoidectomy are not yet available.

Technical considerations

The techniques for incision of the tympanic membrane and insertion of the tube are limited in variety by the small size of the external auditory canal and the exposure of the drumhead. In general, the incision is made in a radial orientation in the anteroinferior quadrant of the membrane. Care is taken to avoid the superficial blood vessels in order to minimize dissection of blood under the epithelium, which may predispose to tympanosclerosis.

Owing to the patterns of epithelial migration, which begins in the anterosuperior quadrant of the tympanic membrane, it is possible to place the tube in a location that predisposes to either retention or extrusion. If placed antero-superiorly and just in front of the malleus, the tube may be retained for a long time. If placed in the anteroinferior quadrant (which is technically easier), epithelial migration promotes extrusion. The median retention time for tubes of the Shepard variety is 7 months (Gates et al 1985a)

Choosing the type of tube from a variety of over 50 types and makes is largely a matter of individual preference. Short tubes generally extrude sooner than long ones and those with flanges stay longer than those with rounded edges. For recurrent cases and those with high risk of recurrence, I prefer the flanged T-tube, which has prolonged retention characteristics and can be removed easily.

COMPLICATIONS

Anatomical

The incidence of anatomical complications following

the extrusion of TT is uncommon. Persistent perforation of the tympanic membrane occurs in less than 1% of cases and surgical repair at a later date is highly successful. Of all the complications, sclerotic plaques in the tympanic membrane are the most common and appear to increase in incidence proportional to the number of tube insertions. Fortunately, these appear to have a limited effect upon hearing and are generally not treated.

Otorrhoea

The most common problem after TT is purulent otorrhoea. The incidence is generally around 25% of cases although Per-Lee (1981) reported that 75% of his patients with his large, long tube experienced otorrhoea on one or more occasions.

Immediate onset otorrhoea is fortunately relatively uncommon and appears to be lessened by measures to sterilize the ear canal and tympanic membrane prior to opening the tympanum and by the use of antimicrobial–corticosteroid drops (Gates et al 1986b).

Recurrence

A vexing problem with any form of therapy of COME is recurrent effusion. As noted above, 75% of children with tubes develop recurrent effusion in the first year after intubation of the tympanum (as opposed to 89% of children treated by myringotomy). Thus, it can be surmised that what we accomplish with tympanostomy tubes is really a form of otological palliation until time and growth bring about the correction of the underlying problem.

Cost

The cost of TT is not trivial. When physicians' fees (otolaryngologist, anaesthetist, pathologist), operating room and recovery room charges, and the costs of supplies are included the total bill is generally between $600 and $1000 depending on local schedules. Not generally appreciated, however, is the cost of repeated medical therapy. An episode of AOM has direct costs of around $150, much of it out of pocket, plus a variety of indirect costs (time away from work, transportation, sitters, etc.) that

are difficult to compute (Gates 1983). Given that the average child receiving TT has been treated medically four or more times, the cost for the surgery does not seem inappropriate, especially in view of the long period of freedom from symptoms that generally follows.

The principal drawback of TT from the family's point of view is the need for water precautions. Although opinion varies, I advise parents to use ear protection during bathing and swimming and prohibit diving. It appears that longer tubes have a lower risk of water contamination of the middle ear and are, therefore, less hazardous in this regard.

Finally, the subject of tube removal comes up. Personally, I do not remove standard TT; they come out within seven months on the average. However, long-term tubes of the Per-Lee or Goode type may stay for several years and one needs to assess each case individually as to whether or when to remove them. In my opinion, age is the key factor. If the child is past the age of 10 years, he or she should have a relatively low risk of recurrence, assuming of course that the tubes have been in for at least a year. Fortunately, at that age most of the long tubes may be simply removed in the office without anaesthesia. The perforation generally heals in three weeks, or, if it is slow, a paper patch may be of assistance in providing a framework for epithelial migration across the perforation.

CONCLUSION

The title of this chapter summarizes my opinion on the value of tympanostomy tubes in the treatment of chronic otitis media with effusion. When integrated into a staged, incremental management plan, tympanostomy tubes are of proven efficacy and utility. Their chief value appears to be aeration of the middle ear and improvement of hearing. The theory that TT help reverse the abnormal mucosa of the middle ear is not substantiated by the early data from our study: the incidence of recurrent effusion is nearly as great after the tubes fall out as after myringotomy (Gates et al 1985a). It is my current opinion that the longer the tubes stay in, the greater the benefit.

TT are not the whole answer to the problem of persistent MEE but, combined with judicious medical therapy, hearing facilitation measures, and, in selected cases, adenoidectomy, they offer the most cost-effective solution to the problem available today. For families with small children who are 'otitis prone', comprehensive management, which includes TT, has contributed greatly to the well-being of both child and parents alike. The low incidence of complications and the generally indolent nature of them attest to the inherent safety of TT.

INTRODUCTION

Secretory otitis media is a worldwide problem, being primarily a condition affecting young children between 1 and 9 years of age (Brooks 1976, Tos & Poulson 1979, Lous & Fiellau Nikolajsen 1981, Casselbrant 1985). The prevalence decreases with increasing age. Suarez Nieto et al (1983) showed a fall from 38.8% at 2 years to 1.1% at 11 years and the pattern fitted a logarithmic regression curve. The condition is multifactorial in origin, the principal underlying cause being a combination of eustachian tube malfunction leading to, or in association with, middle ear cleft infection. A wide variety of conditions may affect eustachian tube function. Holborow (1970) showed anatomical changes from a childhood to an adult form of the eustachian tube at about the age of 7 years. Functional and mechanical obstruction of the tube may occur (Bluestone & Beery 1976). A relationship between postnasal space obstruction by large adenoids and recurrent acute otitis media has frequently been proposed and was demonstrated in children less than 4 years of age by Quarnberg (1981). McNicholl (1983) postulated nasal septal deformities at the vomero ethmoid suture causing turbulence in the postnasal space in children with secretory otitis media. Todd (1984) noted a larger eustachian tube calibre in patients with otitis media and in cleft palate patients compared with controls. However, the tubal diameter was smaller in patients with secretory otitis media and allergic airway disease. The association between cleft and submucous cleft palate conditions with secretory otitis media in children is now well-recognized (Stool & Randall 1967). Mucosal disease involving the eustachian tube may be due to bacterial or viral infections, it may be allergic, or due to conditions affecting the mucociliary system. Whatever the cause of tubal dysfunction, serous or mucoid fluid accumulates within the middle ear cleft where there is a negative pressure. Usually there are no obvious signs of infection, though bacteria can be cultured from the fluid in as many as 30–50% of cases (Senturia et al 1958). However, secondary infection often develops in association with colds, particularly during the winter months, giving rise to symptoms of acute suppurative otitis. The bacteria found in cases of secretory otitis are similar to those cultured in acute suppurative otitis media (Klein 1980) and to those found in the nasopharynx. Otherwise the condition presents as overt or covert hearing loss. In younger children, the latter often manifests as a speech and language problem (Rapin 1979). Later, if the condition persists, there may be learning and behavioural difficulties (Silva et al 1982, Stewart et al 1984). Secretory otitis frequently follows acute suppurative otitis, invariably after two or three months there is spontaneous resolution of the middle ear fluid (Teele et al 1980). One is able to distinguish two clinical subgroups. There is uncomplicated secretory otitis with reversible tympanic membrane changes in which the underlying eustachian tube malfunction is correctable. In contrast, the condition may present as, or progress to, a complicated state with irreversible tympanic membrane changes. These are secondary to persistent and often uncorrectable Eustachian tube malfunction. In the first group there is a high rate of spontaneous resolution of the fluid which makes guidelines for treatment uncertain. Decision-making for treatment is further complicated in that the fluid may be serous or mucoid and unilateral or bilateral. Furthermore, the tympanic membrane appearances are variable (Malcolmson 1969) and do not necessarily reflect the severity or duration of the subjective hearing loss. Spontaneous improvement occurs with increasing age (Suarez Nieto et al 1983) and different age groups do not necessarily require similar treatment. There is no data to confirm whether shorter recurrent episodes of the condition have the same effect as more prolonged unremitting disease. The measurable audiometric hearing loss, impedance change and otoscopic findings do not always correlate with the overall effect on the child's development. Fria et al (1985) have shown the speech awareness threshold in infants aged 7–24 months with secretory otitis to be in the order of 24.6 dB hearing level. Older children 2–12 years of age had mean three frequency pure-tone audiometric and speech reception thresholds of 24.5 dB and 22.7 dB respectively. They found the hearing acuity was not related to age or duration of the history of secretory otitis. Furthermore, there was no relationship between hearing level and the type of impedance curve. It is not surprising, therefore, that recent studies have confirmed considerable differences in the various types of treatment and the rates at which these are recommended for children suffering with secretory otitis. The differences are found to be both national, at regional and district levels, and international (Black 1985).

Current management regimens should include observation and re-examination for spontaneous recovery. Medical treatment with a wide variety of unproven agents has been suggested. These include local and systemic decongestants, antihistamines and antibiotics. As yet, none has been known to effect any long-term cure (Fraser et al 1977, Hayden et al 1984, Hughes 1984). Even after long-term treatment with amoxicillin and clavulanic acid, Thomsen et al (1985) demonstrated only a short-term benefit limited to children more than 5 years of age. Most authors advise control of nasal and paranasal infection and allergy. Quarnberg (1981) showed a relationship between secretory otitis and radiological clouding of the maxillary sinuses; however, it may be the increased susceptibility to respiratory infections found in patients with respiratory allergy which is responsible for their tubal dysfunction rather than the atopic state itself (Clemis 1976). Ultimately, if the condition persists with significant hearing loss, or if there are gradually worsening tympanic membrane changes as seen on pneumatic otoscopy, surgery is usually recommended. This may take the form of myringotomy with or without insertion of a ventilation tube or grommet, adenoidectomy with or without tonsillectomy. A wide variety of ventilation tubes have been manufactured since their introduction by Armstrong (1954). Basically they comprise two groups. The first is designed to effect short-term ventilation and this type stays in place on average for about six months. The second group is designed for longer-term ventilation over a period of years. The individual pattern of the tubes is probably not important, but technique and position of the tube in the tympanic membrane may be relevant to the duration of satisfactory ventilation and the incidence of complications. Unfortunately, current guidelines for use of a ventilating tube vary widely and often relate to the otologist's personal experience and previous training. Frequently they lack scientific validation. The decision to use a tube is usually made after consideration of several variables.

These include the quantity and type of secretion, duration, severity and effects of the hearing loss and the effect on language, learning and behaviour. In view of spontaneous remission it is likely that more than one assessment should be made before recommending treatment. In this respect the age of the child and the seasonal variation of the condition itself should be taken into account.

SHORT-TERM INTUBATION FOR UNCOMPLICATD SECRETORY OTITIS MEDIA WITH REVERSIBLE TYMPANIC MEMBRANE CHANGES

Surgery may be directed to the ears in the form of myringotomy and this may be combined with ventilation tube insertion, either at the first operation or as a treatment for recurrent effusion. Following myringotomy and suction alone there may be an expected recurrence in 25–30% of cases. Combination of myringotomy with a ventilation tube effects more immediate subjective hearing gain, but this is lost once extrusion occurs and this is usually within 6 or 12 months. The reported complications from ventilation tubes have led certain authors to suggest placement of only one tube in bilateral cases (Lildholt 1979).

Immediately following insertion of ventilation tubes there is a noticeable subjective improvement in the child's hearing acuity. Parents often confirm their own and the child's surprise at hearing sounds, such as birdsong and raindrops for the first time. The general level of the child's awareness is increased, the offspring is often said to be a 'different child'. The duration of these effects is dependent on continuation of middle ear cleft ventilation. Gundersen & Tonning (1976) demonstrated an improvement in speech reception thresholds to 20 dB in 97% of their cases. However, bearing in mind the data from Fria et al (1985) this may not represent a worthwhile gain. More recently their follow-up data leads them to question the long-term efficacy of ventilation tube insertion (Gundersen et al 1984). The immediate hearing gain is greater in ears receiving tubes than those treated with a myringotomy and suction alone. After two years no difference in hearing thresholds could be detected, whether or not a ventilation tube had been inserted (Richards et al 1971, Kilby et al 1972). Residual fluid was present in 30% of cases irrespective of initial treatment. Five years postoperatively in the same study group Brown et al (1978) demonstrated tympanosclerosis in 42% of ears treated with ventilation tubes. A final examination of these children after 10 years showed that the incidence had risen to 70% (Miller et al 1982). There was a minimal incidence of tympanosclerosis in the ears without tubes. To et al (1984) showed that the hearing gain following tube insertion did not extend beyond 12 months, but as yet it is not known whether the presence of a functioning ventilation tube will prevent recurrence of further acute suppurative otitis media. It is also not clear whether the tube prevents continued attic retraction and outer attic wall erosion (Tos et al 1984). Retraction of the pars tensa is prevented whilst the lumen of the tube is patent but there are no studies to show that tubes ultimately prevent or reduce the incidence of chronic suppurative otitis media and cholesteatoma formation. In those cases of secretory otitis complaining of imbalance, phonophobia, tinnitus, or pressure sensation there is usually resolution of symptoms whilst the lumen of the tube remains patent and the middle ear clefts remain dry with normal pressures. Quite often there is an early and noticeable effect on speech and language development (Silva et al 1982, Stewart et al 1984). Concurrent with these effects, there is within the middle ear reversal of mucous gland activity, correction of polypoid mucosal change and cessation of the inflammatory process. Combination of surgery to the ears with adenoidectomy and adenotonsillectomy has usually been recommended in the hope of removing a focus of eustachian tube infection or relieving postnasal space obstruction. However, Mawson & Brennand (1969), Dawes (1970) and Mawson & Fagan (1972) reported secretory otitis in 60% of cases where adenoids were either not present or had previously been removed. Unfortunately, these and other studies designed to confirm or refute an effect of adenoidectomy or adenotonsillectomy on the outcome of secretory otitis have certain limitations of design (Lemon 1962, McKee 1963a, 1963b, Roydhouse 1970, Rynell Dagoo 1978, Stroyer Anderson 1979, Roydhouse 1980, Fiellau Nikolajsen 1980). Few, if any, have been designed specifically to evaluate the effect of the operations on chronic established bilateral secretory otitis with significant hearing loss and appropriate impedance change. Not all have been prospective, randomized, adequately controlled or in adequate numbers. Often there has been failure to investigate each operation separately. Bulman et al (1984) demonstrated some benefit from adenoidectomy at 3 and 6 months postoperatively, as judged by pure-tone audiometry, but again design criteria limited longer-term evaluation. Our own investigations (Maw 1983, 1985a, 1985b, Maw & Herod 1985) have assessed the effects of surgical treatment with adenoidectomy, adenotonsillectomy and grommets on highly selected cases of chronic bilateral secretory otitis with significant prolonged hearing loss. Even in these cases there is still a low rate of spontaneous resolution which continues for 12 or more months following initial assessment. One year after adenoidectomy alone, or insertion of a ventilation tube alone, the effusion resolved in 40% of cases with each procedure. However, in those cases treated by adenoidectomy combined with a unilateral grommet, reinsertion was required in 26%. By contrast, in those with only a tube in one ear reinsertion was required in 54% to maintain satisfactory levels of hearing acuity whilst the study progressed. The effect was seen to be dependent both on the child's age and the size of the adenoids, although the latter was shortlived. It probably reflects some degree of nasopharyngeal disproportion, rather than the size of the adenoids themselves. Unpublished discriminant analysis of our data shows that clearance may be predicted in 70% of cases at one year if both age and adenoid size are taken into account. We have shown quite clearly that the addition of tonsillectomy with adenoidectomy confers no extra benefit. There was seen to be only 1 dB hearing gain at 6 and 12 months by the addition of adenoidectomy with a ventilation tube. However, comparison of a ventilation tube alone with adenoidectomy alone produced only a 3 dB gain at 6 months and less than 2 dB at 12 months for the former procedure, neither of which are significant. To achieve this result only one anaesthetic was necessary for the adenoidectomy cases whereas two or more were required in half of the cases treated with only a unilateral grommet. In contrast to adenoidectomy, in the United Kingdom ventilation tube insertion is usually performed as a day-case procedure requiring a short general anaesthetic. The operation is associated with less morbidity and a lower mortality than are found with adenoidectomy.

Adverse effects

Hospitalization of small children, even on a day-case basis, can present problems. After tube insertion there may be serosanguinous discharge for two or three days but this is usually self-limiting. The incidence of discharge has been reported as high as 34% (Barfoed & Rosburg 1980) and 41% (Kokko 1974). Secondary infection may lead to purulent otorrhoea and this was found in 15% of the series by Birck & Mravec (1976) in 2237 ears. The presence of discharge in the meatus may produce additional otitis externa. Fortunately other surgical complications are unusual, though there may be damage to the ossicular chain. Cochlear or vestibular complications can arise either through indirect trauma via the ossicles or as a result of contamination by solutions used to clean the ear canal. There are reports of migration of ventilation tubes into the middle ear and there may be irritation and otalgia from meatal trauma by the wire attached to the tube. Finally there is the question of restriction of swimming activities. This is advisable during the first few days following surgery. However, most studies suggest that swimming need not be limited thereafter although restriction of diving, jumping or underwater swimming may be prudent in some cases. Delayed complications usually occur as a result of the ventilation tube rather than the myringotomy and small triangular scars at the placement site are frequently found. In our own study, tympanosclerosis developed to some degree in 40% of cases at one year and 70% of cases at two years following intubation. This was seen to be entirely due to the tube, and it progressed to involve further quadrants of the drum (Slack et al 1984). Our own unreported studies show no significant effect on audiometric hearing thresholds one year after treatment. However, clinical impressions suggest that later, in a small number of cases where there is complete tympanosclerotic change throughout the drum, a degree of audiometric hearing loss results. Perforation of the tympanic membrane may persist at the site of the tube and in certain cases the ear remains infected and progresses to chronic suppurative middle ear disease. Tos et al (1984) have shown attic retraction, atrophy or tympanosclerosis in 24% of 5-year-old, 37% of 6-year-old and 39% of 7-year-old non-selected healthy children. There was a correlation between the tympanometric profile, the frequency of otitis and eardrum abnormality which did not seem to be corrected with ventilation tubes. In at least 25% of cases the effusions will recur after treatment and repeat intubation may be required (Brown et al 1978).

Treatment strategy

Medical treatment does not seem to effect resolution of the middle ear fluid in the long-term. However, in this group of uncomplicated secretory otitis, surgical intervention should be deferred for at least three months pending a second assessment. Persistent cases, with only mild hearing loss producing little or no subjective ill-effect, may be further observed before surgery is considered. If surgery is contraindicated or unacceptable, provision of a hearing aid may be necessary.

Provided attention has been paid to other factors such as nasal and sinus disease and underlying atopy, and provided the condition is of appropriate duration and severity, it is likely that surgery will be required for this group of cases. From the outset it would be prudent to inform parents that with myringotomy or ventilation tube treatment alone not only will the effect be relatively short-lived and in the order of 6 months, but there will be a significant requirement for revision surgery for recurrence of the effusion and associated hearing loss. This will certainly be required in 25% of cases and may be necessary in as many as 50%. For this reason, combination of surgery to the ears by myringotomy and tube insertion with selective adenoidectomy has been recommended by some otologists in the hope of providing better and longer-term improvement. Our own study (Maw 1983) was not based on selective adenoidectomy but discriminant analysis of the data would support the suggestion that additional benefit from combination therapy may have some validity. This will require a further study prospectively to confirm or refute the analysis. With limited data, Sade (1979) reported no better improvement of secretory otitis after adenoidectomy with insertion of a ventilation tube compared with a tube alone. By contrast, the retrospective study by Marshak & Ben Neriah (1980) showed a statistically non-significant improvement rate (P < 0.3) in secretory otitis after adenoidectomy with myringotomy (74%) compared with myringotomy alone (59%).

It is unlikely that unilateral cases will require intubation unless they are longstanding, or are associated with a deteriorating tympanic membrane appearance. In bilateral cases the use of one, rather than two tubes, may be expected to reduce the overall incidence of tympanic membrane complications at the expense of less certain symmetrical hearing gain.

It is therefore likely that, in order to restore hearing ability in a proportion of this type of case, a ventilation tube or tubes are essential. Undoubtedly, not as many are required as are currently used on a national and international basis at the present time.

LONG-TERM INTUBATION FOR COMPLICATED SECRETORY OTITIS WITH IRREVERSIBLE TYMPANIC MEMBRANE CHANGES

In these cases there is frequently irreversible eustachian tube malfunction. This situation occurs with craniofacial abnormalities such as Down's and Hurler's syndromes. There may be generalized abnormality of the respiratory tract mucosa, as in fibrocystic disease, or where there is an ultrastructural cilial abnormality. Partially correctible tubal dysfunction occurs in cases with cleft palate. From the outset the tympanic membrane change may be so severe that it is obviously impossible to achieve a satisfactory end result. Atelectatic middle ear disease, where there is loss of the middle layer of the tympanic membrane, retraction of the pars tensa and often significant attic disease may be partly treatable but incurable. Studies of these cases with adequate controls do not exist and treatment of this type of middle ear disease is often empirical. Whether such tympanic membrane changes progress to chronic suppurative middle ear disease and cholesteatoma remains unproven, though clinical impression suggests that it is likely. Moreover, the ability of a ventilation tube either to prevent such change, or in the long term to prevent progression of the atelectatic state is also unknown. The obvious desire to

reventilate the middle ear cleft in the hope of controlling disease and improving hearing acuity has led to the quite widespread use of longer-term ventilation tubes. These are frequently referred to as tympanostomy tubes, being based on the concept of a wide flange of flanges which lie intratympanically and are designed to prevent early extrusion. Clinical experience shows that when used for atelectasis this is not the case and extrusion is common. There are immediate and delayed adverse effects as with short-term tubes. However, there is a much higher rate of complications from placement of a tympanostomy tube, probably reflecting the severity of the disease for which the tube was indicated. It is to be expected that a thin two-layered retracted tympanic membrane will not as easily prevent extrusion of the tube as a pars tensa with an adequate middle layer, facilitating firm retention. The high revision rate following use of long-term tubes also reflects the severity of the disease which frequently progresses inexorably to a more advanced stage.

Strategy

Complicated secretory otitis with irreversible tympanic membrane changes and eustachian tube malfunction may be managed by repeated use of short-term ventilation tubes. In children, multiple general anaesthetics would be required. In adults they may be inserted under local anaesthesia. Long-term tympanostomy tubes undoubtedly resolve some problems of middle ear ventilation but in not all cases. However, the acknowledged failure rate and lack of any other effective treatment for this type of disease has led more conservative otologists to recommend provision of a hearing aid in some of these patients.

SUMMARY

Further careful prospective randomized controlled studies are still required to identify those cases of secretory otitis in which ventilation tube insertion should be recommended. Otoscopic, audiometric and impedance studies with psychosocial and linguistic assessments need to be considered before such recommendation is made. Accepting the limitations described above, short-term ventilation tubes are effective in the management of the uncomplicated condition, but may need to be combined selectively with other surgical treatment methods such as adenoidectomy. Unilateral, rather than bilateral, intubation may be preferable. Repeat intubation may be required in a quarter to half of the cases, especially in younger children; longer-term ventila-tion for complicated cases also requires further eva-luation. However, the suggestion that ventilation tubes are over-utilized as a method of treatment seems undeniable. This being particularly the case in secretory otitis of mild degree, of short duration, and with minimal effect on subjective hearing thresholds which might be expected to resolve spontaneously.

In the western world, secretory otitis media (serous otitis media, chronic otitis media with effusion, etc.) is predominantly a disease of the second half of the twentieth century.

While many causative factors have been addressed in depth, its high prevalence among children is somehow related to the therapeutic armamentarium that has emerged to combat inflammatory diseases. Antimicrobial agents either abort or alter the course of the inflammatory disease process, which, in the anatomical site of the middle ear, can produce other problems.

In Third World countries and among native people in the Western World, i.e. North American Indians and Inuit, secretory otitis media is seldom seen unless therapeutic measures are used, either on a prophylactic basis to prevent, or to treat, acute otitis media. For example, 10 years ago among the Inuit children in the Eastern Canadian Arctic, suppurative otitis media was rampant and secretory otitis media was seldom observed. In contrast today, it is commonplace because of the improvement of medical services.

Secretory otitis media, whatever be its cause, can be an insidious process affecting the total development of the individual.

I find nothing conflicting or controversial in the contributions of George A. Gates and Richard Maw. While one titled his discussions, 'Tympanotomy tubes are essential in the management of chronic secretory otitis media', and the other, 'Are ventilating tubes essential in the management of secretory otitis media?', they are complementary. Both acknowledge that ventilating tubes are clinically useful and advocate that they should be used with discretion and only after other modalities of medical treatment have proved to be ineffective. Their chief value appears to be aeration of the middle ear cleft and improvement of hearing. Both acknowledge that ventilating tubes are not the whole answer to the problem of persistent secretory otitis media, that the introduction of ventilating tubes are not without their complications, but combined with medical therapy, hearing facilitory measures andin selected cases, adenoidectomy, this offers the most effective solution to the problem available today.

There is voluminous literature concerning eustachian tube malfunction, the adenoid and nasopharyngeal obstruction, otitis media, etc., and their inter-relationships. I have been impressed over the years that the size of the adenoid is not that important. Inuit children in Northern Canada seldom, if ever, have large obstructing adenoids, but they have a high prevalence of inflammatory middle ear disease. In southern Canada, many Caucasian children have large adenoids, with or without inflammatory middle ear disease. Numerous children present with a history of recurring inflammatory middle ear disease without nasopharyngeal obstruction. On examination of these children they have small to moderate sized adenoids and many have palpable lymph nodes lying along the posterior border of the sternocleidomastoid muscle in the posterior triangle of the neck. Scrutiny of the nasopharynx reveal in many an abundance of lymphoid islets studding the surface of the mucous membranes covering the eustachian cushion and in the fossae of Rosenmuller. These children usually have prominent lateral pharyngeal lymphoid bands.

The lymphoid drainage from the vault of the nasopharynx courses through the fossae of Rosenmuller to the posterior triangle of the neck bilaterally. Histologically, there are submucosal lymphoid collections extending up the eustachian tube and reaction within these collections can reduce the size of the lumen of the eustachian tube. It is the reaction within this lymphatic tissue which is the important factor.

The extent of lymphoid distribution in Waldeyer's ring and the degree of response/hyperplasia within this tissue is individual. The latter is related to a host–microbe interaction, i.e. host defence mechanisms, and in children this is further influenced by the process of acquiring active immunity. We are all the same, but we are all different, as is the individuality of the host–microbe interaction. The ultimate solution to the problem under discussion, perhaps lies in a better understanding of, and an ability to, manipulate the immune mechanism and not in ventilating tubes.

REFERENCES

G A Gates

Armstrong B W 1954 A new treatment for chronic secretory otitis media. Archives of Otolaryngology 69: 653–654

Bluestone C D, Paradise J L, Beery Q C 1972 Physiology of the eustachian tube in the pathogenesis and management of middle ear effusions. Laryngoscope 82: 1654–1670

Bluestone C D, Cantekin E I, Beery Q C Certain effects of adenoidectomy on eustachian tube ventilatory function. Laryngoscope 85: 113–127

Cooper J C Jr, Gates G A, Owen J H et al 1975 An abbreviated impedance bridge technique for school screening. Journal of Speech and Hearing Disorders 40: 260–269

Fiellau-Nikolajsen M, Felding J U, Fischer H H 1984 Adenoidectomy for eustachian tube dysfunction: long-term results from a randomized controlled trial. In: Lim D J, Bluestone C D, Klein J O, Nelson J D, (eds): Recent advances in otitis media with effusion. B C Decker Inc, Philadelphia, p 302–305

Gates G A 1983 Socioeconomic impact of otitis media. Pediatrics 71: 648–649

Gates G A, Wachtendorf C, Hearne E M et al 1985a Treatment of chronic otitis media with effusion: results of tympanostomy tubes. American Journal of Otolaryngology 6: 249–253

Gates G A, Wachtendorf C, Hearn E M, Holt G R 1985b Treatment of chronic otitis media with effusion. Results of myringotomy. Auris-Nasus-Larynx (Tokyo) 12 (Suppl): 264–266

Gates G A, Wachtendorf C, Holt G R et al 1986a Medical treatment of chronic otitis media with effusion (secretory otitis media). Otolaryngology-Head Neck Surgery (in press)

Gates G A, Avery C A, Prihoda T J, Holt G R 1986b Post-tympanostomy otorrhea. Presented at the 1986 Triological Section Meeting, Southern Section, Orlando, Florida, Jan 17

Gebhart D E 1981 Tympanostomy tubes in the otitis media prone child. Laryngoscope 91: 849–866

Giebink G S, Payne E E, Mills E L et al 1976 Experimental otitis media due to Streptococcus pneumoniae: immunopathogenic response in the chinchilla. Journal of Infectious Diseases 134: 595–604

Healy G B 1984 Antimicrobial therapy for chronic otitis media with effusion. In: Lim D J, Bluestone C D, Klein J O, Nelson J D (eds) Recent advances in otitis media with effusion. B C Decker Inc, Philadelphia, p 285–287.

Henderson F W, Collier A M, Sanyal M A, et al 1982 A longitudinal study of respiratory viruses and bacteria in the etiology of acute otitis media with effusion. New England Journal of Medicine 306: 1377–1383

Hubbard T W, Paradise J L, McWilliams B J et al 1985 Consequences of unremitting middle-ear disease in early life: otologic, audiologic, and developmental findings in children with cleft palate. New England Journal of Medicine 312 (June): 1529–1534

Klein J O, Teele D W, Mannos R et al 1984 Otitis media with effusion during the first three years of life and development of speech and language. In: Lim D J, Bluestone C D, Klein J O, Nelson J D (eds) Recent advances in otitis media with effusion. B C Decker Inc, Philadelphia, p 332–335

Liu Y S, Lang R W, Lim D J 1976 Microorganisms in chronic otitis media with effusion. Annals of Otology, Rhinology and Laryngology 85(25): 245–249

Mandel E M, Bluestone C D, Paradise J L 1984 Efficacy of myringotomy with and without tympanostomy tube insertion in the treatment of chronic otitis media with effusion in infants and children: results for the first year of a randomized clinical trial. In: Lim D J, Bluestone C D, Klein J O, Nelson J D (eds) Recent advances in otitis media with effusion. B C Decker Inc, Philadelphia, p 308–312

Maw A R 1984 Chronic otitis media with effusion and adenotonsillectomy: prospective randomized controlled study: In: Lim D J et al (eds) Recent advances in otitis media with effusion. B C Decker Inc, Philadelphia, p 299–302

Maw A R 1985 Age and adenoid size in relation to adenoidectomy in otitis media with effusion. American Journal of Otolaryngology 6: 245–248

Paradise J L 1977 On tympanostomy tubes: rationale, results, reservations, and recommendations. Pediatrics 60: 86–90

Perrin J M, Charney E, MacWhinney Jr J B et al 1974 Sulfisoxazole as chemoprophylaxis for recurrent otitis media. New England Journal of Medicine 291 (Sept): 664–667

Per-Lee J H 1981 Long-term middle ear ventilation. Laryngoscope 91: 1063–1072

Roddey O F, Earle R, Haggerty R 1966 Myringotomy in acute otitis media. Journal of the American Medical Association 197: 127–131

Roydhouse N 1980 Adenoidectomy for otitis media with mucoid effusion. Annals of Otology, Rhinology and Laryngology 89 (suppl 68): 312–315

Sadé J 1979 The natural history of the secretory otitis media syndrome. In: Secretory otitis media and its sequelae. Churchill Livingstone, New York p 89–101

Stangerup S E, Tos M 1985 The etiologic role of acute suppurative otitis media in chronic secretory otitis media. American Journal of Otolaryngology 6: 126–131

Teele D W, Klein J O, Rosner B A 1980 Epidemiology of acute otitis media in children. Annals of Otology, Rhinology and Laryngology 89 (suppl 68): 5–6

Tos M 1974 Production of mucus in the middle ear and eustachian tube: embryology, anatomy and pathology of the mucous glands and goblet cells in the eustachian tube and middle ear. Annals of Otology, Rhinology and Laryngology 83 (suppl 11): 44–58

Tos M, Holm-Jensen S, Sørensen C H et al 1982 Spontaneous course and frequency of secretory otitis in four-year-old children. Archives of Otolaryngology 108: 4–10

A R Maw

Armstrong B W 1954 A new treatment for chronic secretory otitis media. Archives of Otolaryngology 59: 653–654

Barfoed C, Rosborg J 1980 Secretory otitis media. Archives of Otolaryngology 106: 553–556

Birck H D, Mravec J J 1976 Myringotomy for middle ear effusions. Results of a two-year study. Annals of Otology, Rhinology and Laryngology 85 suppl 25: 263–267

Black N 1985 Geographical variations in use of surgery for glue ear. Royal Society of Medicine 78: 641–648

Bluestone C D, Berry Q C 1976 Concepts on the pathogenesis of middle ear effusion. Annals of Otology, Rhinology and Laryngology 85 suppl 25: 182–186

Brooks D 1976 School screening and middle ear effusion. Annals of Otology, Rhinology and Laryngology 85 suppl 25: 223–229

Brown M J K M, Richards S H, Ambegaokar A G 1978 Grommets and glue ear: a five-year follow-up of a controlled trial. Proceedings of the Royal Society of Medicine 71: 353–356

Bulman C H, Brook S J, Berry M G 1984 A prospective randomised trial of adenoidectomy vs grommet insertion in the treatment of glue ear. Clinics in Otolaryngology 9: 67–75

Casselbrant M L, Brostolf L M, Flaherty M R et al 1985 Otitis media in preschool children. Laryngoscope 95: 428–436

Clemis J D 1976 Identification of allergic factors in middle ear effusions. Annals of Otology, Rhinology and Laryngology suppl 25: 234–237

Dawes J D K 1970 The aetiology and sequelae of exudative otitis media. Journal of Laryngology and Otology 84: 583–610

Fiellau Nikolajsen M, Falbe-Hansen J, Knudstrup P 1980 Adenoidectomy for middle ear disorders: a randomised controlled trial. Clinics in Otolaryngology 5: 323–377

Fraser J G, Mehta M, Fraser P M 1977 The medical treatment of secretory otitis media. Clinical trial of three commonly used regimes. Journal of Laryngology and Otology 91: 707–765

Fria T J, Cantekin E I, Eichler A 1985 Hearing acuity of children with otitis media with effusion. Archives of Otolaryngology 111: 10–16

Gundersen T, Tonning F M 1976 Ventilation tubes in the middle ear; long-term observations. Archives of Otolaryngology 102: 198–199

Gundersen T, Tonning F M, Kveberg K H 1984 Ventilating tubes in the middle ear. Long term observations. Archives of Otolaryngology 110: 783–784

Hayden G F, Randall J E, Randall J C, Hendley J O 1984 Topical phenylephrine for the treatment of middle ear effusion. Archives of Otolaryngology 110: 512–514

Holborow C A 1970 Eustachian tubal function. Changes in anatomy and function with age and the relationship of these changes to aural pathology. Archives of Otolaryngology. 92: 624–626

Hughes K B 1984 Management of middle ear effusions in children. Journal of Laryngology and Otology 98: 477–684

Kilby D, Richards S H, Hart G 1972 Grommets and glue ear. Two-year results. Journal of Laryngology and Otology 86: 881–888

Klein J O 1980 Microbiology of Otitis Media. Annals of Otology, Rhinology and Laryngology 89 suppl 68: 98

Kokko E 1974 Chronic secretory otitis media in children. Acta Otolaryngologica suppl 327: 1–44

Lemon A N 1962 Serous otitis media in children. Laryngoscope 72: 32–44

Lildholdt T 1979 Unilateral grommet insertion and adenoidectomy in bilateral secretory otitis media: preliminary report of the results of 91 children. Clinics in Otolaryngology 4: 87–93

Lous J, Fiellau Nikolajsen M 1981 Epidemiology of middle ear effusion and tubal dysfunction. A one-year prospective study comparing monthly tympanometry in 387 non selected seven year old children. International Journal of Pediatrics and Otorhinolaryngology 3: 303–317

McKee W J E 1963 A controlled study of the effects of tonsillectomy and adenoidectomy in children. Brit J Prev. Soc Med 1963; 17: 49–69.

McKee W J E The part played by adenoidectomy in the combined operation of tonsillectomy with adenoidectomy.

British Journal of Preventive and Social Medicine 17: 133–140

Malcolmson K G 1969 Long-term follow up of chronic exudative otitis media. Proceedings of The Royal Society of Medicine 62: 43–46

McNicoll W D 1983 Otitis media with effusion in children and its association with deformation of the vomero-ethoid suture. Journal of Laryngology and Otology 97: 203–212

Marshak G, Ben Neriah Z 1980 Adenoidectomy versus tympanostomy in chronic secretory otitis media. Annals of Otology, Rhinology and Laryngology 89 suppl 68: 316–318

Maw A R 1983 Chronic otitis media with effusion (glue ear) and adenotonsillectomy: prospective randomised controlled study. British Medical Journal 287: 1586–1588

Maw A R 1985 Age and adenoid size in relation to adenoidectomy in otitis media with effusion. American Journal of Otolaryngology 6: 245–248

Maw A R 1985 Factors affecting adenoidectomy for otitis media with effusion (glue ear). Proceedings of the Royal Society of Medicine 78: 1014–1018

Maw A R, Herod F 1985. The effect of adenoidectomy, tonsillectomy and grommets on otoscopic, impedance and audiometric findings in glue ear. In: International symposium on acute and secretory otitis media, Jerusalem

Mawson S R, Brennand J 1969 Long-term follow up of 129 glue ears. Proceedings of the Royal Society of Medicine 62: 460–463

Mawson S R, Fagan P 1972 Tympanic effusions in children. Journal of Laryngology and Otology 86: 105–119

Miller J J, Wilson F, Richards S H 1982 Grommets and glue ear: a ten year follow up of a controlled trial. Clinics Otolaryngology 7: 135

Quarnberg Y 1981 Acute otitis media. A prospective clinical study of myringotomy and antimicrobial treatment. Acta Otolaryngologica (Stockh) suppl 375

Rapin J 1979 Conductive hearing loss effects on children's language and scholastic skills. Annals of Otology, Rhinology and Laryngology 88: suppl 60: 3–12

Richards S H, Kilby D, Shaw J D, Campbell H 1971 Grommets and glue ear: a clinical trial. Journal of Laryngology and Otology 85: 27–32

Roydhouse N 1970 A controlled study of adenotonsillectomy. Archives of Otolaryngology 92: 611–616

Roydhouse N 1980 Adenoidectomy for otitis media with mucoid effusion. Annals of Otology, Rhinology and Laryngology 89 suppl 68: 312–315

Rynnel-Dagoo B, Ahlbom A, Schiratzki H 1978 Effects of adenoidectomy: a controlled two-year follow-up. Annals of Otology, Rhinology and Laryngology 87: 272–278

Sade J 1979 Secretory otitis media and its sequelae. Churchill Livingstone, New York

Senturia B H, Gessert C F, Car C D, Baumann H S 1958 Studies concerned with tubo-tympanitis. Annals of Otology, Rhinology and Laryngology 67: 440–467

Silva P A, Kirkland C, Simpson A, Stewart I A, Williams S M 1982 Some developmental and behavioural characteristics associated with bilateral secretory otitis media. Journal of Learning Disabilities 15: 417–425

Slack R W T, Maw A R, Capper J W R, Kelly S 1984 Prospective study of tympanosclerosis developing after grommet insertion. Journal of Laryngology and Otology 98: 771–774

Stewart I, Kirkland C, Simpson A, Silva P and Williams S 1984 Some developmental characteristics associated with otitis media with effusion. In: Lim D J, Klein J O et al (eds) Recent advances in otitis media with effusion. B C Decker, Philadelphia, p 329–331

Stool S E, Randall P 1967 Unexpected ear disease in infants with cleft palate. Cleft Palate Journal 4: 99–103

Stroyer-Anderson M, Meistrup Larsen U, Meistrup Larsen K I, Peterson E 1979 Acta Oto Laryngologica (Stockh) suppl 360: 195–197

Suarez Nieto C, Malluguiza, Calvo R, Barthe Garcia P 1983 Aetiological factors in chronic secretory otitis media in relation to age. Clinics in Otolaryngology 8: 171–174

Teele D, Klein J, Rosner B 1980 Epidemiology of otitis media in children. Annals of Otology, Rhinology and Laryngology 89: suppl 68: 5–6

Thomsen J, Sederberg Olsen J, Balle V et al 1985 Long-term antibiotic treatment of patients with secretory otitis media. A double-blind placebo controlled study. In: International Symposium on acute and secretory otitis media, Jerusalem

To S S, Pahor A L, Robin P E 1984 A prospective trial of unilateral grommets for bilateral secretory otitis media in children. Clinics in Otolaryngology 9: 115–117

Todd N W 1984 Otitis media and Eustachian tube caliber. Acta Otolaryngologica suppl 404: 1–17

Tos M, Poulson G 1979 Tympanometry in 2-year-old children. Seasonal influence on secretory otitis and tubal dysfunction. Annals of Otology, Rhinology and Laryngology 41: 1–10

Tos M, Strangerup S E, Holm-Jensen S, Sorensen C H 1984 Spontaneous course of secretory otitis and changes of the ear drum. Archives of Otolaryngology 110: 281–289

11

Tests for nasal resistance—are they worthwhile?

D.J. Brain

That great British physicist Lord Kelvin (1824–1907) once said, 'when you cannot measure what you are speaking about and express it in numbers, your knowledge is of a very meagre and unsatisfactory kind. It may be the beginning of knowledge, but you have scarcely in your thoughts, advanced to the stage of a science'.

When a patient complains of a symptom it is highly desirable to make a quantitative measurement of the disability and there is therefore a very strong theoretical argument for performing nasal resistance tests. Nasal resistance cannot be measured directly, but must be calculated using Ohm's law, when the nasal airflow and the pressure difference at the two ends of the nasal cavities are known. This involves the use of rhinomanometry in which the simultaneous measurement of nasal air pressure and flow is made.

$$\text{Resistance} = \frac{\text{Pressure difference}}{\text{Flow}}$$

These tests have been with us for a long time. Of the two basic techniques in use today, posterior rhinomanometry was introduced by Spiess in 1899 and anterior rhinomanometry by Coutade in 1902. Despite, therefore, a history of nearly 90 years, these tests are not widely performed in the UK today. This has been partly due to technical reasons. The earlier mechanical techniques were too slow to follow pressure changes accurately throughout the breathing cycle and it was only with developments in electronics, combined with adequate components for recording and display, that it became practical to construct the necessary equipment. However, similar constraints affected the evolution of diagnostic audiometry, and the progress in this field had been literally gigantic in comparison, audiometry now being universally accepted as an integral diagnostic

element in otology. The relative failure of nasal resistant tests to make a corresponding impact is due to the fact that most otorhinolaryngologists question the usefulness of such tests and are often deterred by the difficulties of performing them.

One of the problems with these tests is the fact that, under normal conditions, the nasal resistance is constantly changing because the nasal cavities are not inanimate rigid tubes, being lined by a labile mucosa. Mackay (1979) has said, 'the target is constantly moving'. The most important intrinsic factor is the nasal cycle, which was first described by Kayser in 1895. This is present in 80% of the population and is characterized by a reciprocal alternate congestion and decongestion of the turbinates, so that although the total nasal resistance remains fairly constant, there are marked differences on the two sides, which Cole et al (1979) have shown in extreme cases to be in the order of 4 : 1. The usual duration of the cycle in most subjects is about 3–4 hours. Holmes et al (1950) have shown that the nasal mucosa can also react to emotional disturbances.

Extrinsic factors include thermal changes, which may be general or local (Drettner 1963), humidity (Salman et al 1971), tactile stimulation (McLean et al 1976), changes in posture (Cole & Haight 1984) and exercise (Dallimore & Eccles 1979) It has been shown that physical exercise has an extremely potent decongestion action on the nasal mucosa and Broms et al (1982) utilize this fact in their test by exercising the patient on an ergometer bicycle before measuring the nasal resistance. Other extrinsic factors include medication (Jackson 1970), exposure to allergens (Mygind 1979) and irritants (Frank 1970).

I started performing rhinomanometry about 15 years ago and abandoned it because I did not consider it to be worthwhile. I have now reconsidered this assessment in view of the progress which has been made. This includes the ready availability of relatively inexpensive equipment commercially and the work done by the committee on the Standardisation of Rhinomanometry (Clement 1984). This stimulated me to acquire a Mercury NR3 rhinomanometer and my personal experience is based on the use of this machine during the past two years, in a practice which is mainly, although not entirely, rhinological.

The technique of anterior active rhinomanometry is used with this equipment and here one gets some limitations, as it cannot be used in cases of:

1. Septal perforations
2. Where one or both nasal cavities is totally obstructed
3. Very young children
4. Very occasionally when it is impossible to obtain a complete seal at the untested nostril

The use of posterior rhinomanometric technique has been greatly limited by the fact that at least 25% of patients are unable to control the position of their soft palate.

To have any credibility, therefore, these tests should be performed under as controlled conditions as possible and the committee report on the standardization of rhinomanometry (Clement 1984) recommends that the patient should be in a sitting position and should have a rest period of at least 30 minutes prior to the rhinomanometry. Previous use of drugs, exercise, or nasal valve dilatation should be mentioned on the graph.

My answer, therefore, to the question, 'tests of nasal resistance—are they worthwhile?' is 'sometimes'. In many of the patients one sees in an ordinary ear, nose and throat outpatient clinic, such as those, for example, with nasal polyposis, I do not think these tests affect the management of the patient. There is, in my opinion, a strong case for directing selected patients to a special 'nose clinic' on the lines that have been developed by McKay (1983), where a battery of investigations, including tests for nasal resistance, are performed.

The main indications for these tests have been:

1. Nasal challenge tests
2. Medicolegal cases

3. Assessment for surgery
4. Research and clinical trials

Nasal challenge tests

In the vast majority of patients with allergic rhinitis, it is possible to make a diagnosis by taking a careful history, clinically examining the nose and performing allergic skin tests. Certain immunological investigations, such as the estimation of the total IgE level and the use of the RAST test, are sometimes of additional help, although the results usually correlate well with those of the skin tests and it is doubtful if the extra expense is justifiable.

There are, however, a small group of patients in whom identification of the causative allergen is not achieved by these methods and this can be of vital importance if it is decided to treat the patient by immunotherapy. It is now generally accepted that a full course of immunotherapy takes up to three years and the investment of this time and effort necessitates that there should be no doubt as to the identity of the causative allergen. In some patients the results of the skin tests do not correlate with the history. For example, in cases of perennial rhinitis there may only be positive reactions to seasonal allergens on the skin tests and here it is necessary to clarify the position by performing nasal challenge tests. These have the advantage that one is testing the response of the actual target organ. When originally described 15 years ago, the response to the delivery of the suspected allergen was assessed by the number of sneezes, the amount of discharge and the sensation of blockage which followed. The test can be further refined by actually measuring the nasal resistance, as has been described by Schumacher & Pain (1979) and Wihl & Malm (1985). This certainly adds an additional recordable parameter to the test.

As well as its diagnostic value, this test can be used to measure the value of drugs in providing protection against the effects of allergen challenge (Mygind et al 1977). It has, therefore, an important role to play when performing clinical trials on the various therapeutic agents used to treat nasal allergy.

Medicolegal cases

The nose is frequently injured and this does often

lead to obstructive problems of a traumatic nature, which, in many instances, progress into the field of medicolegal practice. Here, the assessment of the disability by rhinomanometry provides useful, additional confirmatory evidence.

Assessment for surgery

The main indication for nasal surgery is the relief of obstruction. For this reason, the measurement of this disability is of critical importance in deciding whether or not to operate on the nose. There is usually, but by no means invariably, a fairly good correlation between the symptom of nasal obstruction and the actual nasal airway resistance.

This was certainly confirmed in a study of 1000 patients by McCaffrey & Kern (1970), who found that a total nasal resistance of 3 cm of $H_2O/l/s$ was in most cases associated with a feeling of blockage. There are exceptions to this general rule, and they include both patients complaining of blockage, for which none can be found, and another group who have an obstructed nose of which they are completely ignorant.

The most common exception occurs in the case of the nasal cycle, as most individuals do not notice the often very marked changes in nasal resistance which occur throughout the day, due to this particular factor.

Another example is the so-called 'paradoxical nasal obstruction', which has been described by Arbour & Kern (1975). These patients have a long-standing fixed unilateral nasal obstruction, to which they have become accustomed and of which they are no longer aware. They rather surprisingly complain of an intermittent blockage on the opposite side, which is due to the variations of mucosal thickening associated with the nasal cycle. When the wide cavity is decongested, the total nasal resistance is within normal limits, but during the congested phase there is a considerable increase in the nasal resistance, producing the sensation of blockage on the normally wide side—hence the 'paradoxicaal nasal obstruction'.

Some patients certainly erroneously describe abnormal sensations in the nose as blockage. We are all familiar with cases of atrophic rhinitis in which the patient complains of a feeling of obstruction, despite the fact that the nasal cavity is completely patent and is, in fact, much wider than normal. Here, there may be an atrophy of the sensory nerve supply to the nasal cavity, which prevents the sensation of air passing through the nose, and which the patients invariably describe as a feeling of blockage. Atrophic rhinitis is an extreme example of a not infrequent problem which occurs when patients complain of nasal stuffiness and blockage, when the nasal resistance is within normal limits. It is most important to recognize this factor, as the results of operating on these patients is invariably disappointing and often makes matters worse. Unfortunately, in the past many of these patients have been treated surgically and this has had a damaging effect on the reputation of nasal surgery. The rhinomanometer can help save the surgeon from this disaster.

When definite nasal obstruction is present, this is sometimes due to skeletal stenosis, as occurs in cases of septal deviation, sometimes to mucosal thickening, which often involves the inferior turbinates, and sometimes to both causes. The selection of patients for operative treatment would be greatly facilitated by a test which would differentiate between skeletal stenosis and mucosal swelling. At present most surgeons make their assessment by taking a careful history and then by inspecting the nose. Probably only about 20% of Caucasians have a straight septum (Gray 1978) and it is therefore important to decide whether the septal deviations that are present in a given case are the actual cause of the obstruction. At present the commonest error is to judge the septal deviations too harshly and this undoubtedly results in many unnecessary septal operations being performed. There have been many papers written on the results of septal surgery and, on average, these seem to be disappointing in about 30% of cases. It would appear that the commonest cause of failure is due to mucosal swelling, which may be either in the form of a vasomotor rhinitis (Thomas 1987), or to allergy (Peacock 1981).

Broms et al (1982) claim that the measurement of nasal resistance after decongestion will reliably differentiate between cases of skeletal stenosis and mucosal swelling. They produce decongestion of the nasal mucosa prior to the test, either by physical exertion or topical vasoconstrictor drugs. The findings were repeated and confirmed by Jessen &

Malm (1984), but McCaffrey & Kern were unable to get such clear cut results and came to the conclusion that rhinomanometry was not helpful in establishing the actual cause of the obstruction. Certainly, further work needs to be done before this point can be clarified.

Despite these limitations, I consider the most important clinical use of the rhinomanometer is to identify those cases which are unlikely to benefit from nasal surgery.

Clinical trials and research

Tests of nasal resistance are a vital tool in both research and when assessing the effects of drugs on the nose. They add an essential quantitative element in making the statistical assessment required in this work.

The use of the nasal challenge test in clinical trial has already been mentioned. The nose, in cases of both allergic and vasomotor rhinitis, is hyper-reactive and this can be demonstrated by measuring the response of the mucosa to the administration of a parasympathomimetic agent such as methacholine. This has been developed into a standardized test by Borum (1979). The response is best assessed by measuring the volume of nasal secretions following methacholine challenge, but rhinomanometry can also be incorporated into the test. In addition to its diagnostic value, it can also be used to assess the effects of treatment on the nasal mucosa (Malm et al 1981).

CHOICE OF AVAILABLE TECHNIQUES

We have discussed the main indications for performing tests of nasal resistance and it is now necessary to consider the relative merits of the techniques which are available. The following are the main requirements for any method

1. *Simplicity of operation.* This is both from the point of view of the patient and the technician. This factor is of particular importance when performing tests on children and should be as non-invasive as possible, because any discomfort or unpleasantness will erode the degree of co-operation by the patient and probably result in inaccuracies.

2. *Accuracy.* The results obtained should be reliable and consistent.

3. *Standardization.* It would be desirable to have an internationally agreed standardization of these tests so that workers in different countries could readily compare their measurements, such as occurs in audiology. Unfortunately this has not been achieved, but the work of the European Standardization Committee (Clement 1984) is a major step in this direction and there is a strong case for following their recommendations.

4. *Availability of equipment.* Many papers have been written by workers who have constructed their own equipment. This is not practicable for most of us and the ready commercial availability of an adequate instrument at a reasonable cost is, therefore, essential.

There are many methods available, but none are perfect, and those which I shall consider are:

1. Active rhinomanometry
   a. anterior
   b. posterior
2. Passive rhinomanometry
3. Plethysmography
4. Peak expiratory flow rate

Active rhinomanometry

With active rhinomanometry, the airway resistance of one or both nasal cavities is measured during spontaneous breathing. With the anterior technique, the pharyngeal pressure is recorded via one nasal cavity connected, in an airtight fashion, to the pressure catheter. Meanwhile, the flow through the other open nasal cavity is simultaneously measured. In the posterior technique, the pharyngeal pressure is measured by a catheter inserted into the mouth, the lips being closed. The flow through either one or both nasal cavities is simultaneously measured.

In theory, the posterior method has the advantage of being non-invasive, enabling one to make rapid measurements of the total nasal resistance. In practice, it has the major difficulty that 30% of patients tested are unable to relax their soft palates to obtain accurate measurement of the nasopharyngeal pressure. Patience and instruction will reduce this figure, but there remains a hard core in which the technique is impossible to perform.

The alternative of anterior rhinomanometry also has some limitations. The two nasal cavities must be completely separate and it cannot, therefore, be used in cases of septal perforations. The nasal cavity must not be so badly obstructed that the nasopharyngeal pressure cannot be transmitted anteriorly to the vestibule where the pressure measurements are made. This technique cannot, therefore, be used in cases of very severe or total obstruction. Despite these problems, the anterior method is more generally applicable. It is well tolerated and can be used on children (Georgitis 1985). Several instruments are available commercially at reasonable cost. It is important that the method used to fix the pressure measuring tube to the nostril should not distort the nostril as this can alter the size of the internal nares, thus causing inaccuracies. Adhesive tape is certainly, preferable and can be readily used by paramedical personnel. A transparent mask should be provided so that kinking of the tube or deformation of the nostrils can be readily seen and corrected before the test is commenced. A linear pneumotachograph is desirable, although this can be of either the lamellar or diaphragm type. A simple water manometer should be incorporated into the instrument so that the pressure transducer can be calibrated and this should be carried out at least once a day. As previously mentioned, the conditions of the test should be standardized.

The best method of presenting results is by using an XY recorder. The observer can actually see the curve of flow and pressure during each inspiration and expiration. It is then possible to judge from the shape of the curve if there are any errors in preparing for the test—such as leaks around the tube. The consistency of the curve with 4–6 breaths can be established and then the calculation of the results can be made by a small computer, which will provide a permanent record on hard copy. This particular method has been recommended by the European Standardization Committee, who advise that the rhinomanometric values should be expressed in SI units, (pressure in pascal and flow in $cm^3.s^{-1}$). Preference was also given by this committee for giving expression of the resistance at a fixed pressure rather than a fixed flow, the reference pressure being 150 Pa.

Passive rhinomanometry

Here, air is blown through one or both nasal cavities during the examination and the patient is told neither to breathe or swallow. Most workers in this field agree that it is far better to make measurements of nasal resistance during spontaneous breathing rather than in this atypical fashion. In practice it also has many disadvantages, including:

1. The probe used to blow air into the nose has to fit extremely tightly into the nostril in order to produce a completely airtight seal which does not break down under pressure and thus inevitably cause distortion.

2. There is a possibility of air being blown from one nostril through the nasopharynx and back out through the opposite nostril.

3. Both these factors mentioned above produce extremely variable, inconsistent and inaccurate results.

4. The equipment is not readily available commercially. Several manufacturers of passive systems have appeared from time to time, but have stopped production quite soon.

Plethysmography

Butler (1960), working in the Physiology Department at Birmingham University established that it was possible to measure the nasal resistance by this technique. The whole body plethysmograph makes simultaneous measurement of alveolar pressure and airway flow. The combined nose-mouth airway resistance is first measured and then, by clamping the nose, the mouth airway resistance is measured. From these two readings the nasal airway resistance can be calculated.

The technique is efficient, reliable and makes minimal demands on the patient as regards co-operation or skills. The enormous financial cost of a body plethysmograph precludes its widespread use in most ENT departments. There may be some scope in large centres for the combined use of this equipment with departments of respiratory physiology (Nolte Lüder-Lühr 1973).

Peak expiratory flow rate

Taylor et al (1973) has adapted this last concept by using the much simpler and cheaper alternative of the peak flow meter. The results he obtained compared well with rhinomanometry, but he did encounter some problems, which included:

1. The making of about 12 maximum expirations is exhausting even for young healthy adults.

2. When there was a high degree of nasal blockage, it often resulted in the inflation of the Eustachian tubes, which many patients found alarming and this often deterred them from maximal expiratory effort during the rest of the test.

3. A lot of mucus was blown into the mask during the test.

There are, therefore, advantages and disadvantages in all these methods, and certainly none is anywhere near perfect, but anterior rhinomanometry seems to be generally the most useful technique available to us at present.

SUMMARY

Tests for nasal resistance provide the rhinologist with an additional means of assessing nasal function. It must be emphasized that they supplement, and do not act as a substitute for, the traditional methods, including taking a history and performing a clinical examination of the nose.

They have already become established as an essential tool in research, but their role in routine clinical work is less certain. Despite the limitations and drawbacks of the present tests, I believe that they deserve to be used much more extensively than occurs at present in this country.

INTRODUCTION

The shape of the narrow nasal airways provides a large surface area in relation to airway resistance. This fact makes it possible for the nose to condition the air effectively during inspiration and to recover heat and water during expiration. In these respects the nose is superior to the mouth. We try to breath through the nose in spite of the fact that it requires more energy than oral breathing. Physiological aspects are therefore more important than comfort when choosing to use the nose or the mouth for breathing.

Nasal obstruction is a very common complaint among patients in otorhinolaryngological practice. Objective methods to evaluate nasal obstruction are therefore often required. Rhinoscopy is usually not sufficient to meet such a demand, objective tests being required in order to carry out scientific, physiological, pharmacological or allergological investigations.

Measurements of nasal resistance have been made for many years in order to provide objective assessment of nasal obstruction. Different methods have been used, but, so far, their use has not generally become acceptable. Several factors have contributed to this delay, the main one being the late standardization of rhinomanometry.

METHODS AND PRINCIPLES

Among the different methods for measuring nasal resistance, the following principles have been used: rhinohygrometry, rhinomanometry, peak flow measurement, body plethysmography, oscillation method, rhinostereometry.

Rhinohygrometry

By expiration through the nose towards a cold surface (of metal or glass), the size of the condensing water spots gives an approximate idea of the patency of the two nasal cavities, but no information about total resistance (Zwaardemaker 1925). This method still has a clinical application because it is simple and cheap.

Rhinomanometry

Most of the clinical and scientific investigations have been based on a variety of rhinomanometric measurements. Some of these involved only measurements of pressure in the nose, which gives an approximate value of nasal resistance. The word rhinomanometry is used today in a broader sense, implying measurements both of airflow and pressure through the nose, i.e. rhinorheomanometry. Different procedures have been used.

Air can be blown passively through the nose by a pump. This method is usually considered to be less physiological compared to that using the air flow during ordinary or forced breathing. Passive rhinomanometry has been replaced by active rhinomanometry. However, since passive rhinomanometry usually requires less co-operation by the patient, it is a useful method in children (van Cauwenberge et al 1984).

Furthermore, the apparatus is relatively simple and cheap. Active rhinomanometry can either be performed as anterior or posterior rhinomanometry. Anterior rhinomanometry implies that the pressure is recorded in one nostril while the patient breathes through the other. The pressure in the nostril is the same as the pressure in the nasopharynx, since no air passes through this cavity. The air flow passing through the other nasal cavity can be measured in two different ways, either by introducing a nozzle into the nasal opening or by using a mask with a pneumotachograph. The latter method is usually preferred, due to the fact that the nozzle can interfere with the patency of the nasal cavity. The pressure recording in this system is obtained by using a plastic tube going through the mask and then taped to the nostril, making an airtight seal.

In posterior rhinomanometry the pressure is recorded from a tube in the mouth. This pressure is almost identical to that in the oropharynx. In posterior rhinomanometry a mask is always used covering the nose and most of the face. In order to compensate for the resistance of the mask, the differential pressure between the tube in the mouth and another tube from the mask is measured.

Air flow in both anterior and posterior active rhinomanometry is measured by a pneumotachograph connected to an amplifier and recorder. The results can be evaluated as pressure curves, one expressing the pressure fall over the nose and one the air flow. The results can also be visualized by using an XY recorder, e.g. an oscilloscope showing air flow on one axis and pressure on the other. A third way is to use a digital system expressing a figure for nasal resistance.

Different units have been used for flow and pressure, but today it is recommended using SI units, i.e. pressure (p) in Pascal and flow ($\dot{V}$) in cm^3. s^{-1} (Clement 1984).

Expression of nasal resistance

In pulmonary physiology, the resistance (R) is usually calculated thus:

$$R = \frac{\triangle p}{\dot{V}}$$

This simple relationship refers to laminar air flow in the lower airways. However, in the nose there is more turbulent air flow and this turbulence is variable depending upon air flow. With a complete turbulent air flow, the resistance should be:

$$R = \frac{\triangle p}{\dot{V}^2}$$

In the nose, the exponent is not 2 but about 1.7, indicating that there is not complete turbulence (Drettner 1961). Other ways have also been used to express the relationship between laminar and turbulent air flow. The relationship between pressure and flow varies with flow rate making it necessary to have a defined point on the pressure flow curve where the measurements are taken. This is obvious if the resistance is expressed:

$$R = \frac{\triangle p}{\dot{V}}$$

which is the usual method. Instead of measuring resistance in the nasal airways conductance (C) can be used. Conductance is defined as $1/R$.

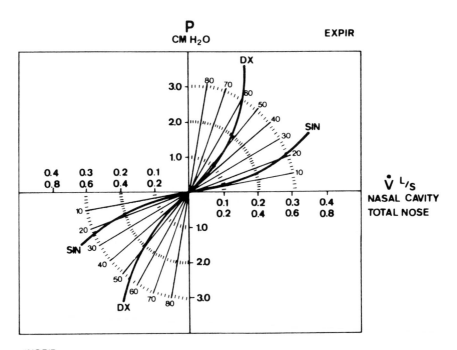

Fig. 11.1 Nasal resistance according to Brooms. There is one flow scale for the nasal cavity and one for the total nose. The curves representing the right and left cavity in a patient are shown. Angles are read from the circular scales. The angle V_2 is 53° for the right and 16° for the left nasal cavity. These values can easily be transformed to resistance. Furthermore the total nasal resistance can be calculated by a special formula. (By permission from Broms et al 1982a.) The values today should be expressed in pascal and cm^3. s^{-1} (SI units).

One way to express resistance is to use the pressure at a certain flow rate, while the flow, at a certain pressure, can be used to express conductance. When the parameter flow at a certain pressure is used, the total conductance of both nasal cavities can be obtained only by adding the flow rates for each nasal cavity.

Rohrer's formula $p = K_1 \times \dot{V} \times K_2 \times \dot{V}^2$ has sometimes been used. This illustrates both the laminar and turbulent part of air flow. The work of breathing is another useful way of expressing resistance by the formula $W = p \times \dot{V}$ (Cole et al 1979).

A new and elegant way of expressing nasal resistance is to use the polar co-ordinates of the pressure–flow relationship (Broms et al 1982a). The polar co-ordinates are obtained on the XY recording by drawing an arc connecting the pressure of 2 cm of water (approximately 200 pascal) and the airflow 200 cm^3 per second (Fig.11.1). The intersection between this arc and the pressure-flow curve is the polar co-ordinate. Broms' method involves a clinical, statistical, as well as a mathematical, model for the calculation of nasal resistance. The latter makes it possible with a simple computer system to calculate total nasal resistance based on the results from each nasal cavity.

Standardization

A standardization committee reported in 1984 (Clement 1984). Different methodological steps for determining nasal resistance have now been standardized and it was decided to give preference to the formula $R = \dfrac{\triangle p}{\dot{V}}$. The choice of a point for measuring resistance has two alternatives. The first is at a fixed pressure of 150 Pa, the other is Broms' model using resistance at radius 200 in a XY co-ordinate system. Both were considered equally good.

Standardization of rhinomanometry should solve many problems in this area. As a result of this standardization, much of the previous criticism of rhinomanometry can probably be eliminated, since results can now be compared as soon as standardization has been generally accepted.

Normal values for nasal resistance measured according to the system of Broms have been published for persons of different height (Broms 1980). Both

mean values and upper limits have been presented, although these do not include children. Furthermore, normal values have only been presented for measurements after decongestion.

Nasal peak flow measurements

Peak flow measurements have been used to measure both expiratory and inspiratory flow rates (Davies 1978). Since these are dependent on pulmonary capacity, the results are usually not considered to be as reliable as more conventional rhinomanometry. However, for evaluation of nasal resistance during repeated examinations, it is helpful, e.g. when doing objective provocation in patients with allergic rhinitis.

Body plethysmography

Body plethysmography is a fairly complicated procedure which is used in pulmonary physiology and also for studies on nasal resistance. The air flow is measured from the changes in thoracic volume and nasal resistance determined as the difference between total air resistance obtained during nose breathing and that obtained during mouth breathing (Niinimaa et al 1979, Graamans 1980).

Oscillation methods

For experimental research, impedance measurements working with a 10 Hz airstream have been used (Berdel et al 1981). Furthermore, a forced random noise technique has been tested (Fullton et al 1984) but these methods have not been commonly accepted.

Rhinostereometry

Stereotactic measurement of one defined point in the nose has been used to observe intermittent changes in the swelling of the mucosa (Juto & Lundberg 1982). This method which uses an adapted microscope is relatively simple.

Errors

There are several errors in measurements of nasal resistance. Rhinohygrometry and peak-flow measurements are considered to be particularly unreliable, the latter being more dependent on the patient's co-operation than other methods.

In rhinomanometry and body plethysmography, different errors are involved. The mask can distort the nasal opening and gives an increased humidity for the nose. A nozzle in a nasal opening can distort the other nasal passage. In posterior rhinomanometry there is a complete failure if the subject obstructs the passage between anterior and posterior part of the oropharyngeal cavity, or if he cannot avoid sucking on the tube. Therefore, posterior rhinomanometry has a failure rate of 10–20%. In anterior rhinomanometry this kind of error is avoided.

Physiological variations in nasal resistance are factors making comparisons unreliable.

It has been estimated that duplicated rhinomanometrical measurements within 15 minutes have an error of 20–25% and day-to-day variation of more than 50% has been reported (Kumlien & Schiratzki 1979, Hasegawa et al 1979). This makes evaluation of changes from one time to another more difficult than for example duplicated audiological tests.

Measurements in children are usually associated with greater errors, although, by using passive anterior rhinomanometry, these are to some extent avoided (van Cauwenberge et al 1984).

Procedures for measurements

The subject should sit quietly for at least 30 minutes prior to rhinomanometry. During measurement the subject remains seated and breathes quietly.

Measurements of the resistance in each nasal cavity are usually performed and the total nasal resistance of both nasal cavities is also measured and/or calculated. Measurement in the recumbent position and when lying on either side is sometimes done in order to study the effect of nasal congestion due to posture. Measurements usually include recording after decongestion either by physical exercise, or by nasal decongestants.

APPLICATION OF TESTS FOR NASAL RESISTANCE

Clinical application

A great number of patients visiting otolaryngolo-

gists complain of nasal obstruction. It is of utmost importance to be able to check this symptom objectively. Subjective nasal obstruction can occur without any real pathological obstruction, e.g. in atrophic rhinitis. Rhinomanometry can show that no increased resistance is present in such cases.

Nasal obstruction can be caused either by deformaties in bone and/or cartilage, or by mucosal swelling. Differentiation between these two kinds of deformities can be performed by carrying out nasal resistance tests before and after decongestion, e.g. topical nasal decongestion drops, or physical exercise. Mucosal swelling will be reduced by such a procedure, while anatomical deformities persist (Bachman 1982, Broms 1982).

Evaluation of rhinomanometry as a test to indicate whether or not septal and/or nasal reconstructive surgery is necessary and to check the results of surgery have been performed in several investigations (Stoksted 1969, Feenstra 1982, Sherman 1977, Bachman & Nieder 1978, Broms et al 1982b, Jessen & Malm 1984). Opinions of the value of rhinomanometry vary in different reports. Some of the more modern papers emphasize that rhinomanometry is of definite value. Broms et al (1982b) showed that those patients, who preoperatively had a high nasal resistance, were mainly satisfied with the result of the operation. Those who, preoperatively, had normal nasal resistance but still complained of nasal obstruction and were operated upon, were not satisfied. Broms et al (1982b), furthermore, made a rhinomanometric analysis of the results of nasal operations. They found that patients who had a high nasal resistance before operation afterwards had a decrease in resistance in the narrower side and in the total nose. Resistance has slightly increased in the wider side. For the group with normal nasal resistance before operation there were no statistical differences pre- and postoperatively. Jessen & Malm (1984) followed up patients who were candidates for nasal surgery, but, due to normal resistance, were not operated upon. Follow-up after five years showed that many of the patients had spontaneously lost their subjective complaints.

Other rarely performed operations in the nose have also been checked by pre- and postoperative rhinomanometry: cryosurgery, vidianectomy (Bachmann 1982).

Rhinomanometry can also be used to reveal the

area in the nose which requires most surgical attention. A high nasal resistance after decongestion is usually indication of an obstruction situated in the valve area, which is the narrowest part of the nose. Furthermore, resistance which is higher during inspiration indicates a collapsed alae where resistance increases during inspiration.

Rhinomanometry is not only of value in pre- and postoperative evaluation. It is also used in clinical practice for allergological investigation. The provocation test used in testing for nasal allergy is usually performed as a subjective test evaluating nasal obstruction, secretion and sneezing. Some authors claim that more exact information can be obtained by combining this with rhinomanometry (Aschan & Drettner 1958, Bachman 1982), or rhinostereometry (Juto 1985), while others have not been able to show such an effect (Wihl & Malm 1985). Rhinomanometry can also be used to check the effect of antiallergic treatment given before a second provocation. In this way, antihistamines, topical corticosteroids and sympatomimetic drugs have been tested objectively.

Other nasal medications have been tested objectively by rhinomanometry. The effect and duration of nasal decongestants have been tested objectively (Aschan & Drettner 1964, Rundcrantz 1969, Broms & Malm 1982). New drugs have been suggested based on the results of such studies (Bende et al 1985).

The effect of different environmental factors, e.g. exposure to cold, has been clarified by using rhinomanometry (Drettner 1961, Cole et al 1983). In some industries, workers are exposed to airborne irritants which cause symptoms. Rhinomanometry has been used in combination with other tests to investigate such occupational factors (Wilhelmsson & Drettner 1984).

Scientific investigations

Modern knowledge of nasal physiology is, to a great extent, based upon studies of changes in swelling of the nasal mucosa. Therefore, nasal resistance tests have to a great extent contributed to scientific development. The nasal cycle, the nasal effect of physical exercise and of changes in posture are physiological variations mainly measured by rhinomanometric tests. Furthermore, nasopulmonary

reflexes have been investigated by using nasal and pulmonary tests (Ogura et al 1964, Cole 1976).

ADVANTAGES AND DISADVANTAGES OF NASAL RESISTANCE TEST

Objectivity and accuracy

Modern equipment for rhinomanometry provides an objective measurement of nasal resistance in which different factors can be analysed. It is, therefore, a complement to a case history and rhinoscopy, sometimes combined with nasoscopy. The value of rhinomanometry to check nasal surgery and carry out objective nasal provocation has been clearly established. The high frequency of error must, however, be recognized in all measurements of nasal resistance.

Standardization

Many different methods have been developed in different clinics, but commercially available apparatus are few. Variations in methods of recording and expressions of nasal resistance has been a drawback which, one hopes, will be overcome.

Earlier instruments for nasal resistance tests were mostly built by combining different instruments not originally intended for rhinomanometric work.

Among the different commercially available instruments used for rhinomanometric measurements is Rhinotest MP (EVG-Vertriebs-GmbH, Ludwigshafen Rhein, West Germany). This is a microprocessor-controlled nasal resistance meter with digital display, a printer and an XY recorder, or computer. The mask covers the whole face. Results are mainly expressed as the flow $\triangle p = 150$ Pa, but also the part of the curve between 150 Pa and 300 Pa is checked.

Another commercially available instrument is Rhinomanometer NR3 and NR4 (Mercury Electronic, Scotland), which has both a digital and an XY recording system. It has a wordprocessing printer and an XY pen-recorder expressing nasal resistance as flow $\triangle p$ 150 Pa.

Computerized instruments will probably be commercially available in the near future (Hamilton & Christman 1977, Cole 1980) and an apparatus using Broms' system has been suggested (Jonsson et al 1983).

FUTURE DEVELOPMENT

It seems likely that rhinomanometry will be more commonly used. In order that the method is generally accepted in clinical practice, it is necessary that a simple, cheap reliable apparatus is available.

Tests to measure nasal resistance are thus of great value and will definitely be used more widely in the near future.

Nasal obstruction is one of the commonest symptoms that bring patients to the rhinologist. Often this is associated with deflection of the nasal septum and it is tempting to assume that the obstruction will be relieved by the apparently simple mechanical expedient of submucous resection.

Yet this procedure is not by any means uniformly successful to the patient, even when the septum, postoperatively, is perfectly straight.

This means that other factors must be at work, and these are usually to be found in the lateral wall of the nose. Some of them, such as polyps, are obvious and call for no further investigation; more commonly it is congestion (or decongestion) of the turbinates, particularly of the inferior turbinates, that determines the degree of discomfort caused by nasal stuffiness.

Even with the healthiest of noses, the nasal resistance is not unvarying. The 'nasal cycle', for example, has been referred to by both Borje Drettner and David Brain and it occurs in 80% of the population; furthermore, there is a whole host of environmental factors which alter the state of the nasal airway. There can be few people who do not breathe more clearly through their noses in the open air than in the dry atmosphere of air conditioning and central heating.

This may be no bad thing and it is probable that the nose would perform its own 'air conditioning' function less well if it were not capable of initiating these changes; yet it is this very variability in the balance between congestion and decongestion in the highly vascular tissues of the 'erectile' inferior turbinates which makes it so difficult to find a really satisfactory way of measuring nasal resistance in a truly meaningful way.

As David Brain points out, attempts have been made for not far short of a century to assess objectively the sensation, sometimes largely subjective, of nasal obstruction. Perhaps the simplest of all is to hold a wisp of cotton wool beneath the nostrils and to observe whether or not it moves up and down with inspiration and expiration. I like the slightly more sophisticated, but equally simple, method described by Gertner and his colleagues in Haifa (Gertner et al 1984), in which the patient is asked simply to breathe on to a polished chrome-coated metal plate, when the pattern produced by the expired air can be recorded graphically. This is but a modification of rhinohygrometry, originally described by Zwaardemaker in 1925.

These methods may not be very scientific, but they do share the virtues of simplicity and cheapness, without any of the distortions that are inevitable when a nostril is invaded or occluded.

Both Drettner and Brain give useful reviews of the various methods used, both of them favour rhinomanometry, especially anterior rhinomanometry, as the most promising method of studying nasal resistance.

Both these authors recognize the limitations of rhinomanometry and, in my opinion, the failure rates are far to high to warrant the use of such a time-consuming procedure in routine clinical practice. Even Drettner, a recognized enthusiast, states that, 'The high frequency of error . . . must be recognized in all measurements of nasal resistance'; and he quotes errors of 20–25% in 'duplicated rhinomanometrical measurement within 15 minutes' and day-to-day variations of more than 50% (Kumlien & Schiratzki 1979, Hasegawa et al 1979). Brain, too, emphasizes that nasal resistance is constantly changing. Furthermore, anterior rhinomanometry is of no value in the presence of a septal perforation, or when one or both nostrils are totally obstructed.

It is true that some of the earlier objections to rhinomanometry have been mitigated by attempts at standardization (Clement 1984), but many variables still remain. As Drettner admits, this makes the evaluation of changes from one moment to another much more difficult than the evaluation of changes in hearing, for instance by audiological tests. Brain also compares rhinomanometry with audiometry. So, too, do Gertner and his colleagues (1984), who state that, 'The state of rhinomanometry is comparable to that of audiometry 40 years ago'.

However, in my view, such comparisons with audiometry are unhelpful: in the first place pure tone audiometry is not an objective test. More importantly, fluctuations in the state of the nasal airway are more wide-ranging, both in normal and in the majority of pathological conditions, than fluctuations in the state of hearing.

If any comparison is to be made between rhinomanometry and audiological tests, it would be more rational to compare it with tympanometry. Both rhinomanometry and tympanometry produce objective responses, in the sense that they are recorded without the active co-operation of the subject under test. Even here comparisons are somewhat spurious, for the parameters measured by rhinomanometry vary sometimes from minute to minute and certainly from hour to hour, whereas those recorded by tympanometry change over much longer time periods, usually of days or weeks and sometimes not at all.

So it is wiser to consider tests for nasal resistance on their own terms and, before attempting to answer the question, 'are they worthwhile?' one must ask, 'are they worthwhile for what?'.

Following the lead of Drettner and Brain, I will comment on these tests separately, in their two main contexts: research and clinical aspects.

RESEARCH

Both Drettner and Brain seem to agree that the main value of tests for nasal resistance lies in the field of scientific investigation, as in studies of the physiological changes which occur during the 'nasal cycle' and of the effects on the nose of physical exercise or changes of posture.

Brain emphasizes that these tests may also be of value in assessing the effects of drugs on the nose, commenting that, 'They add an essential quantitative element in making the statistical assessment required in this work'; and it is to their credit, for instance, that tests of nasal resistance have exploded the myth that menthol is a nasal decongestant. Eccles & Jones (1983) measured the total nasal resistance to air flow in 31 subjects before and after 5 minutes exposure to menthol vapour; they found that the inhalation had no consistent effect on nasal resistance. Although the majority of their subjects reported an increased sensation of nasal air flow, they found no evidence to support any decongestant effect, attributing the apparent relief to the cooling effect of menthol.

Both authors have also staked a claim for the value of rhinomanometry in assessing the results of nasal challenge in allergic subjects and in clinical trials of various decongestant preparations.

It is in this type of work that tests for nasal resist-

ance have their most worthwhile application and any attempt to assess such things in a more scientific way is to be applauded.

CLINICAL APPLICATIONS

Most of the claims that are made for the clinical value of tests for nasal resistance relate to the indications for, and results of, nasal surgery.

Nasal obstruction may result from changes in the skeletal structures of the nose, and particularly of the nasal septum, from changes, either permanent or transient, in the nasal mucosa and, not infrequently, from combinations of these factors.

Brain has said: 'The selection of patients for operative treatment would be greatly facilitated by a test which would differentiate between skeletal stenosis and mucosal swelling'; and two Scandinavian authors (Nicklasson & Sunden 1982) have claimed that, when rhinomanometry is done *after decongestion*, it may be a useful tool in selecting patients whom one may expect to benefit from septal surgery. Ian MacKay and his colleagues (1983) have expressed this succinctly. 'Persistence of increased nasal resistance after decongestion', they write, 'is compatible with a mechanical cause for the nasal obstruction'.

But surely the same information can usually be obtained by careful clinical observation of the effects of decongestion, and so often do skeletal and mucosal changes coexist that examination of the nose before and after spraying it with decongestant solution should be encouraged as a routine part of the assessment of any patient for surgery to the obstructed nose. When surgery *is* recommended, attention should be paid to the common combination of skeletal and mucosal defects.

Drettner further claims that, 'Rhinomanometry can also be used to reveal the area in the nose which requires most surgical attention'. As an example, he states that, when nasal resistance is increased during inspiration, this is indicative of collapsed alae; but surely the dramatic relief usually afforded in such instances by the simple insertion of a nasal speculum will not escape the notice of an observant rhinologist.

Both Drettner and Brain mention that atrophic rhinitis may lead to a complaint of nasal obstruction, both of them mention the use of rhinomanometry in preventing the potential disasters of operating on these patients; but the reasons for the sensation of obstruction in atrophic rhinitis are well enough known and rhinomanometry should really not be required to prevent such a gross error of judgment.

I can see little justification for the routine clinical use of tests for nasal resistance, but it is to be hoped that the reported results of rhinomanometry will encourage all rhinologists to observe more diligently the effects of inserting a nasal speculum or of ap-

plying a decongestant, and to remember that skeletal and mucosal lesions often coexist. In short, to examine their patients more carefully.

In theory, one would expect that a symptom apparently so mechanical as nasal obstruction should yield to the essentially mechanical solution of surgical intervention, but the symptom is so often ephemeral that the patient is likely to remain the final arbiter of the success or failure of our attempts to relieve his stuffy nose.

REFERENCES

D J Brain

Arbour P, Kern E B 1975 Paradoxical nasal obstruction. Canadian Journal of Otolaryngology 4: 333–338

Borum P 1979 Nasal metacholine challenge. Journal of Allergy and Clinical Immunology 63: 253–257

Broms P, Jonson B, Malm L 1982 Rhinomanometry. Acta Otolaryngologica 94: 523–529

Clement P A R 1984 Committee report on standardization of rhinomanometry. Rhinology 22: 151–155

Cole P, Haight S J 1984 Posture and nasal patency. American Review of Respiratory Diseases 129: 351–354

Cole P, Mintz S, Nhimmaa V, Silverman F 1979 Nasal aerodynamics. Journal of Otolaryngology 8: 101–105

Dallimore N, Eccles R 1977 Changes in human nasal resistance associated with exercise, hyperventilation and rebreathing. Acta Otolaryngologica 84: 416–421

Drettner B 1963 Blood vessel reactions in nasal mucosa. International Rhinology 1: 1–7

Frank R 1970 Effects of inhaled pollutants on nasal and pulmonary airflow resistance. Annals of Otology, Rhinology and Laryngology 79: 540–546

Gray L P 1978 Deviated nasal septum: incidence and etiology. Annals of Otology, Rhinology and Laryngology 87 (suppl 50): 3–20

Holmes T H, Goodell H, Wolf S and Wolff H C 1950 The nose. Thomas, Illinois

Jackson R T 1970 Pharmacological responsiveness of the nasal mucosa. Annals of Otology, Rhinology and Laryngology 79: 461–467

Jessen M, Malm L 1984 The importance of nasal airway resistance and nasal symptoms in the selection of patients for septoplasty. Rhinology 22: 157–164

Kayser R L 1895 Über den meg det atmungluft durch die nase. Archiv für Laryngologie 3: 101–110

Mackay I S 1979 Measurement of nasal airflow and resistance. Journal of the Royal Society of Medicine 72: 852–855

Malm L, Wihl J A, Lamm C J, Lindqvist N 1981 Reduction of metacholine induced nasal secretion by treatment with a new topical steroid in perennial non-allergic rhinitis. Allergy 36: 209–214

McCaffrey T V, Kern E B 1979 Clinical evaluation of nasal obstruction. Archives of Otolaryngology 105: 542–545

McKay I S 1983 A nose clinic: initial results. Journal of Otolaryngology 97: 925–931

McLean J A, Mathews K P, Clarkowski A A 1976 Effects of topical saline and isoproterenol on nasal airway resistance. J Allergy Clin. Immunol. Journal of Allergy and Clinical Immunology 58: 563–574

Mygind N J, Johnsen, Thomsen J 1977 Intranasal allergen challenge during corticosteroid treatment. Clinical Allergy 7: 69–74

Peacock M R 1981 Submucous resection of the nasal septum. Journal of Laryngology and Otology 95: 341–356

Salman S D, Proctor D, Swift D L, Evering S A 1971 Nasal resistance. Description of a method and effect of temperature and humidity changes. Annals of Otology, Rhinology and Laryngology 80: 736–743

Schumacher M J, Pain M C F 1979 Nasal challenge testing in grass pollen hay fever. Journal of Allergy and Clinical Immunology 64: 202–208

Thomas J N 1978 SMR—a two year follow up survey. Journal of Laryngology and Otology 92: 661–666

Wihl J A, Malm L 1985 Rhinomanometry in routine allergen challenge. Clinical Otolaryngology 10: 185–189

B Drettner

Aschan G, Drettner B 1958 Nasal obstruction at provocation experiments in patients with hay-fever. Acta Otolaryngology (Stockh) Suppl 140: 91–99

Aschan G, Drettner B 1964 An objective investigation of the decongestive effect of Xylometazoline. Eye, Ear, Nose and Throat Monthly 43: 66–74

Bachmann W 1982 Die Funktionsdiagnostik der behinderten Nasenatmung. Einführung in die Rhinomanometrie. Springer-Verlag, Berlin

Bachmann W, Nieder Th 1978 Der klinische Wert der Rhinomanometrie. Eine Analyse der Diskrepanzen zwischen Anamnese, Befund und Rhinomanometrie. Zeitschrift für Laryngologie und Rhinologie 57: 379–383

Bende M, Andersson K-E, Johnsson C-J, Sjögren C, Svensson G 1985 Vascular effects of pheynlpropanolamine on human nasal mucosa. Rhinology 23: 43–48

Berdel D, Gast R, Huber B 1981 The simplified oscillation method for measuring nasal resistance during provocation with allergens. Clinical Allergy 11: 385–393

Broms P 1982 Rhinomanometry. Procedures and criteria for distinction between skeletal stenosis and mucosal swelling. Acta Otolaryngologica (Stockh) 94: 361–370

Broms P, Jonson B, Lamm C J 1982a Rhinomanometry. A system for numerical description of the nasal airway resistance. Acta Otolaryngologica (Stockh) 94: 157–168

Broms P, Jonson B, Malm L 1982b Rhinomanometry. A pre- and postoperative evaluation in functional septoplasty. Acta Otolaryngologica (Stockh) 94: 523–529

Broms P, Malm L 1982 Oral vasoconstrictors in perennial non-allergic rhinitis. Allergy 37: 67–74 van Cauwenberge P B, de Schynkel K, Kluyskens P M 1984 Clinical use of rhinomanometry in children. International Journal of Pediatric Otorhinolaryngology 8: 163–175

Clement P A R 1984 Committe report on standardization of rhinomanometry. Rhinology 22: 151–155

Cole P 1976 The extrathoracic airways. Journal of Otolaryngology 5: 74–85

Cole P 1980 Respiratory rhinometry, a review of recent trends Rhinology 18: 3–8

Cole P, Niinimaa V, Mintz S, Silverman F 1979 Work of nasal breathing: measurement of each nostril independently using a split mask. Acta Otolaryngologica (Stockh) 88: 148–154

Cole P, Forsyth R, Haight J S J 1983 Effects of cold air and exercise on nasal patency. Annals of Otology, Rhinology and Laryngology 92: 196–198

Davies H J 1978 Measurement of nasal patency using a Vitalograph. Clinical Allergy 8: 517–523

Drettner B 1961 Vascular reactions of the human nasal mucosa on exposure to cold. Acta Otolaryngologica (Stockh) Suppl 166

Feenstra L 1982 Neusweerstandsquotient een maat voor neusobstructie. Thesis, University of Groningen

Fullton J M, Fischer N D, Drake A F, Bromberg P A 1984 Frequency dependence of effective nasal resistance. Annals of Otology, Rhinology and Laryngology 93: 140–145

Graamans K 1980 Neus and Luchtweg. Thesis, Vrije Universiteit, Amsterdam

Hamilton L M, Christman N T 1977 Nasal airway resistance computer. Laryngoscope 87: 1945–1950

Hasegawa M, Kern E B, OBrien P C 1979 Dynamic changes of nasal resistance. Annals of Otology, Rhinology and Laryngology 88: 66–71

Jessen M, Malm L 1984 The importance of nasal airway resistance and nasal symptoms in the selection of patients for septoplasty. Rhinology 22: 157–164

Jonsson B, Malm L, Ivarsson A, Benthin M, Lamm C J 1983 Automated rhinomanometry. Rhinology 21: 265–272

Juto J-E 1985 Rhinostereometry. Thesis, Stockholm

Juto J-E, Lundberg C 1982 An optical method for determining changes in mucosal congestion in the nose in man. Acta Otolaryngologica (Stockh) 94: 149–156

Kumlien J, Schiratzki H 1979 Methodological aspects of rhinomanometry. Rhinology 17: 107–114

Niniimaa V, Cole P, Mintz S, Shephard R J 1979 A head-out exercise body plethysmograph. Journal of Applied Physiology 47: 1336–1339

Ogura J H, Nelson J R, Kawasaki M, Dammkoehler R, Togawa 1964 Experimental observations of the relationships between upper airway obstruction and pulmonary function. Annals of Otology, Rhinology and Laryngology 73: 381–403

Rundcrantz H 1969 Postural variations of nasal patency. Acta Otolaryngologica (Stockh) 68: 435–443

Sherman A H 1977 A study of nasal airway function in the postoperative period of nasal surgery. Laryngoscope 8: 299–303

Stoksted P 1969 Long-term results, following plastic septum surgery. International Rhinology 7: 53–61

Wilhelmsson B, Drettner B 1984 Nasal problems in wood furniture workers. Acta Otolaryngologica (Stockh) 98: 548–555

Wihl J-A, Malm L 1985 Rhinomanometry in routine allergen challenge. Clinical Otolaryngology 10: 185–189

Zwaardemaker H 1925 Die Physiologie der Nase und ihrer Nebenhöhlen. In Denker, Kahler (eds) Handbuch der Hals-Nasen-Ohren-Heilkunde Springer-Bergmann, Berlin Bd I, p 439–484

J Ballantyne

Clement P A R 1984 Committee report on standardization in rhinomanometry. Rhinology 22: 151–155

Eccless R, Jones A S 1983 The effect of menthol on nasal resistance to airflow. Journal of Laryngology and Otology 97: 705–709

Gertner R, Podoshin L, Pradis M 1984 A simple method of measuring the nasal airway in clinical work. Journal of Laryngology and Otology 98: 351–355

Hasegawa M, Kern E B, O'Brien P C 1979 Dynamic changes in nasal resistance. Annals of Otology, Rhinology and Laryngology 88: 66–71

Kumlien J, Schiratzki H 1979 Methodological aspects of rhinomanometry. Rhinology 17: 107–114

MacKay I, Stanley P, Greenstone M, Holmes P, Cole P 1983 A nose clinic: Initial results. Journal of Laryngology and Otology 97: 925–931

Nicklasson B, Sunden L 1982 Rhinomanometry and septoplasty. Journal of Laryngology and Otology 96: 991–995

Zwaardemaker H 1925 Die Physiologie der Nase und ihrer Nebenhöhlen. In: Denker, Kahler (eds) Handbuch der Hals-Nasen-Ohren-Heilkunde. Springer-Bergmann, Berlin Bk I, p 439–484

12

Is surgery the only treatment for recurrent nasal polypi?

A.B. Drake-Lee

INTRODUCTION

The most important precept in understanding the management of any disease, is to have a thorough knowledge of the pathogenesis of the condition. Even if treatments are limited, it will allow advances in therapeutics to be tried and therapy to become a dynamic process. It will also mean that the patient will be managed on scientific and structured lines. Unfortunately, ENT surgeons rely heavily on personal observations and anecdotes: both are notoriously unreliable and unscientific. It is natural that doctors with surgical training will look to this for cures, and perhaps the bigger and more complicated the operation the more likely success will be. Attitudes to the treatment of nasal polyps reflect this conflict and, although it would be absurd to suggest that surgery has no part in the management of the condition, its place must be seen in perspective. Medical treatment has both a definite and increasing place in the management of recurrent nasal polyps.

Surgery

Surgery has been the mainstay of treatment since antiquity. Hippocrates advocated surgical removal by passing a piece of thread through the nose into the oropharynx. This was pulled out of the mouth and a piece of sponge or linen cloth was tied to it. It was then placed into the postnasal space and pulled through the nose, clearing away the polyps in transit. In the Middle Ages and during the Renaissance, instruments similar to those used today were developed (Vancil 1969). Pain-free surgery only came about with the use of cocaine in the nineteenth century and, together with improved illumination,

allowed more satisfactory surgical procedures. General anaesthesia permits more extensive surgery to be performed, or the surgeon to spend all day with the microscope picking out minute pieces of nasal mucosa. Surgical procedures include simple nasal polypectomy, intranasal ethmoidectomy, external ethmoidectomy and procedures on the maxillary sinuses, which include intranasal antrostomies and the Caldwell-Luc operation. All except simple polypectomy are of dubious merit. Supporters of more extensive procedures have never published any worthwhile figures to show their greater efficacy in controlling the condition. Despite the enthusiasms of surgeons, polyps have a great tendency to recur and, plainly, surgery does not cure the disease in the majority of cases.

Another consideration must be the complications that can follow any surgical procedure. Intranasal ethmoidectomy renders the middle turbinate unstable and if it is lost then subsequent surgery is all the more difficult. It makes the cribriform plate more vulnerable and the anterior cranial fossa at risk. The intraorbital structures are always at risk. The long-term sequelae of surgery is the possible development of mucocoeles of the ethmoid and the frontal sinuses.

Recurrence

Only a small proportion of patients with nasal polyps will have severe recurrence. A two-year study of recurrence showed that just over 5% of the admissions had had five or more previous polypectomies whereas over 40% were presenting for the first time. Some of these would obviously go on to develop the more florid manifestations of the disease. It was not possible to determine all the factors associated with recurrence, but the age of onset, the presence of asthma and the presence of aspirin hypersensitivity were important. These patients also had had more extensive sinus surgery and, rather than controlling the condition, appeared to have no impact (Drake-Lee et al 1984b).

Pathogenesis

A more rational approach is needed based on a thorough knowledge of the pathogenesis of the condition. Unfortunately again, the theories of pathogenesis are based on misconceptions. The two main theories are that polyps are either infective or allergic. Other theories, such as an alteration in the ground substance of the nose, can be dismissed when appropriate histological stains are used (Taylor, 1963).

Nasal polyps are a disease almost exclusive to man. Cattle can develop polypoidal changes on the nasal septum, but this is due to irritation and is associated with squamous metaplasia of the surface epithelium. Cats may develop eustacian polyps, but the only animal to have polyps similar to man is the chimpanzee and this is infrequent. It means that man has to be studied since there is no suitable animal model.

Infection

Infection may be present in patients with nasal polyps. Polyps are usually seen when a unilateral pansinusitis is present. They are often small, arise from the ethmoids and resolve once the condition is treated effectively. Polyps may also occur in patients who have either cystic fibrosis or Kartageners syndrome and yet neither of these conditions is primarily infective; infection arises secondarily to the defect in the mucosal defence. Extensive surgery cures neither of these conditions.

When simple mucus polyps are present, the role of infection is more confused. Part of the problem comes from the role of organisms cultured on washouts of the maxillary sinuses and part from the use of the term 'sinusitis' to describe the changes in the lining of the sinuses.

Many surgeons undertake routine irrigation of the maxillary sinuses when performing nasal polypectomy. Well over half the procedures produce no

return. If there is material present, then only one-third will grow a bacterium when cultured (Majumdar & Bull 1982). The commonest organism cultured is a non-capsulated *Haemophillus influenzae*, which is the most frequent commensal in the respiratory tract and is often cultured from the postnasal space. Similarly, its role in chronic bronchitis is difficult to determine and is said to be responsible only if pus cells are present and the condition responds to appropriate antibiotic chemotherapy. Nasal polyps have never been shown to be influenced by antibiotic chemotherapy. The postnasal drip may become less infected. Mistaken belief gives rise to the numerous Caldwell-Luc procedures, where all the offending mucosa is removed from the maxillary antrum. If there was a true infective element then such a procedure should be effective. Unfortunately polyps recur not only in the middle meatus, but also appear in the inferior meatus through the antrostomy. They are most difficult to treat.

One of the great misunderstandings comes from the use of the word sinusitis. During the latter part of the nineteenth century, the term hyperplastic sinusitis was introduced and used frequently in Europe and the United States between the wars (Berdal 1954). It was contrasted with infective sinusitis and used to describe the changes that occurred in patients with nasal polyps and some types of rhinitis. The histological features are the same as those found in nasal polyps. There is gross oedema of the submucosa, but the most striking feature is the tissue eosinophilia. This occurs also in 90% of polyps (Friedman & Osbourne 1982). The terms have been used interchangeably by surgeons. The gross oedema may show up radiologically and is frequently labelled as being consistent with sinusitis by radiologists.

Allergy

It has become increasingly clear that inflammation rather than infection is involved in the pathogenesis of nasal polyps. The nature of the inflammation is uncertain but the commonest view is that polyps are an allergic disease in the majority of cases. This is based on a loose association of facts, which are not causally related. Half the patients have attacks of rhinorrhoea and sneezing and one-third have asthma. The tissue eosinophilia in the majority of polyps would support this view.

Clinically, patients are no more atopic, have the normal incidence of positive skin tests, and hay fever is also only as common as expected by chance. The same applies for penicillin allergy, eczema and infantile asthma, all of which are mediated by IgE (Drake-Lee et al 1984b). The presence of allergy would appear to be coincidental.

The tissue eosinophilia is caused by mast cell degranulation. There are, however, many other causes of mast cell degranulation besides allergic reactions; these include infection, complement activation, chemicals, drugs and trauma. Mast cell degranulation produces a variety of vasoactive mediators, which may be either preformed or generated by the reaction. Histamine, the major preformed mediator in man, is released from the granules and is responsible for the immediate response. Subsequently, arachidonic acid is metabolized from the cell wall by two pathways to produce the prostaglandins and the leukotrienes. The major prostaglandin produced by mast cells is D2, and the leukotrienes were what were previously called slow-reacting substance of anaphylaxis. Together they are responsible for the late response.

Mast cells may be demonstrated in the inferior turbinate and polyps on light microscopy. Ultrastructural examination shows that they are degranulated within the polyp (Cauna et al 1972, Busuttil et al 1976, Drake-Lee et al 1984a). These changes can be seen within the inferior turbinate as well (Drake-Lee, unpublished data).

It appears that, in the majority of cases, mast cell degranulation occurs throughout the nose and results in a loss of homeostasis. This is most evident in the ethmoid sinuses, due to their complex anatomy, and in the sinuses in general because they have a relatively poor blood supply. The vasoactive products from the mast cells are not neutralized and so remain in the oedema: a vicious circle is set up. The eosinophils migrate into the interstitial fluid in an attempt to control the reaction. The process is dynamic. The aim of medical treatment is to break this circle and to reduce the reactions that occur within the nasal mucosa. It is apparent now that a proportion of patients may be managed medically.

Asthma and nasal polyps

Since asthma and nasal polyps coexist in over a third of patients, parallels in treatment may be sought.

The parallels should not be taken to extremes because the bronchioles have both a constricting musculature and a good blood supply, whereas the nose and the sinuses are rigid boxes with a variable blood supply. Treatment aimed at overcoming bronchospasm has little place in the management of nasal conditions and vasoactive sprays should be avoided in the nose.

Asthma is treated entirely medically and most cases which require corticosteroids respond eventually, although some are much more resistant than others. Because the relative risks are much greater in the chest, with the morbidity and mortality being a definite factor in management, systemic corticosteroids have a much greater place in the treatment of patients. Many asthmatic patients who have nasal symptoms do have a dramatic improvement when the chest symptoms require systemic corticosteroids Nasal conditions which respond to treatment include not only allergic and non-allergic rhinitis, but also patients with nasal polyps, which can completely disappear. Moreover, in the management of asthma, most cases are controlled by topical treatment. This usually includes inhaled nebulized corticosteroid sprays that are given regularly and frequently.

MEDICAL TREATMENT OF NASAL POLYPS

Medical treatment may be used in two ways in the management of nasal polyps, the first is to cause the polyps already present to regress, and the second is to prevent the recurrence of nasal polyps in patients who have previously had surgical treatment. Both modes can be used in patients who have had previous surgery, because in many cases no previous medical treatment will have been tried.

Polyps obstruct the nose to a variable degree and will block the passage of sprays to the ethmoid region. This means that there will be inadequate penetration of the nasal mucosa. Topical treatment is best given by nose drops. It is important that the drops reach the ethmoid area and remain in contact with the nasal mucosa for as long as possible. This means that the ethmoids should be below the level of the anterior nares. The head should either be bent forward as in praying to Mecca, or right back over the edge of the bed. Polyps will regress if treated by betamethasone nose drops (Betnasol), two drops each side twice a day for one month. This has been shown in a controlled trial where 6 out of every 10 patients had their polyps disappear (Charlton et al 1985).

Once under control, the condition may be managed by sprays. Since in many departments in the United Kingdom the waiting list for surgical procedures is so long, it would seem sensible to treat all patients medically initially. The additional advantage is that it saves patients from surgery, which in many departments is carried out under general anaesthesia. The small but real risk of complications is increased, since asthma is present in a third of the patients and these are the cases more prone to recurrence.

If polyps do not regress then they may be removed surgically. Since the condition is inflammatory in nature the simplest form of surgery should be undertaken. Polyps may be removed by a variety of simple manoeuvres and the author prefers an avulsion snare on a nose well prepared with cocaine spray and paste. In order to overcome anxiety, an intramuscular premedication with an opiate gives a good patient response. Extensive surgery has never been shown to reduce the recurrence rate and would appear to have no place in the management of these cases.

Once the polyps have been controlled either by medication or surgery, then recurrence may be prevented by medical treatment. Topical treatment with synthetic fluorinated corticosteroid sprays has been shown to prevent recurrence in several series (Mygind et al 1975, Deuschl & Dretner 1977, Dingsor et al 1985). Patients require long-term medication to prevent recurrence. At present, selection of patients for long-term therapy has not been evaluated. It would seem that those most likely to have recurrence should have medical treatment even on first time polypectomy. These are the patients who present at an early age and those with asthma. Any patient who has had a polypectomy within the previous 12 months should also be started on long-term treatment.

There is some evidence from the present studies to suggest that the aqueous sprays are better than the freon ones, but at present the decision is up to the clinician.

Patients may also suffer from the symptoms of rhinitis after their polyps have been removed. The presence of these symptoms is frequent and does not appear to be associated with recurrence (Drake-Lee et al 1984b). These may also be controlled with corticosteroid sprays.

When the condition is exceptionally refractory to treatment then it may be necessary to use systemic corticosteroids for two weeks, assuming that there are no medical contraindications. The minimum dose which will cause resolution should be used and as little as five milligrams a day may be all that is required. Topical treatment may then be started again.

There has been a vogue recently to try diets in medical conditions; many of the claims are inappropriate. There does seem some justification in trying diets in patients who have nasal polyps, asthma and aspirin hypersensitivity. Because there are links between aspirin and tartrazine dyes, the latter should be excluded. Although there are no published reports on symptomatic improvement, many of the patients report that they feel better.

CONCLUSIONS

The inflammatory response that causes nasal polyps may affect not only the nasal mucosa but also the lower respiratory tract. The reactions may be so severe that severe recurrence is a problem in 5% of patients. Medical treatment with topical corticosteroids is aimed at stabilising the homeostatic mechanism, reducing the inflammatory response and consequently either resolving the problem, or preventing polyp recurrence.

INTRODUCTION

The change of emphasis in modern medical education towards a more scientific approach has encouraged trainees to question traditional teachings, many of which have been perpetuated from one generation to the next, largely through the medium of standard textbooks.

With the diversity which exists in current treatment methods, there is increasingly a need to subject these to critical and comparative evaluation if sterility of thought and action are to be avoided. It is not always clear, for example, which form of treatment offers the best results in any given instance and the choice more often than not relates to idiosyncratic whim rather than scientific evidence.

The confusion can be compounded still further if more than one specialty is involved in the management of a particular condition so that treatment methods differ markedly between one discipline and another. Established referral patterns are often the deciding factor as to whom a patient consults, but once a case has been assigned the type of treatment instituted would seem to depend on a number of considerations.

Paramount amongst these is the influence exerted by the specialist's own personal training and background, but others may well impinge on the choice of therapy, and not all are necessarily guided by the best Hippocratic traditions.

Nasal polyposis is an instance in question since it comes under the aegis of allergists, chest physicians and otolaryngologists of varying surgical persuasion, each advocating his own brand of treatment. As a broad generalization, the allergist tends to treat by desensitization, the chest physician with his pharmacopoeia, and the otolaryngologist by one form of operation or another. The value of each method of treatment is not always absolutely clear, nor is the pooling of knowledge and resources from the various interested parties always forthcoming.

RECURRENT NASAL POLYPOSIS

The nature of the dilemma

There is little doubt that, in the contentious debate of how best to manage this intractable problem, surgery would be the option most favoured by otolaryngologists. Moreover, for patients surgical removal has the distinct appeal of providing virtually instantaneous relief, a feature which possibly heightens patient satisfaction to a disproportionate degree.

For that reason, a comparison of the effectiveness of surgery with alternative methods of treatment would only be fair if aspects other than the immediacy of relief are brought into the equation.

The most pertinent of these in relation to the subject under review is the long-term influence of any given treatment on the prevention of recurrence, but secondarily is its therapeutic potency in controlling the symptoms and signs of nasal polyposis.

If the matter were that simple one might perhaps consider the setting up of a controlled clinical trial to compare the effectiveness of surgery with some other unspecified form of treatment, both in respect of the capacity of each modality to prevent recurrence and the overall therapeutic effect vis-a-vis nasal obstruction, hyposmia, sneezing and rhinorrhoea. However, there are a number of variables to compound the issue so that resolution of the dilemma through the medium of a controlled trial remains an elusive objective.

In the first instance there is the problem of patient selection, namely which patients to include in the two arms, for if medical treatment is to compete on an equal footing with surgery it has to be on the basis that the condition to be treated is likely to respond to it. This implies either an allergic or, less commonly, an infective predisposition.

The diagnosis of allergy is not always easy to establish since the guidelines are by no means clear. This is particularly so when patients present with symptoms and signs suggestive of the condition, but to a milder extent.

The building up of a composite picture on the available evidence then becomes the only way of deciding whether a diagnosis of allergy is justifiable or not. In the final analysis the decision is arrived at by looking at all the factors which one normally associates with allergy, such as the family history, the results of skin or nasal provocation tests, the presence of eosinophilia in nasal smears, a raised serum IgE level, and the previous response to treatment, much of which may be indeterminate or frankly misleading. Skin tests, in particular, may falsely suggest an allergic diathesis and the significance of eosinophilia or a raised serum IgE, in the context of how a patient is likely to respond to treatment, is not always clear. Some patients with perennial rhinitis of the allergic type, for example, fail to respond to steroids while others who apparently lack an allergic background seem to benefit (Mygind 1982).

It is possible, therefore, that some patients with recurrent nasal polyps are entered into a trial without the firm conviction that they will respond to appropriate medical treatment. The classical example of a non-responder is the patient with non-specific vasomotor rhinitis whose symptoms and signs are to all intents and purposes identical with those of allergic rhinitis.

The third condition to be associated with recurrent polyposis is chronic sinusitis. Although there is potential for improvement with medical treatment in the form of antibiotics, the response is unpredictable since curability depends very much on the state of the mucous membrane within the affected sinus. If the membrane has been badly damaged by micro-abscess formation to the extent that mucous glands have largely disappeared and the cilia permanently destroyed, the scope for recovery with appropriate antibiotic treatment is marginal. Equally, the type of sepsis and the original cause of the trouble has a bearing on the likelihood of curability. The potential for recovery with surgery is, however, much more predictable if the seat of sepsis is included within the scope of the operation, i.e. if a realistic attempt is made to remove all diseased tissue from the affected sinus and not just the polyps.

The reader may now begin to appreciate the difficulties of the subject at hand, but if anything the reality is even more complex. This is because comparisons of surgery with other methods of treatment for nasal polyposis cannot take into account the wide range of reactivity which exists between one person and another, indeed, the changes which occur in any one individual from day to day.

There may be a wide variation in the level of the provoking factors both temporally and geographically and the disparities may affect people differently. Apart from specific factors, there are a number of additional and coincidental factors which may influence polyp development and these are also subject to a wide degree of variability. They include upper respiratory infections, smoking, alcohol ingestion, anxiety, sinusitis and rhinitis medicamentosa. Of these psychic factors, respiratory infections and smoking may have a greater bearing on the regrowth of polyps than is generally appreciated.

The contribution made by the patients' own immune system must inevitably play a major part in the tendency or lack of it to polyp formation and this in turn comes under the influence of hormonal, biochemical and infective factors.

Finally, there is the imponderable question of how best to judge the effectiveness of treatment. The wide degree of subjectivity in the expression of nasal symptoms is well known and makes for difficulty in assessing the true extent of improvement or otherwise. Equally contentious is the ability to judge the effect of treatment by rhinoscopy, since the nose is a long thin tall cavity and measurement of polyps therefore well nigh impossible. Rhinomanometry is informative to a limited extent in any given patient, but of limited value when comparing one patient with another.

There is also the difficulty of standardizing technique when attempting to assess the results of treatment. On the surgical side, it is possible to select a person of known skills to carry out every operation, although even the best track record cannot be relied upon to provide identical clearance when confronted with septal deflections or excessive bleeding. On the medical side, there is if anything less certainty that the treatment is being carried out in a controlled manner. Studies have shown, for instance, a discrepancy in the responsiveness of polyps to drops or sprays as between the head down and forwards position and the traditional head back position (Chalton et al 1985).

Having accepted that a clinical trial will not disclose whether surgery or medical treatment is the better treatment for recurrent nasal polyps, what then is the evidence to support the contention that medical treatment has any part to play in the management of this problem.

The role of medical management in recurrent nasal polyposis

Systemic steroids are known to cause significant regression of nasal polyps, even to the point of complete disappearance in some cases, and on that basis, if surgery were to be compared with systemic steroids administered over a long period, there would be no contest. However, the known serious hazards of such therapy have precluded its use for nasal polyps in all but the most exceptional cases, namely patients with asthma refractory to conventional treatment.

Although topical steroids are acknowledged to be effective in the control of allergic rhinitis, their role in the management of recurrent polyposis is less clear.

Evidence, however, is mounting that their contribution in this respect is by no means insignificant. The two preparations which stand out by comparison with others are beclomethasone dipropionate (Beconase), administered as a metered aerosol, and betamethasone sodium phosphate (Betnesol) in drop form, the latter being by far the more potent of the two.

Whereas beclomethasone is not considered to be absorbed by the nasal mucous membrane, betamethasone is partially absorbed into the blood stream and this may account in some measure for its increased potency. It also explains the reluctance of many practitioners to use it for all but the shortest periods of time.

Provided that adequate contact takes place between the preparation and the nasal polyps significant regression will occur in a preponderance of cases. In a study which compared betamethasone drops with a placebo there was total disappearance of polyps in 60% of patients who took the active preparation against 13% who took a placebo (Chalton et al 1985).

In another study, the symptoms which one normally associates with nasal polyposis, namely sneezing, rhinorrhoea and nasal obstruction, were significantly reduced by the use of a beclomethasone aerosol and there was objective reduction in the size of the polyps (Mygind et al 1975). However, no mention was made of the total disappearance of polyps, as is the case when betamethasone drops are used and when treatment was discontinued regrowth of the polyps was invariably noted.

Eighty percent of patients were benefited symptomatically by the regular administration of beclomethasone in another trial and regression in polyp size also noted (Pedersen et al 1976). The effect of this preparation on the prevention of recurrence after polypectomy has been the subject of analysis in a group of patients not considered especially to be of allergic type (Karlsson & Rundcrantz 1982).

In 20% of patients the drug did not appear to exert any influence on the prevention of further polyps postoperatively, but in the remainder of the patients' treatment was beneficial in that the need for further surgery was considerably reduced and the interval between operations lengthened.

Patients undergoing ethmoidectomy were assessed for recurrence of polyps under the influence of beclomethasone on the one hand and a placebo on the other. At a year after operation, 60% of the patients receiving the topical steroid were asymptomatic compared with 49% taking the placebo, and there was no visible evidence of polyps in 54% of the former as compared with 13% of the latter (Virolainen Puhakka 1980).

There can be little doubt, therefore, that topical steroids have a significant influence on the growth of nasal polyps, but, with the notable exception of betamethasone preparations which may cause polyps to disappear completely, the response to nonabsorbable steroids such as beclomethasone is subject to some degree of variability and unpredictability. Polyps treated with this preparation rarely disappear completely and the shrinkage of multiple large obstructive polyps tends to be rather limited.

The role of surgery in recurrent nasal polyposis

The question, 'Is surgery the only treatment for recurrent nasal polypi?' presupposes that surgery does in fact confer some benefit on the sufferer from recurrent nasal polyps, but is this in fact the case?

There is little doubt that simple removal is rewarded by symptomatic relief in the majority of patients, but how effective is this type of treatment in the long term? How many patients submitted to surgery remain permanently free of symptoms and of those whose polyps recur, how many times do they have to undergo repeat surgery and what is the interval between operations? The careful notekeeper and regular clinic attender no doubt will have the answer to these questions, but in the absence of precise information the experienced otolaryngologist instinctively knows that nasal polypectomy can only control polyps on a permanent basis in a minority of cases. As to which patients will experience recurrence and which will have the good fortune to escape is a question which might as well be answered by looking into a crystal ball as by any other method of fortune-telling. Some patients may enjoy disease-free intervals of 20 years or more, while in others the gap between recurrences is only a year or two, or even a few months. The sheer unpredictability of nasal polypectomy for recurrent polyposis is perhaps its most noteworthy feature and should prompt caution when discussing prognosis with the patient.

The unsatisfactory long-term outcome must inevitably be tied to the factors which collectively influence the formation of polyps and which have already been touched upon in a preceding section.

The inference so far has been that one type of operation is practised for the control of polyps, namely polypectomy, and although this may be the case in most centres, it is by no means the only operation available. The attraction of polypectomy is its simplicity, its freedom from complications and its low cost in economic terms.

However, there has always been a small body of opinion which favoured the adoption of more radical measures when simple polypectomy has failed to control repeated recurrences.

Ethmoidectomy, when executed with meticulous attention to detail, offers the opportunity of controlling the disease on a permanent basis. The choice between the intranasal and external route is very much a personal one, although in theory the external approach possesses the merits of better exposure and reduced risk. It is argued, for instance, that it allows the surgeon to gain better access to areas which are notoriously difficult to be certain about via the internal route, namely the anterior ethmoid cells, the inner aspect of the lamina papyracea and the sphenoidal sinus. It further provides the operator with a better opportunity to respect the integrity of the orbit and anterior cranial fossa.

Although clinical impressions are notoriously misleading when attempting to draw conclusions about any aspect of medicine, the writer has had reason repeatedly to feel enthusiastic about the capacity of external ethmoidectomy to control nasal polyposis. The impression in this instance is based on a small number of cases performed by one person and judged over a number of years. The emphasis has been on long-term relief of symptoms, rather than on the return of polyps, which in the majority of patients rarely amount to anything more than

miniscule excrescences in the olfactory cleft. Such tiny projections hardly ever grow to obstruct the nose and therefore do not require any further surgical treatment. The effect of ethmoidectomy alone on symptomatology and on the prevention of recurrence has been compared with ethmoidectomy followed by the topical application of beclomethasone aerosol (Virolainen & Puhakka 1980). At the end of a year 60% of the surgery alone group were symptom-free, whereas, as might be expected, the double modality group fared even better.

What is not altogether certain in the writer's mind is whether ethmoidectomy would be as effective if practised primarily as opposed to its usual role as a salvage procedure after failed polypectomy. There is clearly a fundamental need to evaluate its contribution to the long-term control of polyposis, with and without adjunctive topical steroid therapy, and to compare its effectiveness against simple polypectomy. This latter objective could be assessed by treating one side of the nose by the radical operation and the other by polypectomy.

DISCUSSION AND CONCLUSIONS

The theme of this paper has been to ask if surgery is the only treatment for recurrent polyps and the answer therefore has to be in the negative.

It is evident that surgery in the form of ethmoidectomy may have a definite role in the management of recurrent polyps, much more so than simple removal, and equally that topical treatment with steroids has an important part to play. As to the relative merits of surgery versus medical therapy no clear cut answer is likely to emerge in view of the difficulty of comparing like with like. Individual diatheses vary widely from one person to the next and some uncertainty always exists in the extent of response to topical treatment.

The message to emerge is that the ideal policy for the prevention of recurrent nasal polyposis is to embark on treatment initially by ethmoidectomy, preferably via the external route, and thereafter to maintain the status quo by the use of topical beclomethasone, either one puff in each nostril four times a day or two puffs three times a day.

There will be occasions, inevitably, when polyps will reappear to some extent, as a reaction to colds, stress, dust, infections, smoke and exacerbations of an asthmatic tendency. In the ethmoidectomized patient, such recurrences should only be on a minor scale since the bed from which the polyps will take origins has been effectively reduced.

Nevertheless, the threat of further growth once recurrence has taken place should not be dismissed and if symptoms recur under the influence of adverse circumstances the patient should be treated with the stronger topical steroid, namely betamethasone, until the polyps disappear in a matter of days. The patient may then return to the use of the non-absorbable and weaker topical preparation. This technique will not expose him to the dangers of prolonged systemic steroid absorption and will maintain the nose in as trouble-free a condition as possible.

The previous two chapters have outlined the complexities associated with the development of nasal polypi in a masterly fashion, but the precise reason why one nose develops polyps and not another is still not clear.

As has been highlighted, there are a very wide variety of factors involved, but the outstanding feature is that polypi may develop when there is uncontrolled congestion of the mucosa of the nasal cavities and paranasal sinuses. It follows that anything which can be done to reduce persistent or recurrent nasal congestion must have an important influence upon whether or not that nose produces polypi again in the future. The old adage, 'Once a polyp always a polyp' represents the frustration and irritation on the part of the sufferers of this condition, as well as of their medical advisors, and it is still true today. It emphasizes that once a nose has produced polypi, there is an inherent predilection to do so again in the future.

To consider that removal of nasal polypi will solve the problem in the long-term is quite unrealistic, and it has long been recognized that endeavours must be made to reduce the likelihood of more polypi developing.

The complexities concerning the pathogenesis have been thoroughly discussed in the preceding papers, and there is no point in repeating them. As has been emphasized, the confusion and misconceptions concerning the part that infection plays in the development of nasal polypi is real, and the points raised in the discussion in the previous chapters are highly relevant.

Once there is a polyp in the nose, there is impairment of the nasal airway. With progressive enlargement of the polyp and the development of more, as usually occurs, there is increasing impairment of drainage of the normal secretions of the respiratory epithelium which lines the nasal passages and paranasal sinuses. Once there is this obstruction and consequent retention of secretions, secondary infection of the nose and sinuses follows, usually caused by the organisms normally resident in the upper respiratory tract. Alternatively, the presence of polypi disturbs the nasal physiology to render the individual more susceptible to development of upper respiratory tract infections. In either case,

the presence of polypi leads sooner or later to secondary infection, which in turn adds to the degree of congestion of the nasal mucosa, and so the problems are aggravated.

In the presence of an acute infection, the degree of congestion increases markedly, purulent secretions then accumulate under tension, causing pain and discomfort, as well as the general signs of infection. The patient becomes quite ill and he is in need of urgent treatment to deal with his problems. It is hardly surprising, therefore, that infection has assumed a very dominant role in relation to the management of polypi and, in the days before antibiotics, the only means of dealing with these problems was surgical.

Over several decades, antibiotics have enabled infections to be more readily controlled with the result that there has been a substantial reduction in the large numbers of surgical procedures performed to drain the paranasal sinuses.

With less acute infections, the nasal mucosa may become oedematous and this may lead to polyp formation. If these changes can be recognized early, antibiotic and decongestive treatment may induce these changes to resolve and so development of polypi will be aborted.

Many patients attribute the development of their polypi to an acute upper respiratory tract infection, or to an attack of sinusitis, but infection alone is not the sole factor in the production of polypi and, as has been discussed in the preceding chapters, antibiotics have not cured nasal polypi.

The majority of otolaryngologists believe that there is an 'allergic' basis to nasal polyposis and this is probably correct in many cases. If a specific allergen can be identified, so much the better, but the difficulty is that specific allergic causes cannot be found in the majority of cases. Indeed, there is room for the view that positive skin tests may falsely indicate an allergic diathesis in some cases.

It is indeed a matter for regret that the word 'sinusitis' has been allowed to be used so loosely, and this has added considerably to the confusion about the origin of polypi. The problem is compounded even today by radiologists who almost universally attribute mucosal thickening to sinusitis. All these factors contribute to the dilemma of recurrent nasal polypi. We are led, however, to the conclusion that nasal polypi are caused by 'inflammation' and this word needs to be used in its widest sense.

It is a striking feature of modern otolaryngological practice that so many patients put up with a variety of increasing symptoms of nasal congestion for many years without being unduly bothered or concerned, frequently insisting upon aggravating the problems by adding the irritations from tobacco and other pollutants, usually in spite of entreaties by their medical advisors to reduce the sources of irritation of their nasal mucous membranes. There are, of course, enormous variations in environmental, climatic and geographical factors, not to mention the individuals' susceptibility and hypersensitivity, but, overall in the majority of patients, these problems tend slowly to get worse with the passage of time. All experienced otolaryngologists know that the consumption of tobacco inevitably leads to nasal congestion and that mechanical factors, such as enlarged or hypertrophic inferior turbinates and septal deformities, will also lead to increased nasal congestion sooner or later, but climatic and geographical factors play an important part in the time taken for these changes to occur.

After a period of prolonged congestion of the nasal mucosa, some irritation may lead to a bout of prolonged sneezing, or there may be an acute upper respiratory tract infection, and nasal polypi may suddenly develop, much to the dismay of the patient, who suddenly finds his nasal airways completely occluded. Once this occurs, he wants his nose dealt with at once and prolonged decongestive treatment is usually unacceptable—he wants his blocked nose cleared.

Once a true polyp has formed, with the typical appearance of a pendulous mass of oedematous mucosa with a small pedicle, no amount of antibiotic or decongestive treatment is likely to lead to the spontaneous disappearance of the polyp, even when the infection is satisfactorily controlled. This means, therefore, that once a polyp has formed it needs to be removed.

When the nasal polypi have been removed, then the nasal passages need to be restored to as near normal as possible and the medical measures outlined in the previous chapters need to be energetically pursued if the possibility of recurrences is to be minimized. These factors which lead to the development of chronic nasal congestion encompass an exceedingly wides spectrum; they are both inherent with the individual, may be partly anatomical problems and partly related to the sensitivity and irritability of the patient's nasal mucous membrane, rendering it subject to the various noxious influences which cause 'inflammation' in its widest sense. The complexities are so great and the variables so numerous and diverse that controlled studies as to the methods of treatment have not proved satisfactory to date and it is probable that they never will be! Each patient needs to be treated individually and his particular problems identified and eliminated or controlled if his tendency to chronic nasal congestion is to be significantly reduced.

WHAT SURGICAL PROCEDURE SHOULD BE EMPLOYED

The selection of the surgical procedure to deal with recurrent nasal polypi poses a dilemma of considerable magnitude and, after many years of wrestling with this problem, the writer is convinced that the simplest surgical procedure commensurate with complete removal of the polypi is the best method.

Many will advocate that the surgical treatment of choice is the use of nasal snares under local anaesthesia. Undoubtedly, local anaesthesia can provide a satisfactory environment to permit the removal of polyps from many noses, perhaps with the assistance of some sedation, but it is a most unpleasant procedure, and most patients do not accept kindly this type of surgical interference. The result is that frequently the polypi are not removed as thoroughly or as completely as possible, in which case it is hardly surprizing that more polypi develop again after a period of time.

Many otolaryngologists do employ the nasal snare and certainly it is a useful tool to avulse nasal polypi. The problem is that, in many noses, it is difficult to visualize the polyp completely, especially if there are any septal deformities, and in other cases it may be difficult to separate polyp from what is engorged mucosa of the turbinate, especially in the presence of blood after some of the polypi have been removed. In these circustances, it is easy for the loop of the snare to be placed around the turbinate, with consequent partial, or, worse still, total removal and this, of course, is a highly undesirable complication of what should be a simple surgical procedure.

In these days of high costs, shortage of hospital beds and hospital staff, there are compelling reasons to perform as many surgical procedures as possible under local anaesthesia in consulting rooms and in outpatient clinics. However, after 35 years of involvement in otolaryngology, the writer has learned that if the recurrence of nasal polypi is to be minimized, their removal must be complete. To achieve this end there is no susbtitute to having a patient under a general anaesthetic, on an operating table with proper illumination for performing intranasal procedures and with adequate suction to provide the best operative field.

The most satisfactory results are obtained with the minimum surgical trauma and the most efficient means of removal of the nasal polypi is by using the Tilley Henckel ethmoid punch of moderate size and a Killian speculum, or instruments which are very similar.

The removal of polypi must be complete and thorough and, at the same time, oedematous mucosa and polypoidal fringes of the turbinates can be trimmed, or excised; anything less than this will lead to the likelihood of more polypi developing. The less surgical trauma, the quicker the nose recovers and, once the nose has recovered, attention to the causative factors as outlined in the previous contributions needs to be instituted energetically. This regime will lead to the minimum of recurrences of nasal polypi.

There are many who advocate intranasal ethmoidectomy and there are others, equally passionately who would advocate external ethmoidectomy for the eradication of nasal polypi.

In clearing the nasal passages of polypi, if an effort is made to be as thorough as possible, frequently some of the ethmoidal cells may be removed. Whereas this is not necessarily a bad thing, it is at best only a very limited ethmoidectomy and, of course, should be recorded as such.

Persuasive arguments can be developed concerning the complete exenteration of the ethmoidal sinuses for the removal of nasal polypi in order to minimize recurrences and, whether this is achieved by the intranasal or external approach, is a matter for the individual surgeon's choice. However, in these days, antibiotics have reduced the incidence of sinus disease requiring surgical procedures to such an extent that few surgeons perform sufficient numbers of operations to become proficient in intranasal ethmoidal procedures compared with the previous generations and therefore, the external approach is undoubtedly the safer procedure for otolaryngologists these days.

Ethmoidectomy, performed with meticulous attention to detail, will produce apparently excellent results insofar as the recurrence of nasal polypi appears to be eliminated. Sadly, their recurrence is only delayed and, whereas many people will assert that this delay is worthwhile in itself and of considerable advantage, the literature does not contain worthwhile evidence of eradication of nasal polyposis in the long term.

Polypi do have a great tendency to recur and the writer has seen many patients who have had external ethmoidectomy performed by highly competent surgeons, presenting with the nose filled with polypi after a number of years. Then the surgical removal of polypi after an adequate ethmoidectomy is a most hazardous procedure, for all landmarks have been destroyed by the previous surgery. The contents of the orbit, the optic nerve and the anterior cranial fossa are all at risk and to have a complication involving these areas is a high price to pay for the removal of nasal polypi, particularly when the long-term value of these procedures is very much in doubt. All otolaryngologists will be aware that such complications do occur. The incidence may be rare, but blindness or intracranial haemorrhage are unacceptable complications of surgical removal of polypi and have usually occurred when recurrent polypi are being removed from previously exenterated ethmoidal sinuses.

CONCLUSION

Once nasal polypi have formed, they need to be removed, and the most efficient and safest way of accomplishing this and minimizing the likelihood of recurrences is to remove the polypi under general anaesthesia with as little trauma to the nose and sinuses as is possible.

There must always be an emphasis towards restoring the anatomical features of the nasal cavity to as near normal as is possible to reduce the physiological stresses upon the nasal mucosa which, for a wide variety of reasons, may have a tendency to chronic congestion and the subsequent development of more polypi.

As has been outlined in the previous contributions, there is a great deal which can be done to reduce persistent or recurrent congestion of nasal cavities and these measures need to be energetically pursued in each individual's case.

REFERENCES

A B Drake-Lee

Berdal P 1954 Serological examination of nasal polyp fluid. Acta Otolaryngologica suppl 115

Busutill A, More I, McSeveny D 1976 Ultrastructure of the stroma of nasal polyps. Archives of Otolaryngology 102: 589–595

Cauna N, Hindover K, Manzethi G, Swanson E 1972 Fine structure of nasal polyps. Annals of Otolaryngology 81: 41–58

Charlton R, MacKay I, Wilson R, Cole P 1985 Double-blind placebo controlled trial of beclamethasone nose drops for nasal polyposis. British Medical Journal ii: 788–789

Deuschl H, Drettner B 1977 Nasal polyps treated by beclomethasone nasal aerosol. Rhinology 15: 17–23

Dingsor G, Kramer J, Olshot R, Sonderstrom T 1985 Flunisolide nasal spray 0.025% in the prophylactic treatment of nasal polyposis after polypectomy. A randomized, double-blind, parallel, placebo-controlled study. Rhinology 23: 49–58

Drake-Lee A, Barker T, Thurley K 1984a Nasal polyps II. Fine structure of mast cells. Journal of Laryngology and Otology 98: 285–292

Drake-Lee A, Lowe D, Swanson A, Grace A 1984b Clinical profile and recurrence of nasal polyps. Journal of Laryngology and Otology 98: 783–793

Freidman I, Osbourne D 1982 Miscellaneous granulomas and nasal polyposis. In: Pathology of granulomas and neoplasms of the nose and paranasal sinuses. Churchill Livingstone, Edinburgh

Majumdar B, Bull P 1982 The incidence and bacteriology of maxillary sinusitis in nasal polyposis. Journal of Laryngology and Otology 96: 937–941

Mygind N, Pedersen C, Prytz S, Sorensen H 1975 Treatment of nasal polyps with intranasal beclomethasone diproprionate aerosol. Clinical Allergy 5: 159–164

Taylor M 1963 Histochemical studies on nasal polyps. Journal of Laryngology and Otology 77: 326–341

Vancil M 1969 An historical survey of treatments for nasal polyposis. Laryngoscope 79: 435–445

O H Shaheen

Chalton R, Mackay I, Wilson R, Cole P 1985 Double-blind placebo controlled trial of betamethasone nasal drops for nasal polyposis. British Medical Journal 291: 788

Karlsson G, Rundcrantz H 1982 A randomized trial of intranasal beclomethasone dipropionate after polypectomy. Rhinology 20: 144–148

Mygind N 1982 Topical steroid treatment for allergic rhinitis and allied conditions. Clinical Otolaryngology 7: 343–352

Mygind N, Brahe Pedersen C, Prytz S, Sorensen H 1975 Treatment of nasal polyps with intranasal beclomethasone dipropionate aerosol. Clinical Allergy 5: 159–164

Pederson C B, Mygind N, Sorensen H, Prytz S 1976 Long-term treatment of nasal polys with beclomethasone dipropionate aerosol. Acta Otolaryngologica 82: 256–259

Virolainen E, Puhakka H 1980 The effect of intranasal beclomethasone dipropionate on the recurrence of nasal polyps after ethmoidectomy. Rhinology 18: 9–18

13

Place of radiotherapy in the management of juvenile angiofibroma

B.J. Cummings

Controversy over the use of radiation therapy to treat juvenile angiofibromas relates not so much to the ability of radiation to control these tumours as to its potential toxicity. Since angiofibromas are uncommon, most series are small and conclusions must often be supported by limited data. Radiation, surgery and planned combinations of the two modalities have each been championed, and deprecated, at one time or another. However, for angiofibromas, as for many other tumours, there is more than one effective therapy and the choice of treatment frequently does not adversely affect the outcome.

In this account the evidence for the effectiveness of radiation therapy is presented, together with a discussion of possible reasons for some authors considering that angiofibromas do not respond to radiation. The morbidity associated with modern megavoltage radiation techniques is analysed and contrasted with the potential side-effects of resection. Based on these considerations, a philosophy of management is presented.

IS RADIATION THERAPY EFFECTIVE TREATMENT?

The ultimate test of the effectiveness of any treatment is whether it can relieve symptoms and prevent further growth of the tumour.

Radiation therapy was used to treat many angiofibromas prior to the development of modern radiological techniques, which delineate accurately the true extent of these tumours, and prior to the introduction of current surgical concepts supported by blood transfusions, sophisticated anaesthesia and antibiotics. In general, the results obtained by low energy orthovoltage irradiation, or by the insertion of radioisotope applicators into the nasopharynx or into the angiofibroma itself, were not satisfactory. Although the radioresponsiveness of angiofibromas was established, regression was often incomplete, regrowth common and there was considerable morbidity from the high doses and repeated courses of radiation given (Apostol & Frazell 1965, Jereb et al 1970). The emphasis in treatment had swung

Table 13.1 Results of megavoltage radiation therapy (RT)

Reference	Radiation dose (first course)	First course RT	Control by			Follow-up (years)
			Second course RT*	Resection after RT		
Million & Cassisi 1984	30 Gy/4½ weeks	4/4	—	—		2– 7
Cummings et al 1984	30–35 Gy/3 weeks	44/55	8/8	3/5		3–26
Sinha & Aziz 1978	30–35 Gy/3 weeks	4/5	1/1	0/1		4–21
Carvalho et al 1979	35–40 Gy/n.s.	12/25	4/6 (2 not evaluable)	5/7		2–18
Ward 1983	30–45+ Gy/3–4½+ weeks	4/6	1/2 (1 not evaluable)	0/1		n.s.
Biller et al 1974	50–54 Gy/n.s.	3/3	—	—		3– 4
Vadivel et al 1980	10–65 Gy/n.s.	5/5	—	—		2– 7

* Includes patients who received only a second course of radiation and patients who were reirradiated when resection failed to control postradiation recurrence.
n.s. Not stated.

to resection prior to the development of modern megavoltage radiation equipment in the late 1950s.

Several centres have published accounts of patients treated with megavoltage therapy, although from Table 13.1 it will be seen that only the Toronto series has reached even moderate size. In that series, one or two courses of radiation resulted in control in 95% (52/55) (Cummings et al 1984). Ward (1983) reserved radiation for patients with intracranial extension and Biller et al (1974) used it only for incompletely resected tumours, but both found it effective. A group in Brazil (Carvalho et al 1979) did not observe the same level of response and reported control in only 64% (16/25). There is no obvious reason for their lack of success, although it may be remarked that these authors also reported only 9 of 15 tumours (60%) were controlled by resection, a success rate rather less than that commonly described by North American and European surgical centres. Many other reports mention occasional patients treated by radiation with mixed results.

Adequate evaluation of the extent of the angiofibroma is crucial to the planning of appropriate radiation, just as it is planning surgical resection. Computerized tomography with contrast enhancement, combined with conventional coronal tomography, allow excellent vizualization of the tumour mass, and the radiation oncologist rarely gains important additional information from arteriography, which need not be performed routinely if irradiation is to be the primary treatment modality. In the Princess Margaret Hospital series 89% (49/55) of the angiofibromas extended beyond the nasal cavity or nasopharynx. With better understanding and demonstration of the infiltrative nature of angiofibromas, radiation fields can be designed to encompass the tumour more adequately (Cummings et al 1984).

The radiation dose needed appears to be quite low and certainly less than that commonly used for malignant tumours. The Toronto (Cummings et al 1984) and Edinburgh (Sinha & Aziz 1978) groups recommended doses of only 30–35 Gy in 3 weeks. The Toronto group found no difference between these two dose levels with 80% (32/40) control after 30 Gy and an identical level (12/15) after 35 Gy, with no evidence that large tumours had been treated by larger doses. In a smaller series, Ward (1983) reported that two tumours which received less than 35 Gy progressed and required further treatment, whereas none of the 4 tumours which were treated with at least 45 Gy in $4\frac{1}{2}$ weeks recurred. The minimum effective dose is not known, although fractionated doses of 15–20 Gy were apparently without effect (Doyle et al 1977, Patterson 1965). Since the side effects of radiation are dose related, the Toronto philosophy is to use low-dose radiation of 30 Gy in 3 weeks, recognizing that some patients may require further treatment.

An important consequence of this use of low- or medium-dose radiation is that a biopsy should be obtained to confirm a clinical or radiological diagnosis of angiofibroma. The most important differential diagnoses which must be excluded are malignant tumours since the radiation doses and treatment volumes used for angiofibromas are less than those necessary for malignant tumours. Opinions differ on whether such biopsies should be obtained only under general anaesthesia, or whether an office procedure is safe provided conditions allow ready control of any haemorrhage. Chandler (1984) stated that only 5 of the 15 patients biopsied transnasally in his office required anterior packing and only 2 of 36 patients in the Toronto series were transfused after biopsy (Cummings et al 1984). Whichever location is chosen, these biopsies should be taken by the otolaryngologist and not by the radiation oncologist.

The mechanism by which radiation causes angiofibromas to involute is still somewhat speculative. On histological examination these tumours have two main elements, a fibrous stroma containing spindle or stellate fibrocytes and numerous thin-walled vascular channels. It is probable that the critical target cells for radiation damage are both the fibroblasts of the stroma and the endothelial cells of the vascular spaces, since ultrastructure studies show that both contribute to the pool of tumour cells (Stiller et al 1976). The results of radiation therapy and the successful use of cytotoxic chemotherapy to treat advanced angiofibromas (Goepfert et al 1985) indicate that there are exploitable differences between the cellular kinetics of angiofibromas and normal tissues. The response of angiofibromas to relatively low doses of radiation is in some ways similar to the effect of radiation on some congenital haemangiomas, and it may well be that in these tumours radiation acts predominantly by damaging endothelial cells and provoking progressive thrombosis (Denekamp 1984). Several observers have noted that angiograms, obtained within a few months of radiation, sometimes show a decrease in vascularity without a marked change in the size of the tumour (Sessions et al 1976, Ward et al 1974). Also, angiofibromas excised only a short time after treatment may show few histological changes. Radiation acts by damaging DNA and preventing cells from regenerating. Since this damage is normally manifest only when the cell reaches the mitotic phase of the cell cycle, slowly cycling or non-cycling cells may persist for many months after irradiation and acellular material such as collagen is not affected by radiation at all. Consequently, the findings on microscopy shortly after irradiation cannot be used to predict the eventual outcome of treatment.

Many authors have remarked that angiofibromas often regress slowly following irradiation, although symptoms such as epistaxis and nasal obstruction are usually relieved rapidly and long before marked shrinkage of the tumour mass is seen (Cummings et al 1984, Jereb et al 1970, Sinha & Aziz 1978). This slow involution has probably contributed to the impression of some observers that radiation is ineffective. It has led to additional treatment, either surgical or radiotherapeutic, being given to some patients who might otherwise have been observed (Jereb et al 1970). In the Toronto series, there was no visible tumour in the nasopharynx or nasal cavity in 50% of patients within 12 months and in 80% within 24 months, but a few patients had residual asymptomatic masses many years after treatment (Cummings et al 1984). Biopsy of one such mass showed only fibrous tissue. It is likely that, with the availability of computerized tomography, an even greater number of persistent masses will be found. Six of 22 patients who had follow-up computerized tomography had residual soft tissue tumours from 3–15 years after irradiation, and only 2 of these masses were visible on clinical examination (Cummings et al 1984). The finding of such a mass does not mean that radiation treatment has failed. Stable residual asymptomatic masses do not require further treatment and additional therapy should be reserved for the patient with clinically or radiologically progressive disease.

Some authorities who prefer to resect most angiofibromas do use radiation for the 10–20% of patients who have intracranial extension and recommend either radiation alone (Ward 1983), or radiation combined with resection of the extracranial portion of the tumour (Jafek et al 1979). The former approach is predicated on the belief that resection of extracranial angiofibromas carries fewer risks than radiation, but this may not be correct (see below). The second is based on a desire to restrict the volume irradiated. However, it exposes the patient to the risks of haemorrhage from an incompletely resected tumour, to the combined risks of both radiation and surgery and the uncertainties of the completeness of partial extracranial excision do not readily allow the use of small radiation volumes. Despite these theoretical consideration, both approaches have been successful. Using radiation for unresected tumours, Ward (1983) reported control at last follow-up in 5 of 6 patients (the sixth was not evaluable) and Cummings et al (1984) controlled all 9 tumours which extended intracanially. Jafek et al (1979) had no recurrences in 5 patients treated by partial resection followed by radiation of residual intracranial tumour. If radiation can control tumours which have invaded intracranially, it should also be effective against smaller tumours and those with extensive extracranial ramifications and this is indeed what is seen. In addition to their 9 patients with intracranial tumour extension, the Toronto group controlled 43 of 46 (93%) extracranial tumours by radiation (Cummings et al 1984)

The effectiveness of radiation does not appear to be altered adversely by previous resection, although there are theoretical reasons for believing that irradiation of primary angiofibromas might be preferable. Radiosensitivity depends in part on the level of oxygen in the cells irradiated and any procedure, such as surgical manipulation or embolization, which leads to alterations in vascularity and to local hypoxia might be expected to lessen radiosensitivity. This potential problem is best managed by deferring treatment of incompletely resected tumours until regrowth is apparent, since not all residual angiofibromas enlarge and those that do apparently revascularize adequately. In the Toronto series, there was no significant difference in outcome between those angiofibromas treated primarily by radiation and those treated when they recurred following resection (Cummings et al 1984).

Radiation therapy is effective in causing angiofibromas to involute and in releving symptoms.

Radiation therapy does not control every angiofibroma, any more than does surgical resection. Those few centres which do employ radiation either systematically, or in selected situations, report control rates of 80% or better following a single course of low-dose radiation and nearly all failures are controlled by secondary therapy, results very similar to those described in most surgically managed series. Why then is radiation not used more widely? The reasons are two-fold—firstly, surgical resection is also a highly effective treatment for angiofibromas and, secondly, concern is frequently expressed over the potential hazards of radiation.

HOW SAFE IS RADIATION THERAPY?

When two or more treatment methods appear to be equally effective in controlling a disease, any assessment of the relative merits of the different treatments must include a comparison of their toxicity. This is not an easy task when the side effects differ, when the events to be considered are uncommon and when the time during which the patients are at risk varies widely. Green (1977) noted that individuals are typically quite inaccurate in their assessment of probabilities less than 1 in 50. When the incidence of complications is an order of magnitude below this, they tend either to neglect the possibility entirely or to overstate its frequency greatly. It is this phenomenon perhaps which accounts for the appearance in many presentations on angiofibroma of a statement discounting the use of radiation because of potential late sequelae and for the apparent acceptance of general anaesthesia, angiography, embolization and blood transfusion as necessary measures with little if any comment on their possible toxicity. Quantitation of the risks of the various aspects of angiofibroma management is not easy, and the algorithms developed are at best estimates, especially since they must frequently be based on the treatment of conditions other that angiofibroma. An attempt at such quantitation, using the endpoint of a potentially fatal outcome for each procedure, suggested that the order of magnitude of the risk was similar whether the patient was treated by radiation or by surgical resection and was no more than 1% (Cummings 1980).

The complication of radiation therapy over which there is greatest concern is tumour induction. The

Table 13.2 Radiation-associated malignant tumours

Reference	energy,	Radiation dose Gy/fractions/days	Age at first RT (years)	Interval to second tumour	Site of second tumour/histology	Treatment outcome
Batsakis et al 1955	2 mV	60/16/31 30/n.s.	48	10 months	nasopharynx/ fibrosarcoma	surgery NED 7 months
Gisselson et al 1958	165 kV 170 kV n.s.	26/16 d 32/14 d 62/29 d	12 29 33	21 years	nasopharynx/ fibrosarcoma	surgery died 1 year
Conley et al 1968	n.s.	120/n.s.	n.s.	18 years	orbit and face/ squamous cell ca	surgery NED 10 years
Fitzpatrick 1970	nasopharyngeal radium	600/n.s.	18	40 years	nasopharynx/ squamous cell ca	radiation died 6 months
Chen & Bauer 1982	n.s.	325/n.s.	48	18 years	nasopharynx/ fibrosarcoma	surgery/NED 2 years
Cummings et al 1984	^{60}Co	35/17/36	12	14 years	thyroid/papillary- follicular ca	surgery +1-131/ NED 2 years
	^{60}Co	37/16/21	28	13 years	skin/basal cell ca	surgery/NED 2 years
	^{60}Co	30/15/22	36			
Spagnolo et al 1984	n.s. nasopharyngeal radium	48/n.s. 30/20 h	19 19	4 years	nasopharynx/ malignant fibrous histiocytoma	unresectable died 4 months

n.s. not stated.
N.E.D. no evidence of disease.

reported cases in which treatment of an angio-fibroma by radiation has been associated with a subsequent malignant tumour and where sufficient details have been published to allow evaluation, are summarized in Table 13.2. There are several un-usual features about some of these cases. In 1 (Batsakis et al 1955), the interval between irradi-ation and the diagnosis of malignancy was only 10 months, and well below the more usually accepted induction period of several years. In 5 cases (Batsakis et al 1955, Conley et al 1968, Fitzpatrick 1970, Gisselson et al 1958, Spagnolo et al 1984) the doses were very high, and the orthovoltage (Conley et al 1968, Gisselson et al 1958) and intracavitary tech-niques (Fitzpatrick 1970) used have been superseded in modern practice. It is noteworthy that there has been only 1 report of thyroid cancer (Cummings et al 1984), possibly induced by scattered irradiation, since it is tumours in this organ that are discussed most frequently when head and neck irradiation in young people is considered (Hempelmann et al 1975). All of the reported tumours other than this single case of thyroid cancer developed within the irradiated volume. Four were sarcomas (Batsakis et al 1955, Chen & Bauer 1982, Gisselson et al 1958, Spagnolo et al 1984) and it is of interest that there are 2 reports of sarcomas developing in angiofi-bromas which had not been irradiated (Donald 1979, Hormia & Koskinen 1969).

Although the 8 cases listed in Table 13.2 are cited in detail, and there are allusions in the literature to several others, the total number of patients with angiofibroma who have been irradiated is not known and the rate of tumour induction cannot be calcu-lated. Because of the possibly long induction period it will be necessary to continue to study patients who have been irradiated, but one relatively large series in which two-thirds of the patients had been followed for more than 20 years recorded no cases of malignancy (0/69) (Jereb et al 1970). Since any evaluation of the risk of tumour induction from these case reports is impossible, the risk was addressed indirectly from other published data. Estimates of the lifetime risk of death from a radi-ation induced tumour for a teenager who received 30 Gy/3 weeks for an angiofibroma were reckoned to be between 1 in 400 and 1 in 1250 for thyroid cancer, 1 in 3000 for a bone or soft tissue sarcoma, and about 1 in 3000 for a benign tumour (Cummings

1980). To these estimates must be added the risks of general anaesthesia and of any other manoeuvres necessary in diagnosis and management—for example, the risk of death from thyroidectomy is about 1 in 350 (Foster 1978). Even with these ex-panded algorithms the risk level remains small.

Management of an angiofibroma by resection entails the hazards of general anaesthesia, some-times supplemented by hypotensive techniques, of blood transfusion (despite current publicity about AIDS and the risk of transfusion transmitted HIV/LAV virus infection, the greatest risk is still that of transfusion-associated hepatitis—Bove 1986), of arteriography and of embolization (Cummings 1980). The need for blood transfusion has been reduced, but not abolished, by the introduction of selective vessel embolization (Waldman et al 1981, Ward 1983). There is as yet insufficient data to quantitate the risks of embolization, which include neurological sequelae and tissue necrosis (Berenstein & Kricheff 1979, Lasjaunias et al 1980), although the rate appears to be small and within acceptable limits. Transfusion and embolization are not required by every patient who undergoes resection and the criteria used in selecting patients for various pro-cedures differ from series to series. However, the risks of major toxicity from surgical management appear to be similar in magnitude to those of radiation (Cummings 1980).

Radiation can produce side effects other than tumour induction and these are also dose related. For example, the threshold for producing measurable changes in growth hormone levels by pituitary irradiation is about 30–35 Gy and increases with age (Shalet et al 1976, Stone & Cummings 1985), although any such changes do not always correlate with clinical growth patterns. The growth of the face and the development of teeth within the radiation beam may be affected by high dose levels but the effects of low and medium radiation doeses are not well established. The parotid salivary glands in young people recover well from doses up to 35–40 Gy in 3–4 weeks. Other sensitive structures, such as the eye, can usually be shielded from the radiation beam and the tolerance of the central nervous system is above the dose levels generally used for angiofibroma. The connective tissue necrosis described in some early series (Conley et al 1968, Jereb et al 1970) should not occur with modern techniques and doses.

With these potential side effects in mind, a detailed review of the patients treated at the Princess Margaret Hospital was undertaken (Stone & Cummings 1985). One patient had developed clinical hypopituitarism after two courses of radiation (35 Gy/3 weeks plus 30 Gy/3 weeks) for intracranial angiofibroma which involved the cavernous sinus region, but 7 others who received two courses of radiation had no abnormalities. Extensive endocrine testing in 25 patients 3–25 years after treatment showed no significant alterations in pituitary, thyroid, adrenal or gonadal function. Salivary gland secretion, dental development, and facial and skeletal growth were also normal. Three of the patients complained of nasal crusting and occasional epistaxis. Whether regular long-term follow-up is necessary for patients treated by radiation because of the risk of late toxicity is a moot point. It may be argued that serious toxicity is so infrequent that unlimited follow-up is not cost effective, and that significant toxicity carries its own symptoms, which will cause the patient to seek attention. This view is contentious and in Toronto we prefer to maintain follow-up.

It is not possible to compare the less serious side effects of radiation in any quantitative way with those of resection. The latter may include minor facial scarring, nasal crusting and eye or ear symptoms following lateral rhinotomy (Neel et al 1973), and fifth and eighth nerve damage followed the infratemporal fossa approach suggested by Fisch (1983) for some extensive angiofibromas.

There is a danger of becoming bewithched by numbers when attempting to quantitate risk levels. The intent of this analysis, however, is to obtain no more than an estimate of orders of magnitude. Such evidence as there is suggests that the risks of potentially fatal complications, and of less serious side effects, from either irradiation or resection do not differ greatly. Radiation thereapy is not a benign treatment totally free of toxicity. Neither, however, is it so hazardous that it should never be used for angiofibromas.

A PHILOSOPHY OF MANAGEMENT

The resolution of a dilemma requires that a choice be made between two or more alternatives, each equally unfavourable. From this discussion and its companion, it will be seen that both radiation and surgical resection are effective, but neither is devoid of risk. Any complacency by the physician must surely be tempered by the knowledge that those few unfortunate patients who do die from angiofibroma have usually been treated at some time by both radiation and surgery. These young patients should be assessed jointly by an otolaryngologist and a radiation oncologist and the characteristics of each patient and his tumour considered. The experience of the physicians and the evaluation made by the patient and his parents of the information presented to them will influence the choice. In some situations the decision may be easier—for example, because of the increased hazards of resecting intracranial angiofibroma, radiation may be preferred; because of the increased sensitivity of the very young to radiation, surgery may carry fewer risks in the patient under 10 years of age; and if an angiofibroma regrows after a course of low-dose radiation, resection is recommended, if possible, rather than further radiation, since toxicity is related to the total radiation dose.

I prefer to treat most juvenile angiofibromas with radiation therapy, not because radiation gives better results than resection, for it does not, but because it is as effective as resection and poses no greater threat of serious toxicity.

The routine treatment with radiation for most benign lesions in children and adolescents is to be strongly condemned. The histologically benign tumour of the nasophrynx known as juvenile angiofibroma, angiofibroma and nasopharyngeal angiofibroma can behave very aggressively; therefore, the use of radiotheraphy is appropriate in selected cases.

The majority of these tumours arise in the posterior nasal region of the nasopharynx and push into surrounding areas, resulting in bone erosion and encroachment upon important nerves and vital structures. Some of these tumours, while they do not metastasize, behave in an aggressive manner spreading intracranially to involve the cavernous sinus and seem to develop a new blood supply as they expand. The initial primary blood supply is derived from the internal maxillary artery, a branch of the external carotid system. As the tumours grow, they acquire collateral blood supply from adjacent structures, including branches of the internal carotid artery system (Chandler et al 1974, Jafek et al 1973, Ward et al 1974, Goepfert et al 1985).

In the past, the diagnosis of angiofibromas carried with it considerable risk of severe bleeding when attempts were made to biopsy the mass. Many cases were transferred to major medical centres haemorrhaging in and around anterior and posterior packs following biopsy.

The classic presentation of nasal obstruction and bleeding in an adolescent male, combined with the mirror or telescopic finding of a lobulated, violaceous mass in the nasopharynx, is presumptatively diagnostic.

The primary characteristic of these tumours is their predominant occurrence in young males. Only three of the cases in our series were females and in each there is doubt as to the diagnostic validity, since arteriograms failed to reveal the typical tumour stain. The histological appearance in these cases falls within the broadly variable patterns seen in angiofibromas. There are sufficient reports in the literature, however, to validate its occurrence in females. Figi & Davis (1950) reported an 8% incidence in females in the Mayo Clinic series. The highest incidence of female patients was 16% reported by Handousa (1954) in his series of Egyptian patients.

Ages ranged from 10 to 18 with an average of around 14 years, a finding similar to other reported series. The youngest case reported in the literature was discovered in a 5-week-old infant (Handousa 1954) There are reports of the tumour being discovered in older patients, although it is speculated that they had been present for many years in an asymptomatic form. One of the cases reported by Shiff (1959) was found in a 53-year-old-male who has noted nasal obstruction since age 18.

The obscure histogenesis of these tumours has stimulated the advancement of numerous theories of origin. There is some rational support for most of these theories. The almost exclusive occurrence in males suggests an imbalance of the pituitary-adrenogenital system, with neoplastic response of the target tissue in the nasopharynx. There is a widely held theory that the tumour originates from the embryonic chondrocartilage where the basiocciput is joined to the body of the sphenoid by embryonal cartilage during the development of the skull. The closure of this area by ossification during the second decade of life expalins the decreased vascularity with the increase in age (Benschand & Ewing 1941). The origin of the tumour has also been attributed to the periosteum lining of this basicranial area. Ringertz (1938) proposed that the central periosteal layer of the bone arising from the embryonal occipital plate and the anterior aspect of the first and second cervical vertebrae as the target tissue, while Schiff (1959) speculated that the tumours may arise from a desmoplastic response of the nasopharyngeal periosteum to an ectopic hamartomatous nidus of vascular tissue, probably of the inferior turbinate type. Despite the attractiveness of the hormonal target tissue theory, objective measurements of hormonal abnormalities, as shown by measurements of the gonadotrophins, or 17-kelosteroids, have not been consistently demonstrated (Shiff 1959, Henderson & Patterson 1959).

The availability of contrast arteriography and computerized tomography (CT) scan with the classical vascularized blush has eliminated the need for risk of biopsy. In fact, the contrast CT scan is pathopneumonic of angiofibroma. Arteriography is reserved for therapeutic embolization of the operable lesions and has now become an integral part of the operative procedure, resulting in significant reduction of blood loss.

The staging of angiofibromas of the nasopharynx has been proposed utilizing radiographical studies (Sessions et al 1981, Chandler et al 1984, Fisch 1986, personal communication). Most classifications have placed these tumours into four stages. The staging classifications are of questionable value since the tumours are not malignant histologically. This report will make the case for only two stages: 1. those which are operable and can be completely resected with safety, and 2. those which are non-resectable because of their extensive acquired parasellar internal carotid artery blood supply and consequently should be irradiated.

Extension of the tumour into the paranasal sinuses (i.e. maxillary, ethmoid, sphenoid), infratemporal space, or the cheek present no significant technical problems. The tumour is approached by the transpalatal, lateral rhinotomy, Caldwell Luc-Denkers, transmandibular, sublabial retromaxillary, lateral base of skull, or any combination of these approaches. An intracranial, combined with one or more of the latter approaches, has extended the resectabilty of these lesions while further diminishing the surgical risks (Krekoroan & Kato 1977, Jafek et al 1979, Fish 1985).

Serious morbidity and mortality have resulted from severe haemorrhage, injudicious attempts at removal of tumours by surgeons with limited experience, or attempts to remove tumours with intracranial extension (Ward et al 1974). Controversy in the management of nasopharyngeal angiofibromas arises since low-dose external irradiation (Briant et al 1978, Cummings 1981), or a single surgical procedure (Jafek et al 1978, Ward et al 1974) achieves primary control of the tumour in about 80% of the cases. Surgeons (Biller 1978, Jafek et al 1973, Neel et al 1973, Waldman et al 1981) and radiotherapists (Fitzpatrick et al 1980, Cummings 1981) are, for the most part, strong proponents for their respective therapeutic modalities.

Bleeding, palatal fistula, loss of vision, hepatitis, reaction to anaesthesia, recurrence and death are the complications of surgery (Biller et al 1978, Ward et al 1974). Failure to respond (20–48%), radiation-induced carcinomas, sarcomas and osteitis are the complications of radiation (DeGroot et al 1973, Tountas et al 1979). Neither surgeon nor radio-therapist relish complications. It is fair to conclude that if all patients were treated with a single modality the risks, morbidity and mortality would be similar. This being the case, the question arises, 'Is it possible to individualize treatment for each patient and thereby minimize the risks?'

In addition to surgery and radiation, other modalities have been tried, including cryotherapy, electrocoagulation, embolization, injection of sclerosing agents, hormonal therapy, and conservative expectant observation with control of bleeding by repeated nasal packing until the tumour undergoes spontaneous regression. The absurdity of dogma is evident in such statements as 'surgery alone has proven effective' (Conley et al 1968), or the claim that the success rate with surgery at their institution was only 5%, while radiation was successful in 77% of all cases and in 92% of patients receiving this as the primary mode of therapy (Briant et al 1970). The latter authors failed to provide details of the surgical approach to the patients in their series and to elucidate what they meant by 'success' as well as to describe their methods of follow-up evaluation (i.e. angiography, radioisotope scanning, etc.).

The author and his residents have tried most of these techniques only to discard them for lack of effectiveness. The value of hormonal therapy for decreasing vascularity of the tumour is still in the process of evaluation. Our clinical impression is that the effect of oestrogens administered preoperatively is limited. The appropriateness of the approach, the skill of the surgeon and the duration of the operative procedure appear to be more significant factors.

Recently (Goepfeit et al 1985) treated 5 patients with aggressive recurrent nasopharyngeal angiofibromas with a variety of antineoplastic chemotherapeutic agents. These patients had 'failed' surgery and conventional radiotherapy, or implanted Au-198 Gold seeds. The risks of haematological and immunological suppression appear warranted for these cases and need additional evaluation. Since the patients also received irradiation, which may continue to cause shrinkage for 8 months or more (Ward et al 1974, Ward 1983), the actual effectiveness of these toxic drugs still remains to be determined. Chemotherapy may offer a welcome adjunct to the treatment of these aggressive life-threatening lesions, but the risks do not appear indicated for those who can be treated with surgery or with adequate irradiation.

The close working relationship among surgeons and radiotherapists at UCLA over the past two-and-a-half decades has provided us with more than 60 cases of angiofibroma of the nasopharynx upon which intensive study has led to the evolution of a more rational diagnostic and treatment approach (Ward 1983). Few clinicians accumulate sufficient experience in the management of these relatively rare tumours to understand adequately their multi-faceted behaviour. Successful removal of the small angiofibroma confined to the nasopharynx, by any surgical approach or technique, may prove successful and may give the naive clinician a false sense of confidence. In contrast, an encounter with one of the more extensive, invasive tumours that involve the structures of the base of the skull, the middle and anterior cranial fossae may provide a horrendous nightmare-like experience. The author encountered such a case that led to the untimely death of a 16-year-old-boy after 5 operations and 45 units of blood. This unfortunate experience has stimulated repeated review and reassessment of our UCLA experience (Ward et al 1974, 1983). This series of patients, combined with review and comparison of the reports in the literature, has helped develop a rational basis for the management of nasopharyngeal angio-fibromas. Several important conclusions have emerged:

1. The size of the tumour in the nasopharynx does not necessarily represent the true extent and size of the tumour and may be only 'the tip of the iceberg'.

2. Contrast computerized tomography scanning provides a reliable assessment of tumour size and is pathognomonic of angiofibroma without resort to biopsy.

3. Bilateral selective external and internal carotid arteriograms are an unequivocal essential to the diagnostic workup and therapeutic management of patients with angiofibromas.

4. Extension intracranially into the anterior and middle fossae with parasellar feeding vessels from the internal carotid systems are best considered non-resectable.

5. Surgery is the treatment of choice for these young patients, but should be avoided in favour of radiotherapy in cases with cavernous sinus encroachment and when there are parasellar feeding vessels from the internal carotid artery.

6. In all of our cases treated with adequate radiotherapy there has been either a complete response of the tumour, or shrinkage with airway improvement and eradication of the problem of severe recurrent epistaxis.

7. Initially, high ligation of the external carotid saved significant blood. This has now been replaced by embolization of all accessible feeding branches. In the majority of recent cases, after being successfully embolized, blood loss was under one unit and required no replacement.

DISCUSSION

These conclusions deserve further comment. While the massive nasopharyngeal angiofibroma usually is accompanied by expansion into the sinuses, infra-temporal space and even intracranially, this isn't always the situation. Likewise, what appears as a small tumour in the nasopharynx can be much larger than anticipated. Contrast computerized tomography is critical for diagnostic purposes, as well as to provide the initial assessment of the tumour location and size.

Arteriography of the internal and external carotid arteries demonstrated that in 18% of the cases, intracranial parasellar feeding vessels were present. Having previously experienced and reported a mortality in such a case, we decided that in the future those cases deemed non-resectable would be treated by irradiation. Six of the last 36 cases have been treated with 30 to 63 Gy. Four of the 6 cases responded well, marked-to-complete shrinkage of their tumours and no further bleeding. The 2 cases that failed received only 30 to 33 Gy respectively. One case then received a combined intracranial–extracranial surgical resection with the loss of 34 units of blood. The tumour was incompletely removed and grew back over a period of 6 months. A second course of 30 Gy over a 3-week period caused a reduction in the size of the mass and cessation of bleeding. The second case, with failure to respond to irradiation, has recently received a repeat dose of 30 Gy. All of the cases receiving 45 Gy or more in 4 $\frac{1}{2}$ weeks or longer showed shrinkage of the tumour and control of bleeding. It seems reasonable that, if the risks of irradiation are to be elected, more than the conventional 30 Gy should be given. We have resolved this through mutual agreement with our radiotherapist and now give between 45 to 60 Gy for those cases that are irradiated.

Throughout the years covered by this series, we have experimented with blood conservation techniques. A definite correlation cannot be made with arterial ligation or embolization in individual cases. However, overall when we began bilateral external carotid arterial ligation, our average blood loss fell from 3160 ml for non-ligated cases (13 cases) to 2490 ml for ligated cases (34 cases). Initial embolization techniques further reduced the blood loss to an average of 1820 ml. After experience and improved embolization techniques, the blood loss was reduced to an average of 640 ml. There are occasional cases, usually with recognized poor embolization, that require one or more units of blood replacement. Rarely, however, is transfusion necessary for extracranial cases in which the neuro-radiologist has performed a good selective embolization.

The surgical approaches utilized alone, or in combination, were transpalatal, lateral, rhinotomy, Caldwell-Luc-Denkers, sublabial-Denkers, reto-maxillary, lateral base of skull, or simultaneous intra-extracranial.

The following algorithm is now used:

The patient is scheduled for arteriography and surgery the same morning. If the arteriogram shows intracranial invasion with feeding vessels from the parasellar area, the surgery is cancelled and the patient is irradiated. If the arteriogram shows the tumour fed by branches of either or both of the external carotid arteries without paraseller intracranial spread, then the feeding arteries are embolized with gelfoam or plastic discs and the patient is taken to the operating room. Extension of the tumour into the paranasal sinuses, infratemporal space, or the cheek present no great technical problem. The effectiveness of the embolization is believed to be diminished if surgery is delayed more than 48 hours.

There is a place for radiotherapy in patients with juvenile angiofibroma. Individualization of the treatment to each patient diminishes the major risks associated with either surgery or irradiation. Eighty percent of the time, the surgeon can successfully resect these tumours. With the advent of good embolization, blood transfusion is required in only about one-fifth of the extracranial cases. By using adequate radiation (45 Gy or more), the radiotherapist can successfully treat the high surgical risk cases with parasellar intracranial extension. Thus 18–20% of the patients need face the risks of carcinomas or sarcoma secondary to exposure to radiation. Co-operation among surgeons, neuroradiologists and radiotherapists has raised the level of safety and brought new benefits to our patients.

Clinical diagnosis

↓

Contrast CT scan
(pathognomonic)

↓

External and internal carotid
arteriography

↓ ↓

Non-resectable
(intracranial parasellar invasion)　　Resectable
(selective embolization)

↓ ↓

Adequate radiotherapy
45 Gy or more　　Surgery within 48 hours

It is to be expected that the two contributors to the topic on the value of radiotherapy in the management of juvenile angiofibroma, would approach the subject in a varying manner since one is a surgeon, the other a radiotherapist! Surprisingly, it is Cummings who has adopted a rather more flexible approach, whilst Paul Ward, rather disappointingly, has confined himself largely by quoting the 'accepted policy'. This is a pity, since I have always credited him with the realization that these lesions are not nasopharyngeal in origin, but arise in the region of the medial pterygoid plate and sphenopalatine foramen. All 28 patients from my own personal series of 44 cases showed erosion in this region on conventional and computerized tomography. Exposure by lateral rhinotomy, or extensions of this approach, confirm that the base of the lesion is always in this area, with the nasopharynx frequently occupied by expansion since it is the most readily available space. It is interesting to note that secondary vascular attachments are only found when the mass encroaches against mucosa covering bone or cartilage. Consequently, there is rarely difficulty in mobilizing extensions within the pterygopalatine or infratemporal fossa.

One of the few grounds of common agreement is that girls are rarely affected and that the median age at diagnosis is around 14 years. This is perhaps surprising, since despite considerable differences in ethnic maturity, similar ages at presentation are reported worldwide. Although a wide range of age incidence has been reported in the literature—mainly anecdotal, the virtual restriction of the condition to adolescent males has formed the basis for some imaginative and largely hypothetical concepts. Children vary greatly in the rate at which they develop. Although the degree of development of the reproductive system would appear to be the most obvious criteria, skeletal and dental maturity together with shape age are most generally useful. It is only recently that the complex series of hormonal changes underlying the events of puberty have been investigated, utilizing reliable methods of estimating blood and urine levels of pituitary and gonadal hormones. Growth and luteinizing hormones are not secreted at a constant rate throughout the day and some of the earlier reports relating to

gonadotrophin or 17-ketosteroid levels are of little value. The adolescent changes are initiated by the brain and brought about by hormones, each of which act on a set of targets or receptors. The concept that has boys with angiofibromata are sexually underdeveloped has not been confirmed by modern evaluation techniques and even the term 'juvenile' is open to misuse, although legally correct in many counties.

Pathology

It is somewhat surprising that neither of the contributors has emphasized the clinical significance of the variations in histology found within these lesions. Although essentially angiomatous tissue in a fibrous stroma, both the maturity and quantity of these components vary within individual lesions making it impossible to compare random biopsies. Some tumours might well be called fibroangioma, others angiofibroma—although palpation usually allows differentiation of the very vascular soft mass from the hard, largely fibrotic lesion. Such fibrotic lesions are difficult to remove, although it might be expected that regrowth is unlikely since vascularity would be minimal. Very vascular 'soft' tumours can be better excised, although bleeding may result in residual undetected tumour left in situ. Unless the base be narrow it is doubtful if any angiofibroma is ever completely removed and success is more realistically evaluated by recurrence of symptoms rather than clinical or radiological assessment! Response to radiotherapy, which is often variable, is therefore likely to be as related to the underlying structure of the angiofibroma as to dose regime. A similar argument probably applies to rate of growth and degree of expansion, with the more vascular tumours growing more rapidly and extensively.

Radiological assessment has certainly improved dramatically in recent years with conventional tomography now replaced by CT scanning and MRI possibly replacing arteriography unless embolization is contemplated. In my own series, 73% of patients had involvement of the sphenoidal sinus, 60% the infratemporal fossa and 30% the orbit (Lloyd & Phelps 1986).

Although Ward is understandably concerned

about the hazards of attempting surgical removal of intracranial extensions, I wonder if this problem has been perhaps overemphasized! Large tumours at the skull base are always extradural and can be relatively easily removed with adequate access. Involvement of the sphenoidal sinus is common, but attachment to the cavernous sinus appears to be unknown. Extension into orbit is a technical nuisance, but actual involvement of orbital periosteum does not occur. It is growth in the parasellar region that possibly presents the greatest problem. Why should such extensions be removed, for most patients who have died from angiofibromata have done so as a result of treatment? Since it is probable that few tumours are ever completely removed, why not resect all that is feasible and accessible, concerning oneself with any possible residual tissue only if or when it causes symptoms?

Adequate removal is invariably possible via an extended lateral rhinotomy and it is doubtful if any of the present classification systems are of practical value (Chandler et al 1984). All ignore the intrinsic nature of the lesion—(angioma: stroma ratio) and every case has some involvement of the sphenopalatine foramen or pterygoid plates. Displacement of the posterior wall of the maxillary antrum is of little importance, since this region is readily accessible—as is the infratemporal fossa. Probably Ward's own suggestion that some are operable and some inoperable is closest to reality, although in fact *all* are in part removable! Regrowth, producing symptoms, can then be removed again, or possibly become a candidate for radiotherapy.

Arteriography and embolization

Diagnostic biopsy may be safe and useful in cases where fibrous stroma predominates. Obviously, puncture of an angiomatous area could result in severe bleeding and arteriography has been advocated for diagnosis. NMR is certainly safer and equally useful, although in my experience both techniques fail to differentiate angiofibroma from embryonal rhabdomyosarcoma!

Obviously, reduction in blood flow to a vascular tumour prior to surgery is desirable. Effective embolization necessitates the emboli penetrating into the core of the lesion, producing widespread intravascular thrombosis (Lasjaunias 1980).

Examination of histological sections of angiofibroma following embolization rarely shows such a result and reported reduction in expected blood loss may be either from obliteration of main feeding vessels, or representing a relatively avascular lesion.

Unfortunately, success is frequently reported as 'blood loss' rather than 'percentage of total blood volume lost', which is more meaningful and accurate. Arteriography will often show additional supply from the sphenoidal and ophthalmic branches of the internal carotid, ascending pharyngeal and palatine vessels. The distinction between real and false supply from the internal carotid artery is important. Intrasphenoidal extension frequently recruits a supply from the capsular vessels and the posterior ethmoidal vessels from the ophthalmic artery. This looks worse on the arteriogram than in practice (Thompson et al 1979).

Hormone therapy

Some mention must be made regarding preoperative oestrogen therapy, since this has been raised by Ward. The rationale for this therapy is apparently based upon a triological thesis in 1959 (Schiff 1959), where two patients received 15 mg stilboestrol per day for a month preoperatively. Just one patient had a pre- and postmedication biopsy—and it is apparent just how useless this would have been in confirming reduction in vascularity. My own experience with oestrogen therapy in familial haemorrhagic telangiectasia (Harrison 1975) suggests that exogenous oestrogen may produce an improvement in the integrity of the endothelial lining together with an increase in the number of subendothelial microfils. Whether such doubtful benefits justify giving young males synthetic oestrogen in a dosage approximately 15 times that given for prostatic cancer is a matter of some concern, particularly as it is between 9 and 15 years that testicular function is maturing! Testicular atrophy occurs within 1 month in adults taking 1 mg day of ethinyl oestradiol, which is equivalent to 2 mg stilboestrol.

CONCLUSIONS

Paul Ward's paper gives an overall account of generally accepted views regarding this relatively unusual but fascinating condition. Much is stated uncritically, which probably reflects much of the present literature and I have briefly raised a conflicting viewpoint of some of these matters. Unless it is expected that every angiofibroma must be completely removed, which I suggest is both illogical and certainly impracticable, then surgical excision via some modification of the lateral rhinotomy approach is feasible. Even when there is radiological suspicion of intracranial involvement, this is possible, for death has usually followed ill-advised attempts at removing residual angiofibroma which might well have been left safely in situ.

There can be little doubt that Cummings has made a clear and substantial case for primary radiotherapy, although our inability to differentiate the predominantly fibrous lesion from the mainly vascular mass may explain the varying response rate witnessed by most clinicians. This must surely be one of those conditions where centralization of expertise is essential. Since few individuals will have treated more than 50 patients within their professional lifetime, choice of surgical approach and clinical assessment may be faulty in inexperienced hands,

resulting in unjustified morbidity or even mortality.

Despite persuasive arguments, we are concerned at giving any radiation to young patients with benign tumours. Since surgical control is feasible in most patients and resection of local growth possible in those whose recurrence produces symptoms, radiotherapy may well be reserved for those few patients with very vascular lesions who show rapid regrowth. Little information is available as to long-term follow-up of those few patients where radiological assessment has suggested intracranial involvement and primary radiotherapy has replaced surgical excision. In my own experience, possible intracranial residue following surgical excision has been left untreated without apparent symptoms or harm. However, skilled radiotherapy is certainly preferable to unskilled surgery, or possibly adventurous chemotherapy.

Both authors have successfully outlined the problem from their own considerable experience and, in many ways, reached similar conclusions. My own more modest contribution has simply highlighted several of the more controversial issues which perhaps deserve further attention.

REFERENCES

B J Cummings
Apostol J V, Frazell E L 1965 Juvenile nasopharyngeal angiofibroma. Cancer 18: 869–878
Batsakis J G, Klopp C T, Newman W 1955 Fibrosarcoma arising in a 'juvenile' nasopharyngeal angiofibroma following extensive radiation therapy. American Surgeon 21: 786–793
Berenstein A, Kricheff I I 1979 Catheter and material selection for transarterial embolization: technical considerations. Radiology 132: 619–630
Biller H F, Sessions D G, Ogura J H 1974 Angiofibroma: a treatment approach. Laryngoscope 84: 695–706
Bove J R 1986 Transfusion transmitted disease. In: Brown EB (ed) Progress in hematology XIV. Grune and Stratton, Orlando, p 123–147
Carvalho M B, Andrad J, Rapoport A, Fava A S, Magrin J, Scandiuzzi D 1979 Angiofibroma juvenil da nasofaringe. Revista Paulista da Medicina (Sao Paulo) 93: 52–62
Chandler J R, Goulding R, Moskowitz L, Quencer R M 1984 Nasopharyngeal angiofibromas: staging and management. Annals of Otology, Rhinology and Laryngology 93: 322–329
Chen K T K, Bauer F W 1982 Sarcomatous transformation of nasopharyngeal angiofibroma. Cancer 49: 369–371
Conley J, Healey W V, Blaugrund S M, Perzin K H 1968 Nasopharyngeal angiofibroma in the juvenile. Surgery, Gynecology and Obstetrics 126: 825–837
Cummings B J 1980 Relative risk factors in the treatment of

juvenile nasopharyngeal angiofibroma. Head and Neck Surgery 3: 21–26
Cummings B J, Blend R, Keane T et al 1984 Primary radiation therapy for juvenile nasopharyngeal angiofibroma. Laryngoscope 94: 1599–1605
Denekamp J 1984 Vascular endothelium as the vulnerable element in tumours. Acta Radiologica Oncology 23: 217–225
Donald P J 1979 Sarcomatous degeneration in a nasopharyngeal angiofibroma. Otolaryngology and Head and Neck Surgery 87: 42–44
Doyle P J, Riding K, Kahn K 1977 Management of nasopharyngeal angiofibroma. Journal of Otolaryngology 6: 224–232
Fisch U 1983 The infratemporal fossa approach for nasopharyngeal tumors. Laryngoscope 93: 36–44
Fitzpatrick P J 1970 The nasopharyngeal angiofibroma. Canadian Journal of Surgery 13: 228–235
Foster R S 1978 Morbidity and mortality after thyroidectomy. Surgery, Gynecology and Obstetrics 146: 423–429
Gisselsson L, Lindgren M, Stenram U 1958 Sarcomatous transformation of a juvenile, nasopharyngeal angiofibroma. Acta Pathologica et Microbiologica Scandinavica 42: 305–312
Goepfert H, Cangir A, Lee Y Y 1985 Chemotherapy for aggressive juvenile nasopharyngeal angiofibroma. Archives of Otolaryngology 111: 285–289
Green J R 1977 Cost-benefit analysis of surgery: some

additional caveats and interpretations. In: Bunker J P, Barnes B A, Mosfeller F (eds) Costs, risks and benefits of surgery. Oxford University Press, New York, p 70–76

Hempelmann L H, Hall W J, Phillips M, Cooper R A, Ames W R 1975 Neoplasms in persons treated with x-rays in infancy: fourth survey in 20 years. Journal of the National Cancer Institute 55: 519–530

Hormia M, Koskinen O 1969 Metastasising nasopharyngeal angiofibroma. Archives of Otolaryngology 89: 523–526

Jafek B W, Krekorian E A, Kirsch W M, Wood R P 1979 Juvenile nasopharyngeal angiofibroma: management of intracranial extension. Head and Neck Surgery 2: 119–128

Jereb B, Anggard A, Baryd I 1970 Juvenile nasopharyngeal angiofibroma. A clinical study of 69 cases. Acta Radiologica (Therapy Physics Biology) 9: 302–310

Lasjaunias P, Picard L, Manelfe C, Moret J, Doyon D 1980 Angiofibroma of the nasopharynx. A review of 53 cases treated by embolisation. The role of pretherapeutic angiography. Pathophysiological hypotheses. Journal of Neuroradiology 7: 73–95

Million R R, Cassisi N J 1984 Juvenile angiofibroma. In: Million R R, Cassisi N J (eds) Management of head and neck cancer. A multidisciplinary approach. Lippincott, Philadelphia, p 467–474

Neel H B 3d, Whicker J H, Devine K D, Weiland L H 1973 Juvenile angiofibroma—review of 120 cases. American Journal of Surgery 126: 547–556

Patterson C N 1965 Juvenile nasopharyngeal angiofibroma. Archives of Otolaryngology 81: 27–277

Sessions R B, Wills P I, Alford B R, Harrell J E, Evans R A 1976 Juvenile nasopharyngeal angiofibroma: radiographic aspects. Laryngoscope 86: 2–18

Shalet S M, Beardwell C G, Pearson D, Jones P H 1976 The effect of varying doses of cerebral irradiation on growth hormone production in childhood. Clinical Endocrinology 5: 287–290

Sinha P P, Aziz H I 1978 Juvenile nasopharyngeal angiofibroma. A report of seven cases. Radiology 127: 501–505

Spagnolo D V, Papadimitriou J M, Archer M 1984 Postirradiation malignant fibrous histiocytoma arising in juvenile nasopharyngeal angiofibroma and producing alpha-1-antritrypsin. Histopathology 8: 339–352

Stiller D, Katenkamp D, Kuttner K 1976 Cellular differentiations and structural characteristics in nasopharyngeal angiofibromas. An electron-microscopic study. Virchows Archiv Pathological Anatomy and Histology 371: 273–282

Stone E, Cummings B J 1985 Late effects of radiation for juvenile angiofibroma (in preparation)

Vadivel S P, Bosch A, Jose B 1980 Juvenile nasopharyngeal angiofibroma. Journal of Surgical Oncology 15: 323–326

Waldman S R, Levine H L, Astor F, Wood B G, Weinstein M, Tucker H M 1981 Surgical experience with nasopharyngeal angiofibroma. Archives of Otolaryngology 107: 677–682

Ward P H 1983 The evolving management of juvenile nasopharyngeal angiofibroma. The Journal of Laryngology and Otology 98: 103–104

Ward P H, Thompson R, Calcaterra T, Kadin M R 1974 Juvenile angiofibroma: A more rational therapeutic approach based upon clinical and experimental evidence. Laryngoscope 84: 2181–2194

P H Ward

Bensch H, Ewing J 1941 Neoplastic diseases, 4th edn. W B Saunders, Philadelphia, Pa

Biller H F 1978 Juvenile nasopharyngeal angiofibroma. Annals of Otolaryngology, Rhinology, Laryngology 87: 630–632

Briant T D R, Fitzpatrick P J, Book H 1970 The radiological treatment of juvenile nasopharyngeal angiofibroma. Annals of Otolaryngology 79: 1103–1113

Briant T D R, Fitzpatrick P J, Berman J 1978 Nasopharyngeal angiofibroma: A 20-year study. Laryngoscope 88: 1247–1251

Chandler J B, Goulding R, Moskowitz L, Ouencer R M 1984 Nasopharyngeal angiofibromas: staging and management. Annals of Otology Rhinology Laryngology 93: 322–329

Cummings B J 1981 Relative risk-factors in the treatment of juvenile nasopharyngeal angiofibroma. Head and Neck Surgery 3: 21–26

Conley J, Healey W, Blaugrund 1968 Nasopharyngeal angiofibroma in the juvenile. Surgery Gynecology and Obstetrics 126: 825–837

DeGroot L V, Paloyan E 1973 Thyroid carcinoma and radiation. A Chicago endemic. Journal of the American Medical Association 225: 487–491

Figi F A, Davis R D 1950 Management of nasopharyngeal fibromas. Laryngoscope 60: 794–814

Fisch U 1985 Lateral (infratemporal fossa) approach to the base of the skull. In: Cretien et al (eds) Head and Neck Cancer. B C Decker, Philadelphia and C V Mosby, St Louis, p 252–262

Fitzpatrick P J, Briant T D R, Berman J M 1980 The nasopharyngeal angiofibroma. Archives of Otolaryngology 106: 234–236

Goepfert H, Cangie A, Lee Y 1985 Chemotherapy for aggressive juvenile nasopharyngeal angiofibroma. Archives of Otolaryngology 111: 285–289

Handousa F 1954 Nasopharyngeal fibroma. Journal of Laryngology and Otology 68: 647–666

Henderson G P Jr, Patterson C N 1969 Further experiences in treatment of juvenile nasopharyngeal angioma. Laryngoscope 79: 561–580

Jafek B W, Naham A, Butler R N, Ward P H 1973 Surgical treatment of juvenile nasopharyngeal angiofibroma. Laryngoscope 83: 707–720

Jafek B W, Krekorian E A, Kirsch W N et al 1979 Juvenile nasopharyngeal angiofibroma: Management of intracranial extension. Head and Neck Surgery 1: 119–128

Krekorian E A, Kato R H 1977 Surgical management of nasopharyngeal angiofibroma with intracranial extension. Laryngoscope 87: 154–164

Neel H B III, Whicker J H, Devine K D et al 1973 Juvenile angiofibroma. Review of 120 cases. American Journal of Surgery 126: 547–556

Ringertz N 1938 Pathology of malignant tumors arising in nasal and paranasal cavities and maxilla. Acata Otolaryngologica, Stockholm 27: 1–405

Schiff M 1959 Juvenile nasopharyngeal angiofibroma: A theory of pathogenesis. Laryngoscope 69: 981–1016

Sessions R B, Bryan R, Naclerio R, Alford B 1981 Radiographic staging of juvenile angiofibroma. Head and Neck Surgery 3: 279–283

Tountas A A, Fornasier V L, Leung P N 1979 Post irradiation sarcoma of bone. Cancer 43: 182–187

Waldeman S R, Levine H L, Astor F, Wood B, Weinstein M, Tucker H 1981 Surgical experience with nasopharyngeal angiofibroma. Archives of Otolaryngology 107: 677–682

Ward P H 1983 The evolving management of juvenile nasopharyngeal angiofibroma. British Journal of Laryngology and Otolaryngology 8: 103–104

Ward P H, Thompson R, Calcaterra T, Kadin M 1974 Juvenile angiofibroma: A more rational therapeutic approach based upon clinical and experimental evidence. Laryngoscope 84: 2181–2194

D F N Harrison

Chandler J R, Goulding R, Moskowitz L, Quencer R M 1984 Nasopharyngeal angiofibromas: staging and management. Annals of Otology, Rhinology and Laryngology 93: 322–329

Harrison D F N 1975 Use of oestrogen in the treatment of familial haemorrhagic telangectasia. Laryngoscope 101: 246–251

Lasjaunias P 1980 Nasopharyngeal angiofibroma: hazards of embolization. Radiology 136: 119–123

Lloyd G A S, Phelps P D 1986 Juvenile angiofibroma— imaging by magnetic resonance, CT and conventional techniques. Clinical Otolaryngology 59: 675–683

Schiff M 1959 Juvenile nasopharyngeal angiofibroma. Laryngoscope 69: 681–1006

Thompson J N, Fierstien S B, Kohut R I 1979 Embolization techniques in vascular tumours of the head and neck. Head and Neck Surgery 2: 25–34

14

How should recurrent laryngeal papilloma be treated to minimize recurrence and maximize function?

W.S. Crysdale

Laryngeal papilloma, or 'warts in the throat' (Webb 1956), are uncommon, rapidly growing, non-invasive growths of viral aetiology that are located most commonly on the vocal cords and supraglottic structures, but can also involve the oral cavity, trachea and lungs. Pathologically, they consist of connective tissue stalks covered by well-differentiated stratified squamous epithelium and thus are similar in appearance to common cutaneous or genital warts. They are variously referred to as laryngeal papillomatosis, respiratory papillomatosis, papilloma of the larynx, juvenile laryngeal papillomatosis, or papilloma, or aerodigestive tract papillomatosis, etc. The adjective juvenile should be used carefully as it misleadingly implies that the recurrent form is found in the young only; this is not the case as the recurrent form is diagnosed in adults as well, albeit less frequently than in young children. My own preference is the term recurrent respiratory papillomatosis or papilloma (RRP).

Weiss & Kashima (1983) refer to 'juvenile onset group', with onset of disease at 10 years of age or less, versus an 'adult onset group', with presentation of papilloma at age 21 years or greater. Probably the majority of the cases of RRP have their onset prior to the age of 10 years, or are of the juvenile onset group. In one large series of paediatric patients (Cohen et al 1980), 68% of the children were symptomatic prior to 4 years of age. The onset of the disease in the years between 10 and 20 appears to be infrequent (Brondbo et al 1983) and certainly uncommon in old age (Dedo & Jackler 1982). In any case, it is important to realize the RRP is not just a paediatric disease but affects most age groups.

The majority of patients will present with a disturbance of phonation. In the infant, the cry will be abnormal; for that reason, abnormality of cry is a firm indication for diagnostic endoscopy in that age group. Patients may present with stridor—a sign of partial airway obstruction. Airway obstruction may be so severe as to be life-threatening. On one occasion, 10 years ago, I was called urgently to treat a 4-year-old boy with near total airway obstruction. Emergency endoscopy revealed profuse laryngeal papilloma; it was determined postoperatively, when further inquiry was possible, that a lack of language development (aphonia) had been attributed to the fact that he had Down's syndrome! Erroneous diagnosis is common in RRP—Cohen et al (1980) found that less than one-third of patients had the correct diagnosis applied prior to direct laryngoscopy.

Subglottic extension occurs both in the juvenile and adult onset forms and is probably more common than appreciated. Weiss & Kashima (1983) reported that 69% of 39 patients had subglottic involvement. In that same group of patients, there was a 20% rate of tracheal involvement. Dedo & Jackler (1982) reported similar statistics with 18.3% of 109 patients having tracheobronchial involvement. The juvenile form of the disease seems more 'virulent' clinically, as cases with lung involvement have been reported occurring just in the paediatric age group fortunately in less than 1% of cases (Weiss & Kashima 1983, Kramer et al 1984, Kawanami & Bowen 1985). Malignant change is rare, but was reported by Bewtra et al (1982), presenting, with a fatal outcome, in a 26-year-old female who had onset of the disease at 6 years of age.

RRP resembles other virus infections involving epithelium (such as herpes simplex) in that it is potentially a lifelong disorder. The variability and unpredictability of the clinical course has been noted by most authors and that fact is a major problem, both when counselling patients and/or parents about

RRP and when assessing the efficacy of any form of therapy. For instance, Cohen et al (1980) reported a series of 90 paediatric patients (with mainly multiple lesion disease) who had an average of 11.8 procedures; however, 1 patient required only two procedures while another had 110 procedures! Bergstrom (1982) reported recurrence after a 33-year remission in a male patient who had originally presented with a juvenile onset form of RRP.

Death is uncommon in this disease, but morbidity is significant. Dedo & Jackler (1982) had no deaths in their series of 109 patients, but Cohen et al (1980) reported a mortality rate of 3.3% in his series of 90 paediatric patients. Persistent dysphonia or aphonia as a consequence of the disease process or its treatment is common. Tracheotomy is necessary in 2–4% of patients (Dedo & Jackler 1982, Cohen et al 1980). Rinne et al (1983) reported 3 patients with total laryngeal obliteration following prolonged repeated endoscopic treatment. Robbins & Howard (1983) reported 2 patients who underwent laryngectomies for the treatment of chronic disabling disease. However, perhaps Brondbo et al (1983) touch upon the most significant morbidity of RRP—the social economic effects. These authors made these observations with particular reference to adult patients whose ability to work or maintain employment was severely threatened by the presence of dysphonia and the frequent absences necessitated by the disease process and treatment procedures. The psychological well-being and academic progress of the paediatric patients is compromised in a similar fashion.

Many forms of therapy have been advocated for RRP, which is really indicative of a lack of uniform success with any particular method to date. Robbins & Woodson (1984), in a succinct review of the treatment modalities utilized in RRP, divided them into broad categories of medical methods, immunotherapy, physical methods and surgical measures. Many patients will receive more than one form of treatment in the course of their disease.

Medical methods listed include the use of many topical medications, in particular podophyllum and 5-fluorouracil. Medications administered systemically have included antibiotics and magnesium and calcium replacement therapy. Dedo & Jackler (1982) painted the raw surfaces in the larynges of their patients with podophyllum after CO_2 laser excision

and felt that this combined modality approach was responsible for the good results with low morbidity reported in their series. Smith et al (1982), in their report, use 5-fluorouracil (5-FU) as an adjuvant to CO_2 laser treatment; they found that the major limitation to the effectiveness of this approach was the need for frequent administration. At present, forms of medical treatment, systemic or topical, appear to play an adjunctive role only.

Forms of immune-orientated therapy have involved the use of vaccines, lavamisole, transfer factor and interferon (IFN). Strauss et al (1982) reported the use of BCG in 19 patients with RRP (one of the documented effects of BCG administration is the release of IFN); they felt that no conclusions could be made regarding the efficacy of this approach. Schouten et al (1981) felt that, although the administration of a drug such as lavamisole is simple compared to some forms of immune therapy, their results of treatment in three patients do not justify a formal clinical trial. Interferons are polypeptides with potent antiviral, antiproliferative and immunomodulative effects and the efficacy of this treatment approach will be discussed in greater detail separately.

Physical methods have included cauterization, ultrasound, cryosurgery and irradiation. The author has no experience with any of these methods and did not encounter any recent reports advocating their usage. At this time, external irradiation for benign disease is not acceptable.

Surgical measures used have included local excision, tracheotomy, laryngofissure and laryngectomy. Endoscopic surgical excision had usually been accomplished with cup forceps until the development of the CO_2 laser, which is probably more widely used. Brophy et al (1982) reported the use of the argon laser in two patients with RRP; however, concern was expressed by Dedo (1982) that the depth of the burn may be excessive. Tracheotomy is to be avoided, but may be required for the relief of airway obstruction in proliferative disease; Tucker (1980) reported an unusual case involving a 2-year-old child with virulent and rapidly progressive disease in whom he maintained a double-barrelled or diversionary tracheostomy for almost 5 years until the disease was in remission. Robbins & Howard (1983), in their report of 2 adults who underwent laryngectomy from a series of 63 patients with RRP, state that the prime reason that their 2 patients underwent laryngectomy was their concern for morbidity and possible mortality of repeated surgical procedures under difficult conditions in the face of aggressive disease. Previously reported laryngectomies for this condition have been related to the development of malignant disease.

So the clinician of the mid-1980s is faced with the problem of treating a relatively uncommon but troublesome problem with recognized variability of clinical course knowing that none of the different modalities used by his predecessors or present colleagues has successfully eliminated RRP. How should RRP be treated so that recurrence can be minimized and yet best maintain the airway and phonation? I believe the answer is the judicious combination of surgical excision using the CO_2 laser, plus the administration of exogenous interferon in selected cases.

SURGICAL EXCISION

Removal with cup forceps was for years the method of choice for surgical excision and this approach is still preferred when debulking large amounts of papilloma from a larynx which usually is obstructed. However, the cup forceps should not be used to define clearly the structures within the larynx; this task should be done with the aid of the operating microscope and carbon dioxide laser, which is ideally suited for this task because of the precision it affords, the minimal damage to surrounding tissue and the haemostatic effect (Fried 1984). In fact, it is dangerous to use the laser for debulking, as a continuous mode of operation will be necessary and too much heat will be generated. This results in second and third degree burns to the underlying tissues within the larynx and cicatricial stenosis of the larynx may be the end result.

The carbon dioxide laser is used surgically; the tissue to be removed is grasped by forceps and a plane of cleavage between papilloma and normal tissue in Reinke's space is produced with the laser (using the pulsed mode). Although he does not state why, Vaughn (1983) feels that Reinke's space should not be invaded and that muscles should not be exposed. Instruments are now available to protect the contralateral cord. However, care must be taken not to cross the anterior commissure for fear of cre-

ating a web in that area. With diffuse disease, a number of procedures scheduled at 4–8-week intervals may have to be scheduled to clear out and maintain a low incidence of endolaryngeal disease. Low morbidity and good function will result if removal is scheduled routinely, without waiting for the onset of symptoms of airway obstruction of dysphonia (Dedo & Jackler 1982).

In fact, there are many facets to this surgical technique that are crucial. Ideally the patients should be under general anaesthesia ventilating spontaneously; the Venturi jet method is contraindicated as that technique is most likely associated with distal tracheobronchial seeding of viral particles and the subsequent development of pulmonary lesions (Kramer et al 1985). For similar reasons, traumatic instrumentation of the subglottic airway is to be avoided. Tracheotomy is associated with a higher incidence of tracheal involvement (Weiss & Kashima 1983) and should be avoided or eliminated as quickly as possible (Cohen et al 1980). Properly used, laser treatment seems to be associated with a lower incidence of laryngeal scarring or stenosis, although Wetmore et al (1985) reported that the incidence of anterior glottic webs and laryngeal oedema was relatively high in those patients requiring six or more laser laryngoscopies. Perhaps the largest series of laser laryngoscopies is that of Healy et al (1985). They reported 9 complications (0.2% complication rate) in 4416 cases during an 11-year period. There were 6 airway fires, 1 facial burn and 2 haemorrhages with no fatalities. Thus, while the development of the CO_2 laser undoubtedly represents an advance in the surgical treatment of RRP, it is essential to pay meticulous attention to all details of proper technique if complications are to be avoided.

Early identification and elimination of all detachable papilloma is fundamental to the prevention of spread and Weiss & Kashima (1983) advocate gentle telescopic examination of the tracheobronchial tree at the time of each endoscopy. How effective this approach may be is thrown into question by the report of Steinberg et al (1983), who determined the presence of latent infection in the adjacent 'normal' tissue of patients with papilloma and in the 'normal' tissue of patients in remission. These authors confirmed what we know; removal of all papilloma tissue during surgery does not eliminate infected tissue and therefore new papillomas will grow.

INTERFERON

Interferons, as previously stated, are polypeptides with potent antiviral, antiproliferative and immunomodulating effects that compromise part of the cellular defence mechanisms. Interferons may induce regression of papillomas in several ways (Schouten et al 1982): they might inhibit the replication of viruses, activate host mechanisms against the papillomas, or inhibit cell division in the papillomas. The observation that IFN is effective in RRP may also mean, as suggested by Naiman et al (1984), that RRP patients are deficient in their ability to produce IFN in response to viral infections, or that an IFN-regulated antitumour immune response is deficient in these patients. The human papilloma virus responsible for RRP may not induce IFN production and exogenous IFN is needed to control their disease. In fact, when these authors studied natural cytotoxicity (NK activity) and IFN production in 9 patients, they demonstrated that the NK-IFN system was intact in untreated patients with RRP, but the production of IFN alpha in RRP on IFN therapy was low.

Variation in the history of RRP makes interpretation of treatment difficult but IFN therapy does seem to change the pattern of recurrence of RRP and supplements surgical treatment (Bomholt 1983). Resurgence or regrowth of papilloma after cessation of therapy is a reported problem (McCabe & Clark 1983). McCabe & Clark (1983) identified a group of 'poor responders' that they could not explain, nor did they find a predictable relationship between response, level of toxicity or side effects. In light of these cases of poor response or RRP regrowth, more studies are needed to gain more experience to determine what dosage, type of IFN and route of administration is most effective (Goepfert et al 1982).

For the administration of IFN, it is best to have a protocol and involve the assistance of other medical personnel familiar with its use. Pretreatment evaluation may have to be done in hospital and tests to be completed include WBC count with differential, platelet and reticulocyte counts, liver and renal function tests, immunoglobulin quantitation, chest X-ray and records of the patient's height and weight. Prior to IFN therapy, laryngoscopy plus possible bronchoscopy is required and, at the time of the endoscopy, particular care should be taken to document the distribution of the lesions. If possible, the status of the larynx should be documented photographically. As IFN therapy progresses, the pretreatment tests should be repeated periodically (usually monthly) depending on the side effects, dosage and timing of treatment.

The amounts of IFN administered and timing of administration varies from report to report. McCabe & Clark (1983) used human leukocyte IFN i.m. 3 times per week in variable quantities—children received 3 000 000 units per injection, while older patients received 4 000 000 and 10 000 000 units. Every 3 months they decreased the dose by about one-third until a maintenance dose of one-third the pretreatment dose was reached. Sessions et al (1984) administered type I alpha human leukocyte IFN i.m. at a dosage of 2 000 000 units per square metre of body surface area daily—the frequency of administration was reduced to 3 times weekly when reduced rate of papilloma growth was documented. Schouten et al (1982) used two types of IFN—human fibroblast IFN (Hu IFN beta) and human leukocyte IFN (Hu IFN alpha). These drugs were injected subcutaneously 3 times per week in 2 different patients. Other authors (Sessions et al 1983, Goepfert et al 1982, Lundquist et al 1984, Bomholt 1983) have also reported their experience with exogenous (human) leukocyte interferon (IFN alpha).

No mortality reports attributable to IFN therapy for RRP were found. It seemed that most patients experienced fever, chills, anorexia and vomiting during the early weeks of treatment. Sporadic and transient temperature elevations throughout treatment and temperature elevation on the day of injection also seem common. Sessions et al (1984) reported SGOT elevations in 4 of 11 patients which all responded to dose modification. Goepfert et al (1982) had to discontinue IFN therapy in 1 of 14 patients (a 9-year-old boy) because of continued toxicity (primarily SGOT elevation), despite dose modifications. Another of their patients (an 8-year-old girl) had treatment discontinued at parental request because of early signs of liver toxicity. McCabe & Clark (1983) modified dosage schedule in their patients if the WBC count dropped below 4000, platelets below 75 000, or if the SGOT is above 100 iu per litre.

At present, IFN therapy should be considered in

patients with aggressive and troublesome RRP (Sessions et al 1984), when surgical excision is required more often than every 6 weeks for maintenance of the airway, or when aphonia persists. In this type of case, endoscopic treatment will be required less often (perhaps 1–3 times per year, as suggested by Lundquist et al 1984) and there will usually be a return of vocal function. My only personal experience with IFN involves such a case—a 4-year-old girl requiring 11 endoscopies in 15 months (life-threatening obstruction on 3 occasions) with aphonia. Now, after 6 months of IFN treatment, she has had only 2 endoscopies (both elective) and is talking normally! Interferon should also be considered in cases with significant tracheal, broncheal or pulmonary involvement. McCabe & Clark (1983) feel that patients requiring a tracheotomy should be considered for IFN therapy.

Whether RRP can be prevented by advocating Caesarian section in those women with vaginal condyloma is still debatable. Vaginal condyloma and RRP do seem to be epidemiologically related (Quick et al 1980). Between 2 and 10% of American women of child-bearing age have vaginal papillomavirus infection and yet RRP is relatively rare. These facts indicate that, either the condyloma virus is only slightly infectious, or that, a subset of condyloma viruses is responsible for RRP, or that most infections are 'silent' and are never expressed as RRP (Steinberg et al 1983).

Morrell Mackenzie introduced the term laryngeal papilloma in 1871. He was the first to differentiate the lesions clinically from other laryngeal masses and described multiple small papillary growths causing hoarseness and varying degrees of dyspnoea. He described cases in both children and adults and, although subsequent literature has tended to concentrate on the problem in children, some published series contain a high proportion of patients over 16 years of age (Holinger et al 1968, Strong et al 1976). Alberti & Dykun (1981) reported 52 patients over the age of 16 years, 12 of whom had residual childhood papillomata and 40 who developed papillomata after the age of 16. Of the adult-onset group, 28 presented with multiple, rather than solitary, papillomata. It is not possible histologically to differentiate between papillomas from children or adults, whether multiple or solitary, though important clinical differences, which have a direct bearing on management, are apparent.

In the child-onset group, the tumour is almost always multiple, affects predominantly the glottic area and recurs more frequently after excision. In children there is no clear sex predominance, whereas in adult disease many series show a male:female preponderance of 2:1 (Alberti & Dykin 1981, Capper et al 1983, Strong et al 1976).

There is a widely held view that hormonal factors may play a part in this change of incidence and that the disease often regresses during puberty. However, the evidence for this is poor and no particular pattern of clinical behaviour has been observed which allows prediction of pubertal regression, indeed many cases continue into adult life. Capper et al (1983) found the same sex ratio in juvenile papillomas continuing on into adult life and Strong et al (1976) and Marjoros et al (1964) failed to link the age of remission with puberty. Bjork & Webber (1956) found only 2 out of 37 patients with juvenile papillomas who regressed during puberty. Treatments with oestrogens and testosterone have also proved unsuccessful.

Cases may relapse years later and certainly a minimum follow-up of 5 years, beyond supposed remission, is necessary to obtain an accurate picture. Unfortunately this situation rarely exists.

In adults, relatively more of the lesions present as solitary papillomas and, whereas the lesions in children rarely undergo malignant change, in adults solitary papillomas may merge in an ill-defined manner with carcinoma in situ and verrucous carcinoma. The literature on the subject of malignant change in juvenile multiple papillomatosis contains many pitfalls, but if the guidelines laid down by Kleinsasser & Glanz (1979) are adhered to then the number of 'genuine' cases in the world literature remains in single figures. For a true diagnosis of spontaneous malignant degeneration in juvenile multiple papilloma, there should be an interval of at least 5 years between primary diagnosis of the multiple, recurring, nonkeratinized papilloma, and malignant change. Radiotherapy should not have been received and there should be histological proof of invasive carcinoma, which may be difficult to distinguish from severe dysplasia. Different degrees of atypia in juvenile laryngeal papillomas are not an uncommon finding.

Few reported cases have fulfilled these criteria (Barth 1898, Justus et al 1970, Toso 1975, Zehnder 1975, Lyons 1978, Kleinsasser & Glanz 1979, Oloffson et al 1980, Bewtra 1982). Only 1 was a child, a boy aged 12 years, the others occurring between 35 and 64 years of age. Four of these patients were heavy smokers and the possibility that the malignant change was caused by this carcinogenic factor cannot be ruled out. In conclusion one can say that, although there is a remote possibility of spontaneous malignant change in multiple papillomas, it does not affect treatment choice in the great number of patients.

Solitary adult papillomas have an undeserved reputation for being more likely to undergo malignant change, but this is not substantiated if initial histological diagnosis is correct, a point demonstrated by Capper et al (1983) when they reviewed 63 cases of squamous papillomas of the larynx in adults. When criteria described by these authors is strictly adhered to, the diagnosis of papilloma presents little difficulty. Although verrucous squamous carcinoma may show papillomatous areas, markedly distorted, elongated, and branching ridges are present quite unlike papillomatosis. Papillomatous change may also occur in the region of a true squamous cell carcinoma, but the correct diagnosis is made clear by the dysplastic cells of the malignant neoplasm. Their studies showed adult papillomas to be histologically identical to juvenile papillomas and to show similar clinical behaviour. Furthermore, the patients overlapping from juvenile to adult life showed many similarities to the purely adult group.

Aetiology

Therapeutic modalities must reflect aetiological possibilities and greatest effort has centred round the possibility of a viral agent. Mackenzie (1871b) noted the common coexistence of papillomas and skin warts and this has been confirmed by subsequent authors. Uhlman (1923), in his classical experiment transplanted a papilloma from the larynx of a 6-year-old boy to his arm and then successfully implanted this onto canine vaginal mucosa, an experiment which has only been duplicated successfully by Ishikawa in 1936.

Despite electron microsopic evidence of papova virus particles in papilloma tissues (Boyle et al 1973, Arnold 1979), no actual isolation of human papilloma virus has so far been achieved, possibly due to the lack of a satisfactory culture system. Extensive examination of laryngeal papillomas have not confirmed the presence even of virus particles, but without the keratin layer of cutaneous warts to 'trap' the maturing virians it is not surprising that EM identification of virus in laryngeal papilloma has been at best serendipitous (Quick et al 1980). Five different human papilloma viruses have been found in cutaneous papillomas in man. Immuno-histochemical techniques have recently suggested that viruses of a common subgroup may be responsible for laryngeal papillomas and some cutaneous papillomas (Quick et al, 1978). Laryngeal papillomas in children have also been linked to maternal anogenital warts by Cook et al (1973) and Quick et al (1980), an important point when considering prevention.

Clinical features

The most common presenting and persisting symptom is hoarseness. In young infants an abnormal cry may be the first indication. Whilst respiratory distress symptoms are more common in children, Alberti & Dykun (1981) found respiratory symp-toms in no less than 20% of their adult series. There is no doubt that the typical course is one of extensive growth and rapid recurrence in the children with predominant respiratory symptoms, necessitating frequent surgery. It must be remembered that the considerably smaller size of the infant or young child's larynx makes it more vulnerable to even moderate encroachment by papilloma.

Papillomas are commonest on the true cords and frequently extend into the ventricles. Fortunately, because of the superficial nature of lesions the cords remain mobile unless the disease is very extensive or complications from surgery intervene. Occasionally other areas of the larynx may be the only site, but usually in advanced cases the lesions may involve the supraglottis, subglottis, trachea and bronchi. Dissemination into, or initial presentation in the other areas is of poor prognostic significance.

A variety of theories have been proposed to explain the maximal incidence of papillomas on the vocal cords. The glottis obviously presents the site of greatest airflow and constriction, therefore inhaled viruses are most likely to be implanted there. The vocal cords are also the most likely site of mucosal trauma, particularly the anterior two thirds, where indeed most papillomas occur. A break in the mucosa is undoubtedly important as seeding of papillomas will occur in areas of trauma, most notably tracheostomy sites, and this is obviously relevant when considering the various methods of surgical excision and the possibility of tracheostomy.

The vocal cords do not have any notable sub-mucosal lymphatics and may therefore be relatively deficient in immunological protection. Certainly the cords appear to act as a reservoir of recurrent papillomas in many cases, even after careful and apparently total removal of all papillomas.

Prevention

As it is probable that laryngeal papillomas are caused by an infective viral agent, this aspect deserves more attention. An aetiological relationship between laryngeal papilloma in children and maternal anogenital warts, condylomata acuminata, has long been suspected and the maximal incidence occurs in children before the age of 7 years. The earliest reports were those of Hajek (1956) and Kaufmann & Balogh (1969). Cook and co-workers (1973) reported an analysis of 13 patients with laryngeal papillomas and found that the mothers of 9 children had condyloma at the time of delivery. Quick et al (1980), in a survey of 31 papilloma patients, found 21 with a definitive history of condyloma. Frequently the presence was initially denied by the mother, but on further investigation the information was found to be forgotten or the individual was unaware of the presence of the lesions. In some instances the vulva and vagina were free of clinical condyloma but small flattened lesions were reported on the cervix.

A prospective trial involving 31 infants born of mothers with condylomata acuminata at parturition, or during pregnancy, was reported in 1981. It proved disappointing in that none of the 19 children followed for between 1 and 5 years developed papillomas and leaves the question to be answered as to the true risk of acquiring the disease in this manner. In the area of America where this study was done, the incidence of condylomata acuminata in women of child-bearing age was estimated as 1 in every 100. No figures were available for the overall incidence of laryngeal papilloma, but it is obviously important that this epidemiological research is continued.

Unfortunately, at this stage there is no way to predict which infants will develop papilloma. Perinatally acquired viral infections are certainly well recognized and the acquisition of human papilloma virus during passage through the contaminated birth canal seems plausible.

Various factors, such as suction of meconium, may help to implant virus. It is known that human papilloma viruses can remain dormant for long periods and re-emerge after trauma. Condylomata are certainly spread easily by sexual contact and Strong et al (1976) suggested that the male predominance in adults may be related to orogenital contact from infected females.

Hopefully in the future the situation will be clarified so that possible alternative methods of delivery, such as caesarean section, may be considered by informed obstetricians and patients.

In addition to initial prevention of the disease, avoidance of spread of existing disease around the upper respiratory tract is obviously important. There is no doubt that clinical spread is induced by excessive surgical trauma, particularly tracheostomy. This can readily be appreciated in the light of the recent immunohistochemical evidence of viral par-

ticles in the superficial layers of the papilloma, which are easily dislodged (Quick et al 1980).

It also calls into question the most appropriate anaesthetic technique. Endotracheal intubation is associated with a small, but definite, risk of seeking into the trachea, and endolaryngeal venturi techniques may aid dissemination of papillomas down the trachea and bronchi.

From a theoretical point of view, high frequency jet ventilation, via a narrow bore needle, placed through the neck into the trachea below the larynx, would be the best technique.

ASSESSMENT OF TREATMENT RESULTS

The literature is abundant with reports of methods to treat the condition and the remainder of this chapter will review these treatments in the hope of providing some perspective on current management.

A number of factors compromise therapeutic assessment and the natural history of the disease is variable, both between patients and in the same patient over a long period of time. There is a natural tendency for remission, but usually no indication of when this is going to occur. These factors are relevant when small series of patients are presented (as with the recent 'crop' of reports related to interferon). Unless the study is a properly designed prospective controlled trial, the results may be invalid. Because of the relative infrequency of laryngeal papillomas, prospective trials are difficult to set up and large numbers of patients treated by the same doctor are a rarity.

In many cases an initial report is published endorsing a particular method in a small number of patients, which is not followed by a satisfactory long-term report. Assessment of treatment must involve a realistic long-term follow up and, at present, only complete resolution of lesions over a period of several years represents cure.

Surgical methods of treatment

The commonest complications of laryngeal papillomata are the complications of treatment and, to minimize recurrence due to 'seeding', it is important that any surgery be carried out atraumatically.

Complications of disease, notably respiratory obstruction, are more common in florid cases, so a fine balance is required to keep the patient's symptoms to a minimum without undertaking an unnecessary amount of surgery.

As no definite evidence exists that any form of surgery alters the natural history of the disease in an individual patient, it is principally required to control symptoms, particularly respiratory obstruction.

In most large series, the commonest complications are laryngeal webbing and stenosis. The need for a tracheostomy commonly occurs in association with problems encountered postoperatively and not as an emergency on presentation of the disease. All complications are more common with florid disease in small children and in those who continue from childhood to adult life requiring multiple procedures over many years.

However, there is little doubt that, even with relatively mild adult onset disease, significant webbing can be produced after only minimal procedures. In the milder forms of the disease it is important not to be overenthusiastic, as minimal symptoms can easily be replaced by more difficult, and sometimes irreversible, complications of surgery. It is, of course, tempting to think that repeated attempts at complete removal will in some way shorten the natural history of the disease—there is no good evidence that this is the case.

Local excision—for many years the endoscopic removal of papillomas using a variety of forceps—has been the most widely used surgical technique. Since the early 1960s microlaryngoscopy and its associated instrumentation has improved the accuracy of this method. With the development of the laser, precise endoscopic excisions are now possible, with excellent haemostasis, little damage to healthy laryngeal tissue, and minimal postoperative oedema. However, there is no evidence that the laser significantly alters the recurrence rate and those surgeons practised and skilled over many years of microlaryngeal surgery need not forsake their instruments for the CO_2 laser. Certainly, in the adult larynx there is little to choose between the two methods. In the small child haemostasis and lack of postoperative oedema give the laser an undoubted advantage, particularly in those children with florid disease likely to cause respiratory obstruction. There have been many reports of laser treatment of papilloma, but the yardstick remains the first large series of 110 cases treated by this method in 1976 by Strong et al. One-third of the cases achieved remissions lasting one or more years. The high cost of the CO_2 laser is often cited, but in those centres dealing with significant numbers of patients it is quickly offset by the resultant shorter hospital stay.

Suction-diathermy is an inexpensive and efficient compromise between the above two methods. It allows selective cauterization of papilloma with haemostasis and minimal damage to the surrounding mucosa. As with any other modality, excessive use can result in scarring, stenosis and webbing. The details of this method are well described by Frootko & Rogers (1979).

Earlier articles described the use of chemical cauterizing agents such as acids, arsenicals and bismuth (del Villar et al 1956). These agents will destroy papillomas, but their use is haphazard, with precise application difficult and significant scarring possible. They are not part of the modern armamentarium.

Cryosurgery was initially reported with enthusiasm in the early 1970s, Singleton & Adkins (1972) describing the largest series of 21 patients. They postulated that freezing may decrease the infectivity of any viruses present in sloughing papillomas. However, other authors have reported only moderate success with cryosurgery, noting that the recurrence rate is unaltered and that scarring may still occur. In addition, the technique is time-consuming and individual freezing of each papilloma may be difficult. In the small child's airway postcryosurgery oedema may be considerable and the method is not recommended for this group.

Tracheotomy—it is not always clear whether this predisposes to dissemination of laryngeal papillomas into the tracheobranchial tree, or whether the actual severity of the disease predisposes them to tracheostomy. Undoubtedly the papillomas do 'seed' at the site of a tracheostomy in some patients. If a tracheostomy is necessary to relieve severe dyspnoea, then its omission is unwise. It may render anaesthesia for urgent papilloma removal a major hazard and each case must be carefully assessed on its individual merits. A policy of avoiding a tracheostomy at all costs is to be discouraged. A significant percentage of children still undergo tracheotomy, usually as a temporary measure, and decannulation is advisable when the airway is restored.

Laryngofissure procedures have occasionally been undertaken in difficult cases of laryngeal papillomatosis (Holinger et al 1968). A wide exposure with thorough excision of the lesions is possible, and a keel may be used to inhibit web formation. The good exposure allows intraluminal grafting and both split-thickness skin grafts and vein grafts have been used. Tabb & Kirk (1962) reported good results in two adults and two children using vein grafts to cover the excised papilloma areas. There have been no long term follow-up reports of this procedure, so it merits further evaluation, particularly in persistent cases.

Laryngectomy—the exact number of laryngectomies carried out for severe laryngeal papillomatosis is unknown. There are only three reported cases in patients who had not undergone malignant transformation. Fechner et al (1974) reported one case undertaken for extension of the papilloma into the prelaryngeal soft tissues. Robbins & Howard (1983) reported two cases, both performed for severe refractory disease. The procedure should be considered for those cases whose larynx is a large reservoir of papilloma and is entirely functionless, i.e. they are aphonic and breathing via a permanent tracheostomy. It may diminish the likelihood of any tracheobronchial spread.

Radiotherapy

During the 1930s many articles described effective control of laryngeal papillomatosis with various methods of irradiation, e.g. Cohen (1933), Foster (1933), New (1938). However, the complications of radiotherapy have subsequently declared themselves. Arrested laryngeal development, radionecrosis, chronic laryngeal stenosis, hypothyroidism and malignancy have all been documented. These complications have meant that radiotherapy is contraindicated in children and young adults, although it may still have an occasional place in older adults with unremitting serious disease.

Ultrasound

In 1953, Newton & Kissel reported fragmentation of the tobacco mosaic virus and almost total loss of its infectivity following ultrasound. In 1959 Kent reported the successful treatment of plantar warts with ultrasound. Assuming a viral aetiology in laryngeal papillomatosis, reports of treatment by ultrasound appeared in the 1960s, (Birck & Manhart 1963, Jenkins 1967). These initial reports used an externally applied energy source and involved only 5 and 6 patients respectively with short-term follow-up. Initial encouraging reports were not confirmed by larger long-term studies. A report of 12 cases, using an intralaryngeal probe for application, by White et al in 1974, also lacked definitive evidence and subsequent long-term analysis. There have been no recent reports of note and one can only conclude that the method does not produce satisfactory control during a longer follow-up period.

Medical methods

Topical medications of many types have been used in the past and, on occasions, small numbers of patients have been enthusiastically reported. However, none of these substances has been effective in the long-term and many have obvious disadvantages. The list includes alcohol, arsenic, bismuth, castor oil, podophyllum, formaldehyde, lactic acid, nitric acid and trichloroacetic acid.

Systemic medications also tried, but of dubious benefit include heavy metals, steroids, magnesium, calcium, potassium iodide and antibiotics. A good example is that of tetracycline. Holinger et al (1950) reported 7 cases given aureomycin, with 5 initially improved. However, in a subsequent article in 1968, Holinger et al did not propose this as an effective treatment. A similar fate has no doubt befallen many other medications. I am, at present, assessing the possible benefit of the antiviral drug acyclovir in these patients, but the numbers are small and as yet no dramatically beneficial effect can be convincingly demonstrated.

Hormones are perhaps worthy of separate mention although the initial rationale for their use, that perhaps a hormonal factor played a part during puberty, has not been substantiated in recent studies. Broyles (1948) reported the first use of oestrogen in 5 cases. There was no subsequent report and a similar pattern occurred with stilboestrol. However Szpunar (1967) published a trial of 107 children treated over a 17-year period by intralaryngeal injections of oestradiol. This excellent report included a long follow-up period, good functional results and complete disappearance of papilloma in 70% of cases. Szpunar postulated that the favourable effects were due to changes at cellular level in the local ground substance induced by the oestradiol, making the tissue more resistant to viral infection. In a later report in 1977, he reported a 42.6% cure (5 years without recurrence) in 136 children. The injections follow endoscopic removal of the papillomata and routine endoscopic oestradiol injection three times a year was recommended, even in quiescent disease, until a 3-year disease-free period was reached. Of the supplementary measures to endoscopic removal so far evaluated, this method deserves further attention.

Chemotherapy—in the 1960s Kiviranta (1966) reported with enthusiasm the benefits of treatment using methionine and Bunting, in a personal communication quoted by Holinger et al (1968), obtained benefit using methotrexate. Neither of these approaches seem to have been reported later. In 1980 Smith et al reported the use of 5-fluorouracil in 8 patients with severe papillomatosis. The medication was instilled by spray or solution and 6 patients showed a notable decrease in the lesions; Pritchard et al (1980) reported similar improvement in 6 children given the anti-DNA virus agent adenine arabinoside.

The use of these powerful drugs in children is not without complication and further careful work is required to evaluate potential improvement against inherent dangers. For the moment it would seem appropriate to use these drugs only in patients whose disease was uncontrolled by endoscopic removal.

Immunotherapy

Vaccines as a treatment for laryngeal papillomatosis were reported with varying results during the 1960s. Moffitt (1959) reported four cases using bovine wart virus with encouraging results, but a later report by Irvine & Moffitt (1962) in 29 patients showed 45% having varying reactions, such as abscess formation at the site of injection. There have been no further reports since then.

Smallpox and bacille Calmette-Guérin vaccinations were also tried during the 1960s, but intralaryngeal injections produced mucosal ulceration and there have been no satisfactory reports since.

Holinger et al (1962), Shipkowitz (1967) and Strome (1969) have all reported on the use of autogenous vaccine. Apart from Shipkowitz's group, the numbers of patients were small and the results variable. There have been no further long-term reports.

Transfer factor has been administered to small numbers of patients by two groups of workers, Quick et al (1975) and Lyons et al (1978), without convincing improvement.

Interferon therapy has recently generated considerable interest and Haglund et al (1981) reported 7 cases of severe juvenile papillomatosis treated with exogenous leukocyte interferon. During treatment the papillomas decreased in size, but recurred rapidly in 5 cases when the treatment was discontinued. Subsequently, similar reports of small numbers of patients by Bomholt (1983), Goepfert et al (1982) and Sessions et al (1984) have all shown that inferferon can produce a good response in severe disease, but required prolonged sustained treatment to maintain a remission. The treatment is expensive and requires frequent injections. It appears to be the latest in the long line of medications which will not provide a definitive cure.

CONCLUSIONS

The inevitable conclusion is that, at present, laryngeal papillomatosis is still best controlled by endoscopic microsurgical removal. The technique used must be safe and atraumatic and, although laser excision is very effective, forceps removal and selective suction diathermy are as good in experienced hands. It must always be borne in mind that most of the complications of the disease are iatrogenic. Overenthusiastic and too frequent removal is likely to produce more problems than it solves. There is no evidence that one form of surgery has any distinct advantage in terms of altering the natural history of the disease. In order to maximize function and minimize complications, surgery should only be undertaken when symptoms are sufficient to warrant it. Although tracheotomy is best avoided, arrangements should always be made to undertake it whenever endoscopy is carried out.

Ideal adjunctive measures to cure or control the disease have yet to be developed and research into this sphere requires reasonable groups of patients with accurate and long-term follow up.

This has been a problem for the laryngologist since the specialty began to develop in the early to middle years of the last century. Both contributions emphasize that there have been many attempts to solve the difficulties encountered, but that, as yet, no obvious definitive treatment is available. The development over the past 40 years of a subspecialty of paediatric otolaryngology could be the first stage in the evolution of a more academic approach, which, over the years, may lead to a more rational management of the disease.

Both contributions refer to the often observed fact that recurrent papillomatosis is not confined to any particular age group. In this author's personal series the youngest patient was 5-months-old when referred for advice and the oldest 84 years. Both Crysdale and Howard distinguish between the occurrence of a single papilloma, which is unlikely to recur after removal, and multiple papillomatosis, which has a marked tendency to recurrence, particularly in children. Recurrence in adults is seen from time to time but this appears to be more likely to occur in those patients whose treatment began in childhood. Thus, the old lady of 84, who presented for the first time at that age, required just three treatments to clear the larynx of disease, whereas Mrs W.H., who had been attending hospital since the age of 4 years, continued to attend at the age of 42, by which time she had four healthy children of her own.

Natural history of the disease

The surgeon of today approaches disease from three aspects, when considering how any particular patient should be managed. The topography of the organ involved, together with its physiology, are of fundamental importance. Today's medical student is encouraged to regard anatomy and physiology as one subject rather than separate disciplines. This approach is of particular value in multiple papillomatosis, for the difficulties of treatment are compounded by the need to preserve both the anatomy and physiology both locally in the larynx and in the lower respiratory tract. Careful consideration must therefore be given to the nature of the disease process and to the effect that this may have in distorting the anatomy and disturbing the physiology.

The view that recurrent papillomatosis is of viral origin is widely accepted by laryngologists. However, there has as yet been no convincing demonstration as to the precise virus which is responsible. Viruses which are known to produce cutaneous papillomas in man have never been isolated from recurrent papillomatosis of the respiratory tract. There are, however, recorded cases of parents and doctors developing cutaneous papillomata when involved in the care of children with recurrent respiratory papilloma. Quick has been interested for many years in the association between vulval and perineal condylomata in the mother and recurrent respiratory papillomatosis. However, although Quick was able to find some association, 19 children whose mothers had such condylomata were followed up and failed to develop papillomatosis. For over 50 years the tendency for respiratory papillomata to implant on traumatized areas and to spread from those areas has been recognized. This was recorded in the pioneer textbook of otorhinolaryngological pathology by Eggston and Wolff. This is one of the most significant clinical observations which must affect the laryngolotologist's approach to the management of the condition. Limitation of local trauma to epithelial surfaces discourages the spread of the condition.

The hope has been expressed already that the development of a subspecialty of paediatric otolaryngology will lead to a better appreciation of the factors peculiar to children which affect management. Because there are no discernable microscopic differences between the papillomata found in adults and those found in children, there has been a tendency to feel that the problems to be solved are identical in both age groups. However, experience shows that children have many more crises in the management of the disease than adults. Deaths from respiratory obstruction may occur and the papillomata flourish and require removal more frequently in the child than they do in the adult. Why is this? The paediatric otolaryngologist recognizes that he is dealing with an immature individual. This immaturity affects, not only structure and function, but also immunity and the processes of repair. It is now well recognized that children born in hospital should be sent home at the earliest possible opportunity because of their susceptibility to endemic hospital infections. They have no proper defence in the early weeks of life. In the same way, the child with papillomata does not produce the same vigorous immune response, seen in the adult, which helps to localize the condition to the larynx.

MANAGEMENT

Since the cause of the disease has not been identified, it is not possible to discuss the relative merits of specific treatments which have been found to be effective. The problem of the patient with recurrent respiratory papillomatosis is a problem of management. The laryngologist's role is to support the patient in development of a resistance to the disease, while at the same time preserving the functions of the laryngotracheobronchial tree and the overall physical and psychological development of the patient. Whereas, in the case of the adult, it may be possible to carry out treatment at long intervals of perhaps months or years, it is often necessary to keep the child in hospital because of the rapidity with which new papillomata may form, leading to respiratory obstruction. Prolonged hospitalization of a young child can lead to emotional deprivation and educational retardation. The child needs both parents and siblings to develop normally. If possible, therefore, children who require prolonged hospitalization should be treated in children's hospitals where they will be in the company of other children and where the parents will be allowed to spend as much time as they are able with their child. There is no substitute for the home and school environment for normal development but open visiting and a hospital school is the most effective alternative. Crysdale finds medical treatment to be of some value. Howard feels that the best chance of cure is by early surgical removal.

Medical treatment

Over the years, a variety of remedies have been tried. In the 1940s and 1950s the vogue was for such topical applications as podophyllin and aureomycin paste. Some centres still use podophyllin, but al-though it may be effective in debulking the larynx of papillomata, its use can lead to an unacceptable degree of scarring and even web formation. In more recent years attention has been directed to parenteral treatment with such powerful agents as Ara-A and interferon. There can be no doubt that both can affect significantly the course of the disease in a particular child. One or two courses of Ara-A may lead to a dramatic death of papillomata, which can be removed with a sucker with no bleeding. A successful outcome can be predicted from the clinical appearances. The papillomata lose their blood supply and become transparent, pale and jelly-like. Interferon too has its protagonists. In the author's experience it has proved to be less effective than Ara-A. However, the disadvantage of both treatments appears to be that it is impossible to predict the case which is likely to respond favourably. A case could be made out for a single course of treatment with Ara-A, followed by endoscopic examination. Failure to respond would appear to be an absolute indication for the resort to other methods. Crysdale recommends a trial with interferon before resorting to surgery.

Surgical treatment

This must be considered under two headings: local removal of papillomata and relief of airway obstruction.

Local removal of papillomata

The objective to be attained by surgical removal is the removal of the papilloma, the whole papilloma and nothing but the papilloma. This is, of course, a counsel of perfection and takes no account of the site, size or accessibility. A further problem, which confronts the surgeon bent on removal by cold excision, is bleeding. Simple removal with cup forceps may be effective, but all too often the field becomes obscured by blood and it becomes difficult to ensure that small pieces of the tumour do not fall into the lower respiratory tract. For this reason, the author developed the suction diathermy in the 1960s. The bell mouth of the sucker ensured a broad face for the attachment of the tumour, which could then be held away from healthy tissue and, by the application of a diathermy current, be destroyed in situ.

Other modalities employed at that time included cryosurgery and ultrasonics. Both had some success, but both had disadvantages which made their application difficult. Difficulty was found in developing a cryoprobe of sufficiently small dimensions which could be applied to small tumours and, at the same time, in which it was possible to reverse the freezing process when required. Ultrasound, if applied from the outside, could not always be focussed where required and, from the inside, was complicated by the need to accompany the application with irrigation to prevent overheating.

The development of the CO_2 laser, attached to the operating microscope by Strong and others in the 1970s, proved to be a real advance in the selective destruction of the tumours as they formed. There was significantly less postoperative oedema and the subepithelial damage was minimal due to the small degree of penetration (0.2 mm). Crysdale speaks of scarring and third degree burns of the larynx. It would be interesting to know how many other surgeons have this experience. Two forms of application are available, pulsed and continuous. Pulsed application has proved to be significantly safer in use. Furthermore, the laser can now be delivered via the tracheoscope and bronchoscope and so it has become possible to deal effectively with tumours which seed themselves down into the lower respiratory tract.

Relief of airway obstruction

Because there is no specific therapy for recurrent laryngeal papillomata and because, ultimately, success depends on tipping the balance in favour of the patients' immunity, complications are likely to occur along the route towards achieving this goal. Each patient and every age at which the disease occurs affects the pattern which will emerge.

The complication to be feared most is the development of a sufficient degree of lower airway obstruction to make it necessary to create an artificial airway. A tracheostomy will certainly provide relief in the short term. However, tracheostomy affects normal respiratory physiology in three ways: 1. it diverts the normal inspiratory and expiratory airflow, 2. it removes the ability to clear the lower respiratory tract by coughing and 3. it disturbs the mucus transport from the lower respiratory tract. Each of these factors has to be taken into account. In terms of the spread of the disease from the larynx, the loss of

expiratory thrust and the effect of that thrust on the ciliary transport of mucus means that pieces of necrotic papilloma can fall into the lower respiratory tract and implant there in any site where the condition of the mucosa is degraded by repeated trauma or infection.

The price of unobstructed breathing may be the development, in the longer term, of iatrogenic disease remote from the primary site. The use of the carbon dioxide laser is accompanied by little or no postoperative oedema. A decision to open an artificial airway should be taken only after the most careful appreciation of the current status of the patient under treatment. Crysdale speaks of papillomata seeding down the trachea before a tracheostomy has been made. It is possible that this is due to obstruction to the expiratory thrust and mucus transport as a result of tumour bulk in the glottis.

Where it is found necessary to open an artificial airway, the use of a valved tracheostomy tube is strongly recommended, because, by its use, the expiratory thrust and ability to cough are restored. Clearly this helps to limit the dissemination of the disease down the airway.

CONCLUSIONS

The management of recurrent papillomata in the larynx and trachea has always presented a challenge to the laryngologist. The last 40 years has seen the introduction of powerful new modalities of treatment which can assist the surgeon in fighting the disease process. Advances in technology have not been matched by advances in the isolation of the cause of the condition and in the understanding of the way in which the disease process varies according to the age of the host. The current position is complicated further by the dangers inherent in the use of the new technology. Failure to monitor the haemopoietic status when chemotherapy is used, or to take the precautions necessary to prevent damage to healthy tissue when either diathermy or laser are used, may lead to a permanent degradation of the quality of life or even to death of the patient.

In the last analysis, only the final isolation of the causative factor and the development of specific therapy will solve the dilemma of the laryngologist who undertakes the care of these patients.

REFERENCES

W S Crysdale

Bergstrom L 1972 Laryngeal papillomatosis: recurrence after 33-year remission. Laryngoscope 92: 1160–1163

Bewtra C, Krishnan R, Lee SS 1982 Malignant changes in nonirradiated juvenile laryngotracheal papillomatosis. Archives of Otolaryngology 108: 114–116

Bomholt A 1983 Interferon therapy for laryngeal papillomatosis in adults. Archives of Otolaryngology 109: 550–552

Brondbo K, Alberti P W, Crowson N 1983 Adult recurrent multiple laryngeal papilloma: laser management and socioeconomic effects. Acta Otolaryngologica 95: 431–439

Brophy J W, Scully P A, Stratton C J 1982 Argon laser use in papillomas of the larynx. Laryngoscope 92: 1164–1167

Cohen S R, Geller K A, Seltzer S et al 1980 Papilloma of the larynx and tracheobronchial tree in children: a retrospective study. Annals of Otology, Rhinology and Laryngology 89: 497–503

Dedo H H 1982 Discussion. Laryngoscope 92: 1167

Dedo H H, Jackler R K 1982 Laryngeal papilloma: results of treatment with the CO_2 laser and podophyllum. Annals of Otology, Rhinology and Laryngology 91: 425–430

Fried M P 1984 Limitations of laser laryngoscopy. Otolaryngology Clinics of North America 17: 199–207

Goepfert H, Sessions R B, Gutterman J U et al 1982 Leukocyte interferon in patients with juvenile laryngeal papillomatosis. Annals of Otology, Rhinology and Laryngology 91: 431–436

Healy G B, Strong M S, Shapshay S et al 1984 Complications of CO_2 laser surgery of the aerodigestive tract: experience of 4416 cases. Otolaryngology, Head and Neck Surgery 92: 13–18

Kawanami T, Bowen A 1985 Juvenile laryngeal papillomatosis with pulmonary parenchymal spread: case report and review of the literature. Pediatric Radiology 15: 102–104

Kramer S S, Wehunt W D, Stocker J T et al 1985 Pulmonary manifestations of juvenile laryngotracheal papillomatosis. American Journal of Radiology 144: 687–694

Lundquist P, Haglund S, Carlsoo B et al 1984 Interferon therapy in juvenile laryngeal papillomatosis. Otolaryngology, Head and Neck Surgery 92: 386–391

McCabe B F, Clark K F 1983 Interferon and laryngeal papillomatosis: the Iowa experience. Annals of Otology, Rhinology and Laryngology 92: 2–7

Naiman H B, Doyle A T, Ruben R J, Kadish A S 1984 Natural cytotoxicity and interferon production in patients with recurrent respiratory papillomatosis. Annals of Otology, Rhinology and Laryngology 93: 483–487

Quick C A, Watts S L, Krzyzek R A et al 1980 Relationship between condylomata and laryngeal papillomata: clinical and molecular virological evidence. Annals of Otology 89: 467–471

Rinne J, Grahne B, Sovijarvi A R A 1983 laryngeal stenosis following papillomatosis—a report of three severe cases. International Journal of Pediatric Otology, Rhinology and Laryngology 5: 309–316

Robbins K T, Howard D 1983 Multiple laryngeal papillomatosis requiring laryngectomy. Archives of Otolaryngology 109: 765–769

Robbins K T, Woodson G E 1984 Current concepts in the management of laryngeal papillomatosis. Otolaryngology, Head and Neck Surgery 6: 861–866

Schouten T J, Bos J S, Bos C E et al 1981 Levamisole in the treatment of juvenile laryngeal papillomatosis. International Journal of Pediatric Otology, Rhinology and Laryngology 3: 365–369

Schouten T J, Weimer W, Bos C E et al 1982 Treatment of juvenile laryngeal papillomatosis with two types of interferon. Laryngoscope 92: 686–688

Sessions R B, Dichtel W J, Goepfert H 1984 Treatment of recurrent respiratory papillomatosis with interferon. Ear, Nose and Throat Journal 63: 26–32

Sessions R B, Goepfert H, Dichtel W J et al 1983 Further observations on the treatment of recurrent respiratory pappilomatosis with interferon: a comparison of sources. Annals of Otology, Rhinology and Laryngology 92: 456–461

Smith H G, Vaughan C W, Healy G B et al 1980 Topical chemotherapy of recurrent respiratory papillomatosis: a preliminary report. Annals of Otology 89: 472–478

Steinberg B M, Topp W C, Schneider P S et al 1983 Laryngeal papillomavirus infection during clinical remission. New England Journal of Medicine 308: 1261–1264

Strauss M, Conner G H, Harvey H A et al 1982 Aerodigestive tract papillomatosis: bacille Calmette-Guérin (BCG) immunotherapy. Laryngoscope 92: 971–975

Tucker H M 1980 Double-barreled (diversionary) tracheostomy in the management of juvenile laryngeal papillomatosis. Annals of Otology, Rhinology and Laryngology 89: 504–507

Vaughn C W 1983 Use of the carbon dioxide laser in the endoscopic management of organic laryngeal disease. Otology Clinics N A 16: 849–864

Webb W W 1956 Papillomata of the larynx. Laryngoscope 66: 871

Weiss M D, Kashima H K 1983 Tracheal involvement in laryngeal papillomatosis. Laryngoscope 93: 45–48

Wetmore S J, Key J M, Suen J Y 1985 Complications of laser surgery for laryngeal papillomatosis. Laryngoscope 95: 798–801

D J Howard

Alberti P W, Dykun R 1981 Adult laryngeal papillomata. Journal of Otolaryngology 10: 463–470

Arnold W 1979 Tubular forms of papavo viruses in human laryngeal papilloma. Annals of Otology, Rhinology and Laryngology 225: 15–19

Bomholt 1983 Interferon therapy for laryngeal papillomatosis in adults. Archives of Otolaryngology 109: 530–552

Barth E 1898 Zus casuistik des uebergangs gutartiger kehkopfgeschwülse in bösartige. Archives of Laryngology 7: 287–302

Bewtra C 1982 Malignant changes in non-irradiated juvenile laryngotracheal papillomatosis. Archives of Otolaryngology 108: 114–116

Birck H G, Manhart H E 1963 Ultrasound for juvenile papillomatosis. Archives of Otolaryngology 77: 603–608

Bjork H, Webber C 1956 Papilloma of the larynx. Acta Otolaryngologica 46: 499–519

Boyle W F, McCoy E G, Fogarty W A 1971 Electron microscopic identification of virus-1ke particles in laryngeal papilloma. Annals of Otology, Rhinology and Laryngology 80: 693–698

Broyles E N 1984 Treatment of laryngeal papillomata in children. South Medical Journal 34: 239–242

Capper J W R, Bailey C M, Michaels L 1983 Squamous papillomas of the larynx in adults. Clinical Otolaryngology 8: 109–119

Cohen L 1933 Treatment of intractable laryngeal papilloma in adults with case report. South Mediterranean Journal 26: 621–625

Cook T A, Brunschwig J P, Butel J S, Cohen A M, Goepfert H, Rawls W E 1973 Laryngeal papilloma: etiologic and therapeutic considerations. Annals of Otology, Rhinology and Laryngology 82: 649–654

del Villar R, Echverria E, de Acosta V M, Dibildox J C, Diaz F L 1956 Laryngeal papillomatosis. Archives of Otolaryngology 64: 480–485

Fechner R E, Goepfort H, Alfort B R 1974 Invasive laryngeal papillomatosis. Archieves of Otolaryngology 99: 147

Foster J H 1933 Papillomatosis laryngis. Annals of Otology, Rhinology and Laryngology 42: 548–559

Frootko N J, Rogers J H 1979 The treatment of laryngeal papillomatosis by suction diathermy. Journal of Laryngology and Otology 9: 373–381

Goepfert H, Gutterman J H, Dichtel W J, Sessions R B. Cangir A, Sulek J 1982 Leukocyte interferon in patients with juvenile laryngeal papillomatosis. Annals of Otology, Rhinology and Laryngology 91: 431–436

Haglund S, Lundquist P G, Cantell K, Strander H 1981 Interferon therapy in juvenile laryngeal papillomatosis. Archives of Otolaryngology 107: 329–332

Hajek E 1956 Contribution to the aetiology of laryngeal papilloma in children. Journal of Laryngology and Otology 70: 166–168

Holinger P H, Johnson K C, Anison G C 1950 Papilloma of the larynx. A review of 109 cases with a preliminary report of Aureomycin therapy. Annals of Otology 59: 547–564

Holinger P H, Johnston K C, Conner B R, Conner G H, Holper J 1962 Studies of papilloma of the larynx. Annals of Otology, Rhinology and Laryngology 71: 443–447

Holinger P H, Schild J A, Manizi D G 1968 Laryngeal papilloma a review of aetiology and therapy. Laryngoscope 78: 1462–1474

Irvine E W Jr, Moffit O P Jr 1962 Further studies in treatment of laryngeal papillomas with bovine wart vaccine. Cancer 13: 1221–1223

Ishikawa K 1963 Experimentalle studien uber die transplantatian des papilloma. Fukuoka Otol 8: 68–76

Jenkins J C 1967 Preliminary report on the treatment of multiple juvenile laryngeal papillomata by ultrasound. Journal of Laryngology and Otololgy 81: 385–390

Justus J, Baerthold W, Preibisch-Ettenberger R 1970 Juvenile larynx papillomatose mit Ausbreitung über das Tracheobronchialsystem und maligne Entartung ohne Stahlentherapie. HNO 18: 349–354

Kaufmann R S, Balogh K 1969 Verrucas and juvenile laryngeal papillomas. Archives of Otolaryngology 89: 748–749

Kent H 1959 Plantar wart treatment with ultrasound. Archives of Physical Medicine 40: 15

Kiviranta 1966 Methionine treatment of laryngeal papillomatosis. Duodecim 82: 435–440

Kleinsasser O, Glanz H 1979 Larynxpapillome spontane kanzerisiening nicht begrahler juvenile laryndpapillome. Laryngology

Lyons G D, Schlowwer J V, Lansteau R, Marney D F, Benes E N 1978 Laser surgery and immunotherapy in the management of laryngeal papilloma. Laryngoscope 88: 1586–1588

Mackenzie M 1871a Essay on growths in the larynx. Churchill, London

Mackenzie M 1871b Essays on growths in the larynx, with reports and analysis of one hundred consecutive cases treated by the author. Lindsay and Blakiston, Philadelphia

Marjaros M, Parkhill E M, Devine K D 1964 Papilloma of

the larynx in children. A clinico-pathological study. American Journal of Surgery 108: 470–475

Moffitt O P Jr 1959 Treatment of laryngeal papillomatosis with bovine wart vaccine. Laryngoscope 69: 1421–1426

New J B, Erich J B 1938 Benign tumours of the larynx. A study of seven hundred and twenty-two cases. Archives of Otolaryngology 28: 841–910

Newton N, Kissel J W 1953 Biophysical studies of the ultrasonic fragmentation of tobacco mosaic virus. Archives of Biochemistry 47: 424

Oloffson J, Bjelkenkrantz K, Grontoft O 1980 Malignant regeneration of a juvenile laryngeal papilloma—a follow up study. Journal of Laryngology 9: 329–333

Pritchard J, Eggerding D, Evans J G N et al 1980 Treatment of laryngeal papillomatosis. Lancet 1383

Quick C A, Behrens H W, Brinton-Danell M, Good R A 1975 Treatment of papillomatosis of the larynx with transfer factor. Annals of Otology 84: 607

Quick C A, Farns A, Crzyzek R 1978 The aetiology of laryngeal papillomatosis. Laryngoscope 88: 1789–1795

Quick C A et al 1980 Relationship between condylomata and laryngeal papillomata. Annals of Otology, Rhinology and Laryngology 89: 467–468

Robbins K T, Howard D J 1983 Laryngeal papillomatosis requiring laryngectomy. Archives of Otolaryngology 109: 765–769

Sessions R B, Dichtel W J, Goepfort H 1984 Treatment of recurrent respiratory papillomatosis with interferon. Ear, Nose and Throat Journal 63: 488–493

Shipkavitz N L, Holper J C, Worland M C, Holinger P H 1967 Evaluation of an autogenous laryngeal papilloma vaccine. Laryngoscope 77: 1047–1065

Singleton G T, Adkins W Y 1972 Cryosurfical treatment of juvenile laryngeal papillomatosis. Annals of Otology, Rhinology and Laryngology 81: 784–790

Smith H G, Vaughan C W, Healy G B, Strong M S 1980 Topical chemotherapy for recurrent respiratory papillomatosis. Annals of Otology, Rhinology and Laryngology 89: 474–477

Strome M 1969 Analysis of an autogenous vaccine in the treatment of juvenile papillomatosis of the larynx. Laryngoscope 79: 272–279

Strong M S, Vaughan C W, Healy G B, Cooperband S R, Clemente M P, 1976 Recurrent respiratory papillomatosis. Annals of Otology, Rhinology and Laryngology 85: 508–516

Szpunar J 1967 Laryngeal papillomatosis. Acta Otolaryngolica 63: 74–86

Szpunar J 1977 Juvenile laryngeal papillomatosis. Otolaryngologic Clinics of North America 10: 67–70

Tabb H G, Kirk R L 1962 Vein grafts in the management of laryngeal papillomas. Laryngoscope 72: 1228–1238

Tosa G 1971 Epithelial papillomas-benign or malignant? Interesting findings in laryngeal papilloma. Laryngoscope 81: 1524–1531

Uhlman E V 1923 On the aetiology of the laryngeal papilloma. Acta Otolaryngologica 8: 317–334

White A, Halliwell M, Fairman H D 1974 Ultrasonic treatment of laryngeal papillomata. Journal of Laryngology and Otology 88: 249–260

Zalin H 1948 The treatment of laryngeal papillomata in childhood. Journal of Laryngology and Otology 62: 621–626

Zehnder P R, Lyons G D 1975 Carcinoma and juvenile papillomatosis. Annals of Otology, Rhinology and Laryngology 84: 614–618

15

When is surgery the best treatment for recurrent laryngeal paralysis?

P. McKelvie

A flaccid, palsied vocal cord arrested in a lateralized position may leave the patient virtually speechless with nothing more than a faint whisper. For the last two decades conventional treatment has been to implant such a cord with a deposit of Teflon paste to give bulk and rigidity so that the functioning vocal cord can reach across and phonate against it. This makes a larynx continent and produces a voice of virtually normal volume, but with the timbre of a vocal cord palsy. Various refinements have included the implantation of the cord at various points along its free margin to make a relatively straight vocal cord rather than the fusiform enlargement arising from a single deposit in the middle of the mobile portion. Early workers did this under local anaesthetic, with the aid of indirect laryngoscopy and a long, curved, injection needle. This enabled them to put in only the amount required to restore the voice and to obtain an optimum effect. It also required a fair amount of dexterity and a tolerant patient. The advent of microlaryngoscopy has, in many places, supplanted this method; this is not without benefit since the deposit of Teflon paste (shredded Teflon suspended in glycerine) is not the same shape and size as the final bulk. Such an injection first of all invites an oedematous reaction, a reabsorbtion of the glycerine, a granuloma which forms around the Teflon granules and the final organization in which the Teflon occupies a smaller volume than that implanted initially. At best, fine voices can be achieved. Marked improvement in many voices can be achieved by this means, allowing the patient to conduct all normal activities, including public address with reasonable ease. It is not, however, compatible with singing, loud or prolonged shouting and other major demands made on the human voice.

Some limitations in the benefits to be gained have become apparent over the years and it is probable that certain patients should be excluded from this mode of therapy. Firstly there are those patients who have made, as many do, a marked improvement in voice over a period of some months following initial palsy, no matter what the origin. These patients present complaining that their voice is still abnormal, tires easily and is weak. Yet in the consulting room they can carry on normal conversation, raising the voice reasonably, can quite obviously carry on their business, including shopping and even teaching. They are correct in complaining that their voice is not as it used to be, since both they and the onlooker with a keen ear can detect the timbre of a vocal cord palsy. For all that on examination the cord is easily reached by the functioning one, the larynx is continent, the patient can cough and certainly is not producing a whisper. Under these circumstances there is little gain for the patient in having the flaccid vocal cord implanted; in other words, the better the voice presentation in the clinic the less gain there is to be had from Teflon implantation. Moreover, there is no guarantee that the quality achieved from implantation no matter how carefully placed, will result in a louder or more easily produced voice, nor one that tires less, or is marginally louder. It may be offset by the disadvantage of a poorer quality, including gruffness, growling, or a more marked timbre typical of the cord palsy.

Secondly, there are those patients who quite clearly, despite the existence of a cord palsy have an overlay of functional dysphonia. These patients quite commonly have had thyroid surgery and may well be seeking some resort in the courts. They may well produce a much poorer, indeed whispering, voice after implantation than the voice that they have had before. Those with an ability to cough well, to hum and in whom the voice is known from time to time to be excellent, would appear to be poor subjects for implantation. The advice of a speech therapist, experienced in the results of Teflon implant, are invaluable in assessing these patients.

The third patient in whom Teflon implantation has very well marked limitations are those in whom there is a vocal cord palsy arising from a total vagal disruption. This, resulting in a loss of the superior laryngeal nerve and the cricothyroid muscle, may well have an asymmetrical larynx in which cricoid is slewed round on thyroid, with one long cord and one short cord. Asymmetry of cord tensing in such a situation appears to make Teflon implantation of the flaccid cord less effective. It is possible that the voice gained will have an even more marked cord palsy timbre, with only a moderate gain in the volume.

All these should not be absolutely precluded from receiving cord implant, but they should be warned to have lesser expectations of the result when compared to their more fortunate colleagues with unilateral recurrent laryngeal nerve palsy.

Patients may well suffer a recurrent nerve palsy postoperatively after major cardiothoracic surgery especially on the left-hand side. There are good reasons for implanting the cord in such patients postoperatively to give them the ability to cough, although, in general, the use of Teflon implantation to make a larynx continent and able to withstand aspiration and overspill from the pharynx has limited value. It is the ability to cough which this procedure offers and is widely practised with varying success, but has become established in only a limited number of centres. The practice of implanting these patients at extubation after a cardiothoracic operation, in which the left recurrent laryngeal nerve is known to have been divided, is one with obvious appeal. Most would wait to ascertain if the cord palsy produced a faint whisper and is incontinent. Occasionally physicians, neurologists in particular, present the frail, the elderly and those with a range of neurological syndromes affecting the laryngopharynx. Provided that the lesion is unilateral and the patient has a poor voice, there is a prospect of restoring voice and continence to the larynx with Teflon implant. The greatest care has to be exercised to ensure that there is no vestige of contralateral palsy. Prognosis, as

regards making the larynx continent and proof against overspill, has to be extremely guarded in these patients. Moreover, even the slightest suggestion of stridor precludes such a bulking implant, since some patients may be precipitated into respiratory obstruction by this otherwise extremely harmless procedure.

Examination of the implant in patients who have died reveals that the Teflon granules have not travelled far from the sight of implant and, in particular, have not gone into the tissues in the neck, nor migrated into the regional lymph node. The possibility of these implants being carcinogenic is an extremely remote one; from time to time they have been put into vocal cords in which malignancies are afterwards detected; it would appear that the cord palsy was probably a fixation of the cord by an occult carcinoma.

The totally palsied laryngopharynx presents quite separate problems. The patient's life is imperilled by the aspiration of pharyngeal contents and a wide range of procedures have been proposed for closing off the larynx from the upper air and food passages. This has always been against a background of the belief that the neurological condition may abate, may be subject to neurosurgical or medical rescue, or that the progress of the neurological condition is extremely slow and may well be confined to the laryngopharynx for many years. A considerable number of patients with motor neurone disease and other neurological conditions have died of inhalation bronchial pneumonia and an assortment of laryngeal operations have been devised to counteract this. Among them have been exteriorization of the trachea below the larynx, closing up the subglottis so that the patient breathes through an endtracheostome for the rest of his natural life. This of course, could reasonably be expected to be reversible should the neurological condition abate, but involves, the larynx in being flooded and not self-cleansing during a potentially extremely long period. Total laryngectomy serves the same purpose, but of course is not reversible. Laryngofissure, coupled with cord suturing, affords a means of occluding the larynx. This involves baring of the margins of the vocal cords and also of the false vocal cords; these can be sutured together with long-stay sutures, resulting in obliteration of the laryngeal lumen and sparing the lower respiratory tract from aspiration.

In much the same manner, large implants of Teflon paste injected in the conventional manner will bulk both vocal cords to clamp them firmly against each other, occluding the laryngeal lumen and also obliterating the lumen. This has to have carefully metered doses of implant, since considerable pressure is required to close the larynx against the force of pharyngeal pressure. Too little will allow fluids to be injected into the larynx and yet prevent the patient coughing through them; a tracheostomy, of course, is essential in this type of procedure. Overambitious deposition will produce ulceration because of pressure inside the cord. It is not readily reversible.

Epiglottopexy may be carried out through a lateral pharyngotomy usually from the right-hand side (non-dominant carotid, no thoracic duct), with baring of the laryngeal surface of the epiglottis and also of the aryepiglottic folds. The epiglottis is then stitched down tightly over the top of the larynx in the manner of the lid of a German beer mug. A tiny lumen can be left in the interarytenoid space so that the patient can both cough and phonate. It is readily reversible endoscopically, if and when the happy occasion presents.

Naturally, all of these procedures involve the patient in leading a tracheostomy life; a tragic situation in the face of conditions which are so often terminal. However, life may be prolonged by these manoeuvres, since a rapid demise produced by inhalation bronchial pneumonia is an early feature of the neurological condition.

Such patients learn to cope with a tracheostomy over the months and indeed years made available to them. Those with multiple sclerosis have been most remarkable in coping well with this unpleasant burden.

The problems associated with bilaterally palsied vocal cords are of an entirely different nature. Commonly arising from thyroid surgery, but occasionally from other penetrating or space-occupying lesions in the root of the neck, the major difficulties are those of airway obstruction. The early recourse to intubation followed by tracheotomy, the establishment of a tracheostomy with a speaking valve, the attempts to extubate over the months and the wait for spontaneous resolution of the palsy in one or both cords, is all well documented. So also is the varied positioning of the flaccid palsied vocal cord,

both at the time of palsy and in the subsequent months. The incidence of this type of surgical disaster has been much reduced following increased expertise and training of the thyroid surgeons. There are some measures in the perioperative period which can well be taken with the finding that the patient has bilateral palsies. This is usually discovered at extubation after thyroidectomy and there is commonly a resort to immediate reintubation. At this point it is worthwhile re-exploring the thyroidectomy wound, preferably by an ear, nose and throat surgeon used to the operating microscope, with otological or cimino shunt instruments. Sutures, ties and diathermy burns may be discovered, involving the trunk or branches of the recurrent laryngeal nerve on one or both sides. Ties and sutures can be removed—the earlier the better. Diathermy burn wounds should be cleared of surrounding tissues, but steroids, antibiotics and cover with plastic sheeting should not be applied. It is conventional to graft lengthy defects in the recurrent laryngeal nerve, but the results in obtaining meaningful functional movements in the palsied vocal cord are poor in the extreme.

All too commonly, the debate centres around the procedure for lateralization of one of the palsied vocal cords. This is after a 6-month wait in the hope of there being a recovery of at least one of them. The wide range of procedures for lateralization may be divided into three groups:

1. Primarily endoscopic, involving arytenoidectomy, the application of lateralizing clips, or a cordectomy with the aid of a laser beam.

2. Lateralization through one of the lateral approaches behind, or through, the thyroid cartilage on one side in a King or De Graaf Woodman manner; this latter operation has received widespread recognition and, until recently, has been a firm favourite.

3. Those procedures done through a laryngofissure with direct visualization of the lumen of the larynx route in which arytenoidectomy, or other cord lateralization procedure, is carried out. In addition these procedures may well place one vocal cord at a different height in the larynx to its fellow producing a better airway.

A fourth group has to be mentioned; a number of procedures for introducing musculature into the posterior end of the cord suspended on its innervation (e.g. a portion of strap muscle on the ansa hypoglossi) have been extensively discussed, examined and, on occasion, practised. There may be some value in it, but for the most part it is fanciful! The value of the movements, if any, are in doubt and the airway improvement may well be associated with setting the cord at a different level in the larynx.

The elderly and the obese would often be well advised to accept the valved tracheostomy tube. This is associated with excellent voice production and, while the burden of a stoma is rejected or accepted in so many variable ways, it is often the best of a bad job. Any cordopexy or cord lateralization procedure trades voice for airway; the latter is far from being assured and the elderly and obese may still have difficulty in dispensing with the tracheostomy. If and when they do so, they may have a degree of stridor and indeed dyspnoea. Promises of excellent voice/airway are rash indeed.

Laser cordectomy has its enthusiastic adherents. It is a microlaryngoscopic procedure, the best results closely resemble those of the finest cordopexy/cord lateralization operations. It closely resembles in principle those cordectomies done endoscopically with the aid of knife and diathermy, which result in a strand of scar tissue bow stringing into exactly the same position as a medially placed palsied vocal cord and has the associated airway problems. This current spate of laser cordectomies remains to be assessed. The choice between the lateral approaches, e.g. De Graaf Woodman or the laryngofissure approaches, remains much the province of the enthusiasm and experience of the individual operator. Certainly, the laryngofissure procedure gives a much better view of the end result desired without recourse to endoscopy.

Those bilateral vocal cord palsies of central origin, or due to disruption of vagi high in the neck, give problems of a much more intractable nature, associated as they are with pharyngeal losses, sensory denervation of the supraglottis and overspill. They do not lend themselves to cordopexy procedures.

The aetiology and treatment of vocal cord paralysis is a subject that has courted the interest of the otolaryngologist since the earliest days of the specialty. No other discipline in the field of medicine has the privilege to observe as closely the anatomical, physiological and psychological ramifications of laryngeal paralysis, or has the opportunity to evaluate the results of therapy as easily as does the practising head and neck surgeon. As with most areas of patient care, the more complex the problem the more approaches and solutions are generated. Otolaryngology has traditionally been in the forefront of specialities devising experimental and clinical procedures to alleviate the potentially life-threatening sequelae of vocal cord paralysis.

In 1916, Dr. Charles Baker of Bay City, Michigan, described the case of a 9 year-old boy with abductor paralysis, whom he had successfully treated by removing the right vocal cord and arytenoid cartilage via a laryngofissure (Baker 1916). Apparently the results were excellent. Jackson (1922) expanded this technique by removing the ventricle with the cord in an attempt to further enlarge the airway. Ten years later, Hoover 1932 described the submucosal resection of the vocal cord following laryngofissure and, in 1936, Lore further improved access by elevating the mucous membrane and resecting the internal portion of the thyroarytenoideus muscle and part of the cricoarytenoideus lateralis muscle leaving the perichondrium behind (Lore 1936). In the meantime, in 1928, Dr T Lahey had reported the successful repair of a recurrent laryngeal nerve 6 months after the injury (Lahey 1928).

In 1939, King, an orthopaedic surgeon, advocated the transfer of the omohyoid muscle (anterior belly) to the muscular process of the arytenoid cartilage. Kelly (1941) diplomatically reported that perhaps King's impressive results were more related to his complete mobilization and outward displacement of the arytenoid cartilage than to any function of the omohyoid. Subsequently, Kelly devised a procedure whereby a window was created in the thyroid cartilage and an arytenoidectomy carried out. He was also the first to point out that an endotracheal tube helped to 'fix' the arytenoid cartilage in one position and acted as a point of counterpressure when cutting the arytenoid cartilage free from the articular surface of the cricoid. If the patient had a tracheotomy, a bronchoscope could be substituted with similar results.

The concept of arytenoidectomy evolved and Woodman (1946) reported a technique which became the mainstay of bilateral abductor paralysis therapy. Arytenoidectomy was performed via a posterior–lateral extralaryngeal approach and lateralization was accomplished by anchoring the vocal process to the inferior corner of the thyroid cartilage. Shortly thereafter, Thornell (1948) described an endoscopic arytenoidectomy which employed electrocoagulation to promote scarring, retraction and, it was hoped, a larger airway. (Anyone who has had experience with this procedure can appreciate the amount of finger strength required.)

Nerve muscle transposition, a new technique improving the treatment of abductor paralysis, was introduced by Tucker in 1976. This work was supported by Tucker's follow-up reports (Tucker 1978, 1980) and by May et al (1980). An adequate airway with good quality of voice may be created with this procedure. Failure does not preclude other surgical procedures of lateralization.

Modification of the endoscopic approach of Thornell was first published by Ossoff & Sisson in 1983 and again in 1984. Endoscopic laser arytenoidectomy was successfully performed on 10 of 11 patients and provided a new application for the technology of laser medicine.

Vocal cord paralysis, because of various circumstances, can be classified in several ways. The basic divisions of unilateral or bilateral, central or peripheral, symptomatic or asymptomatic are acceptable systems to use when classifying these problems. In this discussion, vocal cord paralysis will be addressed on the basis of whether or not it is unilateral or bilateral.

The decision to perform surgery is usually determined by clinical findings and the patient's psychological state, not necessarily the aetiology. Surgeons are observers and manipulators of nature and we should be aware of the various ramifications a disease process can have for a given patient. A condition that is crippling for one may, psychologically, be merely an inconvenience for another. The decision for or against surgical intervention can be difficult.

The factors are usually complex and challenging, philosophical as well as scientific.

With these considerations in mind, let us discuss the Northwestern approach to vocal cord paralysis.

All patients with vocal cord paralysis deserve a thorough investigation. The cause of the paralysis should be determined, a careful history should be taken, a physical examination made and a laboratory evaluation, including chest X-ray, base of skull films, lateral neck films, oesophagram, thyroid scan, blood studies and endoscopy must be performed unless the cause is obvious. If aetiology is not uncovered, 6–9 months should elapse before an anatomically irreversible procedure is planned, since 40–50% of patients with unilateral paralysis will show improvement during this time.

Unilateral vocal cord paralysis is most often treated because the patient's voice is weak and breathy, not because aspiration is a problem. The prudent surgeon will allow 6 months for the return of function, or contralateral compensation, before resorting to definitive and non-reversible intervention. Options consist of medialization injection or reinnervation. We prefer to inject Gelfoam first as a test procedure. If we are convinced there is improvement, we then inject Teflon to obtain permanent improvement and a solution of the problem. We always under inject the needed volume (usually 0.9 to 2.2 ml), adding more if necessary. Local and topical anaesthetic is preferred. Using a Brunning syringe, the standard technique is injection of Teflon just lateral to the thyroarytenoid muscle. The anterior, middle and posterior cord are injected to a depth of 5 mm so that the free margin touches the opposing cord. Additional Teflon is injected into the posterior third of the cord. One must be cautious and avoid infusing too deeply, since subglottic injection will change the level of the cord and subperichondrial injection may cause perichondritis. If is far better to be conservative and repeat the procedure than to introduce too much Teflon and compromise the airway.

Bilateral recurrent nerve paralysis, particularly if iatrogenic, is psychologically difficult for a patient and frequently a life-threatening situation. Whether manifested immediately after thyroid surgery or more subtly after exertion, decisions must be made which will have a long-term effect on the patient. It is imperative that the problem be approached in an orderly fashion so the expectations of both physician and patient will be satisfied.

Historically, the airway insufficiency of bilateral cord paralysis has forced the surgeon and patient to make some degree of compromise between retaining voice quality and an adequate airway without a tracheostomy. Since a laryngeal pacemaker is not yet available for human use, the options for long-term management include either vocal cord lateralization (intra- or extralaryngeal), or nerve muscle pedicle transposition.

May I repeat again, before embarking upon definitive therapy, one must have determined the cause of the paralysis and the likelihoood of recovery. Occasionally, as in viral diseases, recovery could be within 6 to 9 months.

The mainstay of basis of treatment has been arytenoidectomy, either endoscopic or transcervical, with nerve-muscle pedicle transposition being reserved for the patient with extraordinary needs and a surgeon with particular interest and experience with the procedure.

Endoscopic laser arytenoidectomy is the procedure of choice for most patients with bilateral abductor paralysis. We have found this technique reliable and precise. It has a low rate of complication. We employ the procedure as described by Ossoff & Sisson (1984). An operating microscope and CO_2 laser are employed to ablate the arytenoid cartilage, including the vocal process and the adjacent portion of the vocalis muscle. A remnant of the muscular process and attached arytenoideus muscle are preserved. This procedure is so precise that it may be tailored to meet the needs of the individual patients. Repeat surgery, if necessary, is equally uncomplicated. Problems usually are related to the injudicious use of the laser (skin or mucosal burns), or insufficient precaution so as to prevent endotracheal or tracheotomy tube ignition. Venturi insufflation will obviate this problem and facilitates better exposure of the posterior chink during surgery.

When a surgeon does not have access to a CO_2 laser, the transcervical extralaryngeal arytenoidectomy and lateralization of Woodman is the most frequently employed approach to bilateral vocal cord paralysis. This procedure creates a good, or at least acceptable, voice in most instances. As was pointed out by Woodman and Pennington, the tracheostomy should be performed at least one week prior to lateralization to reduce the cough reflex and an endotracheal tube or bronchoscope should be placed through the larynx to provide stability for the dissection. We agree that patients who have undergone previous surgeries in unsuccessful attempts at lateralization, or those who have had prior laryngeal surgery or trauma, should be operated via laryngofissure approach.

The nerve muscle tranposition of Tucker, whereby a portion of respiratory muscle and its innervation is transposed to reinstitute abductor function of the larynx, is an effort to restore an adequate airway and maintain a high quality of voice. Tucker's results have been supported by both May (1980) and Applebaum (1979). The senior author has had experience with the technique and states that it is physiologically sound. However, in general, long-term follow-up has been disappointing and he currently reserves the operation for the exceptional case.

In treating vocal cord paralysis, it is always important to remember that decannulation and quality of voice are not a purely physical or mechanical phenomenon. No matter how earnest a patient appears, his sincere desire for improvement may be questioned. There are, at times, underlying social and/or emotional benefits gained from a handicap of which even the patient is unaware, or is unable to address. Occasionally this possibility must be considered, especially when the quality of voice or airway do not improve after excellent objective surgical results and intensive speech therapy.

CONCLUSION

Vocal cord paralysis is a complex problem affecting a patient's ability to communicate, breathe and eat. Obviously, this can have far-reaching effects on emotional well-being, social interaction and economic potentials. Only after the cause of paralysis and the potential for return of function have been assessed can a reasonable course of treatment be proposed. The options for surgical treatment are well established and usually represent some degree of compromise between adequate airway and voice. Until the development and perfection of some sort of laryngeal pacemaker, the previously mentioned procedures will remain the basis of therapy.

These two papers present excellent reviews and judgements regarding surgery for unilateral and bilateral vocal cord paralysis.

There are differences of opinions presented; the major difference being the assessment of vocal cord reinnervation. McKelvie indicates that reinnervation of the vocal cord is 'fanciful', while the Northwestern group states that 'an adequate airway with good quality voice may be created with this procedure'. They then go on to state that it is reserved for patients with 'extraordinary needs'.

At the same time as indicating that this procedure is successful, the Northwestern group indicates that laser arytenoidectomy is the procedure of choice. Finally, the authors admit that long-term follow-up for reinnervation has been disappointing and, therefore, is reserved for the exceptional case.

The reinnervation procedure as described by Tucker, electrophysiologically may demonstrate activity, but has been uniformly a functional failure when performed for bilateral vocal cord paralysis in humans. Therefore, until this procedure is modified and is demonstrated beyond any doubt that it will lateralize the vocal cord, the operation is not indicated and should not be performed.

The aetiology of unilateral vocal cord paralysis has been stressed by both authors. The typical historical investigation of a unilateral vocal cord paralysis can be abbreviated with the performance of a CT scan extending from base of skull to mediastinum. This procedure eliminates the necessity for base of skull and lateral neck films, oesophagram and thyroid scan. Similarly, routine laryngoscopy, bronchoscopy and oesophagoscopy is no longer indicated in the diagnostic evaluation of the patient with a unilateral vocal cord paralysis if an accurate CT scan is obtained. If the CT scan is inadequate, or if there is any question regarding interpretation, endoscopy is required.

The treatment of the unilateral vocal cord paralysis by Teflon injection or cartilage implant should be deferred for 12 months. The Northwestern group indicates 50% will show improvement within this time, although the authors do not indicate whether this improvement is with voice or return of motion of the paralysed cord. The majority of patients do not have recovery of motion, but do have improve-ment in voice. This improvement can be enhanced with speech therapy. Even though the majority of patients do not recover motion, recovery can occur up to 12 months, therefore permanent medialization of the paralysed vocal cord should not be performed until 12 months have elapsed from the onset.

In the interim, if the voice is poor, temporary improvement with a Gelfoam injection can be utilized. If, after 12 months, the voice is poor because of lack of cord apposition, Teflon can be injected. In those patients in whom for anatomical reasons, laryngoscopy and Teflon injection cannot be performed, the subperichondral insertion of a piece of cartilage between the paralysed cord and adjacent thyroid cartilage will medialize the vocal cord. Those patients who complain of inability to project the voice, or fatigue with speaking, but in whom glottic closure is present on examination, probably have insufficient force on closure. In these patients, a trial injection with Gelfoam to increase mass of the paralysed cord may alleviate the symptoms. If the symptoms are alleviated then Teflon may be utilized.

Contrary to McKelvie's opinion, it has not been documented that the final volume of Teflon is smaller than the original. If the Teflon is deposited submucosally or subglottically, migration may occur and then the original volume site would be less. McKelvie also indicates that Teflon injection is less effective in patients with loss of the recurrent and superior laryngeal nerves. Teflon in these patients has to be assessed carefully, but usually will have an excellent result in phonation. The amount of Teflon required is greater than with isolated recurrent laryngeal nerve paralysis. Occasionally, the aryepiglottic fold and anterior displacement of the arytenoid will prolapse into the lumen on inspiration, resulting in a decreased airway. Teflon is contraindicated in these cases until the prolapsed tissue has been removed.

Treatment for the 'totally palsied laryngopharynx' secondary to neurological disease, postneurosurgical, or base of skull resection, requires accurate assessment for successful rehabilitation. Reversibility of the disease is not necessary for treatment. Deglutition without aspiration and maintenance of phonation should be our aim. This cannot be obtained in all patients! At the time of presentation, these patients usually have a cuffed tracheostomy tube and a gastrostomy.

Patients with a bilateral paralysed palate may be helped by a palatroprosthesis. Patients with bilateral 12th nerve paralysis will not be able to swallow without total airway occlusion or diversion. Bilateral 19th nerve paralysis may require similar techniques. Patients with postsurgical cranial nerve loss, Parkinson's disease, neurological or neuromuscular disease can be best assessed with cine swallow. These patients frequently obtain benefit with Teflon injection and a myotomy of the cricopharyngeus muscle. Even if the 10th nerves are intact, myotomy of the cricopharyngeus may be helpful, since its relaxation phase either lacks co-ordination or fails to relax because of decreased pharyngeal pressure. If these ancillary procedures do not correct aspiration, then laryngeal protection is required. Diversion and obliterative procedures eliminate phonation. Partial supraglottic obstruction by approximating the aryepiglottic folds or epiglottopexy can preserve phonation if a 1 cm opening remains at the most superior aspect of the approximation. A cricopharyngeal myotomy should be performed in all cases. Even though these procedures require a pharyngotomy, the results are excellent in eliminating aspiration and maintaining voice. Peroral reversibility is maintained.

The authors described the various procedures for bilateral vocal cord paralysis. Although the Northwestern group is enthusiastic for laser arytenoidectomy, McKelvie correctly indicates that the result of laser arytenoidectomy 'remains to be assessed'. The reported success of 10 of 11 patients by the Northwestern group should not necessarily be considered a reason for advocating this procedure! The report indicates a follow-up period of 6 months to 3 years, but the authors do not indicate how many patients were followed for less than 1 year. Assessment of arytenoidectomy, either by the transoral route, extralaryngeal or by thyrotomy, demonstrate that there are a considerable number of patients in whom early success is followed by late failure. Examination of these patients indicate that the airway obstruction is secondary to medialization of the previously lateralized vocal cord. Early failures can be secondary to subglottic or interarytenoid scar tissue, as was present in the one failure reported by the Northwestern group. The late failures who do not have intralaryngeal scar tissue must be explained by either interarytenoid or lateral cricoarytenoid muscle shortening. If this is the circumstance, then one would anticipate that the majority of early successful laser arytenoidectomies would return ultimately as failures. The Northwestern experience, therefore, will have to be reviewed after a 5-year follow-up.

Submucosal laser cordectomy has an advantage in that the arytenoid is undisturbed and, therefore, if sufficient bulk of vocalis muscle is removed, an airway would be obtained. The other major detraction of endoscopic procedures is the unpredictability of the degree of cord lateralization and, therefore, the unpredictability of the resultant voice.

The early widespread acceptance of endoscopic laser procedures is related to the ease of performance. Although the endoscopic procedures have enthusiastic proponents, caution in widespread adoption is indicated.

The standard by which lateralization procedures are measured is the extralaryngeal procedure described by Woodman. This should be reserved for bilateral vocal cord paralysis secondary to nerve injury. Patients with arytenoid fixation or intralaryngeal abnormalities should not be treated by an extralaryngeal approach.

The major advantage of the Woodman procedure is the ability to determine accurately the amount of vocal cord abduction. This is assessed by direct laryngoscopy before the procedure is terminated. The degree of lateralization, therefore, can be assessed and determined in millimetres. This procedure is technically difficult and, therefore, is readily replaced by easier endoscopic or thyrotomy procedures. Late failures are avoided by: 1. avoiding interarytenoid mucosal perforation, 2. performing an extraperichondrial resection of the arytenoid, 3. sectioning the muscular insertions attached to the arytenoid.

The voice is preserved by lateralization of the vocal cord 3 mm and tying the suture to the inferior thyroid cornu, thereby lowering the level of the posterior aspect of the lateralized cord.

Arytenoidectomy performed through a thyrotomy is indicated whenever there is a possibility of pre-existing intralaryngeal abnormality or arytenoid joint fixation. Since the vocal cord is lateralized through a thyrotomy, the degree of lateralization cannot be accurately assessed. As a result, the lateralization is usually maximal, and therefore the resultant voice is poor when compared to the extra-laryngeal approach.

Bilateral arytenoidectomy should not be performed by any method because of the increased possibility of aspiration!!

REFERENCES

H J Pelzer Jr, G A Sisson

Applebaum E L, Allen G W, Sisson G A 1979 Human laryngeal reinnervation: the Northwestern experience. Laryngoscope 89:1784–1787

Baker C H 1916 Report of a cases of abductor paralysis with removal of one vocal cord. Journal of the Michigan Medical Society 15: 485

Blau J W et al 1969 Idiopathic palsy of the recurrent laryngeal nerve: a transient cranial mononeuropathy. British Medical Journal 4: 259–260

Hoover W B 1932 Bilateral abductor paralysis: operative treatment by submucous resection of the vocal cords. Archives of Otolaryngology 15: 339–355

Jackson C 1922 Ventriculocordectomy: a new operation for the cure of goitrous paralytic laryngeal stenosis. Archives of Surgery 4: 257–274

Kelly J D 1941 Surgical treatment of bilateral paralysis of the abductor muscles. Archives of Otolaryngology 33: 293

King B T 1939 A new and function-restoring operation for bilateral abductor cord paralysis. Transactions of the American Laryngology Association 61: 264

Lahey F H 1928 Suture of the recurrent laryngeal nerve for bilateral abductory paralysis. Annals of Surgery 87: 481

Lore J M 1936 A suggested operative procedure for the relief of stenosis in double abductor paralysis: an anatomic study. Annals of Otology, Rhinology and Laryngology 45: 679–686

May M, Lavorato A S, Bleyaert A L 1980 Rehabilitation of the crippled larynx: application of the Tucker technique for muscle-nerve reinnervation. Laryngoscope 90: 1–18

Ossoff R H, Sisson G A et al 1984 Endoscopic laser arytenoidectomy for the treatment of bilateral vocal cord paralysis. Laryngoscope 94: 1293–1297

Schramm V L, May M, Lavorato A S 1978 Gelfoam paste injection for vocal cord paralysis: temporary rehabilitation of glottic incompetence. Laryngoscope 88: 1268–1273

Thornell W C 1948 Intralaryngeal approach for arytenoidectomy in bilateral abductor vocal cord paralysis. Archives of Otolaryngology 47: 505–508

Tucker H M 1976 Human laryngeal reinnervation. Laryngoscope 86: 769–779

Tucker H M 1978 Human laryngeal reinnervation: long-term experience with the nerve-muscle pedicle technique. Laryngoscope 88: 598–604

Tucker H M 1980 Vocal cord paralysis—1979: etiology and management. Laryngoscope 90: 585–590

Woodman D 1946 A modification of the extralaryngeal approach to arytenoidectomy for bilateral abductor paralysis. Archives of Otolaryngology 43: 63–65

16

The T3 glottic cancer—diagnosis and management?

B.W. Pearson

Management decisions in the treatment of advanced (T3 and T4) laryngeal cancer are seemingly made in an atmosphere of conflict. In the 1970s the conflict was between radiation and surgery, and perhaps the notion of conflict was valid. Radiation was advocated by some to spare the voice, but it now appears to have cost more in terms of life (Desanto 1984). Surgery, a total laryngectomy, was usually offered to save life, but it probably cost too many voices (Stewart 1975). Innovators on each side developed sophisticated strategies to deal with the shortcomings of each approach; salvage surgery protocols after primary radiation (Harwood et al 1980) and fistula speech operations after total laryngectomy (Asai 1972). But the basic ingredient of both programmes remained the same, primary or salvage surgery by total laryngectomy.

Little has been made of the fact that the historical basis for total laryngectomy was not oncological. The acceptance of total excision of the organ of voice for cord-fixing laryngeal cancer derived from the observation that the crippled laryngeal remnant that remained after partial excision of this organ led to aspiration and pneumonia. Total laryngectomy was, in fact, a wide ablative procedure, which was excused of its mutilating disadvantages by its efficacy in separating the airway from the foodway. This protected the vulnerable pulmonary system of patients with a high burden of chronic obstructive pulmonary disease, which was probably related to the tobacco abuse that led to their cancer in the first place.

In recent years our own efforts have centered around a reconciliation of this conflict, by attempting to combine the curative potential of surgery with the voice preservation of successful radiation. The detailed studies of advanced laryngeal cancer undertaken in whole-organ serial section laboratories around the world (Kirchner 1969, Tucker 1974, Pearson 1975, Norris et al 1980) have given us a tentative foundation on which to build new treatment strategies. If the vocal cord is fixed by cancer, the muscle is invaded and the paraglottic space is at risk. So is the cartilage framework (Olofsson et al 1973, Kirchner & Som 1971).

We know from numerous clinical reports that T3 (cord fixing) glottic cancer is highly curable (Desanto 1984, Harwood 1980, Ogura et al 1975). This is not surprising for the total volume is small, the diagnosis is often made early, prior to metastasis, and a highly developed expertise exists for treatment.

DIAGNOSIS

The problem is not the histopathological recognition of squamous cell cancer so much as the determination of the extent of the disease. Sophisticated training in clinical laryngology, microlaryngoscopy and biopsy, and the development of better laryngoscopes and anaesthesia, has greatly reduced the likelihood of missed diagnosis which plagued this field in the past (McInnes et al 1976). The parameters which define the entity of 'recurrent glottic cancer after radiation' are better understood now, also, and the appropriateness of a deep biopsy in the face of persistent postradiation oedema is widely recognized.

In recent years, improved imaging techniques have been applied to laryngeal cancer. It was hoped that computerized tomography would improve our ability to recognize paraglottic involvement and cartilage invasion especially. CT scans (Manusco et al 1978) do occasionally document these findings well, but they tend to fall down in the equivocal case, where the clinician is most in need of help. Unfortunately, the CT scanner is unable to define precisely the axial transition from the true to the false cords. When bulky tumours displace the true and false cords, they make it appear as if the displaced tissue is infiltrated with tumour when it is not. Of course, superficial mucosal abnormalities are not seen; motion cannot be evaluated; the pyriforms are rather unclear on a CT scan; even the status of the laryngeal cartilage is in doubt. A good scan can diagnose the presence of cartilage invasion, but its absence can never be proven or assumed.

The older radiological studies still have a place in the determination of extent (Jing 1978). Frontal tomography can silhouette laterally situated subglottic extensions, but when the ventricle is obliterated the superior extent is indeterminate. Contrast laryngography can reveal the extent of an anterior subglottic component and it is probably the best radiological study for mobility (detected during formal inspiration and phonation manoeuvres). Once again, however, the extent of surface disease is unclear. All in all, it is doubtful that we can learn much more from roentgenograms and scans than can be appreciated from careful clinical evaluation, supplemented by fibreoptic nasopharyngolaryngoscopy.

MANAGEMENT DECISIONS

Management decisions in the treatment of 'advanced' (by which I mean T3 and T4) glottic cancer continue to be debated as if there is a fundamental dichotomy between the goal of cure and the hope of voice (McNeil et al 1981). In the discussion of treatment, I will try and show that:

1. The cure-versus-voice concept is flawed. For advanced glottic cancer, a promising strategy for voice is not necessarily a poor strategy for cure, and vice versa.

2. Once beyond T1 and T2 lesions, we overemphasize the importance of site when we discuss treatment. The extent of a tumour should be our primary consideration. The specific features that characterize a cord-fixing cancer of glottic origin versus one of supraglottic, transglottic, or even pyriform origin are minimal (Pearson 1981). Making the site of origin, rather than extent, the principle basis for classification, we tend to obscure the

common principles that might well guide the treatment of any of these lesions. Each of them replaces the glottic musculature, extends upwards from the subglottic to the supraglottic level, probably involves the paraglottic space and must be considered to involve cartilage since, in the individual case, it is virtually impossible to prove otherwise.

3. Neither radiotherapy backed up by salvage surgery, nor total laryngectomy backed up by vocal fistula surgery are rational treatments for cord-fixing cancers. When radiation is given as initial treatment in advanced laryngeal cancer, too many lives and larynges are ultimately lost (Desanto 1984). When total laryngectomy is employed initially, the excision is inappropriately extended to encompass the organ rather than the cancer (Pearson et al 1980). The obvious cost, in terms of voice, is not balanced in terms of cure by a proven gain over slightly less extensive operations.

Conservation surgery in cancers grouped T1 or T2

Conventional 'conservation' operations refer to vertical hemilaryngectomy and its modifications and, of course, supraglottic laryngectomy and its extensions. In the majority of T3 cases, it is generally recognized that conventional conservation operations will fail. It is also admitted that total laryngectomy will work (produce local cure) and radical radiation with surgical salvage will keep a few larynges that would otherwise be lost.

When cancers of similar volume to T3 glottic lesions (but confined to the next site up) are present, supraglottic laryngectomy has frequently been employed. The regional problem in supraglottic disease, i.e. metastatic spread of cancer to the cervical lymph nodes, should not obscure the important observations about the local disease. Supraglottic laryngectomy is an operation which rarely fails locally (Coates et al 1976)!

In early glottic disease, a high local control rate is achieved as well. Cordectomy almost always cures properly selected T1 cases (Neel et al 1980). These observations appear to suggest that close margins are tolerable in the larynx. The clinical evaluation of the tumour's extent must be sound and intraoperative frozen section histopathology must be readily available, but when these criteria are met conservation surgery and close margins (by comparison with the margins required in other mucosal sites) do produce excellent local control.

In T3 glottic cancers, as noted above, the oncological grounds for total extirpation of the larynx are questionable. In laryngeal cancer of all sites, when all of the cancer is removed surgically, the local control rate is around 80–85%. The Mayo Clinic experience of glottic cancer certainly shows that the cure rate of surgery alone exceeds the cure rate of either radiation alone or radiation and salvage surgery in T3 disease by a clear margin (Desanto 1984).

Less well documented, but probably also true, is the fact that a single curative operation followed by an aggressive rehabilitation programme is usually able to produce a satisfactory voice, whereas a lengthy radiotherapy programme followed by failure and salvage surgery, and perhaps wound complications or extensive reconstruction, reduces the likelihood that a patient will succeed in establishing oesophageal voice (Skolnik et al 1975). The weeks and months of practice, instruction, and enthusiasm necessary to reach this goal are harder to come by after a complex, multimodality treatment experience.

Vocal rehabilitation operations

A good deal of information has accumulated in recent years on the various vocal rehabilitation operations after total laryngectomy (Miller 1976, Leipzig 1980). All a patient requires in order to speak is a fistulous connection between the airway and the foodway. Unfortunately, after a total laryngectomy, a speaking shunt must be crossed by a reconstructive suture line. Inevitably, there is a percentage of patients whose shunt will stenose. Worse, if it remains adequately patent for voice, but adynamic during swallow, the patient will usually aspirate. One solution to the problems of stenosis and aspiration is Blom and Singer's one-way prosthetic valve (Leipzig 1980) (a host of other valves are also available— Panje 1981). However, connecting the foodway to the airway with a plastic tube introduces two new problems.

The first is the dual burden assumed by the patient of maintaining both a mechanical prosthesis and an unstable tracheo-oesophageal fistula. The second relates to the physiology of the speech itself. When air is introduced into the oesophagus instead of the pharynx, reflex spasm of the pharyngo-oesophageal segment impedes its upwards release into the mouth (Blom et al 1985). These problems are not without their attempted solutions. However, these involve further procedures and an incidence of failure. Wouldn't it be better if prostheses and their problems could be avoided wherever possible? The fact is, they usually can be, if the concept of near-total laryngectomy is properly applied (Pearson et al 1980).

The trouble with near-total laryngectomy is that if a laryngologist hasn't done one he may not really know what it is and, conversely, to know what it is, he often has to do one. Surgeons who are able to do this procedure may decline, because they know the cost of failure in cancer is death. This knowledge cautions any prudent surgeon from embarking on a new procedure without strong evidence of efficacy.

When the technique of near-total laryngectomy is clear, its appropriateness for a particular case is also clear. The indications and limitations are obvious when the technique is adequately described. If a surgeon knows what is to be excised, he knows exactly what can be cured. If he knows what must necessarily be left behind, he knows when a lesion should not be subjected to near-total laryngectomy.

The indications for near-total laryngectomy

A fixed cord is the basic indication for a near-total laryngectomy (Pearson 1981). In not only T3 glottic cancers, but in transglottic, T3 and T4 supraglottic and even pyriform cancers, a great deal of the larynx, namely the paraglottic space and its surrounding tissues, will have to be removed. The lymphatics in the paraglottic space communicate to the neck nodes; the neck is clearly at risk and ought to be treated too.

When one side of the larynx is infiltrated with cancer, fixed at the glottic level and clearly beyond cure with so-called 'conventional' partial operations (vertical/partial laryngectomy, supraglottic laryngectomy, or partial laryngopharyngectomy), a near-total laryngectomy will usually encompass the cancer. When it cannot (extensive posterior and/or bilateral disease reaching both arytenoids), the contraindications will be apparent. In the uncommon case of uncertainty, intraoperative frozen sections will tell.

Vocal cord fixation by cancer is the indication for near-total laryngectomy—the site of origin is only important in suggesting slight variations. A mobile cancer-free posterior glottis and contralateral arytenoid is an essential condition for this operation to be applicable. Fortunately, this condition is usually satisfied in T3 and T4 laryngeal carcinoma.

T3 glottic tumours and beyond

It is impossible to discuss T3 glottic carcinoma, recommend near-total laryngectomy for the majority and not digress beyond the rather artificial focus on the glottic site.

Typical tumour candidates for near-total laryngectomy are: 1. transglottic cancers which fix the hemilarynx but leave the opposite cord mobile, 2. supraglottic cancers too big for a conventional supraglottic laryngectomy, and 3. the rare exophytic unilateral subglottic cancer that has spread upwards to fix one vocal cord, sparing the opposite subglottis.

Certain paralaryngeal cancers, originating in the hypopharynx or the base of the tongue, are also candidates for near-total laryngectomy. These include: 1. pyriform carcinomas without postcricoid involvement, 2. vallecular carcinomas that require extensive loss of the supraglottic larynx and the base of the tongue, and 3. combinations of this type of involvement. In cases in which hypopharyngeal cancer extends to the tongue or oropharynx, it is assumed the patient will not be able to sustain an extended supraglottic laryngectomy, or a partial laryngopharyngectomy with its attendant requirements for pulmonary function and its difficulties relating to aspiration and dysphagia.

Where does near-total laryngectomy fit in the spectrum of treatment for T3 glottic carcinoma?

Near-total laryngectomy offers the cure rate of total laryngectomy without the loss of voice (Pearson et al 1980). It appears to offer a better cure rate than radiotherapy, without the high prospect of re-treatment and the loss of voice, through the loss of any meaningful conservation surgery option after radiation has failed.

Total laryngectomy and, of course, radiotherapy are still widely performed. Both have a very broad distribution network. The availability of near-total

laryngectomy on the other hand is limited to centres where the operating team has studied the surgical anatomy and carefully anticipated the intraoperative judgements that may be required. A physician who clearly understands the sequence of surgery and a surgical pathologist who produces reliable intraoperative histopathological frozen sections are essential.

The introduction of near-total laryngectomy into the spectrum of treatment for T3 laryngeal carcinoma offers additional advantages besides voice preservation and a high cure rate.

1. All other adjuncts to the best management of the case at hand can still be applied, such as neck dissections, flap reconstructions of the pharynx, postoperative radiotherapy, etc.

2. Surgical brinksmanship, the ill-advised surrender to the temptation to extend a hemilaryngectomy or a supraglottic laryngectomy just beyond its bounds, is no longer encouraged. The major problems of dysphagia, aspiration, fistualization, or incomplete tumour removal that follow extended conservation procedures can be eliminated from the surgeon's experience.

3. The patient's need to learn the care and maintenance of an unstable tracheo-oesophageal fistula and its prosthetic obturator and valve is obviated.

4. Oesophageal voice, which offers only about 90 ml of breath support for speech as opposed to the 450 ml the lungs provide, is not required.

What is a near-total laryngectomy?

We define near-total laryngectomy as the resection of the entire larynx except for a narrow strip that connects the airway and the pharynx over an uninvolved arytenoid. This strip contains the mucosal, muscular and neural elements necessary for the creation of a reliable speaking shunt. It will not permit breathing, but it prevents aspiration. When a near-total laryngeal resection is performed, voice is rehabilitated by closing the laryngopharyngeal tissue that remains into a simple tube. The object is to use a strip of tissue still connecting the trachea to the normal pyriform over an uninvolved arytenoid to create a composite tracheopharyngeal fistula sphinctered by residual laryngeal elements. There is little justification for discarding readily identified normal laryngeal tissue when T3 glottic cancer so rarely involves the entire larynx. This is even more particularly the case when the normal tissue discarded is the sine qua non for a reliable speaking tracheopharyngeal shunt. It is true that the uninvolved laryngeal tissue is small, but the size of a body component is little guide to its significance.

The word 'composite', in reference to the tracheopharyngeal shunt associated with near-total laryngectomy, indicates the shunt is derived from two sources. One is the laryngeal remnant which provides the mucosal continuity, the muscles for sphincter action and the solitary recurrent laryngeal nerve innervation required to drive the antiaspiration sphincter. The second is a small upper hypopharyngeal flap, which is rotated down into the defect to add mucosa to the laryngeal strip. This permits an adequate shunt diameter despite the extent of resection of the larynx, an extent which is after all dictated by the cancer and an extent which must pay little attention to the reconstructive requirements.

In the cancers of laryngeal origin, the hypopharyngeal flap is used to bring the shunt diameter up to 0.5 cm. It augments the laryngeal remnant. In the case of cancers of pyriform origin, there is no pharynx available to make such a flap after an adequate excision. On the other hand, more larynx remains (about half) after excision in pyriform cases. Thus, fortunately, there is little need to augment the shunt with additional tissue. Enough larynx remains to make a satisfactory speaking shunt with the laryngeal remnant alone. A near-total laryngectomy avoids the major drawback of total laryngectomy—loss of the voice—but it does not avoid the necessity for a tracheal stoma for breathing. Experience shows that patients who are cured of their cancer, but assured of their powers of communication, adjust to the management of a tracheal stoma relatively well.

A composite shunt is rendered dynamic by its residual laryngeal musculature. This is innervated by the 'good side' recurrent laryngeal nerve. This structure from the side opposite the site of cancer involvement would otherwise have been discarded in a total laryngectomy. Without this innervation, a tracheopharyngeal fistula patient will aspirate. This is perhaps why the lengthy record of disappointment with post-total laryngectomy fistula reconstructions does not seem to extend to patients who have undergone near-total laryngectomies.

Safety

The safety of total laryngectomy is well-known, especially when it is carried out in the unirradiated patient. Near-total laryngectomy is probably just as safe, but it does imply a slight increase in operating time and a slightly more troublesome postoperative stoma than the end-on tracheal stoma that follows a total laryngectomy. Radiation and salvage surgery perhaps provides the least safety. The incidence of salvage surgery after radiation is high in T3 and T4 cases.

Near-total laryngectomy is only safe when the extent of the tumour is clinically discernible. Atypical patterns of spread and ill-defined margins are so characteristic of radiation failure that we have avoided using this operation in cases initially treated with radiation at the T3 stage. On the other hand, near-total laryngectomy has been successfully used to salvage cases which were initially T1 failed radiation and then recurred as T3 cases.

Technical factors

There has been little change in the technique of total laryngectomy or radiation for T3 glottic cancer in the last 10 years and it is assumed these treatment modalities have plateaued.

In the performance of near-total laryngectomy, the operative sequence is planned to maintain the tumour under direct vision at all times. The larynx is entered initially through the laryngeal ventricle on the uninvolved side. This ventricle is a reliable landmark. It can be inspected for the absence of cancer at the direct laryngoscopy. Its destruction does not damage the proposed shunt. It provides a safe entry point suitable for every case in which a near-total laryngectomy is indicated.

With the tumour under direct vision, the excision can centre on the cancer rather than the entire larynx. A near-total laryngectomy specimen consists of the entire hemilarynx, trachea to tongue, along with most of the front of the larynx and all of the paralaryngeal tissue as well. The entire paraglottic space and the pre-epiglottic space are included. So is the arytenoid on the involved side and the subglottis and cricoid on the involved side as far down into the trachea as the tumour requires.

A small portion of the larynx that would have been

discarded in a total laryngectomy is preserved to maintain union between the airway and the foodway. This tissue is a better bridge between these two systems than the one provided by a plastic valve. Once this vital mucosal link has been discarded, as it is in a total laryngectomy, the pathway back to a serviceable voice becomes difficult and uncertain. Most patients without this mucosal bridge are forced to rely on oesophageal mechanisms powered by air gulped into the mouth, or admitted from the lungs through the artificial tracheopharyngeal prosthesis.

As long as one pyriform fossa is salvageable into which the upper end of the laryngeal shunt can continue, a composite shunt can be created. Thus, the patient can tolerate extensive loss of the pharynx. Near-total laryngectomy has been used successfully in patients undergoing pharyngeal reconstruction with a pectoral myocutaneous flap, a Bakamjian flap, or a free jejunal transplant.

Total laryngectomy for T3 glottic cancer

Total laryngectomy is still viable. Near-total laryngectomy does not compete with total laryngectomy or total laryngopharyngectomy when cancer invades the posterior larynx or involves both arytenoids. This is also true when cancers permeate both sides of the larynx from the anterior commissure and epiglottis, or invade the interarytenoid region and posterior larynx from the pharynx. In these cases, total extirpation of the larynx is an oncological necessity, so near-total laryngectomy is not an option. The conventional techniques of vocal rehabilitation, such as oesophageal speech and tracheo-oesophageal puncture and prosthesis, also retain their place. Again we emphasize that near-total laryngectomy simply seeks to avoid discarding functional components of the larynx that we have repeatedly shown are reliable for rehabilitation of the voice when their sacrifice is not oncologically required.

The reacquisition of voice

Reacquisition of a voice after total laryngectomy is quite variable. Widely differing estimates on the successful acquisition of oesophageal speech have been published (Horn 1962, King et al 1968). The same is true of puncture and prosthesis techniques, such as Singer & Blom's (McNeil et al 1981) or Panje's (Panje 1981). Purely surgical voice rehabilitation techniques like those introduced by Staffieri, have been so widely plagued with aspiration or stenosis that their superiority over oesophageal speech or puncture and prosthesis techniques has never been solidly established (Leipzig 1980).

Voice quality after near-total laryngectomy is not acoustically superior to that observed after total laryngectomy and the acquisition of good oesophageal speech. However, if the criterion is predictability of acquisition, near-total laryngectomy, which seems to produce voice in virtually every case, is clearly superior. If speech is not acquired after near-total laryngectomy, it can usually be produced later by the application of several trivial postoperative manoeuvres (dilatation, for example).

Speech after near-total laryngectomy does not require a prosthesis and it avoids inflating the oesophagus. The innervated laryngeal musculature underlying the mucosa of a composite shunt after near-total laryngectomy must be relaxed by the patient. The value of the muscle lies in its contractile role during swallowing. The problem of aspiration, which has traditionally plagued biological vocal rehabilitation operations, is overcome by this automatic intrinsic sphincter-like activity during deglutition.

For a few near-total laryngectomy patients, the acquisition of shunt speech is no more complicated than learning to occlude the stoma when they wish to talk. However, for the majority of cases, communication rehabilitation is greatly enhanced by professional counselling. Prior to surgery, the speech pathologist can learn much of importance about the patient's personality, his needs. and his anxieties before the voice is temporarily lost. Later, by providing a mechanical instrument in the immediate postoperative period, the speech pathologist bridges the communication gap until the stoma is healed. This must occur before the patient can valve. Once it does, the speech pathologist proves invaluable again in helping the patient achieve good finger placement, the best stomal tube, optimal articulation, a proper speaking rate and appropriate phonation.

ONE VIEW OF THE FUTURE IN THE TREATMENT OF T3 AND T4 GLOTTIC CARCINOMA

Of every 10 patients presenting at the Mayo Clinic with an initial diagnosis of laryngeal carcinoma, 7 have a lesion small enough to be treated with conventional conservation techniques. These are T1 and T2 cancers amenable to cordectomy, supraglottic laryngectomy, radiation therapy, hemilaryngectomy, or some therapeutic strategy that does not threaten the voice or require a permanent stoma.

The other 3 out of 10 have extensive cancers. In former times we would have applied a total laryngectomy with, or without, a partial or total pharyngectomy. When any of these patients underwent radiation, surgery was usually still required. Vocal rehabilitation after total laryngectomy may be of excellent quality in a motivated patient. These patients are usually also the best cases for tracheo-oesophageal puncture.

But there were always laryngectomy patients where the motivation or physiology was lacking and satisfactory communication was never achieved. Near-total laryngectomy has essentially eliminated this problem. It has enabled us to steer clear of the overextended conventional conservation operations with their poor swallowing and fear of inadequacy. It has eliminated the intraoperative conversion of a supraglottic laryngectomy to a total laryngectomy.

We have had to rethink our classifications, re-examine our basic strategies in the larger laryngeal cancers and pay closer attention to the intricacies of laryngeal anatomy and physiology in each individual case. However, modern laryngologists are well-trained in the anatomy of physiology of the larynx and the patterns of spread of laryngeal cancer. Our literature is replete with histopathological reports documenting behaviour of this disease and contrasting its predictability in the pristine state to its unpredictability in the postirradiated state. As we see no promising chemotherapy on the horizon for laryngeal squamous cell carcinoma and we have perhaps reached the patients' limits of tolerance of radiotherapy for this disease, it seems reasonable to encourage young laryngologists to apply their hard-won anatomical and pathological knowledge of its true extent. If we accept the slight increase in the complexity of our surgical techniques for the treatment of laryngeal cancer, in the name of preservation of life, the avoidance of unnecessary irradiation of normal tissues and the predictable rehabilitation of voice, we will have met the challenge and promise of treating advanced glottic carcinoma in the 1980s and 1990s.

INTRODUCTION

A dilemma is the choice between two alternatives, both of which are unfavourable. The treatment of glottic T3 carcinoma is thus not a true dilemma, rather it poses several unanswered questions, beginning with the definition of what is meant by a T3 glottic carcinoma. Thereafter, the main controversial point is whether patients with such a tumour (squamous carcinoma alone will be considered), with no palpable lymph node metastases, should be treated by radical surgery or by irradiation: it can safely be assumed that the treatment of such a carcinoma with cervical lymph node metastases is surgical. Other controversial areas include the place of emergency laryngectomy for patients who present with stridor, the value of prophylactic neck dissection for patients with no palpable lymph node metastases, the role of adjuvant chemotherapy plus radiotherapy and, finally, the possible advantages of fast neutrons compared to conventional radiotherapy.

Before reasonable conclusions can be drawn, we must first define what we are discussing.

DEFINITIONS

The glottis

The glottis is defined by both the American Joint Committee on Cancer (AJCC) and The International Union Against Cancer (IUCC) systems as the true vocal cords and the anterior and posterior commissures. The IUCC does not define any of the three structures or the extent of the vocal cord, nor does the AJCC, except to say that the lower boundary of the vocal cord is the 'horizontal plane' 1 cm below the apex of the ventricle.

Anatomists define the vocal cord as being that part of the larynx in which the mucous membrane is very thin and firmly adherent to the subjacent ligament, which is the part normally covered by squamous epithelium and bounded above and below by the superior and inferior arcuate lines. Other definitions have been suggested and used by some: Ogura (1963) says that the glottis includes that part of the undersurface of the vocal cord extending for a distance of 1 cm below the free edge of the cord,

whereas Kirschner (1971) states that the glottis extends down to the superior surface of the cricoid cartilage. The latter two definitions in particular include a fairly large part of the subglottic space with its relatively rich lymphatic drainage. This variation in definition can produce enormous variation in results.

A further minor criticism is that the mucosa covering the vocal processes of the arytenoid cartilage, which constitutes almost half of the glottis, is not included in the definition of either the IUCC or the AJCC. Thus, tumours arising from this part of the glottis, although uncommon, cannot be classified.

T3 glottic tumour

A T3 glottic tumour is defined by both the AJCC (1983) and IUCC (1978) as being a tumour confined to the larynx with 'cord fixation'. A major criticism of both systems is that this term covers at least two and, quite possibly, three distinct entities:

1. A tumour confined to one vocal cord which is fixed.

2. The so-called transglottic or multiregional carcinoma that crosses the vocal cord to invade the supra- and subglottic compartments. The origin of such a tumour is in dispute, but it is unlikely that such a tumour is simply a glottic carcinoma which has spread upwards and downwards. Indeed it may represent two distinct entities:

a. A tumour of all laryngeal compartments due to simultaneous widespread field change.

b. A tumour arising in the ventricle and spreading medially onto both true and false cords. Such a tumour is seldom described or discussed, indeed van Nostrand (1974) says that he has never seen such a tumour. However, there seems to be no reason why tumours should not arise from this part of the larynx, and 20% of laryngeal carcinomas were thought to be ventricular in a series from the Gustav Roussy Institute in Paris (Micheau 1976). They found that such tumours spread up and down to invade both the false and true cords with obliteration of the ventricle, a fairly common clinical finding. About half these tumours invade the base of the epiglottis, and about one-quarter cross the glottis. Most invade the paraglottic space and then spread further to destroy the conus elasticus and the thyroid cartilage.

Clearly a useful modification of the TNM system would be the creation of a separate category for transglottic tumours.

Thus the term glottis means different things to different people, and the term T3 glottic tumour is used to describe at least two distinct entities. Furthermore, we must consider inconsistencies in assigning a T stage to any particular tumour.

All classification systems are subject to error, and the classification of the T3 glottic tumour is the most prone of all head and neck sites to such error. The cause is the difficulty in detecting invasion of the thyroid cartilage, found in 20% of patients with a tumour confined to the cord, and in 50% of trans-glottic tumours, an event which changes the classification to T4. Kirschner (1984) found a 40% error rate in prediction of cartilaginous invasion before operation. It might be thought that a CT scan would resolve this problem but sadly this is not so. A series in which a preoperative CT scan was compared with pathological findings showed a high proportion of false positives, i.e. the CT scan showed convincing evidence of cartilaginous invasion which would demand radical surgery, but this finding was not borne out by subsequent pathological findings (Hoover et al 1984).

RADIOTHERAPY

The Toronto school have been the main proponents of primary radiotherapy for glottic T3 carcinoma. Bryce (1972) showed that the 5-year survival is similar, at about 55% for the three main forms of treatment: total laryngectomy, total laryngectomy plus preoperative radiotherapy, and radical radiotherapy with salvage surgery for failure. The great advantage of the third policy is that about half the patients retain a functioning larynx. One criticism of a more recent report from the same school (Harwood 1980) is that the authors do not define the type of tumour they are treating; furthermore it is impossible to discern how they treated patients who presented with stridor. They must have been confronted with such patients if they were dealing with multiregional tumours, which presumably they were because 30% of their patients were women. This is a similar sex incidence to our multiregional tumours, whereas over 90% of patients with purely glottic carcinoma are men (Stell et al 1982).

If patients treated by radiotherapy are broken up into two groups, regional tumours and tumours confined to the cord, it is found that the results do differ: tumours confined to the true cord have an 80% actuarial survival rate at 5 years, and about 65% of them retain their larynx (Stell et al 1982). The figure for survival of 50%, with 50% of patients retaining their larynx, appears to be most applicable to the multiregional group.

One of the main complications of treatment of glottic T3 carcinoma by radiation is the resultant oedema and its assessment. An oedematous larynx may harbour recurrence, but unfortunately a laryngoscopy and biopsy can often precipitate cartilaginous necrosis, which has its own special symptoms and complications, yet the patient has no recurrence of his tumour. In one series (Fu et al 1982) 20% of patients undergoing radiotherapy for T3 glottic carcinoma developed oedema persisting for more than three months. In about half of these patients, the laryngeal oedema was associated with persistent or recurrent disease. The incidence of oedema increased significantly with increase of minimum tumour dose above 70 Gy, being 46.2% with a minimum tumour dose above 70 Gy and 13.7% with minimum tumour dose below 70 Gy. When laryngeal oedema is progressive and unresponsive to conservative measures the authors felt that multiple biopsies should be performed to establish the presence of persistent or recurrent disease before salvage surgery is attempted. However, if it is mild, stable, with no visible sign of recurrence, and especially if it is limited to the arytenoids, biopsy should not be attempted because of the risk of inducing cartilaginous necrosis. They do not say what to do when biopsies were negative and where there was a clear clinical suspicion of recurrence. It is recommended by many authorities, e.g. Ward et al (1975), that a total laryngectomy should be carried out if oedema persists or progresses after six months. At least a third of these larynges will be found not to contain tumour.

Further progression of this leads to necrosis of the larynx. Necrosis can affect as many as 7% of patients with T3 tumours subjected to radiotherapy

(Hunter & Palmer 1980), but this event can almost always be managed successfully, whereas recurrence is often fatal. The recurrence rate is significantly higher in men than in women, and in young men compared with older men (Harwood et al 1981). The dose in young men should be higher to reduce the risk of recurrence, despite the risk of necrosis.

Finally, fast neutrons are mentioned only to be dismissed. Good results reported initially by a few enthusiasts have not been substantiated by controlled trials. Indeed a large European multicentre study has shown that the cure rate for laryngeal cancer treated by neutrons is significantly lower than that achieved by conventional radiotherapy (Duncan et al 1984).

SURGERY

The primary tumour

Few reports of the results of surgery alone can be found in the literature, yet it is almost certainly the commonest form of treatment for these tumours. Some (Kazem 1984, Woodhouse 1981) claim high cure rates—up to 80%—but it is impossible to compare different series for two reasons: firstly, patients in many series received preoperative radiotherapy; secondly, no attempt is made to distinguish true cord tumours from multiregional tumours.

The rate quoted by most authors is around 55%—including the present authors with 54%. DeSanto, however, claimed a 5-year actuarial survival of 91%, from which it would appear that T staging of glottic cancer is irrelevant if advanced tumours do as well as early ones! Based on this survival, he claims that surgery is the treatment of choice and that the compromise of radiotherapy followed by salvage surgery, although it might preserve the voice in a lot of patients, does so at the cost of the 25% of patients who needlessly lose their life. Not for the first time one is left wondering why the same treatment on the same type of patient produces results two or even three times better in North America than those achieved in Europe!

In the past, the only surgical option was total laryngectomy. More recently the classical hemilaryngectomy and the newer near-total techniques have been used (Pearson 1981).

Evidence is accumulating that vertical hemilaryngectomy is safe for highly selected glottic T3 carcinomas with a good cure rate, as described by Shumrick and his colleagues (Mohr et al 1981). They describe a series of 57 patients with glottic carcinoma who underwent vertical hemilaryngectomy: only 5 had a T3 lesion but they all survived 5 years with a voice. The great advantage of this paper is that it is one of the very few which describes exactly what the authors were treating and how. They restricted vertical hemilaryngectomy to glottic lesions which could have impaired cord mobility, or fixation due to the bulk of the tumour, or invasion of the vocalis muscle, and which could have recurred after irradiation. The anatomical limits were:

1. Extension to not more than one-third of the opposite cord
2. Extension to the ventricle
3. Not more than 5 mm of subglottic extension posteriorly
4. Not more than 10 mm subglottic extension anteriorly
5. Excision of the entire hemithyroid to 1 cm beyond the midline and up but not more than one-half of the ipsilateral cricoid cartilage

One great advantage of vertical hemilaryngectomy is that it can be performed on patients who have failed radiotherapy with minimal complications and a good salvage rate (Sorensen 1980, Biller 1970, Stell & Dalby 1983). Biller & Lawson (1986) describe an extended variant which can be used to excise the subglottic margin. Half the cricoid cartilage is resected and replaced by a cartilage graft and a muscle flap.

The great worry about vertical partial laryngectomy is that all the tumour may not be removed. Cartilage invasion occurs in as many as 50% of patients with T3 lesions and there is no known method of detecting this before operation, even with CT scans. Kirschner's pathological studies (1984) have shown that the operation is safe for small lesions with a fixed cord not extending below the inferior edge of the thyroid ala or 1 cm below the level of the glottis. A danger signal is the bulge sometimes seen on tomography of the subglottic area representing spread of cancer under the conus elasticus, allowing the tumour to escape from the laryngeal framework through the cricothyroid membrane.

Another procedure gaining in popularity is the

subtotal laryngectomy in which the supraglottic larynx and one vertical half of the glottic and sub-glottic compartments are removed. A strip of endolarynx on the opposite side is preserved and this can be used to form a valvular speaking shunt (Pearson 1981). Pathological studies (Robbins & Michaels 1985) have shown this method to be safe.

In the author's experience, 25% of patients with multiregional tumours present with stridor and there is controversy about what form of treatment is best for this. If a patient with stridor is treated initially by tracheostomy (followed by surgery or radiotherapy) it has repeatedly been shown that there is a high chance of stomal recurrence, which is virtually always fatal (Keim 1965, Stell & van den Broek 1971). The alternative is emergency laryngectomy, which is not as hazardous as might be thought, but which has the ethical objection that it is not possible to obtain a truly informed consent from a patient who cannot breathe. Furthermore, it has yet to be shown convincingly by large studies that this policy reduces the incidence of stomal recurrence. The author has carried out 20 emergency laryngectomies, the 5-year actuarial survival being 60%. No patient died of a stomal recurrence, but it is not possible to draw conclusions because the series is relatively small, which is inevitable because of the comparative rarity of this event.

The cervical nodes

In the author's experience 25% of patients with multiregional tumours have palpable cervical nodes at presentation. These clearly require radical neck dissection. For patients with no palpable nodes, another point of controversy is a prophylactic neck dissection. The incidence of occult (i.e. invaded but not palpable) nodes in glottic T3 carcinoma is fairly low—17% in Bocca's series for example (Bocca et al 1984). Whether prophylactic neck dissection improves the survival compared to a policy of 'wait and see' has never been clarified by a controlled trial for laryngeal carcinoma. In the author's experience

only 2.5% of patients with advanced disease treated initially by surgery die solely of recurrence in the neck; these are the only patients who could benefit from this procedure, so that the scope for improvement of survival is modest.

ADJUVANT CHEMOTHERAPY

Chemotherapy as an adjuvant to radiotherapy is currently very popular. Huge numbers of phase II studies (that is where the criterion is response of the tumour) have shown that quite high response rates can be obtained, the best being obtained by regimens including cisplatin. Sadly, the few phase III trials (i.e. where the criterion is survival) show that response does not equate with an increase in survival and so far these regimens have produced no effect on cure rate (Jacobs et al 1984).

SUMMARY

Because of difficulties in classification, lack of clarity in exactly what tumours are being treated and omission from analysis of patients unsuitable for radiotherapy, it is difficult to draw any firm conclusions. Patients presenting with stridor and/or palpable lymph node metastases should be treated by total laryngectomy and radical neck dissection.

For the other two-thirds of these patients, i.e. those without stridor or palpable lymph node metastases, it appears that the three policies of radical radiotherapy with salvage surgery for recurrence, radical surgery, or preoperative radiotherapy plus radical surgery give equal 5-year cure rates of about 60%. The great advantage of radical radiotherapy with surgery in reserve for recurrence is that about half the patients retain their larynx. However, until a classification system is defined that allows us to describe exactly what is being treated, the main question of the relative merits of radiotherapy and surgery will remain unanswered.

Because of his training, the surgeon is probably motivated towards cutting, whereas the radiotherapist may be more conservation minded.

In order that the patient may benefit from the expertise of both modalities, it is important that treatment is discussed at joint consultative clinics by specialists of comparable experience. The decisions regarding treatment of this disease, as well as other oncological problems, is one for the senior and not the junior staff to decide.

It is accepted that it is important but difficult to define the extent of the tumour. Although both main classifications agree that in T3 glottic cancer the tumour is confined to the larynx, in practice it may spread to the supra- or subglottis or both, the latter resulting in the transglottic tumour. This can result in a change in the pattern of the disease and what may be appropriate treatment for one group may not be for another for the causes of fixation are varied (Belson et al 1976). The most favourable group appears to be where the bulk of the tumour has caused mechanical fixation and the most unfavourable where there is deep infiltration of the tissues. In the first instance radiotherapy is likely to be successful, in the latter less so.

Although Pressman's work (Pressman et al 1960) has shown the extent to which laryngeal tumours may remain confined within the compartment of origin and that the deep lymphatic vessels do not cross the midline, by the time fixation has occurred it is likely that, in some cases the disease will have spread microscopically, even if not macroscopically, contralaterally. This must cause problems in deciding whether or not patients are suitable for limited surgery, even when extensive use is made of frozen sections. Radiotherapy is certainly useful in treating microscopic disease, but it is difficult to understand why the sophisticated machines now available cannot always destroy deeply infiltrating tumours, particularly when one considers the bulky tumours of the breast and cervix which can be cured by radiotherapy alone. It has been suggested that it is related to the presence of anoxic cells, in which case one would have expected dramatically better results in patients treated with radiotherapy under hyperbaric oxygen but this has not proved to be so (Henk et al

1977). Nor had the addition of the radiosensitizer misonidazole improved results (Medical Research Council 1984). However, treating patients under hyperbaric oxygen was a rather crude attempt to increase oxygenation in the tumour and misonidazole was almost the first generation of that type of radiosensitizer. There are many other means of trying to make radiotherapy more effective and they will be discussed later.

Perhaps this is the place to mention one cause of failure that can now usually be excluded, the 'geographical miss'. Any radiotherapist treating laryngeal cancer must be able to perform an adequate indirect laryngoscopy and the use of simulators, together with simple techniques of head immobilization, have made it virtually impossible to miss the macroscopic extent of the tumour. However, it is not a matter of simple mechanics, but also a knowledge of the natural history of the disease that is important, raising questions such as whether the whole of the supra- and subglottis should be treated irrespective of the macroscopic spread and what should be the policy regarding lymph node irradiation. Since it is technically easy to treat a large volume with external radiation, this might be desirable even as a 'prophylactic' measure, but the larger the volume treated the more severe the reaction, both general and local, and the greater the possibility of complications if subsequent surgery is needed.

Most surgeons consider that the ideal combined treatment is surgery followed by radiotherapy, but unfortunately using the latter postoperatively is seldom very effective, probably because of impaired blood supply and at this site it results in the patient losing his larynx.

While total laryngectomy gives a chance of complete removal of disease no surgeon can promise an absolute cure because of such factors as spread of disease beyond the confines of the larynx, unsuspected lymph node metastases together with the, admittedly small, possibility of operative mortality. Although realizing possible difficulties caused by preoperative radiotherapy, it is nevertheless necessary to decide whether they outweigh advantages to the patient in terms of survival and quality of life. There are many different combinations that can be used, but it is essential that preliminary radiation should never be used in such a way that it is impossible to operate afterwards.

Preoperative radiotherapy can be applied in various ways. One seldom used for the larynx, but occasionally in sites such as the rectum, is to give one large dose, such as 10 or 20 Gy a few days before surgery, on the assumption that peripheral cells will be damaged but no major reactions will have time to develop. The larynx does not seem an appropriate site for this approach.

More commonly, a dose of about 40 Gy will be given in 3–4 weeks and the situation reassessed. In some centres an operation will be done, however good the response! In others, therapy will be continued to between 60 and 70 Gy if there has been a marked decrease in the tumour and, above all, if mobility has improved. Most radiotherapists would agree that if mobility has not improved after 400 Gy it is unlikely to change with a higher dose. Although there are many centres in different countries using one or other of these regimes, the experience of the Princess Margaret Hospital in Toronto is particularly useful since they have used both methods. This has meant that the surgeons and radiotherapists and, therefore, the techniques are the same in both groups. Perhaps the statistical continuity is even more important since the results can differ so dramatically from one centre to another that one wonders if it is the same disease that is being treated! From this hospital, Harwood et al (1980) reports on 112 patients treated by radiotherapy with surgery for salvage and 28 patients treated by combined preoperative irradiation and laryngectomy. In each group half the patients were alive and well at 5 years. Results were better in females and older men, but the most significant finding was that half the larynges removed in the combined treatment group contained no tumour and were therefore removed unnecessarily. The authors are now following this policy in all suitable patients, provided good follow-up facilities are available.

After 40 Gy given in 4 weeks it is usually possible to operate within a month. If a full course is given it will take longer for the resection to settle and the response of the disease to be assessed. This is the difficult and potentially dangerous time when there is uncertainty whether or not tumour is still present

and there is reluctance to biopsy an oedematous larynx. This delay in diagnosing persistent disease may account for the difference in survival quoted in some series. Certainly, a persistently fixed larynx, even with healed mucosa, should be regarded as containing disease. However, it is oedema which causes the greatest problem in assessment. There is no doubt that the larger the fractions of radiation and the shorter the time over which they are given, the more severe it is likely to be. Infection makes it worse, as does smoking and drinking, though the latter is often secret and denied. In these cases the oedema is likely to be bilateral, but unilateral oedema on the diseased side is likely to be due to persistent tumour and biopsy is indicated. The risk of causing perichondritis may be mitigated by the use of antibiotics, steroids and the skill of the surgeon.

In the past it was not uncommon in some centres, where high doses were given over a short time, for laryngectomies to be needed for radionecrosis and even quoted a 'minimal permissible necrosis rate'. This has been virtually obviated by the use of modern equipment and more individualized fractionation.

If radiotherapy preceding total laryngectomy causes difficulties, they may be even worse if one or other of the less radical operations is performed. Yet it is precisely in this group that it would appear to be needed, even though surgeons in various parts of the world have shown that, where the larynx is concerned, it is possible to operate successfully with much smaller margins of safety than in most other sites (Lesinsky et al 1976). Pearson is the inventor of an ingenious new method of subtotal laryngectomy. However, the patient still needs a stoma and also digital pressure to produce a voice. Unfortunately, many patients have a tremor or arthritis making precise movements difficult. It is really not possible to consider this result as equal to that of a successful postradiation patient without a stoma and with a good voice. It is easy to comment on radiation failures, but patients referred for treatment are often unfit and with unfavourable tumours (Mittal et al 1984). One wonders how many T3 tumours are suitable for this operation and what will be the long-term results. It is also probable that a surgeon with a reputation for doing a particular type of operation will have more patients referred to him and thus gain an inaccurate impression of the frequency of suitable cases.

It is not uncommon for patients with advanced disease to present with stridor and some consider this to be an indication for immediate surgery. However, as it is an emergency procedure, there is little time for the usual investigations and assessment to be made so that the operation may be performed on a patient with virtually inoperable, and sometimes disseminated, disease. Radiotherapy may be successful in treating such a patient while assessments are being made.

It needs to be supplemented with antibiotics and steroids while the patient must be examined at least once daily for the dose to be decided. Facilities for an immediate tracheostomy must be available and, if the airway has not increased substantially after 20 Gy it is unlikely that an operation will be avoided. However, during this time it will have been possible to assess both patient and disease. Adopting this procedure may also avoid a stomal recurrence since Keim (Keim et al 1965) considers that these are related to a previous tracheostomy, although others such as Modlin (Modlin & Oguea 1969) and Wang (1973) do not agree. Such recurrences are difficult to treat by surgery or radiation. External radiation is seldom effective and, although interstitial radiation using radon seeds or gold grains may give better palliation, there is always the risk of cartilage necrosis.

In the past 40 years external radiation has been the main method of applying radiotherapy. It may be, however, that if radiation were more localized it might be both more effective and easier to combine with surgery. One of the earliest methods of applying local radiation to the larynx was the Finzi Harmer operation (Harmer & Finzi 1930) where, following a fenestration of the thyroid cartilage, radium needles were applied to the tumour and left in place for up to about 7 days. The results were good in some cases and the complications in the hands of Sir Stanford Cade minimal, a tracheotomy being seldom required even in those preantibiotic days (Cade 1940). This procedure was eventually abandoned with the advent of effective external radiotherapy, but interstitial radiation is still extremely useful in treating cancers of the oral tongue and lip, quite apart from sites elsewhere in the body. It might, therefore, be worthwhile reassessing this operation and perhaps modifying it according to modern types of irradiation. It could be a simple method where dose and duration could be varied according to the type of tumour, a bulky one being treated more slowly than an infiltrative one, but both would complete treatment in 7–10 days. A high dose could be given, which seems necessary for some of these tumours, but, as the volume would be small by comparison with that included in external fields, there should be fewer problems if subsequent surgery was needed and assessment should be quicker than after external treatment. This might obviate the criticism of those who consider the long delay elapsing between unsuccessful radiation and salvage surgery to be a possible cause of failure.

As Stell and Pearson have mentioned, T3 glottic cancer is in clinical practice not just one disease. If localized to the glottis the possibility of lymph node metastases is small (Woodhouse et al 1981). Even spread to the subglottis, with its rich lymphatic network, does not greatly increase their incidence, although it is often a cause of failure in treating the primary disease (Rose et al 1983). However, once the supraglottis is involved, the percentage of metastases increases (Miltal et al 1984). The differing distribution of the various subgroups in reported series probably accounts for the differing incidence of nodes reported in the literature. Mittal, reporting on transglottic disease of all stages, quotes 26% nodes at initial presentation, with 19% developing in untreated necks, while Woodhouse quotes 18 out of 323 glottic cancer (all stages), of which 14 occurred in the transglottic group. Most surgeons are not convinced that radiation is effective in treating cancer in lymph nodes and, admittedly, it is often more difficult than in the primary site and also differs according to the origin of the primary tumour. However, the use of fine-needle aspirates proving disease to be present (although a negative result may be false) has increased accuracy.

The use of hyperbaric oxygen and misonidazole have been mentioned, but radiotherapy itself can be modified, particularly with regard to fractionation. In most centres, the same fractionation is used for all tumours, although it is unlikely that cellular metabolism is always the same. Perhaps one of the reasons for the success of local continuous irradiation is that it gives a better chance of damaging more cells at the most sensitive part of their cycle. In the early days, Coutard improved results by treating patients twice a day and deciding, by clinical observations, what the next dose should be. However, as it became possible to give treatment more quickly with newer apparatus and as more patients were referred, it became more practical to give single daily prescribed treatments. Over the last few years interest has revived in changing this regime. Harvard found that it seemed more effective to treat malignant melanomas with large fractions, such as 5 and 6 Gy twice a week for 3–4 weeks, while Svoboda (1984) has been experimenting with giving 2–3 treatments a day, finishing the whole course in 2–3 weeks. It, therefore, does not yet seem appropriate to write off radiotherapy as having 'plateaued', quite apart from the fact that combination of chemotherapy with radiotherapy has not been finally assessed, nor the use of newer radiation particles such as fast neutrons and pi-mesons. Although fast neutrons radiobiologically appeared to offer so much in clinical practice, they have been disappointing, producing very severe reactions which make subsequent surgery almost impossible. Duncan (1986), however, suggests that, if higher energy beams are developed, then the therapeutic ratio may be significantly increased with improvement in results and decrease in reaction.

The use of hyperthermia as a potentiator of radiation sometimes results in success in individual cases, but no long-term results are yet available. As carcinoma of the larynx is a comparatively rare disease, it is difficult to find enough patients to take part in all the necessary clinical trials.

The rather paternalistic approach of doctor to patient in the past has often led to the latter having little choice in his treatment and alternatives were seldom put to him as the doctors were convinced that their choice was the right one! It has been suspected that many patients presented only with the possibility of total laryngectomy would, in fact, prefer to try to save their larynx, even if it made treatment more prolonged and the chances of survival slightly less. McNeil et al (1981) tried to investigate this very problem of patient's choice of treatment for T3 glottic cancer by putting the various possibilities to 37 healthy volunteers comprising 25 executives and 12 fire fighters. Each group showed a large percentage who would trade 14–17% of their full life expectancy in order to retain their natural voice. As the article says, 'Patients' attitude towards morbidity are important and survival is not their only consideration . . . attempts should be made to incorporate patients' attitude toward quality and quantity of life into decision making process'.

REFERENCES

B W Pearson

Asai R 1972 Laryngoplasty after total laryngectomy. Archives of Otolaryngology 95: 114–119

Blom E D, Singer M I, Haymaker R C 1985 An improved esophageal insufflation test. Archives of Otology 111: 211–212

Coates H L, DeSanto L W, Devine K D, Elveback L R 1976 Carcinoma of the supraglottic larynx. Archives of Otology 102: 686–689

DeSanto L W (1984) T3 glottic cancer: options and consequences of the options. Laryngoscope 94: 1311–1315

Harwood A R, Bryce D P, Rider W D 1980 Management of T3 glottic cancer. Archives of Otolaryngology 106: 697–699

Horn D 1962 Laryngectomy survey report. Eleventh Annual Meeting International Association of Laryngectomees, Memphis, Tennessee

Jing B-S 1978 Malignant tumors of the larynx. Radiology Clinics NA 16: 247–260

King P S, Loweks E S, Pierson G A 1968 Rehabilitation and adaptation of laryngectomy patients. American Journal of Physical Medicine 97: 192–203

Kirchner J A 1969 One hundred laryngeal cancers studied by serial section. Annals of Otology, Rhinology and Laryngology 78: 689–709

Kirchner J A, Som M L 1971 Clinical significance of a fixed vocal cord. Laryngoscope 81: 1029–1044

Leipzig B 1980 Neoglottic reconstruction following total laryngectomy: A reappraisal. Annals of Otology, Rhinology and Laryngology 89: 534–537

McInnes W D, Egan W, Aust J B 1976 The management of carcinoma of the larynx in a prominent patient, or did Morell MacKenzie really cause World War I? American Journal of Surgery 132: 515–522

McNeil B J, Weichselbaum R, Pauker S G 1981 Speech and survival: Trade-offs between quality and quantity of life in laryngeal cancer. New England Journal of Medicine 305: 982–987

Manusco A A, Calcaterra T C, Hanafee W N 1978 Computed tomography of the larynx. Radiology Clinics NA 16: 195–208

Miller A H 1976 Experiences with the Asai technique. In: Alberti P W, Bryce D P (eds) Workshops from the centennial conference on laryngeal cancer. Appleton-Century-Crofts, New York, p 557

Neel H B, Devine K D, DeSanto L W 1980 Laryngofissure and cordectomy for early cordal carcinoma: Outcome in 182 patients. Otolaryngology, Head and Neck Surgery 88: 79–84

Norris C W, Tucker G T, Kuo B F, Pitser W F 1980 A correlation of clinical staging, pathological findings, and five-year end results in surgically treated cancer of the larynx. Annals of Otology, Rhinology and Laryngology 79: 1033–1048

Ogura J H, Sessions D G, Spector G J 1975 Analysis of surgical therapy for epidermoid carcinoma of the laryngeal glottis. Laryngoscope 85: 1522

Olofsson J, Lord I J, Van Nostrand A W P 1973 Vocal cord fixation in laryngeal carcinoma. Acta Otolaryngologica 74: 496–510

Panje W R 1981 Prosthetic vocal rehabilitation following laryngectomy: the voice button. Annals of Otology, Rhinology and Laryngology 90: 116–120

Pearson B W 1975 Laryngeal microcirculation and pathways of cancer spread. Laryngoscope 85: 700–713

Pearson B W 1981 Subtotal laryngectomy. Laryngoscope 91: 1904–1912

Pearson B W, Woods R D, Hartman D E 1980 Extended hemilaryngectomy for T3 glottic carcinoma with preservation of speech and swallowing. Laryngoscope 90: 1950–1961

Skolnik E M, Martin L, Yee K F et al 1975 Radiation failure in cancer of the larynx. Annals of Otology, Rhinology and Laryngology 84: 804–811

Stewart J G, Brown J R, Palmer M K et al 1975 The management of glottic carcinoma by primary irradiation with surgery in reserve. Laryngoscope 85: 14–77

Tucker G F 1974 The anatomy of laryngeal cancer. Canadian Journal of Otolaryngology 3: 417–431

P M Stell, D A Bowdler

Manual for staging of cancer 1983 Philadelphia: Lippincott, p 37

TNM classification of malignant tumours 1978 Geneva, UICC, p 33

Biller H F, Barnhill R F, Ogura J H 1977 Hemilaryngectomy following radiation failure for carcinoma of the vocal cords. Laryngoscope 80: 249–253

Biller H F, Lawson W 1986 Partial laryngectomy for vocal cord cancer with marked limitation or fixation of the vocal cord. Laryngoscope 96: 61–64

Bocca E, Calearo C, De Vincentiis I, Marullo T, Motta G 1984 Occult metastases in cancer of the larynx and their relationship to clinical and histological aspects of the primary tumor: a four-year multicentric research. Laryngoscope 94: 1086–1090

Bryce D P 1972 The role of surgery in the management of carcinoma of the larynx. Institute of Laryngology and Otology 86: 669

De Santo L W 1984 T3 glottic cancer: options and consequences of the options. Laryngoscope 94: 1131–1315

Duncan W, Arnott S J, Battermann J J, Orr J A, Schmitt G, Kerr G R 1984 Fast neutrons in the treatment of head and neck cancers: The results of a multi-centre randomly controlled trial. Radiotherapy and Oncology 2: 293–300

Fu K K, Woodhouse R J, Quivey J M, Phillips T L, Dedo H H 1982 The significance of laryngeal edema following radiotherapy of carcinoma of the vocal cord. Cancer 49: 655–658

Harwood A R, Bryce D P, Rider W D 1980 Management of T3 glottic cancer. Archives of Laryngology 106: 697–699

Harwood A R, Deboer G, Kazim F 1981 Prognostic factors in T3 glottic cancer. Cancer 47: 367–372

Hoover L A, Calcaterra T C, Walter G A, Larsson S G 1984 Preoperative CT scan evaluation for laryngeal carcinoma: correlation with pathological findings. Laryngoscope 94: 310–314

Hunter R D, Palmer M K 1980 An analysis of the fate of patients treated radically for glottic carcinoma of the larynx. Clinical Radiology 31: 449–452

Jacobs C, Wolf G T, Makuch R W, Vikram P 1984 Proceedings of ASCO 708 (abstract C) p 182

Kazem I, Van Den Broek P 1984 Planned preoperative radiation therapy vs definitive radiotherapy for advanced laryngeal cancer. Laryngoscopy 94: 1355–1358

Keim W F, Shapiro M J, Rosen H D 1965 Study of postlaryngectomy stomal recurrence. Archives of Otolaryngology 81: 183

Kirchner J A, Som M L 1971 Clinical significance of a fixed vocal cord. Laryngoscope 81: 1092

Kirchner J A 1984a Invasion of the framework by laryngeal cancer. Acta Otolaryngologica (Stockh) 97: 392–397

Kirchner J A 1984b Pathways and pitfalls in partial laryngectomy. Annals of Otology, Rhinology and Laryngology 93: 301–305

Micheau C, Luboinski B, Sancho H, Cachin Y 1976 Modes of invasion of cancer of the larynx. Cancer 38: 346–360

Mohr R M, Quenelle D J, Shumrick D A 1983 Vertico-frontolateral laryngectomy (hemilaryngectomy). Archives of Otolaryngology 109: 384–395

Ogura J H, Mallen B W 1963 Carcinoma of the larynx. Postgraduate Medicine 34: 493

Pearson B W 1981 Subtotal laryngectomy. Laryngoscope 91: 1904–1912

Ramadan M F, Morton R P, Stell P M, Pharoah P O D 1982 Review. Epidemiology of laryngeal cancer. Clinical Otolaryngology 7: 417–428

Robbins K T, Michaels A 1985 Feasibility of subtotal laryngectomy based on whole-organ examination. Archives of Otolaryngology 111: 356–360

Sorensen H et al 1980 Partial laryngectomy following irradiation. Laryngoscope 90: 1344–1349

Stell P M, Dalby J E 1985 Treatment of early (T1) glottic and supraglottic carcinoma: does partial laryngectomy have a place? European Journal of Surgical Oncology 11: 263–266

Stell P M, Van Den Broek P 1971 Stomal recurrence after laryngectomy: aetiology and management. Journal of Laryngology and Otology 85: 131–140

Stell P M, Dalby J E, Singh S D, Ramadan M F, Bainton R 1982 The management of glottic T3 carcinoma. Clinical Otolaryngology 7: 175–180

Van Nostrand A W P 1974 Centennial conference on laryngeal cancer. New York: Appleton-Century, p 61

Wang C C 1973 Treatment of glottic carcinoma by megavoltage radiation therapy and results. American Radium Institute 120: no 1

Ward P H, Calcaterra T C, Kagan A R 1975 The enigma of postradiation edema and recurrent or residual carcinoma of the larynx. Laryngoscope 85: 522–529

Woodhouse R J, Quivey J M, Fu K K, Sien P S, Dedo H H, Phillips T L 1981 Treatment of carcinoma of the vocal cord: a review of 20 years experience. Laryngoscope 91: 1155–1162

V M Dalley

Belson T P, Duncavage J A, Toothill R J, Lehman T P 1976 Vocal cord fixation in laryngeal carcinoma. Archives of Otolaryngology 102: 281–283

Cade S (ed) 1940 Harmer's method. In: Technique of radium

treatment. Fenestration of the larynx. Malignant disease and its treatment by radium.

Duncan W 1986 In: Correspondence. International Journal of Radiation Oncology, Biology and Physics 12: 11, 2053

Harmer, Finzi 1930 Cancer of the larynx—treatment by radiation. In: Crookshank F9, Cruchet R (eds) Anglo-French library of medical and biological science.

Harwood S R, Beale F A, Cummings B J, Hawkins N V, Keane T J, Rider W D 1980 T3 glottic cancer: an analysis of dose time-volume factors. International Journal of Radiation Oncology, Biology and Physics 6: 675–680

Henk J M, Kunkler P B, Smith C W 1977 Radiotherapy and hyperbaric oxygen in head and neck cancer. Lancet ii: 101–105

Keim W F, Shapiro M J, Rosin H D 1965 Study of postlaryngectomy. Stomal recurrence. Archives of Otolaryngology 81: 183–185

Lesinsky S G, Bauer W C, Ogure J H 1976 Hemilaryngectomy for T3 (fixed cord) epidermoid carcinoma of the larynx. Laryngoscope 86: 1563–1571

McNeil B J, Weichselbaum & Pauker S G 1981 Speech and survival. Special article. New England Journal of Medicine 305: 17, 982–987

Medical Research Council 1984 A study of the effect of Misonidazole in conjuction with radiotherapy for the treatment of head and neck cancer. British Journal of Radiology 57: 585–595

Mittal B et al 1984 Transglottic carcinoma. Cancer 53: 151–161

Modlin B, Ogura J H 1969 Post-laryngectomy tracheal stomal recurrences. Laryngoscope. 2: 239–250

Mohr R M, Quenelle D J, Shumrick D A et al 1983 Vertico-frontolateral laryngectomy (hemilaryngectomy). Indications, technique and results. Archives of Otolaryngology 109: 384–394

Pressman J J, Simon Mildred B, Monell C 1960 Anatomical studies related to the dissemination of cancer of the larynx. 64th annual session of the American Academy of Ophtalmology & Otolaryngology, Oct 1959: 628–637

Svoboda V H J 1984 Accelerated fractionation. The Portsmouth experience, 4th varian meeting

Wang C C 1973 Treatment of glottic carcinoma by megavoltage radiation therapy and results. American Journal of Roentgenology and Radium 120: 1, 157–163

Woodhouse R J, Quivey J M, Fu K K, Sien P S, Dedo H H, Phillips T L 1981 Treatment of carcinoma of the vocal cord. A review of 20 years experience. Laryngoscope 91: 1155–1162

17

How are patients chosen for conservation surgery of the larynx?

C.B. Croft

Conservation surgery of the larynx has evolved over a surprisingly long period of time. Gordon Buck performed the first laryngofissure for intrinsic carcinoma of the vocal cord in 1851 (Buck 1853) and Billroth had already performed the first vertical 'hemilaryngectomy' by 1878 (Schwartz 1978). Subsequently, the use of lateral pharyngotomy to approach tumours of the epiglottis and aryepiglottic fold was established by the outstanding contributions of Wilfred Trotter amongst others (Trotter 1920). Not surprisingly, early attempts at conservation surgery in the larynx were attended by poor results, mainly due to attempts to control extensive lesions with subglottic spread by partial surgery. However, increasing awareness of the surgical anatomy and pathology of the larynx and its embryological derivation led to a resurgence of interest in conservation surgery. The studies of Pressman (1956) demonstrating the highly compartmentalized nature of the larynx and the pioneering work of Alonzo, Ogura and Som led to the successful evolution of conservation procedures and to their general acceptance.

Consequently, it is no longer a question of how to do it, but the more important issue of when to do it.

There are important differences in treatment philosophy for early laryngeal carcinoma between North America on the one hand and the UK and Northern Europe on the other. It is fair to say that early glottic and supraglottic squamous cell carcinomas are often treated by partial laryngectomy in North America, whereas radiotherapy is more frequently employed in the UK and Europe. These important differences in management of early laryngeal carcinoma are difficut to reconcile, but the author, having trained on both sides of the Atlantic Ocean, is about to try!

This discussion will concentrate on the use of vertical partial (hemilaryngectomy) and horizontal partial (supraglottic) laryngectomy. The author considers these operations appropriate treatment for T1 tumours of the supraglottic larynx, with or without nodes, and for T1 and early T2 tumours of the glottis. The available figures which allow us to compare the effectiveness of radiotherapy and surgery in controlling early disease at these sites show that both modalities are very effective. A 5-year actuarial survival of 95% after surgery for cordal cancer was achieved by Neel et al (1980) and a recent series of patients with T1 glottic carcinoma treated with radiotherapy reported 5-year survival of 95% (Stewart et al,1975).

Early supraglottic squamous cell carcinomas are also apparently equally well handled with either primary radiotherapy or surgery and Stell & Dalby (1985) recently reported 5-year survival for T1 No supraglottic cancer treated by radiotherapy of 79%, against an historically comparable group treated by supraglottic laryngectomy and prophylactic neck dissection with a 77% 5-year survival. If radiotherapy and surgery are equally effective treatments when deployed in the best hands, how are we to decide between them? Radiotherapy certainly has an advantage in preserving better voice in glottic carcinomas and better swallowing in supraglottic carcinomas—why then should we choose conservation surgery for our patients? I believe the answer to this question lies in considering three issues:
1. The nature of the host
2. The stage, site and type of the tumour
3. Treatment options that are really available.

PATIENT SELECTION

As Harrison (1985) has pointed out in a recent discussion paper dealing with conservation surgery of the larynx, assessment of the 'whole patient' is vital in deciding on the role of conservation surgery in a particular patient.

In this respect, the patient's age is of some importance. Evidence of the long-term carcinogenic effects of radiotherapy continues to accumulate and, over the long-term, the possibility that a new malignancy may be promoted in the treatment field must be very real. A risk factor of somewhere between 2% and 10% is established in the reports of Harwood and Lawson.

A further problem arises in respect of the possibility of a second primary carcinoma arising in the area of 'field change'. This appears to be more of a problem in tumours of the supraglottic larynx (Wagenfield et al 1981) and again makes the point that 'using up' a valuable treatment modality such as radiotherapy in a young patient severely limits the treatment options if a second primary develops in the area. The author feels that in younger patients with early laryngeal carcinoma, appropriate conservation surgery should be the treatment of choice.

There is some evidence that patients with chronic laryngitis and long-standing keratosis do badly with radiotherapy (Stell & Dalby 1985). They tolerate treatment poorly and follow up is often complicated by the development of persistent laryngeal oedema.

Laryngeal oedema which persists for longer than 6 months has a high correlation with persistent tumour activity (Ward 1975) and it may be very difficult to exclude this possibility with a biopsy. Tumour may be spreading under an intact and apparently uninvolved mucosa and overaggressive biopsies in such cases are fraught with the danger of initiating perichondritis of the larynx. The difficulties in managing such cases are substantial and I can only agree with Stell (1985) in feeling that conservation surgery, where appropriate, is a better first-line treatment in patients with long-standing laryngeal keratosis.

On the other hand 'whole patient assessment' will mitigate against the use of conservation techniques in certain patients.

Recovery of deglutition after horizontal partial laryngectomy in particular takes a deal of effort and endurance on the part of both patient and surgeon. A substantial number of these patients will aspirate and all require adequate pulmonary function if they are to avoid the complication of aspiration pneumonia (Leonard Litton 1971). Simple tests, such as the 'two flight test', are helpful but the author favours pulmonary function tests on all patients being considered for supraglottic laryngectomy.

A number of patients, either by virtue of age, personality or cultural background, will find the management of the compromise of airway, voice and swallowing attendant on conservation surgery impossible to deal with. The case quoted by Donald (1984), in which a 72-year-old man recovering from a vertical partial laryngectomy for T1 carcinoma of the vocal cord, insisted that he could not swallow or breathe—in spite of objective evidence to the contrary—is precisely reproducible in this author's experience. Older patients or those in poor general health, lacking flexibility of mind and adaptability, are really not candidates for conservation laryngeal surgery.

THE STAGE, SITE AND TYPE OF TUMOUR

Laryngeal cancer is not one disease, but rather several diseases occurring in a wide variety of hosts. If one considers T1 glottic carcinoma, the spectrum extends from a localized 'microinvasive' carcinoma to a horseshoe lesion extending around the anterior commissure and extensively involving both vocal cords. Both are T1 lesions but what is the ideal treatment in such cases? A further difficulty relates to the staging of tumours, which is of fundamental importance in assessing patients' prospects and deciding on appropriate treatment. How often is a crucial initial endoscopic assessment and biopsy performed by an inexperienced or junior surgeon? There is no doubt that recording of tumour site and extent can be of variable quality and some of the treatment failures we all see could be attributed to an initial underestimate of tumour size and spread. Furthermore, a lesion can be staged only in two dimensions, the third dimension is missing, and although CT scanning may help in identifying deep spread within the larynx in large lesions, it is of little use in identifying infiltration in early tumours.

The principles applied to conservation laryngeal surgery are those that apply in tumour surgery at any site. Namely, the tumour has to be totally excised with an adequate margin of normal tissue. Fortunately for patient and surgeon alike, an adequate margin in the larynx can be measured in millimetres. It is also interesting to note that not all tumour excisions with positive margins lead to recurrence (Bauer et al 1975) in the larynx. Obviously, the problem should be strenuously avoided by the use of frozen section control, but if positive margins are identified, postoperative radiation is often effective in preventing local recurrence (Bauer et al 1975).

Intraepithelial carcinoma T1$_s$

Although classical conservation surgery is not going to be employed in the primary treatment of this disease, there are several points which are germaine to this discussion.

Although there is some debate about the malignant potential of carcinoma in situ, most pathologists and clinicians agree that here is potential for invasion from in situ carcinoma. There is also marked correlation with carcinoma in situ and coexistent invasive carcinoma of the larynx (Bauer et al 1978). Clearly, a thorough search for an area of invasive carcinoma must be made in such cases. The treatment of patients with localized or multicentre carcinoma in situ does create a controversy. Should these lesions be treated by radiotherapy or surgery? When one considers that endoscopic surgery with cord stripping, with or without the CO_2 laser, may in itself be curative, then recourse to radiotherapy is clearly overtreatment in every sense of the word. Radiation is not always effective in controlling in situ cancer and Miller & Fisher (1971) reported a substantial failure rate using radiotherapy of 51%. The author's experience with radiotherapy is equally disappointing and optimal therapy would be careful microlaryngoscopy with supravital staining, followed by stripping of the affected cord or cords. Repeat stripping is resorted to six weeks later and subsequent careful follow up is mandatory. Only if follow-up is likely to be inadequate, or the problem recurs, is radiotherapy indicated. The benefits to the patient of this approach in terms of missing out on the complications of irradiation—and the overall cost effectiveness of such treatment—are apparent. It is, of course, vital that these patients cease to smoke and that pressure on this point is maintained at each review.

Glottic carcinoma T1

The glottic carcinomas confined to the membraneous vocal cord respond well to primary irradiation and this is considered the treatment of choice by most authorities. Cure rates of 85–95% are obtainable and cannot be bettered by surgery (Stell & Dalby 1985). Irradiation has the distinct advantage of leaving an intact pair of vocal cords and normal voice in most patients. Conservation surgery in T1 vocal cord carcinoma can be equally effecive (Neel et al 1980) with 95% 5-year survivals achieved using laryngofissure and cordectomy. However, the voice is impaired following vertical partial resections of the larynx and the better functional results achieved with radiotherapy make it the treatment of choice.

Irradiation failures in T1 glottic carcinoma can be managed safely and effectively by conservation techniques (Stell & Dalby 1985, Silver 1981). Clearly, the recurrent lesion should have been suitable for conservation surgery before irradiation commenced and, ideally, the treating surgeon should have seen the patient throughout. The minimum operation for postradiation recurrence would be a vertical partial laryngectomy or 'hemilaryngectomy', using frozen section control of resection margins. Although the complication rate escalates after irradiation, particularly in relation to maintaining an adequate glottic airway, the operation is effective and presents us with a valuable salvage procedure if irradiation fails.

Controversy exists about ideal primary treatment of carcinomas extending across the anterior commissure and those involving the vocal process of the arytenoid. The point being made that such cases are more likely to recur following radiation due to the possibility of cartilage invasion. However, there is no firm evidence to substantiate this claim and Kirchner has shown that, as long as the tumour remains confined to the level of the glottis, invasion of the laryngeal framework is extremely unlikely (Kirchner 1984) However, Kirchner also clearly demonstrated that those lesions with gross tumour extending upwards onto the base of the epiglottis will frequently invade the thyroid cartilage and these more aggressive lesions may be more suitably dealt with by conservation laryngectomy via an anterior commissure technique.

T2 carcinoma of the vocal cord

Those cases amenable to vertical partial laryngectomy with arytenoid resection include those cases with tumour extending posteriorly into the vocal process and anterior face of the arytenoid and extending laterally onto the floor of one ventricle.

Contraindications to partial surgery include tumours extending onto the posterior surface of the arytenoid, or crossing the ventricle laterally to reach the ventricular surface of the false cord. These extensions raise the strong probability of involvement of both cricoarytenoid joint and thyroid cartilages, and partial surgery is contraindicated—similarly, subglottic extension of more than 10 mm anteriorly or 5 mm posteriorly. Although the surgical cure rate for T2 glottic carcinomas range from 69% to 82% (Biller et al 1971, Ogura et al 1975) and cure therefore less likely, the author feels that primary radiotherapy is still probably the treatment of choice with conservation surgery reserved for radiation failures and younger patients, as already described in T1 tumours. Of course, the criteria of tumour extent already discussed should apply to the lesion prior to radiotherapy treatment.

T3 glottic carcinoma

Some authorities maintain that glottic tumours with cord fixation (Ogura & Thawley 1980) can be managed safely by conservation techniques, such as extended vertical partial laryngectomy, and there are certainly occasional cases in which this sort of approach can be successful. However, Kirchner and others have shown these tumours may extend well into the subglottis, with tumour spreading under the conus elasticus and escaping from the larynx via the cricothyroid membrane. These lesions are not suitable for conservation operations in the classical sense and the fact that one or two leading laryngologists have been able to manage them conservatively does not mean that the rest of us will do as well. Attempts at partial laryngeal surgery in this situation are really examples of surgical brinkmanship!

CONSERVATION SURGERY IN TUMOURS OF THE SUPRAGLOTTIC LARYNX

The development of the operation of supraglottic subtotal laryngectomy is well described by Silver (1981). The great problem with this operation was, and remains, securing surgical closure of the larynx

and pharynx and then getting the patient to swallow again. The work of Som and Ogura has contributed greatly to perfecting surgical reconstruction after this technique and it has become a widely accepted and oncologically sound procedure.

Although there have been many extensions described to the classical supraglottic partial laryngectomy, the operation basically consists of resection of the epiglottis, hyoid bone, thyrohyoid membrane and upper half of the thyroid cartilage with supraglottic soft tissues and mucosa. This excision completely removes the entire pre-epiglottic space. The operation is therefore suitable for carcinomas of the laryngeal surface of the epiglottis and false cords, provided the true vocal cords are uninvolved and mobile and the arytenoid region clear. Involvement of the epiglottis below the petiole is a problem area and, although we know that narrow resection margins of area 2.0 mm are adequate in this region (Silver 1981), it may be difficult to assess this area adequately preoperatively. The use of laryngography may help, but cannot eliminate the possibility of tumour reaching the anterior commissure and invading the thyroid cartilage. This is a particular danger in ulcerating, poorly differentiated carcinoma and contraindicates the use of supraglottic partial laryngectomy.

The operation of supraglottic laryngectomy has been extended to include lesions invading the valleculae and tongue base and certain limited lesions of the related hypopharynx (Silver, 1981). However, such extensions greatly increase the technical difficulties of securing adequate surgical closure and of restoring deglutition. Furthermore, only early and limited lesions involving these related areas are suitable for conservation surgery and few such cases seem to present themselves in the UK.

CHOICE OF TREATMENT IN T1 N0 SUPRAGLOTTIC TUMOURS

The practice in the United Kingdom is to irradiate early tumours of the supraglottic larynx, which might otherwise be amenable to conservation techniques. A recent review by Stell & Dalby (1985) of their cases treated by both supraglottic laryngectomy and prophylactic neck dissection and radiotherapy showed comparable 5-year survival of 77% and 79%

respectively. Similar results obtained from either surgery or radiotherapy mean that optimal treatment will depend on the patient's age and fitness. Surgery is preferred for younger patients who then have irradiation held in reserve, in case of further problems as already discussed.

Patients with cervical node metastases

Thirty percent of patients with supraglottic tumours will have palpable metastases at presentation. These patients are more likely to do well with primary surgery and a radical neck dissection (Stell & Dalby 1985). The use of radiotherapy is unlikely to control disease in patients with nodes greater than 2 cm and evidence is available that shows combinations of surgery and radiotherapy do not appear to affect outcome (Snow et al 1978). Significantly, some postoperative radiotherapy after supraglottic laryngectomy can result in laryngeal oedema and airway obstruction (Bocca et al 1968, Silver 1981), although it is possible to get away with postoperative irradiation at this site if treatment is taken slowly and carefully. Postoperative irradiation should only be considered if excision margins are positive or if the patient has multiple positive nodes in the neck.

Surgery of failed radiotherapy in the supraglottic larynx

Considerable controversy exists about the advisability of using conservation techniques in the supraglottic larynx after irradiation has failed. As Silver has noted, 'Greater difficulties can be encountered in performing surgery in previously irradiated cases'. Stell (1985) advises total laryngectomy for radiation failures in this site and Sorensen et al (1980) reported a 40% pharyngeal fistulae rate after supraglottic resection in irradiation failure. Only 20% of their patients were able to swallow without aspiration following surgery. However, Burns et al (1979) reported a 55% success rate following partial supraglottic laryngectomy after failed radiation—all these patients apparently swallowed well, although conversion to total laryngectomy was required in 25% of their patients who could not swallow. The author's view is that if supraglottic laryngectomy is to be considered following irradiation failure, then the patient must be counselled most carefully about all

the eventualities. The tracheostomy may have to remain for a prolonged period and conversion to total laryngectomy a possibility. Patients may even require temporary gastrostomy feeding to allow recovery of adequate deglutition. When one considers the very real difficulties and risks in this situation and the recent developments in speech rehabilitation following total laryngectomy using an internal fistula and either a Blom Singer or Panje prosthesis, then one's doubts about attempting conservation surgery in supraglottic tumours after irradiation increases. The author feels that conservation operations in this situation can only be contemplated in young, fit and fully informed patients.

TUMOUR TYPE

The discussion so far has centred on the management of squamous cell carcinoma of the larynx. There are other rare tumour types, which, by virtue of their poor response to irradiation, are better treated with primary surgery. If the site and extent of tumour allows a conservative operation, then certain of these lesions can be managed conservatively.

Verrucous carcinoma

This well-differentiated keratinizing squamous cell tumour has an exophytic warty appearance and fingerlike projections which slowly push into surrounding tissues. The tumour rarely metastasizes but grows relentlessly and destructively within the larynx.

There has been considerable debate about the ideal treatment of this tumour, most authorities believing that surgery is the ideal primary treatment in view of the evidence of radioresistance and anaplastic transformation after radiotherapy (Biller & Bergman 1975). Although the Toronto Group (Burns et al 1976) feel that radiotherapy is equally effective as surgery in treating this tumour, my experience tends to confirm the radioresistance of this tumour and I believe that surgery is the treatment of choice, with conservation surgery an option, if tumour site and extent allow.

Other rare tumours include adenocarcinoma and minor salivary gland tumours, together with tumours of the cartilaginous framework of the larynx. All are exceedingly rare and radioresistant and, if circumstances permit, can be managed by conservation techniques.

WHAT TREATMENT OPTIONS ARE REALLY AVAILABLE?

The discussion thus far presupposes that treatments available to all patients are the same in all centres and that all centres have surgeons who are trained in conservation laryngeal surgery and who are experienced in managing both the procedures and coping with the inevitable complications and difficulties. This is probably not the case, and, furthermore, the practice of submitting all early tumours of the larynx to radiotherapy inevitably means that the failures will come to total laryngectomy. There are several studies which tend to support the view that this policy leads to the sacrifice of larynges in patients in whom conservation surgery would have been possible (Russ et al 1978). To put it simply, if skills are not available or practised, it is highly unlikely that they will be deployed in cases in which difficulty can be anticipated. This is certainly the case in irradiation failure and, to return to the original question, conservation surgery is an appropriate and effective treatment, but it can only be the treatment choice in centres where the necessary skills are available and maintained.

INTRODUCTION

During the past 20 years, we have witnessed the remarkable evolution of conservation laryngeal surgery (CLS). Once thought to be a drastic departure from traditional thinking, it has gradually become essential in the treatment of laryngeal cancer; and the surgeon unskilled in this methodology lacks an important technical versatility. Fifty to seventy percent of laryngeal malignancies are amenable to conservation methods, while the balance are better treated by total laryngectomy and/or radiation (Tucker 1977). Recent years have also been characterized by the development of sophisticated radiation therapy (RT) techniques necessary for the treatment of laryngeal cancer. At times, laryngeal cancer therapy was somewhat hindered by a spirit of territoriality, in which surgeons and radiotherapists each sought dominance. Simultaneously, there existed an ongoing discussion between proponents and opponents of CLS techniques. Expectedly, oncologists have learned which lesions are best suited for which surgical methods and which are as effectively treated with RT. Survival figures for early stage laryngeal cancer (American Joint Committe on Cancer 1980) are essentially comparable with surgical or RT methods (Dickens et al 1983).

The process of selecting the most appropriate method for treating laryngeal cancer is not always simple and a number of factors should be taken into consideration. Patient health and reliability, the availability of skilled radiotherapist and surgeons and, finally, certain tumour characteristics enter the decision process.

BASIS FOR CLS

The larynx is compartmentalized in such a manner that its individual parts can be thought of almost as separate structures, both from an oncological, as well as a physiological, standpoint. In this regard, the organ itself is uniquely suited for tailored surgical methods. Between the supraglottic and the glottic-infraglottic larynx there exist a certain relative barrier to tumour spread from one area to the other. Additionally, lymphatics are distributed so that there is quadrant drainage. The epiglottis, however, should be viewed as a midline structure with a more complex drainage pattern; thus, lesions here demonstrate a propensity for bilateral metastasis. Lateralized supraglottic lesions are more likely to demonstrate ipsilaterally oriented metastatic patterns, but even these must be viewed critically for contralateral spread (Biller et al 1971). Within the supraglottic larynx itself, individual structures do not present the same barriers to tumour spread that exist in other laryngeal regions (McDonald et al 1976). For example, cancers of the false cords and aryepiglottic folds often involve deep structures, and lesions of the infrahyoid epiglottis frequently invade the pre-epiglottic space (Kirchner & Som 1971). With these facts in mind, the surgeon must exercise great caution in removing less than the entire supraglottic larynx.

The lymphatics of the true vocal cords (TVC) are sparse and, except for mucosal channels, there is little connection between left and right. Lesions here are partially confined by the conus elasticus, and, as such, are usually slow to escape the larynx. TVC cancer, therefore, lends itself nicely to CLS techniques. An exception to this is the posterior TVC, where cancer behaves less predictably, because of the abundance of lymphatics.

CLASSIFICATION OF CLS

Any surgery for laryngeal cancer that allows preservation of glottal voice production is conservation

Table 17.1 Classification of conservation laryngeal surgery

I. Endolaryngeal procedures
  A. Epiglottectomy
  B. Cordectomy
II. Extralaryngeal procedures
  A. Horizontally oriented procedures
    1. SGL
      a. partial-supraglottic
      b. standard SGL
    2. Partial laryngopharyngectomy
    3. Near-total laryngectomy
  B. Vertically oriented procedures
    1. Cordectomy via laryngofissure
    2. Hemilaryngectomy
    3. Frontal laryngectomy
    4. Frontolateral hemilaryngectomy

surgery. In the jargon of 1986, the term usually refers to variations on either supraglottic laryngectomy (SGL) or hemilaryngectomy; however, for the sake of thoroughness, our classification of conservation surgery is shown in Table 17.1.

SPECIFIC FACTORS INFLUENCING THE DECISION

Patient factors

When part of the larynx is removed, there is invariably some challenge to the lower airway. How much difficulty that follows depends not only on the particular part and extent of the removal, but also on the state of pulmonary health, i.e. the ability of the lungs to deal with chronic insult. Regardless of their general health and/or mental capabilities, patients usually cope well with the surgical treatment for isolated TVC cancer. Endoscopic laser cordectomy, or a variation of the hemilaryngectomy, are usually tolerated quite well unless the arytenoid cartilage is removed. With an intact arytenoid, the pseudocord often has adductive capabilities that help glottic closure, but even when the pseudocord is immobile, it forms a midline buttress onto which the mobile opposite cord can touch. Overall, about 20% of patients have some degree of aspiration after hemilaryngectomy, although it is usually mild (Schecter 1986).

Such is not the case for the SGL. With this operation, rehabilitation can be difficult. The instincts and reflexes inherent in swallowing and vocalization are primitive and profound. When altered by surgery, the rhythm associated with these voluntary acts can be lost and a significant part of this disruption relates to the alteration of supraglottic sensory nerves. In effect, the loss of supraglottic sensation alters the 'early warning' system and when this deficiency is added to the actual alteration of the anatomic lid over the laryngeal vestibule, food is dumped onto the glottic structures without adequate glottic preparation. Mastery of both swallowing and speech is enhanced by the patient's willingness and capacity to understand specific instructions given him. If the patient cannot be trained voluntarily to inspire, close the glottis, forcefully swallow and lastly cough, in that order, rehabilitation is difficult, sometimes impossible. The comprehension and concentration

on this sequence of voluntary acts is even more important in those patients in whom glottic closure has been compromised. Because older people do not usually adapt to such changes easily, special consideration must be given to age during the selection process for this operation. That is not to say, however, that age itself should be a contraindiction to SGL (Tucker 1977). Actually, given the right circumstances, older people fare surprisingly well with head and neck surgery; however, SGL is unique and presents a special challenge with which older patients have particular difficulty. Much of what is needed in the rehabilitative effort following SGL involves confidence—a state of mind that results from early success with swallowing efforts. Conversely, the rehabilitative process is thwarted when early attempts to swallow are associated with coughing, laryngospasm and aspiration. Additionally, because of the confidence factor, time does not necessarily correct the problem; one problem begets others.

Regarding the patient's health, the respiratory tract is most affected by partial laryngectomy and, especially in the elderly, careful consideration should be given to this system. Even when bilateral vocal cord motion is normal, many, if not most, patients who have had a SGL aspirate to some degree. How well they handle the varying amount of foreign material in the upper airway is the important issue. Patients with substantial obstructive lung disease have a limited ability to cough and the muscular debilitation of the thoracic cage that is associated with the perioperative period often makes matters worse. The astute clinician generally is able to estimate the relative functional pulmonary capability of a patient by watching him breath, talk and respond to modest exercise. The patient who cannot tolerate a brisk walk that includes the climbing of one flight of stairs will generally have significant difficulty with SGL; the person who does tolerate this activity is not usually troubled by the operation. A more sophisticated evaluation can and should be accomplished with pulmonary functions test (PFT) (Murray 1976). These should include flow loop studies to evaluate the upper airway. Although there is no absolute value marking a point of contraindication, those patients with substantial impairment (PFTs less than 50% predicted normal) should not have SGL. Less severe disease (PFTs 50–70%

predicted normal) are marginal candidates and it is with this group in which clinical judgement is so important.

Facility and logistical factors

Often non-medical factors are important in deciding between CLS and RT. Several authors (Schechter 1986, Thawley & Ogura 1979) have described the extensive network of support and expertise needed for sophisticated laryngeal RT, and many patients do not have access to radiation oncology centres that can produce optimal results. Also, the patient must be able to travel back and forth for RT and, if this is not possible, hospitalization for treatment is rarely practical given the current economic climate in the USA. Obviously, access to a surgeon capable of dealing with the nuances of contemporary laryngeal surgery is equally important. Whatever the treatment, a surgeon with appropriate endoscopic skills should be involved actively with the patient from the start. The honest appraisal of local capabilities must enter the decision of surgery versus RT and in this regard the integrity of those making the decision is paramount. Regarding cost, even when transportation and other expenses are considered, the cost of treating a vocal cord lesion with RT is probably less than that of having a hemilaryngectomy (Thawley & Ogura 1979).

There are those patients who are clearly better treated by surgery and then a group that are clearly better treated with RT. Finally, there exists that marginal group in which either modality is acceptable and it is this circumstance in which those factors such as logistics, expenses, specialty availability and patient bias become important to the decision process.

Tumour factors

Although there is some disagreement among surgeons regarding the individual tumour characteristics that preclude CLS, and while some surgeons are more aggressive than others in pursuing a conservation philosophy, there has been established a reasonably consistent set of guidelines that influence this decision. There are some absolute contraindications to CLS and some relative ones; with the latter, clinical judgement and experience are often critical in making the correct decision. Although modern imaging techniques have helped greatly in the three-dimensional analysis of laryngeal cancers, indirect laryngeal examination remains the cornerstone of the evaluation process. This method provides more valuable information to the astute diagnostician than any other. Subtle contour or colour changes of surface mucosa, or slight alterations in the movability of various portions of the larynx often reflect important factors about underlying disease. Often, pathology is clearly defined and treatment options straightforward; however, in some marginal situations, it is for the CT scan and direct laryngoscopic examination to answer the final question.

The most common of laryngeal cancers, glottic lesions, are usually placed into a therapeutic category without difficulty. All other factors such as logistics and specialty availability aside, early vocal cord lesions are effectively managed by either CLS or RT. We usually manage carcinoma in situ and some superficially invasive TVC lesions with laser vaporization, reserving RT for persistence. Laser systems have assumed a realistic place in the surgical armamentarium and are now correctly looked upon as merely another surgical tool, rather than an exotic technology. It is axiomatic, in utilizing the CO_2 laser, that the disease be accessible with a direct line of vision. Deflection techniques of laser light on reflective surfaces, while alluring, are somewhat uncertain and, when possible, should be avoided. With the aid of modern amplification, the directly visible lesion is effectively controlled by vaporizing down to the appropriate depth. If necessary, vocalis muscle is exposed and often partially vaporized. During follow-up observartion, small areas of recurrent cancer can even be revaporized without added jeopardy, provided, of course, an exact appreciation of the disease extent is possible. There are those who advocate endoscopic laser cordectomy for limited invasive cordal lesions (Blakeslee 1984). It is our feeling, however, that lesions involving more than superficial extension are best managed with RT, a modality that yields a high cure rate and outstanding voice quality.

With reference to evaluation, while CT imaging is helpful in measuring gross disease in the vocalis muscle, more subtle surface changes of superficial cancer escape today's technology. The clinical appraisal of surface motion and contour is more important than any image available today. Surface disease can alter the fluidity of mucosal motion, even though the gross excursion of the cord remains normal. The edge of such a vocal cord may appear stiff. On the other hand, if the abductive excursion is not brisk, we feel that the disease is usually too deep for vaporization.

With the exception of those superficial T1 lesions treated with laser, we treat T1 and many T2 vocal cord cancers with RT. T2 lesions with a large tumour volume are sometimes treated by hemilaryngectomy. Those T2 lesions, in which the inferior extent is questionable, usually are operated rather than radiated. Conservation surgery remains possible in most patients failing RT, provided the recurrence is found early (Biller et al 1970).

There are several glottic cancers that are uniquely deceptive and present special hazards with treatment. Those lesions located posteriorly can be troublesome because of the more abundant and less regular lymphatic drainage of that area. Additionally, there is less room here for inferior extension, and posterior lesions that extend subglottically are not only difficult to evaluate, but are also difficult to remove by partial laryngectomy. In general, those posterior lesions that can be completely visualized indirectly and are thought to be superficial are best treated with RT, even when they are onto the body of the arytenoid. If the lesion cannot be completely visualized, however, we perform an extended hemilaryngectomy—a procedure that includes arytenoid and possibly inferior extension. Just as tumour on the arytenoid is not a contraindication to RT, neither does it preclude hemilaryngectomy (Sessions 1980). The key to selecting the appropriate method is, in our view, more related to tumour depth. A good surgical margin is usually possible with hemilaryngectomy, if tumour involvement is limited to the vocal process and anterior half of the arytenoid body. However, in circumstances in which the entire arytenoid is involved, or in which there is any restriction of vocal cord motion, one must assume that there is tumour in the lateral musculature; thus the effectiveness of CLS would be less certain. Kirchner (1975b) and others (Mancuso et al 1982) have shown that, in posterior glottic lesions, invasion around the cricoarytenoid joint is the major cause of motion restriction. Evaluation of

the appearance and function of this area is best done by indirect laryngoscopy; the sophisticated laryngologist can usually distinguish between fixation of the arytenoid and impairment of motion that results from tumour bulk in adjacent membraneous cord. In most cases, the CT scan adds little to the clinical evolution of this area, usually serving only to confirm what is obvious to the laryngologist. Enough emphasis cannot be placed on the value of indirect laryngeal examination of the awake patient.

Another troublesome lesion is that cordal cancer extending onto the anterior commissure, or, less commonly, that begins primarily in the anterior commissure. Again we ascribe significance to the depth of the lesion. The anterior commissure ligamentous tissue is a sturdy barrier that influences the natural history of cancers in this area (Kirchner & Som 1975); accordingly, deep penetration into the adjacent cartilage, while possible, is not commonplace. In general, depth is best appreciated by endoscopic appraisal plus CT scan. We feel that easily visualized superficial anterior commissure lesions should be treated with RT. The repeated references in the older literature to a flawed isodosimetry that results in a 'cold spot' anteriorly is, in our view, a reflection of the inadequacies of radiotherapy techniques of the past. In effect, we have confidence in the ability of the therapist to deliver the appropriate dosage to the anterior commissure of the larynx. On the other hand, anterior cancers with extension onto the epiglottic petiole are viewed with the same concern given to infrahyoid epiglottic lesions. We are loathe to treat these tumours radiotherapeutically. Anterior commissure lesions with greater than 1 cm of caudal extension are at higher risk for escape through the cricothyroid membrane and should be treated with a frontal hemilaryngectomy. This particular lesion is especially difficult to evaluate and, for that reason, excision is desirable. Those membraneous VC lesions that happen to extend onto the anterior commissure are looked upon with the same concerns for depth and overall tumour bulk and, if deemed surgical lesions, an extended frontal hemilaryngectomy is done (Bailey 1971).

Lesions of the TVC that extend subglottically are removed by hemilaryngectomy, or an extended version of same, provided the disease does not exceed 1 cm in the anterior larynx or 5 mm posteriorly.

CT scanning is helpful in evaluating the subglottic larynx. We do not recommend radiating patients with this degree of subglottic disease.

Finally, there is that subgroup of TVC lesions in which there is motion restriction or even fixation. The subject of TVC motion restriction often involves subjective analysis—the excursion of many vocal cords designated as 'fixed' is often, in reality, only limited by adjacent tumour bulk. The recent literature has correctly emphasized the difference between 'impaired motion' and 'fixation'. Also, staging systems now underscore this difference by including those TVC lesions with some impairment of motion in the T2 grouping (American Joint Committee on Cancer 1980). Actual fixation does not always preclude the employment of hemilaryngectomy; however, such factors as invasion of the thyroarytenoid joint, transglottic extension, or subglottic extension posteriorly that fixes the cord to the cricoid, are not reliably managed with CLS techniques (McDonald et al 1976). For example, when fixation results from transglottic tumour extension, there is a 50% local failure rate associated with hemilaryngectomy (Biller & Lawson 1984). On the other hand, glottic cancers that result in cordal fixation because of vocalis muscle invasion can be encompassed acceptably with hemilaryngectomy, provided the tumour is limited to the endolarynx, does not have significant subglottic extension, or does not cause cartilage destruction (Lesinski et al 1976). Modern imaging is helpful in precisely delineating the periphery of such tumours and, especially in the non-radiated patient, CT scan and tomography enhance the selection process for hemilaryngectomy. Prior to the development of such technology, the imprecision of hemilaryngectomy on T3 glottic cancer was substantial.

The 'near-total laryngectomy' is an extended hemilaryngectomy that is designed to treat T3 lesions. In effect, the technique utilizes a preserved laryngeal remnant that is used for voice, although it cannot accommodate breathing without the aid of tracheostomy (Pearson et al 1980). Further application and data analysis are needed to delineate exactly the role of this clever technique in laryngeal cancer surgery.

Verrucous carcinoma is a controversial lesion that, because of concern for radiation-induced malignant transformation, is generally treated sur-

gically. Some radiotherapists (Burns et al 1976), on the other hand, have treated 'several' patients with this lesion that have responded favourably and not recurred. We have also seen two such laryngeal lesions treated satisfactorily with radiation therapy. We do, however, continue to have sufficient concern about malignant transformation to favour surgery whenever possible. Most laryngeal verrucous carcinomas are well managed by either laser vaporization for the smaller lesions, or hemilaryngectomy for more substantial tumours. When CLS is not possible, the patient should be appraised of the reluctance to employ RT; however, rather than remove the entire larynx, we recommend that modality, reserving laryngectomy for salvage. In such a situation, it is essential that the patient be closely followed, lest early detection of unfavourable change be missed. The biological behavior of verrucous carcinoma is locally less aggressive than standard squamous carcinoma, and one is able to extend the margins of CLS; thus a substantial portion of the larynx can be preserved with relative oncological safety (Schechter 1983).

We manage the majority of supraglottic carcinomas surgically, either by total or SGL. In general, those patients with smaller, i.e. more favourable, supraglottic cancers are usually treatable with either radiation therapy or SGL. On the other hand, more advanced lesions with TVC fixation are better treated with total laryngectomy. These are seldom eligible for RT as a primary treatment modality. Smaller supraglottic lesions that involve only the suprahyoid epiglottis, while unusual, are well managed with radiation therapy. Also, a small percentage of patients who are technically suitable for SGL are rejected for medical reasons, and are treated with radiation therapy—laryngectomy is reserved for salvage. Unless medical circumstances dictate otherwise, T2 lesions that involve the lower part of the supraglottis are managed with SGL. In such lesions, one should assume pre-epiglottic space invasion until proven otherwise; however, pre-epiglottic space involvement in itself, does not preclude SGL. In T2 lesions in which the arytenoid is involved with tumour, but in which the vocal cord motion is unchanged, the SGL can be extended to include the arytenoid cartilage (Ogura et al 1975).

Lesions of the suprahyoid epiglottis that involve the base of tongue (BOT) and lesions of the aryepiglottic folds that spill into the pyriform sinus are often problematic because these areas are not characterized by the barriers to spread seen in other parts of the larynx. Additionally, such cancers are often poorly differentiated and are characterized by ill-defined margins. These features, when combined with the lymphatic abundance characteristic of these areas, compromise local surgical control and increase the probability of cervical metastasis (McGavran et al 1961). These facts impact on the feasibility of employing CLS techniques, both from an oncological as well as a rehabilitative standpoint. Under such circumstances, the appropriate employment of these techniques tests the clinical judgement of the surgeon.

Those supraglottic lesions involving the BOT that are characterized by a clear anterior line of demarcation well posterior to the circumvallate papillae can be managed with a SGL extended anteriorly. The undifferentiated tumours, on the other hand, are not safely encompassed surgically, despite modern clinical and imaging techniques. Such lesions should be managed primarily with radiation therapy; total laryngectomy is reserved for salvage. It should also be mentioned that resection of the BOT in conjunction with SGL is probably the most challenging circumstance for swallowing rehabilitation. The posterior tongue provides an important shelf over the newly constructed larynx, and the amount of aspiration is directly proportional to the amount of tongue base removed. This must be considered in patient selection.

Primary pyriform sinus cancer is not often detected in the early stage, but when the opportunity does occur and when the disease occupies the medial wall exclusive of the apex, a variation of SGL known as a partial laryngopharyngectomy can be utilized for removal. Although CT scan gives some information of value, only endoscopy is consistently reliable for determining the lower extent of such lesions (Schechter 1986). In addition to direct visualization of tumour in the apex, a tell-tale sign of tumour involvement here is oedema of the adjacent subglottic area. At best, doing this operation for pyriform sinus cancer is fraught with oncological hazards and the occasional laryngeal surgeon should be discouraged from such an undertaking. The small pyriform sinus lesion suitable for RT techniques is the

exception. More often than not, these cancers require a total laryngectomy (Kirchner 1975a).

The status of the neck, while not in itself responsible for the method of managing laryngeal tumours, has a significant influence on that decision process. If the laryngeal primary is a small suprahyoid lesion and the neck is clinically negative, we usually treat the primary and neck by RT. Even in smaller supraglottic lesions, the incidence of neck metastasis is high enough (Lindberg 1972) to warrant its inclusion in the radiation portals. On the other hand, if a suprahyoid lesion is to be treated surgically and if the CT, as well as the clinical examination, of the necks are negative, we would do bilateral modified neck dissections (MND), harvesting the nodes at highest risk. Since we do not view the modified procedures as therapeutic, the presence of histological disease in the neck specimens would dictate radiation of the necks. We observe the N0 necks in only the very small suprahyoid epiglottic lesion. If a T2 supraglottic lesion is associated with clinical neck disease, we combine SGL with appropriate neck surgery and administer postoperative RT to the necks. In summary, irradiation and SGL are both highly successful modes of therapy for the early lesions, and it is seldom necessary to combine the two for initial management of the primary site; however, combined treatment seems indicated to control neck disease. We believe that dealing with the N0 neck in general, and especially the N0 neck with supraglottic laryngeal cancer, is less problematic since the popularization of the family of MND. Different sites within the supraglottis have different propensities for inapparent neck disease (Ogura et al 1971) and the utilization of the appropriate MND, while not absolute, provides a staging method that enhances the overall treatment plan.

The status of the neck can have a more direct effect on the decision process for the primary. An example is the very small suprahyoid lesion with clinical neck disease, bilaterally or unilaterally. Since combined therapy would be necessary for control of neck disease, we might elect to avoid partial laryngectomy, instead relying on radiation alone to the primary and surgery plus RT for the necks.

With reference to glottic cancer, the status of the neck usually has little bearing on the selection of the type of operation or RT. Practically speaking, glottic cancer is slow to metastasize and those lesions associated with neck disease are usually not amenable to CLS techniques anyway. Now that hemilaryngectomy is employed for selected T3 glottic cancers, however, this issue will become more relevant.

CONCLUSION

It is hoped that this overview of a rather extensive topic is viewed with the realization that indications and methods are dynamic and, as radiation oncologists have gradually refined their skills, alternative and equally effective methods for management of early laryngeal disease have evolved. We work in an era of multidisciplinary management of cancer and it is especially relevant to this atmosphere that laryngeal cancer treatment methods be selected that are oncologically, economically, physiologically and emotionally tailored to the particular problem and patient. As is true so often in such writing, scholarship must be blended with a certain dogma so that a specific direction is suggested to the reader. This is not to claim, however, that variations of this treatment are necessarily less than valid; rather they represent legitimate difference on how to manage complex problems.

INTRODUCTION

Treatment plans to a degree, for patients with carcinoma of the larynx, can be taxing and must be individualized. A simple algorithm is not possible. The goals are clear: as surgical oncologists we wish to rid the patient of disease and as reconstructive surgeons to minimize morbidity by performing functional conservation surgery.

Today's laryngeal surgeon is faced with a vast array of information and technical options with which he must be thoroughly familiar. He must have complete confidence in his expertise, otherwise he may consciously or subconsciously shelve a surgical option inappropriately.

Laryngeal surgery and radiation therapy are currently the two accepted methods of treatment. Both have similar cure rates reported for specific stages of disease. Either radiation or surgery may be the only primary therapy necessary, leaving the other option for salvage in the event of failure.

The Disease

One must first consider the disease process. The biological characteristics of the tumour must be evaluated. Is the cancer growing rapidly? Has the immunological response of the patient failed? Is the lesion exophytic and superficial, or deep and invasive? These characteristics can be assessed by history and physical, as well as other, diagnostic techniques including computerized axial tomography and magnetic resonance imaging. Histology, although not necessarily an indicator of long-term survival, may indicate the initial biological behaviour of the tumour. The patient's age, general health, pulmonary status, personality traits, family support and desire are all important considerations.

The physician

The expertise and ability of the medical personnel greatly influence the outcome of any treatment plan. The radiotherapist must set the most appropriate portals and administer the correct type and dose of radiation to both the primary and high-risk metastatic sites to irradicate effectively either occult or overt disease. Harwood et al (1979) reported a sizeable reduction in the number of local failures of early laryngeal carcinomas (TIS, TI) from 18% to 9% by changing the portal size from 5×5 cm to 6×6 cm. Likewise, by altering the total dose and daily fraction, Kim et al (1978) demonstrated much improved local cancer control. Similarly, the conservation laryngeal surgeon must exercise skill and good judgement in removing the tumour and reconstructing the defect so as to maximize cure rates and minimize morbidity.

The patient

Additional criteria, providing a basis for case selection besides the stage and location of the lesion, include the age and general health of the patient. We have been more surgically inclined in younger patients in order to avoid possible future development of radiation-induced tumours. The long-term cumulative effects of radiotherapy in the formation of a new malignancy seem to be very real. The incidence reported by Harwood and Lawson reveals statistics between 2% and 10% (Harwood et al 1979). The general health of the patient and pulmonary status play a significant role in the decision. Adequate pulmonary function is essential if partial laryngectomy is comtemplated. Lastly, we feel that patients with transportation problems, either to and from the radiotherapy treatment centre, or to and from the hospital for follow-up, are better treated by surgery if possible.

MANAGEMENT

Vocal cord carcinoma in situ

In our discussion of conservation laryngeal surgery, the objectives are to cure the patient and preserve vocal function. First let us consider cordal carcinoma in situ. It is known that carcinoma in situ may occur either as an isolated entity, or in association with invasive carcinoma. Bauer (1976) has stated that in a study involving 354 laryngeal cancer specimens, carcinoma in situ was also noted in 49%.

The actual definition and histological characteristics of carcinoma in situ remain controversial. The terms dysplasia, atypia and carcinoma in situ are at times used interchangeably. Clinically, carcinoma in situ looks granular, erythematous and seems to have an inflammatory component. Various pathologists have attempted to formulate rigid criteria in an effort to consistently characterize carcinoma in situ. Ultimately, this disorder is best treated by laryngoscopic excision at the time of biopsy. A 95% cure rate with only a 5% local recurrence rate was reported in a multiyear follow-up study (Lillie & DeSanto 1973).

The use of radiation therapy for in situ carcinoma of the larynx is controversial. Although most centres report cure rates exceeding 90%, Miller & Fisher (1971) have reported significant failures in approximately 50% of their patients. Other investigators have also reported failure rates of 11% and 26% following radiation (Aine & Fletcher 1976, Hintz et al 1981).

Glottic carcinoma

Glottic carcinoma is the most common site of involvement and fortunately produces early symptoms and rarely metastasizes. There are three therapeutic options: endoscopic removal using microlaryngeal or laser surgery, excision via an open approach, or external beam radiotherapy. Each of these modalities is effective and all report 5-year survival rates of approximately 95% (Neel et al 1980, Stewart et al 1975).

For lesions that are more extensive, but still with a mobile cord, Lawson & Biller (1981) have stated that, 'while radiotherapy is preferable to total laryngectomy in the management of these more extensive unilateral mobile cord lesions, the better local control provided by hemilaryngectomy ultimately results in more retained larynges and makes it the preferred mode of treatment'. Although the literature does not significantly confirm this statement, it does not refute it. It is the opinion of the authors that this rational is appropriate and thus surgery is preferred over radiotherapy, providing no circumstances preclude surgery.

Supraglottic carcinoma of the larynx

These tumours tend to be larger at the time of diagnosis, primarily because of their early asymptomatic behaviour. It is well known that these cancers metastasize more often and at an earlier stage than glottic carcinomas, because of the lymphatic pattern.

The patient's age and general pulmonary condition contribute the most important information influencing the decision to operate or radiate. A supraglottic laryngectomy is the preferred treatment modality if the patient's general health can tolerate the procedure. If the patients are elderly and in poor general health, they seem to better tolerate either radiotherapy or total laryngectomy.

Sorenson and others have reported a significant complication rate following partial laryngectomies on patients with previously irradiated supraglottic carcinomas (Sorenson et al 1980). Total laryngectomy is often the result of radiation failures in an effort to avoid this higher complication rate (Sorenson et al 1980, Stell & Dalby 1985). The inherent difficulty in examining the larynx following full course radiation therapy is well known. The larynx seems forever oedematous, appears inflamed, and tumour may grow undetected submucosally and insidiously throughout the radiated larynx. Tumour growth is difficult to assess and perhaps the increase in tumour bulk resulting from a possible delay in diagnosis may necessitate a more radical initial surgical procedure following radiotherapy. Ward has stated that persistent laryngeal oedema for more than 6 months following radiation therapy may be a prelude to the discovery of recurrent tumour (Ward et al 1975, Ogura et al 1975). Conservation laryngeal surgery remains a viable, albeit guarded, option following radiotherapy, since it is more often associated with an increase in morbidity due to postoperative fistulization. There may also be a dilemma in the determination of margins in radiated tissue if submucosal tumour is present. In addition, there remains the possibility of a second upper aerodigestive tract primary in 10–15% of the cases for which radiotherapy should perhaps be reserved. In general, however, if the patient with a supraglottic carcinoma is not a candidate for supraglottic laryngectomy, then radiation therapy for voice preservation is the next best choice, despite the possible necessity for a total laryngectomy, should radiotherapy fail.

Advanced laryngeal carcinoma

After focusing our attention on smaller and more manageable lesions of the larynx, we shall now discuss radical attempts to preserve the glottic mechanism in more advanced cancers.

Let us first consider the indications for horizontal subtotal supraglottic laryngectomy with arytenoid-ectomy and horizontal subtotal supraglottic laryngectomy with ipsilateral true vocal cord resection (three-quarter laryngectomy). Contraindications to these procedures include cancer invasion through the paraglottic space into the thyroid cartilage and involvement of the apex of the pyriform fossa, post-cricoid, or interarytenoid area. If only one arytenoid is involved, it may be removed. Arytenoid involvement implies no alteration of long-term survival; it does, however, increase morbidity. Glottic incompetence will likely result unless the vocal cord remnant is sutured posteriorly to the cricoid in the midline (Ogura et al 1975).

Indications for a three-quarter laryngectomy include a transglottic carcinoma that crosses the ventricle and involves both the false and the true vocal folds. The initial site of origin may be supraglottic with extension inferiorly onto the true cord, or, inversely, the tumour may originate on the true cord and extend superiorly. This procedure cannot be recommended for patients with extensive paraglottic space involvement. Likewise, those with vocal cord fixation, significant subglottic extension, cartilage invasion, or a history of prior radiotherapy are not appropriate candidates.

Reconstruction of the 'three-quarter laryngectomy' defect is challenging and several methods of reconstruction have been described. Utilization of the laryngeal cartilage as a 'fold-over' technique is one option (Ogura & Dedo 1965). Pearson has described reconstruction of the vocal cord using a muscle flap (Pearson & Donald 1984); the drawback tends to be muscle atrophy resulting in glottic incompetence. Other means of reconstruction include use of the contralateral superior cornu of the thyroid cartilage or the posterior aspects of the ipsilateral thyroid cartilage (Blaugrund & Kurland 1975).

Despite the development of these more radical and innovative techniques for the restoration of glottic mechanism following cancer ablation in the supraglottic larynx, there is, as yet, no consensus on the preferred way of treating more advanced supraglottic cancer.

In general, radiation alone provides relatively poor results for large lesions. Hansen (1975) reported less than a 50% cure rate with radiation as the sole modality of treatment. Radiation for T3 and T4 supraglottic lesions results in control rates of 36% and 15% respectively (Vermund 1970). It is our opinion that the role of radiotherapy in controlling advanced carcinoma of the supraglottic larynx remains unclear.

Numerous studies appear to question the efficacy of combined therapy. In these studies it seems that combined therapy offers no distinct therapeutic advantage over surgery alone and appears not to influence long-term survival (Goepfert et al 1975, Snow et al 1978, Schuller et al 1979). The concept of combined therapy does not appear to improve survival and in some cases may actually cause harm by exposing the patient to excessive unnecessary radiation. In a study of 236 patients which were treated by surgery alone, DeSanto (1985) demonstrated that the local recurrence rate was 3.3%. With a recurrence rate of this magnitude combined therapy does not seem warranted. To subject 90% of the population at risk to needless radiation appears unnecessary and is certainly not cost-effective. The reasons for attrition are more commonly regional and distant metastases and the concept of controlling disease in these areas utilizing radiotherapy is more appropriate.

Radical radiation for cure with surgical salvage (RRSS)

The intention of the radical radiation approach is primarily to save the larynx and preserve voice in a greater number of patients without compromising overall survival rates. Treatment failures are anticipated, however, if followed closely, early detection of recurrence is likely. Surgical salvage for recurrent cancer then, is said to provide an overall rate comparable to other treatment protocols (Halwood 1982, Hendrickson et al 1975). The net result is a larger yield of surviving patients with good glottic voice. Again, the problem is not so much local control, but regional control, primarily in the neck. DeSanto stated that when one compares a 5% probability of death from cancer in patients with N0 cervical staging treated by surgery alone, with a 42% probability in those with N0 neck disease treated by the RRSS approach, the difference is strikingly significant. If patients present with nodal disease, the difference is less; 53% probability of death with the RRSS approach compared with a 40% probability of those treated by surgery alone (DeSanto 1984).

The pendulum seems to swing back from the concept of radiating the N0 neck to, now, performing a functional neck dissection in patients at greater risk for occult cervical disease. The probability that radiation sterilizes occult metastases in the cervical lymph nodes is a controversial issue. In addition, the theory that one can carefully observe and wait for metastases to develop is likewise a risky process. We believe that an aggressive approach to more advanced carcinomas of the supraglottic larynx will yield, in the future, more satisfying results. Surgery in this area of advanced carcinoma of the supraglottic larynx continues to be our most encouraging therapeutic option.

DeSanto feels that the RRSS protocol is inappropriate in patients with early supraglottic cancer. The radical radiation concept is more attractive in the patient with T3 glottic carcinoma, because the alternative has historically been total laryngectomy.

Lastly, let us consider definitive therapy for a T3 carcinoma of the true vocal folds which implies, quite often, fixation of one of the vocal cords. As with carcinoma of the supraglottis, the concept of radical radiation with surgical salvage (RRSS) as compared to surgery alone should be considered.

Following analysis of the data, it appears that, in an effort to salvage glottal speech, RRSS offers a reasonable alternative to radical surgery. If after consultation the patient's primary desire is to preserve speech at the risk of possibly diminishing long-term survival, then the concept of RRSS should receive serious consideration. However, if the ultimate goal is to maximize long-term survival, then surgery including either partial or total laryngectomy seems to be the most appropriate recommendation.

also be considered in the above argument (Pearson et al 1980). The concept of near-total laryngectomy concerns approximately 50–60% of the patients who would have previously required total laryngectomy. Many carcinomas causing vocal cord fixation can be treated in this manner. Because a permanent tracheostoma is necessary with this procedure, we hesitate to call it a classic conservation procedure and yet because of the preservation of a pulmonary powered glottal speech, the procedure does fall within the realm of this discussion. Long-term survival does not appear to be compromised as is the case with radical radiotherapy and surgical salvage (DeSanto 1975, Pearson et al 1980). Data from a variety of sources will be helpful in eventually validating what appears to be an attractive alternative.

Improvement in long-term survival for these cancer patients is the major goal. Achieving this goal while limiting the morbidity and continually improving functional results through innovative techniques is of paramount importance.

REFERENCES

C B Goft

Bauer W C, Leonski S G, Ogura J H 1975 The significance of positive margins in hemilaryngectomy specimens. Laryngoscope 85–1

Bauer W C 1978 Concomitant carcinoma in situ and invasive carcinoma of the larynx. Canadian Journal of Otolaryngology 3: 533

Biller H, Ohura J H, Pratt L 1971 Hemilaryngectomy T2 glottic cancers. Archives of Otolaryngology 93: 238

Biller M F, Bergman J A 1975 Verrucous carcinoma of larynx. Laryngoscope 85: 1898

Bocca E, Pignataro O, Mouciaro D 1968 Supraglottic surgery of the larynx. Annals of Otology, Rhinology and Laryngology 77: 1005

Buck G 1853 On the surgical treatment of morbid growths within the larynx. TransAmerican Medical Association 6: 509

Burns H P, Van Nostrand A W, Bruce D P 1976 Verrucous carcinoma of the larynx: management by radiotherapy and surgery. Annals of Otology, Rhinology and Laryngology 85: 538

Burns H P, Bryce D P, Van Nostrand P A W 1979 Conservation surgery in laryngeal cancer and its role following failed radiotherapy. Archives of Otolaryngology 105: 234–239

Donald P J 1984 Management of the difficult case. In: The larynx in head and neck cancer. W B Saunders, Philadelphia

Harrison D F N 1985 Head and neck surgery in the 1980s: the role of more or less. Head and Neck Cancer 1: 27

Harwood A R, Hawkins N V, Keanes J 1980 Radiotherapy of early glottic cancer. Laryngoscope 90: 465

Kirchner J A 1984 Pathways and pitfalls in partial layngectomy Annals of Otology, Rhinology and Laryngology 93: 301

Lawson W, Som M 1975 Second primary cancer after irradiation of laryngeal cancer. Annals of Otology, Rhinology and Laryngology 84: 771

Leonard J R, Litton W B 1971 Selection of the patient for conservation surgery of the larynx. Laryngoscope 81: 232

Miller A H, Fisher H R 1971 Clues to the life history of carcinoma in situ of the larynx. Laryngoscope 81: 1475

Neel H B, Devine K D, De Santo L W 1980 Laryngofissure

and cordectomy for early cordal carcinoma: outcome in 182 patients. Otolaryngological Head and Neck Surgery 88: 79

Ogura J H, Sessions D G, Spector G J 1975 Analysis of surgical therapy for expidermoid carcinoma of the laryngeal glottis. Laryngoscope 85: 1522

Ogura J H, Thawley S E 1980 Treatment for early carcinoma of the larynx. Surgery is the treatment of choice. Controversy in Otolaryngology. W B Saunders, Philadelphia

Pressman J 1956 Submucosal compartmentation of the larynx Annals of Rhinology, Laryngology and Otology 65: 766

Russ J E, Sullivan C, Gallager H J, Jesse R H 1979 Conservation surgery of the larynx: a reappraisal based on whole organ study. American Journal of Surgery 138: 588–596

Schwartz A W 1978 Dr Theodore Billroth and the first laryngectomy. Annals of Plastic Surgery 1: 513

Silver C E 1981 In: Surgery for cancer of the larynx. Churchill Livingstone, Edinburgh

Snow J B, Gelber R D, Kramer S et al 1978 Evaluation of randomized pre operative and postoperative radiation therapy for supraglottic carcinoma. Annals of Otology 8: 686–691

Sorensen H, Hansen H S, Thomsen K A 1980 Partial laryngectomy following irradiation. Laryngoscope 90: 1344–1349

Stell P M, Dalby J E 1985 The treatment of early (T1) glottic and supraglottic carcinoma: does partial laryngectomy have a place? European Journal of Surgical Oncology 11: 263

Stewart J G, Brown J R, Palmer M R, Cooper A 1975 The management of glottic cancer by primary irradiation with surgery in reserve. Laryngoscope 85: 1477

Trotter W 1920 A method of lateral pharyngotomy for the exposure of large growths in the epilaryngeal region. Journal of Laryngology and Otology 35: 289

Wagenfield D J H, Harwood A R, Boyce D P, Van Nostrand A W P, de Boer G 1981 Second primary respiratory tract malignant neoplasms in supraglottic carcinoma. Archives of Otolaryngology 107: 135–137

Ward P H, Calcaterra T C, Ragan A R 1975 The enigma of post irradiation oedema and recurrent residual carcinoma of the larynx. Laryngoscope 85: 522

R B Sessions, R Parish

American Joint Committee on Cancer 1980 Manual of staging of cancer of head and neck sites and melanoma

Bailey B 1971 Conservation surgery in carcinoma of the anterior commissure. Southern Medical Journal 64: 305

Biller H, Lawson W 1984 Partial laryngectomy for transglottic cancer. Annals of Otology, Rhinology and Laryngology 93: 297

Biller H, Barnhill F, Ogura J, Perez C 1970 Hemilaryngectomy following radiation failure for carcinoma of the vocal cords. Laryngoscope 80: 249

Biller H, Davis W, Ogura J 1971 Delayed contralateral cervical metastasis with laryngeal cancers. Laryngoscope 81: 1499

Blakeslee D 1984 Excisional biopsy in the selective management of T1 glottic cancer. Laryngoscope 94: 488

Burns H, Van Nostrand A, Bryce D 1976 Verrucous carcinoma of the larynx: Management by radiotherapy. Annals of Otology, Rhinology and Laryngology 85: 538

Dickens W J, Cassissi M, Million R, Bova F 1983 Treatment of early vocal cord carcinoma. Laryngoscope 93: 216

Kirchner J 1975a Pyriform sinus cancer. Annals of Otology 84: 793

Kirchner J 1975b Staging as seen in serial sections. Laryngoscope 85: 1816

Kirchner J, Som M 1971 Clinical and histological observation in supraglottic cancer. Annals of Otology, Rhinology and Laryngology 80: 638

Kirchner J, Som M 1975 Anterior comissure technique of partial laryngectomy. Laryngoscope 85: 1308

Lesinski S, Bauer W, Ogura J 1979 Hemilaryngectomy for T3 epidermoid carcinoma of the larynx. Laryngoscope 86: 1563

Lindberg R 1972 Distribution of cervical lymph node metastases from squamous cell carcinoma of the respiratory and digestive tracts. Cancer 29: 1446

McDonald T, DeSanto L, Weiland L 1976 Supraglottic larynx and its pathology as studied by whole laryngeal sections. Laryngoscope 86: 635

McGavran M, Bauer W, Ogura J 1961 The incidence of cervical node metastases from epidermoid carcinoma of the larynx. Cancer 14: 55

Mancuso A, Harrafee W 1982 CT of the head and neck. Baltimore, Williams & Wilkins, p 1–65

Murray G 1976 Pulmonary complications following supraglottic laryngectomy. Clinics in Otolaryngology 1: 241

Ogura J, Biller H, Witte R 1971 Elective neck dissection for pharyngeal and laryngeal cancers. Annals of Otology, Rhinology and Laryngology 80: 647

Ogura J, Sessions D, Ciralsky R 1975 Supraglottic carcinoma with extension to the arytenoid. Laryngoscope 85: 1327

Pearson B, Woods R, Hartman D 1980 Extended hemi-laryngectomy for T3 glottic carcinoma. Laryngoscope 90: 1950

Schechter G 1983 Epiglottic reconstruction and subtotal laryngectomy. Laryngoscope 93: 729

Schechter G 1986 Conservation laryngeal surgery. In: Otological head and neck surgery, vol 3. C V Mosby, St Louis, ch 109, pt 4, p 2095

Sessions D 1980 Extended partial laryngectomy. Annals of Otology, Rhinology and Laryngology 89: 556

Thawley S, Ogura J 1979 Health care costs of laryngeal surgery. Laryngoscope 89: 595

Tucker H M 1977 Conservation laryngeal surgery in the elderly patient. Laryngoscope 87: 1995

J M Fredrickson, R L Brubaker

Aine F, Fletcher G H 1976 Results in irradiation of the in situ carcinomas of the vocal cords. Cancer 37: 2586

Bauer W C 1976 Concomitant carcinoma in situ and invasive carcinoma of the larynx. In: Workshops from the Centennial Conference on Laryngeal Cancer. Appleton-Century-Crofts, New York

Blaugrund S M, Kurland S R 1975 Replacement of the arytenoid following vertical hemilaryngectomy. Laryngoscope 85: 935

DeSanto L W 1984 T3 glottic cancer: Options and consequences of the options. Laryngoscope 94: 1131

DeSanto L W Cancer of the supraglottic larynx: A review of 260 patients. Otolaryngology Head and Neck Surgery 93: 705–711

Goepfert H, Jesse R H, Fletcher G H, Hamberger A 1975 Optimal treatment for the technically resectable squamous cell carcinoma of the supraglottic larynx. Laryngoscope 85: 14–32

Hansen H S 1975 Supraglottic carcinoma of the aryepiglottic fold. Laryngoscope 85: 1667

Harwood A R 1982 Cancer of the larynx: the Toronto experience. Journal of Otolaryngology 11 (suppl 11): 10–13

Harwood A R, Hawkins N V, Rider W D, Bryce D P 1979 Radiotherapy of early glottic cancer. International Journal of Radiation Oncology Biology Physics 5: 473

Hendrickson F R, Kline T C Jr, Hibbs G G 1975 Primary squamous cell carcinoma of the larynx. Laryngoscope 85: 1650–1666

Hintz B L, Kagan A R, Nussbaum H et al 1981 A 'watchful waiting' policy for in situ carcinoma of the vocal cords. Archives of Otolaryngology 107: 746

Kim J C et al 1978 Carcinoma of the vocal cord. Cancer 42: 1114

Lawson W, Biller H F 1981 Cancer of the larynx. In: Sven J Y, Meyers E N (eds) Cancer of the head and neck. Churchill Livingstone, New York, 456

Lillie J C, DeSanto L W 1973 Transoral surgery of early cordal carcinoma. TransAmerican Academy of Ophthalmology and Otolaryngology 77: 92

Miller A W, Fisher H R 1971 Clues to the life history of carcinoma in situ of the larynx. TransAmerican Laryngology, Rhinology and Otology Society 96: 666

Neel H B, Devine K D, DeSanto L W 1980 Laryngofissure and cordectomy for early cordal carcinoma: outcome in 182 patients. Otolaryngology Head and Neck Surgery 88: 79

Ogura J H, Dedo H H 1965 Glottic reconstruction following subtotal glottic-supraglottic laryngectomy. Laryngoscope 75: 865

Ogura J, Sessions D G, Spector G J 1975 Conservation surgery for epidermoid carcinoma of the supraglottic larynx. Laryngoscope 85: 1808

Pearson B W, Donald P J 1984 Larynx. In: Donald P J (ed) Head and neck cancer management of the difficult case. W B Saunders, Philadelphia

Pearson B W, Woods R D II, Hartman D E 1980 Extended hemilaryngectomy in T3 glottic carcinoma with preservation of speech and swallowing Laryngoscope 90: 1950

Schuller D E, McGuirt W F, Krause C J, McCabe B F, Pflug B K 1979 Symposium: Adjuvant cancer therapy of head and neck tumors. Increased survival with surgery alone vs. combined therapy. Laryngoscope 89: 582–594

Snow J B Jr, Gelber R D, Kramer S, Davis L W, Marcial V A, Lowry L D 1978 Evaluation of randomized preoperative and postoperative radiation therapy for supraglottic carcinoma: Preliminary report. Annals of Otology, Rhinology and Laryngology 87: 686–691

Sorenson H, Hansen H S, Tomsen K A 1980 Partial laryngectomy following irradiation. Laryngoscope 90: 1344–1349

Stell P M, Dalby J F 1985 The treatment of early (T1) glottic and supraglottic carcinoma: does partial laryngectomy have a place? European Journal of Surgical Oncology 11: 263

Stewart J G, Brown J R, Palmer M R, Cooper A 1975 The management of glottic cancer by primary irradiation with surgery in reserve. Laryngoscope 85: 1477

Vermund H 1970 Role of radiotherapy in cancer of the larynx as related to the TNM system of staging. Cancer 25: 485

Ward P H, Calcaterra T C, Ragan A R 1975 The enigma of postirradiation edema and recurrent residual carcinoma of the larynx. Laryngoscope 85: 522

18

The role of primary surgery for oral cancer?

G.B. Snow

Squamous cell carcinomas make up the great majority of malignant tumours of the oral cavity. For squamous cancers in most parts of the mouth and certainly at the sites most frequently involved like the mobile tongue and floor of mouth, the status of the cervical lymph nodes is the single most important prognostic factor (Harrold 1969, Hibbert et al 1983) The behaviour of these tumours with regards to their metastases to regional lymph nodes is of utmost importance in establishing any plan of therapy.

Depending on the policy of the institution, the primary cancer is treated either surgically or by radiotherapy. In locally advanced tumours it has been the common practice over the last 15 years to apply radiation therapy as a pre- or postoperative adjuvant to surgical resection. Solid evidence to support the validity of this combined approach, however, is lacking. Treatment of metastatic neck nodes has traditionally been by surgery, although elective irradiation of the neck has been recommended for the management of occult metastasis.

In this chapter a management policy for oral cancer will be reviewed that is based on primary surgery. It is important to note that this policy has been developed over the years in an institution where the team approach to the problem of management is considered mandatory and where radiotherapists and surgeons work closely together. Management of the primary tumour and that of the neck, although intimately associated, for reasons of clarity will be discussed separately. Firstly, selection of patients will be considered. Finally, combined radiation and surgery.

SELECTION OF PATIENTS

During the past decade sophisticated techniques of reconstruction have become available, which allow for repair of almost every defect. Furthermore, oral cancer is rarely inoperable on account of its local, regional or distant spread, whereas the mortality rate for major head and neck surgery has steadily declined to 1–3% (Beahrs 1973, McGuirt et al 1979). However, when the magnitude of the resection will be such that the patient will be left with a functional deficit resulting in a poor future quality of life, the question arises whether the patient is better off left untreated by surgery. An example of this problem is when total removal of the tongue is required to eradicate the disease. No general advice can be given to this problem; the solution should be individualized for each patient, philosophy and psychology of both patient and doctor playing an important role.

Anaplastic carcinomas usually behave aggressively in a diffuse way and, therefore, should not be treated surgically but by radiotherapy. This also holds true for most of the poorly differentiated squamous cell carcinomas. Both histological types of tumours, however, are rare in the oral cavity. Rapidly progressing well-, or moderately differentiated squamous cell carcinomas—also an unusual situation—should probably better not be attacked by surgery as the first modality of treatment.

Finally, of course, are medical contraindications for surgery. Although, in general, biological age has to be taken into account, it appears from the studies of Williams & Murtagh (1973) and McGuirt et al (1977) that the age of 80 marks the limit for major head and neck surgery.

MANAGEMENT OF THE PRIMARY TUMOUR

The surgical management of primary tumours is different for the various anatomical sites within the mouth. A detailed account of surgical treatment relative to site of primary tumour would be beyond the scope of this chapter. This review, therefore, will be limited to the most frequently involved sites: the mobile tongue and the floor of the mouth. These two sites also happen to be the areas of controversy when choice of treatment is considered. In tumours close to bone or invading bone, like carcinoma of the gums, it is generally agreed that radiotherapy is usually less successful than surgery (Lee & Wilson 1973, Henk 1985), whereas for carcinoma of the cheek mucosa Vegers et al (1979) found, in one of the few large series of patients published, that surgery was superior over radiotherapy for each T- and N-stage.

The importance of successful treatment of the primary tumour is apparent from the poor results almost invariably obtained in the treatment of locally recurrent disease. Cancers of the mobile tongue and floor of the mouth, particularly, may spread easily along submucosal, muscular and neural planes. Except for the small (< 1 cm) T1 lesions with minimal invasion, generous margins should be taken. Westbury (1981) states that a margin of 2 cm in all three dimensions is required for all deeply invasive cancers of the tongue. Byers et al (1978) emphasize the value of frozen section microscopic studies for the determination of the extent of the surgical margins. The author of this chapter has found electrocoagulation of the tumour before the excision has begun very helpful in determining the extent of the lesion (Snow 1984).

For practical reasons, management of the primary tumour will be considered first for small tumours, T1 and T2, less than 4 cm in greatest diameter and then for more extensive lesions.

Treatment of small tumour

Small cancers of the mobile tongue situated anteriorly can be excised readily through the mouth. The defect is usually closed primarily; this does not impair tongue mobility, because the floor of the mouth is stretched out. Large superficial defects resulting from excision of minor invasive carcinoma with extensive areas of leucoplakia are resurfaced with a split skin graft (McGregor & McGrouther 1978). Partial glossectomy requires only a few

hospital days and the effect on articulation and swallowing is usually minimal.

In T1 and T2 tumours of the mobile tongue, partial glossectomy results in a high percentage of control at the primary site in the order of 90% and 80%, respectively (Spiro & Strong 1971, Marks et al 1981). Similarly, excellent control of the primary lesion is possible with radiation therapy. Interstitial irradiation of the primary tumour by implantation is generally agreed to be considerably better than external beam therapy alone (Pierquin et al 1971, Fu et al 1976, Decroix & Ghossein 1981). The question then, whether one of the two methods of treatment—surgery or radiotherapy—is superior, focuses on the morbidity associated with these treatments rather than on their results. The morbidity is obviously different for the two methods, whereas measures of quality of oral function after treatment are either lacking or imprecise (Teichgraeber 1985). After surgery there is always loss of oral function, though usually to a small degree. In contrast, the main complication associated with radiotherapy is radiation-induced ulceration, manifesting as painful recurrent ulceration after initial healing. This causes considerable discomfort and pain and may present a diagnostic dilemma during follow-up. Meikle et al (1985) recently reported that this complication developed in one-third of their cases. Although most of these radiation-induced ulcers heal eventually, some never do. Concern about this complication has led us to abandon interstitial radiotherapy for oral cancer at our institution and we prefer surgery as primary treatment. Also, we could not reproduce the excellent results with interstitial irradiation as reported above and this has been the experience of many others (Marks et al 1981, Leipzig et al 1982, Frazell & Lucas 1962).

Treatment of large tumours

As the lesions increase in size and become more infiltrative, the results of surgery are considerably better than those obtained by radiation therapy (Hirata et al 1975, Guillamondegui et al 1980, White & Byers 1980). The cosmetic and functional loss which result from the commando type surgery that is needed for these advanced tumours, naturally increase directly with tumour size. However, surgical techniques of both resection and repair, have improved considerably during the last 15 years and have resulted in a considerable reduction in both the funtional and cosmetic difficulties which the patient faces after major surgery.

An important point in this regard is the management of the mandible which is considered in three categories: those with gross invasion where resection is inevitable, those with a degree of involvement and those in whom there is still a measurable distance of several millimetres of normal mucosa between the gross edge of the lesion and the mandible. It has been held that the mandible, although uninvolved by tumour, should be resected in large tumours of the tongue and the floor of the mouth to get better access to the primary tumour and to facilitate primary closure. With the availability of adequate procedures of exposure, like the mandibular 'swing' approach (Spiro et al, 1981) and of the methods of reconstruction discussed below, this view is certainly obsolete. It has also been stated that the lymphatic channels draining the tongue and floor of mouth communicate with the periosteal lymphatics of the mandible and this necessitates resection of bone. This view, too, is to be discarded since Marchetta et al (1971) and Carter et al (1980) have clearly demonstrated that involvement of the periosteum or underlying bone is by direct extension of tumour and not through periosteal lymphatics. In most patients belonging to the two last categories mentioned above, a more conservative management of the mandible, marginal mandibulectomy, can be considered and indeed has been proved feasible (Guillamondegui & Jesse 1976, Callery et al 1984).

Many notable advances have been made in the field of reconstructive surgery in the last decade (Daniel & Taylor 1973, McGregor & Morgan 1973, McCraw et al 1977). For oral lining and replacement of soft tissue loss the reconstructive surgeon today has a wide variety of methods available in his armamentarium, ranging from local (Cohen & Theogarj, 1975) and regional flaps (Ariyan 1979) to microvascular free flaps (Soutar et al 1983). A major advantage of these methods over those used in the past is that these can be used as a single stage procedure and this has considerably reduced the average stay in hospital. The pectoralis major myocutaneous flap is safe and can reach all areas of the oral cavity (Tiwari & Snow, 1983). It has the disadvantage,

however, that it is a bulky flap, which in general makes it less feasible when mandible has been preserved. When mandible has been resected, and it is felt that it should be replaced as in an anterior arch defect, bone can be included in a regional or free flap (Franklin et al 1980, Panje & Cutting 1980) at the time of immediate reconstruction. Alternatively, mandibular reconstruction can be carried out as a secondary procedure provided measures to prevent mandibular drift are being taken at the initial operation (Snow et al 1976).

From the literature, it is clear that at least 50% and probably 75% of the patients with large tumours require surgical treatment after initial irradiation and that surgery controls approximately 30% of these cases (McQuarrie 1986). The extent of residual or recurrent disease after radiation therapy is often difficult to assess. As a result, much wider excisions are needed than had been carried out if initial surgery would have been preferred. Marginal mandibulectomy, for instance, is rarely feasible in salvage surgery for large tumours. The complication rates of salvage surgery for irradiation failures are high (Joseph & Shumrick 1973), whereas reconstruction is associated with special problems. Finally, it is important to note with regards to the small proportion of patients in whom radiotherapy might be successful in eradicating local disease, that radiotherapy is often associated with major complications (Larson et al 1983) and xerostomia.

MANAGEMENT OF NECK NODES

The clinically negative neck

Although Vandenbrouck et al (1980), reporting on the results of a randomized clinical trial on elective versus therapeutical radical neck dissection in oral cancer, concluded that it is justified to delay neck dissection until a node becomes clinically palpable, controversy has remained regarding the treatment policy of the N0 neck. Long-standing, continuing discussion as to the indications for elective neck dissection, is furthermore complicated by the more recent publications that elective irradiation of the neck might be equally effective in eliminating microscopical nodal disease (Fletcher 1972, Million 1974, Mendenhall et al 1980). In general, elective treatment of regional neck nodes is considered indicated when there is a high likelihood of occult nodal metastasis, when the status of the cervical nodes cannot adequately be assessed, as in patients with short muscular necks, when the patient will not be available for regular follow-up visits, or when the neck must be entered for access to and/or resection of the primary tumour, as is nearly always the case in advanced carcinoma of oral tongue and floor of mouth. The question of the likelihood of microscopical nodal metastasis therefore focuses on T1 and T2 tumours.

It has been reported that the incidence of false-negative neck nodes depends on the extent of the primary tumour (Mendenhall et al 1980). However, others (Hibbert et al 1983, Ali et al 1985) could not find any relationship between the T-stage of the primary tumour and the incidence of false negative nodes. Even patients who have a T1 lesion of the mobile tongue and whose nodes are initially disease-free will have a nodal metastasis develop in the neck in 19–36% (Spiro & Strong 1971, Mendelson et al 1976, Becker et al 1986). Nodal conversion rates for T2 and T3 lesions are equally high. Treatment of late-onset cervical metastasis carries a poor prognosis: not more than 35% of these patients can be cured (Lee & Litton 1972, Marchetta et al 1977, Whitehurst & Droulias 1977, Johnson et al 1980). Based on this indirect evidence, an aggressive management policy as to the clinically negative neck is being carried out in most institutions (Spiro & strong 1971, Mendelson et al 1976, Whitehurst & Droulias 1977, Leipzig & Hokanson 1982, Lldstad et al 1983). The author recommends that all patients with deeply invasive (> 0.5 cm) tumours have elective treatment of the neck. This includes virtually all T2 (and larger) tumours and a fair proportion of T1 lesions.

To the author's knowledge, a randomized prospective trial comparing elective neck dissection to elective irradiation of the neck has not been carried out. Both modalities have their morbidity. If an 11th nerve-sparing operation is done (Bocca et al 1980, Jesse 1981) morbidity is minimal. Elective irradiation avoids initial tissue loss, but is associated with xerostomia (Cummings 1984). An important advantage of surgery over radiotherapy is that surgery allows for histopathological examination and staging of the neck nodes and identification of un-

favourable histological factors, such as extranodal spread. It has been demonstrated that extranodal spread is present in 14–22% of nodes that are less than 1 cm in diameter and thus can easily be missed by clinical palpation. When extranodal spread is found, postoperative irradiation is applied (see below).

The clinically positive neck

For any patient who has clinical evidence of cervical node involvement, a radical neck dissection is carried out. The feasibility of preservation of the spinal accessory nerve in each individual case has to be carefully evaluated during dissection. For those patients in whom the spinal accessory nerve has to be removed, Jones & Stell (1985) developed a modified technique of radical neck dissection preserving the cervical spinal nerves to the trapezius muscle. Comparison of patients undergoing this modified radical neck dissection with patients undergoing a classical radical neck dissection shows them to have better shoulder function.

When nodal metastasis is present on admission, the neck operation is performed in continuity with excision of the primary tumour because viable tumur cells may be present in the lymphatics between primary and regional nodes. However, Spiro & Strong (1971) have demonstrated that the principle of incontinuity neck dissection may be abandoned in selected patients without affecting the cure rate.

COMBINED RADIATION AND SURGERY

Combined radiation and surgery became popular in the 1960s for advanced head and neck cancers at certain sites, such as in the oral cavity. This multimodality approach attempts to increase the effectiveness of therapy to these problem areas. The philosophy behind this treatment is that surgery fails at the periphery and radiotherapy at the poorly oxygenated centre of the tumour and that, hopefully, a combination of the two might do better than either alone.

Radiotherapy can be administered either preoperatively or postoperatively; both methods have their advantages and disadvantages (Cachin &

Eschwege 1975). Preoperative radiation is supposed to sterilize the tumour cells at the margin of the tumour and to reduce the risk of implantation of metastasis within the surgical field and of iatrogenic metastasis beyond the head and neck. However, it entails the disadvantage of increasing the complication rate of surgery. Furthermore, it limits the possibility of more effective postoperative radiation when this is desirable. Another disadvantage of preoperative radiotherapy is that it may obscure tumour margins, which may render it difficult for the surgeon to determine the adequacy of resection. Postoperative radiotherapy carries three advantages: on the basis of the histopathological report of the surgical specimen, radiation can be justified and planned more selectively, it has no influence on surgical complication rates and it is usually better tolerated by the patient than preoperative radiation therapy. However, at least on theoretical grounds, radiotherapy is assumed to be less effective when vascularization of the tissues has been disrupted by previous surgery. Furthermore, postoperative irradiation may be delayed by complications in wound healing. Finally, it obviously has no influence on iatrogenic metastasis to distant sites.

Most experiences have been gained with preoperative radiation therapy. Terz & Lawrence (1981) reviewed all literature reporting the results of clinical experience with preoperative radiation for head and neck cancer between 1969 and 1979. Regarding retrospective studies the evidence is conflicting. Initial studies in selected patient populations have reported a beneficial role of radiation therapy as a preoperative adjunct. In contrast, later studies (Carpenter et al 1976, Schuller et al 1979) could not establish that combined therapy offers improvement over surgery alone. More importantly, all three randomized prospective clinical trials (Strong et al 1978, Hintz et al 1979, Terz et al 1981) failed to demonstrate any higher survival for those patients receiving preoperative radiation when compared with control groups treated by surgery alone. The question regarding the role of preoperative radiotherapy in the management of head and neck cancer finally appears to have been answered by the outcome of these randomized trials. To this conclusion the objection might be raised that the low doses of irradiation used in two of these three randomized studies might not be as effective as higher doses given over a longer period of time. The higher incidence of postoperative complications associated with higher doses, however, may well preclude the feasibility of such a preoperative radiation approach.

An increasing number of reports advocate postoperative rather than preoperative irradiation (Jesse & Lindberg 1975, Vandenbrouck et al 1977, Marcus et al 1979, Vikram et al 1980, Bartelink et al 1983, Mantravadi et al 1983). The histopathological information on the resected specimen can be used to select the patients who are most likely to benefit from combined treatment, i.e. those patients with a significant probability of local and/or regional failure after surgery alone. Patients with tumour close to, or at, the surgical resection margins are at high risk of recurrent malignancy. Looser et al (1978) reported a 71% tumour recurrence rate in patients with inadequate margins as compared to 32% in patients with tumour-free margins. Similarly, Byers et al (1978) found a local recurrence rate of only 12–18% in patients with tumour-free margins as compared to 80% of patients in whom free margins could not be achieved. With the addition of immediate postoperative radiotherapy in patients with tumour at surgical margins, Vikram et al (1980) reported a significant decrease in relapse rates from 50–75% to 18%. Similarly, Mantravadi et al (1983), in their study on the value of postoperative radiotherapy for persistent tumour at the surgical margins, reported a 31% tumour recurrence rate for patients with microscopical tumour at resection margins versus 50% for those with macroscopical tumour. These results indicate an improved prognosis for patients with advanced tumours with persistent tumour at the margin using combined surgery and postoperative radiotherapy over that achieved with surgery alone.

The value of postoperative irradiation therapy has been demonstrated particularly in regards to failure in the neck. The reported recurrence rate in the neck after radical neck dissection alone varies from 14–30% (Beahrs & Barber 1962, Strong et al 1966, Jesse & Fletcher 1977). Such recurrences depend directly on the extent of metastatic disease present at the time of surgery. Histopathological examination of the neck dissection specimen has been shown to be far more accurate than nodal palpability in the assessment of the extent of metastatic disease in the neck. Particularly when extranodal spread and multiple histologically positive nodes are present there is a high risk of recurrence in the neck (Kalnis et al 1977, Micheau et al 1978, Cachin et al 1979, Johnson et al 1981, Snow et al 1982). In these cases, surgery should be followed by radiotherapy, as it has been demonstrated that postoperative radiation therapy is effective in reducing the number of recurrences in the neck (Jesse & Fletcher 1977, Vikram et al 1980, Bartelink et al 1983, Arriagada et al 1983, Goffinet et al, 1984, Snow et al, 1986).

If irradiation is given postoperatively, it must cover the entire operated area that is at risk. When there is a substantial risk of contralateral neck node metastasis, postoperative radiation is given to the opposite side of the neck as well. An important point in postoperative radiotherapy is that it should be started within 3–4 weeks after the surgical procedure (Jesse & Lindberg 1975) and not later than after 6 weeks as it has been demonstrated that further delay in the start of postoperative radiation therapy might indeed affect the results adversely (Vikram 1979, Mantravadi et al 1983). It should be realized that radiation therapy adds significantly to the patient's permanent disability (Schuller et al 1983).

SUMMARY

In small oral cancers surgery is at least as effective as radiotherapy in eradicating tumour at the primary site. In this situation the effect of surgery on oral function is minimal, whereas radiotherapy, apart from the usual xerostomia, is quite often associated with radiation-induced ulceration, causing considerable discomfort. In large tumours the results of surgery are considerably better than those obtained by radiation therapy, whereas improvements in techniques of both resection and repair have resulted in a considerable reduction in the functional and cosmetic difficulties which the patient faces after major surgery. Spread to regional lymph nodes is common and, accordingly, the neck is usually treated in continuity with the excision of the primary tumour. Patients with inadequate surgical margins, extranodal spread or multiple histologically positive nodes should have immediate postoperative radiotherapy.

To consider the case for primary surgery in the management of oral cancer is to review a treatment option out of context. It is more appropriate to discuss a philosophy of management which allows the flexibility of a multidisciplinary approach. Identifying the impact of any one method of treatment of cancer is difficult, since the traditions of management, availability of other specialists, patterns of referral and definitive expertise vary from centre to centre. The established trend of multimodality management in head and neck oncology makes strict comparisons a problem because important nuances of patient and disease variation may not be reflected in staging.

Oral cavity cancers comprise cancer of the lips, floor of mouth, oral tongue, buccal mucosa, upper and lower gingiva, hard palate and the retromolar trigone. The most common of these are cancers arising in the floor of the mouth and the tongue, and it is on those that the discussion of this chapter will concentrate.

The absolute mortality from cancer of the oral cavity has decreased rapidly over the last 20 years (OPCS Cancer Statistics Registrations 1982). This is due to a fall in incidence and not to improved results from therapy. Advances in public health measures, in dental hygiene, nutrition and the more effective treatment of syphilis can take some of the credit for this declining incidence. However, smoking, although decreasing, and the excessive intake of alcohol, are aetiological factors which still persist. When discussing the management of oral cancer, it must be remembered that patients with this disease are frequently in poor general condition and often will not tolerate the radical procedures of surgery, radiotherapy and chemotherapy which could be appropriate.

Disappointingly for those of us using newer techniques, both of surgery and radiotherapy, in the management of patients with carcinoma of the oral cavity, the relative mortality has not changed over a 30-year period. This finding has been documented by Strong (Callery et al 1984) in America and by Stell (Stell & McCormick 1985) in the UK. At the Memorial Hospital in New York, there was a definite improvement in cure rate from 1927 to 1957 but from 1957 to 1978 there was no significant improvement in cure rate although the overall dis-

tribution of patients by clinical stage had remained constant. It must, therefore, be remembered that the impact of newer surgical techniques and radiotherapy apparatus has not been on mortality, but on morbidity. During this time there was considerable reduction in morbidity with less patients having the aggressive commando type surgery. The cosmetic and functional result which follows the use of jaw-sparing procedures, such as marginal mandibulectomy and mandibulotomy with paralingual extension, is readily apparent. The advent of supervoltage radiotherapy produced a marked decrease in morbidity from radiation. A high dose in the area of the tumour with relative sparing of the surrounding tissues and a much reduced biological dose to bone was achieved. Complex arrangements of supervoltage fields prevent excessive radiation to the parotid glands. This avoids the dry mouth, which resulted from irradiation of the whole oral cavity, when widespread gum retraction and dental caries ensued. Improved awareness of the necessity for good oral hygiene and a close assessment of teeth prior to radiotherapy also results in many patients completing their treatment with useful and effective dentition. The impact of primary surgery must be considered against the background of this developing expertise in all fields.

The importance of historical studies of mortality cannot be overestimated and make it difficult to be overconfident about recent advances. The head and neck area is not the only field of cancer management where mortality is remaining the same in centres of excellence, but morbidity is decreasing (Spittle 1984). This is no small achievement. However, reduction in mortality must continue to be the goal. It is probable that parallel centres with less experience will have improved standards of management, reflecting the expertise publicized from larger centres. Reduced morbidity will only be achieved where there is multidisciplinary management of the patient with oral cancer. Fortunately, in the head and neck field there has been a long-standing tradition of combined management clinics with otolaryngologists, radiotherapists, oncologists, pathologists, dentists and radiologists. This is particularly important since the techniques, both surgical and radiotherapeutic that are employed, are often at the extreme limit of tolerance of the tissues involved. If therapies are combined in this context, a close working relationship with a knowledge of other fields of management is essential. It is also only by staging patients accurately that comparison within and across series may occur. The problems of assessing advances in this field make it the responsibility of those who see large numbers of patients to ensure adequate documentation and correct staging. The latter can be achieved using the staging system proposed by the American Joint Committee on Cancer (AJCC) (Beahrs & Myers 1983), or the International Union against Cancer (IUCC) (Union International Contre le Cancer 1978).

Without effective combined clinics, the management of patients with cancer of the oral cavity can all too readily be determined by the specialist to whom they present. This may not be in the patient's best interest. Early lesions of the tongue, particularly those occurring on the tip, can readily be treated by local excision. Primary surgery is ideal in this situation, although such small tumours are rare. However, even when surgery has been performed and histological clearance has been demonstrated, local recurrence may occur because of the small size of the incisions practicable and the difficulty of judging disease at this site. Excision or irradiation produce similar control rates and the choice of treatment is determined by the morbidity produced.

Radiotherapy by interstitial implant is an excellent treatment for early cancers, particularly of the lateral border and dorsum of the anterior two-thirds of the tongue. A well-performed two-plane implant should be adequate radical treatment. The radioactivity implanted may be left for 5–8 days to achieve a tumouricidal dose and, since the tongue is vascular and forgiving of radiation damage, radiotherapy complications should not ensure (Larson et al 1983). However, the tip of the tongue is technically difficult to implant and is the most suitable site for surgery.

A small radiotherapy implant to an early lesion in the floor of the mouth is also well tolerated with minimal long-term side-effects. However, the proximity of bone makes the adequacy of the implant more critical and, although rare when using interstitial treatment, may result in an incidence of osteonecrosis (Marks et al 1983). This is seen occasionally with external beam radiotherapy. The incidence of osteonecrosis increases in patients with poor dental condition and, particularly, with very advanced disease. Superficial limited lesions of the floor of mouth may be succesfully treated by excision, with or without rim resection of the mandible.

The decision between primary surgery or radiotherapy for management of these small lesions of the tongue and floor of the mouth is not really of over-riding importance since such lesions are readily cured by either method. The radiotherapist's cynical view that 'early lesions are too early for surgery and late lesions are too late for surgery' may be voiced about cancers of the oral cavity. The trend away from management either by surgery or radiotherapy and towards joint management is often a result of combined oncology clinics. Although occasionally 'management by committee' may lead to unconventional or muddled decisions, in general the added expertise results in more perceptive treatment regimes.

The early trend away from surgery to combined management raises the question of whether surgery or radiotherapy should be the first in this combination. Despite the inability to support the argument with facts, aficionados of either regime are convinced of its effectiveness. The arguments for primary radiotherapy revolve around the importance of a maintained blood supply, since radiotherapy injury is greatest to cells which are well oxygenated (Belli et al 1962). An area which has been operated is likely to have a parlous, or at least prejudiced, blood supply to areas of residual tumour. Likewise, the radiotherapist feels that a relatively wide area can be treated by a method that largely ignores anatomy and may thus be able to sterilize the periphery of a tumour, leaving the surgeon faced with a more appropriate field for his surgery. However, it is certain that radiotherapy itself will gradually impair the vasculature of the area treated and the fact that surgery relies for its success on a good blood supply is also true. The well vascularized flaps used now for major surgery in the head and neck area mobilize and bring with them an excellent, reliable blood supply and are well able to withstand radical irradiation. The problem arises with the possibility of tumour remaining in the often less robust periphery of the flap at the site of initial disease. The important unanswered question is whether a lesion, initially inoperable and therefore incurable by virtue of its extent, can ever be made curable by preoperative radiotherapy—although it can frequently be made technically operable.

The surgeon dealing with otolaryngological malignancies should be competent to operate following full radical doses of radiotherapy. Any proposed surgery which compromises the dose of radiotherapy which can be given will produce an ineffective result and be useless. Therefore, that combination of radical radiotherapy and surgery which can be tolerated by a stoical patient and administered by co-operating specialists, offers the patient with moderately advanced carcinoma of the oral cavity the best chance of cure. Where initial radiotherapy has been given, surgery may either be contemplated as part of a predetermined treatment programme initiated at the outset, or it may be utilized when it has become clear that the radiotherapy treatment has failed to cure. The complications of surgery following radiotherapy are undoubtedly more than when radiotherapy has not been employed. The dual injury of radical radiotherapy and radical surgery to an area already compromised by tumour may be sufficient to cause necrosis of bone and flaps. However, it is also true that there are many problems encountered by the radiotherapist when treating an area that has been the site of radical surgery. It seems illogical to give high-dose irradiation to suture lines and anastomoses, which may be initially tenuous, or to a flap which has been brought in from elsewhere and is, therefore, not at risk for recurrence and yet forms the major part of the tissue irradiated postoperatively. Although the question of whether surgery or radiotherapy is given first has not been answered, there is clearly enough information in the literature to realize that neither one nor the other is the clear answer to improved mortality in these patients.

Following development of supervoltage irradiation and improvement in investigations, including CT and other scans, in helping to delineate the extent of disease, the thrust of management has commonly been towards combined treatment—radiotherapy followed by surgery. However, the advent of newer flaps, such as myocutaneous (McCraw et al 1979) and free flaps (Sharer et al 1976) and more competent anaesthetics and parenteral feeding has lead to a recent reconsideration of initial surgery. Any improvement in survival should first be seen in the moderately advanced lesions—too advanced for single modality treatment and yet not inoperable. Here, radical initial surgery, with or without complimentary irradiation, must prove its worth. The poor choice of cases for initial surgery—especially operating on the incurable—would bring such decisions into disrepute. The radiotherapist is then often faced with a complicated operative site plus gross residual disease.

It is important to be sure that, in giving patients radiotherapy and surgery in any combination, they are being offered the best of both worlds rather than the worst. It would be unfortunate if they were subjected to the complications of both modalities with the advantages of neither. If, in advanced disease, inoperable is incurable, then palliative irradiation must also fail to cure. However, this does not mean an operation should have been performed. Recognition of the incurable is one of the most difficult and important judgemental skills in head and neck cancer.

High-dose radiotherapy to the tongue and floor of mouth inevitably produces an initial reaction, with severe mucositis, dryness and pain in the treated area. The dose which can be achieved in patients who are debilitated, diabetic, or alcoholic is often reduced. However full dose is readily reached in most patients and the late complications include altered taste, fibrosis, dryness of the mouth and the dreaded osteonecrosis. The latter is more common where surgery has also been part of initial management and where disease involves bone from the outset. Extensive initial investigations, elegant anaesthetics and flaps with more energetic prosthetic replacements have helped to ensure that the morbidity from extensive surgery is minimal. The radiotherapist has explored other avenues to improve the local results of treatment, including neutron therapy, hyperfractionation and, of course, the much discussed area of combined treatment with chemotherapy.

The theoretical advantage of neutron therapy is that irradiation treatment is as effective in the poorly vascularized cells of a tumour as it is in the well vascularized normal tissue. This, for once, prevents the normal tissue from being placed at a disadvantage in the radiotherapeutic field. The series from centres such as the Hammersmith Hospital in England (Catterall 1977) have shown that, particularly in carcinomas of the floor of the mouth which were readily treated by the limited depth neutron beam, there is an excellent local response rate (Aygun et al 1984). The floor of the mouth is ideally suited to such a method where there has been some insecurity as to the relative biological efficiency of the dose achieved. Apart from the mandible, which is a potent cause of osteonecrosis, there are no other tissues that are of important radiotherapeutic sensitivity in the treatment field. The difficulty with which a method of treatment, which precludes salvage surgery, is considered in patients with carcinoma of the head and neck has resulted in a lack of enthusiasm for use of neutron therapy. Strict trials are in progress and their results are eagerly awaited. The effect that neutron treatment will have on subsequent surgical management should the patients' lesions fail to respond will be critical.

Hyperfractionation of radiotherapy is another way of optimizing radiotherapy treatment, tailoring it to suit the growth kinetics of a particular tumour (Wang 1971). Head and neck cancers are usually squamous, tend to be of the more rapidly proliferating type and, therefore, should respond better to multifraction treatments per day. Multiple fractions of radiotherapy may be given to shorten the overall treatment time, but are particularly useful in the head and neck area when given as two or three treatments in one day over approximately the same total treatment time. This should increase the therapeutic ratio allowing for more repair of normal tissue damage. In the head and neck area the radiotherapy and indeed surgical treatment is always close to what can be tolerated by the normal structures. Hyperfractionation should theoretically lessen morbidity and—since a higher effective dose could be given if the normal tissues would tolerate it—hopes of increased cure rates may be entertained. The results of hyperfractionation studies have suggested an increased local response rate but, as yet, no effect on mortality (Kramer 1975).

An important aspect of management is the assessment of the neck in both carcinoma of the tongue and floor of mouth, as even early lesions will have involved neck nodes on presentation in up to 30% of cases (Jesse et al 1970). Midline cancers are notorious in that they have lymphatic drainage to both sides of the neck. With early primary disease, no attempt is made by surgeon or radiotherapist to treat adjuvantly the ipsilateral neck. However, with

more advanced lesions, even in the absence of palpable disease, radiotherapists may well elect to irradiate the neck at risk. Likewise, the surgeon may remove locally placed nodes en bloc at the time of surgery, particularly for carcinomas of the floor of the mouth. Clearly, mobile involved nodes in the neck should be treated surgically by an elective block dissection. Bilateral nodes, if they are mobile, should still be managed surgically, although a bilateral dissection is often accompanied by many problems for the elderly patient. Inoperable large fixed nodes are treated by radiotherapy on the grounds that the patient may be incurable and that the nodes cannot be removed satisfactorily.

The role of chemotherapy in the management of advanced cancer of the head and neck is still contentious and therefore its role as a complement to surgery or radiotherapy in the primary management of the cancer of the oral cavity is difficult to define. Occasionally, exceptionally good response occurs when drugs with the greatest reputation in this disease—cisplatin, methotrexate, bleomycin, 5-fluorouracil—are used. This makes it difficult to accept the results of most randomized trials, which, in general, show that although local control may be improved with the addition of chemotherapy in early disease, the effect on survival is nil (Vogl et al 1986). Remarkable regression can often be seen in oral cancers when treated with combinations of chemotherapy (Ensley et al 1986). There have been no biological predictors of cytotoxic response yet determined. It is therefore impossible to distinguish between patients who would respond to chemotherapy and those for whom the addition of multiple toxic agents to an already toxic and complicated treatment regimen would be unsuccessful. Extrapolating from the frequent good results seen with chemotherapy in advanced disease, chemotherapy has been combined with both primary surgery and with primary radiotherapy. Cytotoxic agents may be delivered by the intravenous route, or infused via a catheter into the local blood supply of the tumour. Intra-arterial chemotherapy for head and neck cancers has had waves of popularity (Klopp et al 1950). The protagonists feel that increased doses may be administered locally to the tumour. An enhanced local response may be achieved without the systemic toxicity associated with the drugs. Many suggest that the blood supply of a large tumour is rarely derived from one artery, and that catheter-associated problems, such as embolism, infection and impairment of the blood supply to the tumour, may compromise subsequent treatment without offering the patient any survival advantage. The problem associated wih chemotherapy treatment of head and neck tumours is that, although the lesions may be moderately sensitive to the cytotoxic agent, partial response is all that can be realistically achieved. Since only complete response is associated with cure, combination with surgical or radiotherapeutic management is necessary. It has never effectively been shown that the response of the tumour to chemotherapy has resulted in either a decreased volume of tissue needing to be eradicated by surgery, or a reduced field size for radiotherapy. Induction chemotherapy in head and neck cancer has given some promising results. Spaulding et al (1986), using historical controls, showed an increased disease control in patients treated with a multiagent cytotoxic regime for two courses prior to definitive surgery. Radiotherapy was given only where margins were positive, or where there was tumour in the soft tissue of the neck. However,this was not a controlled comparison and even in a disease where survival rates have remained static, historical controls, because of inequality of investigatons or an inconsistent referral pattern, are not reliable. It is argued that giving a short course of chemotherapy prior to surgery will not compromise the clinical status of the patients and that reduction in tumour bulk in responding patients will make subsequent surgery easier.

The failure to change the pattern of recurrence in head and neck cancer over many years and the fact that these tumours do respond to cytotoxic chemotherapy have made oncologists strive to find the exact place of combined management in the treatment of patients with early cancers of the head and neck. It is disappointing that, in many early controlled trials, no survival advantage was seen. Frequently, the local control rate was enhanced and recently there has been more optimism in this field, with some suggestion of mortality advantage (Rooney et al 1983).

The thrust of management of patients with head and neck cancer must be towards answering the many remaining questions by the use of controlled trials. Sadly, few centres are large enough to be able to conduct these alone. Groups of collaborators, who work consistently together, are necessary so that pooled data may contribute useful results.

The state of the art in head and neck cancer is that combinations of existing methods of management are failing to have an increased impact on survival. The patient should be offered the best treatment available for his malignancy, whether or not this is primary surgery. At the same time greater effort should be concentrated on prevention and early diagnosis.

I have been given the privilege of judging the case for primary surgery for oral cavity cancer. The deposition for the initial management of oral cancer with surgery is given by two formidable giants in the field of head and neck oncology. Professor Snow and Dr Spittle offer their respective bias as to how oral cavity cancer patients should be treated. They agree that small oral cancers (4 cm in diameter) may be cured with either surgery or radiotherapy, whereas larger cancers require multimodality therapy. Both agree at least about smaller neoplasms, that morbidity is the chief issue in deciding what form of therapy should be selected.

For smaller cancers, Snow concludes that the effect of surgery on oral function is minimal, whereas radiotherapy, apart from the usual xerostomia, is quite often associated with radiation-induced ulceration and oral discomfort. Dr Spittle tends to be cautious in suggesting radiotherapy over surgery in treating small oral cavity cancers. She tells us that a multidisciplinary team consisting of otolaryngologists, radiotherapists, oncologists, pathologists, dentists and radiologists is important in reducing morbidity, regardless of selected therapy. She suggests that xerostomia, osteoradionecrosis, radiation-induced ulceration and dental deterioration, associated with irradiation of oral cavity cancers, has been reduced significantly in recent years. Supervoltage and interstitial radiotherapy, as well as multidisciplinary care, are offered as the reason for reduced morbidity.

I tend to support the viewpoints of both authors! That is, both forms of therapy, surgery or irradiation, can effectively cure small oral cavity cancers. Debating which form of therapy is best for cure thus seems less of an issue than what subsequently happens to the patient following surgery or irradiation.

Successful surgical treatment of small oral cavity cancers can be done either transorally, or transgressing the neck (Barton & UcMakli 1977, Strong et al 1979). Transorally, the tumour can be removed by knife, but CO_2 laser offers an excellent method of removing small tongue and/or floor of mouth cancers. The tumour can be stained with the vital dye Toluidene Blue to identify what needs to be removed. CO_2 laser intensity can be controlled so that minimal tissue damage occurs. In addition, with the CO_2 laser the tumour can be removed for histopathological examination with minimal postoperative discomfort, excellent haemostasis, reduced scarring, preservation of oral anatomy and without dispersing cancer cells. Because of oral cavity exposure and tongue control, utilization of a knife to transorally ablate the cancer offers a greater chance of cutting across tumour, bleeding and oral cavity mutilation. Electrocoagulation and cryotherapy are effective in controlling carcinoma in situ and superficially invasive cancers; neither mode of therapy provides information as to whether or not the cancer has been removed. The problem with transoral surgical removal of oral cavity cancers does not appear to be oral dysfunction, but the relatively high recurrence rate that requires re-excision (Berkett & Miller 1979). There is also a greater chance of oral mutilation. Another problem with primary surgery of the oral cavity, as opposed to irradiation, is the 'variability' factor. All otolaryngology, head and neck surgeons, although highly trained and skilled in their work, do not operate the same. What one surgeon feels is a curative intent, another may feel is too radical. Westbury (1981) states that a 2 cm tumour-free margin circumferentially is required for tongue cancers (Westbury 1981). Assuredly, significantly oral cavity dysfunction will be induced when this much tissue is removed from the tongue (Fuller et al 1987). Thus, irradiation might be favoured as primary therapy in cases where the surgeons might be inexperienced, difficult location for adequate removal, or when significant oral dysfunction might be induced by an appropriate excision. For example, to remove 5 cm of tongue to ablate a 1 cm tumour will produce significant speech, chewing and deglutition problems, regardless of the patient's habitus, age, occupation and mentation. To remove such an amount of tongue tissue from a lawyer, teacher, professor, or any person that requires speech for their occupation, might finish with that patient disabled but cured. In this situation, it might be considered prudent to offer irradiation and some xerostomia, decreased taste and fibrosis.

Radiotherapy in general offers the capability of delivering a constant amount of irradiation to a specified area of the head and neck. Thus similarity of treatment exists whether given in the UK or in the USA. Treatment fields and dosimetry can be compared and standardized for radiotherapy of a tongue or floor of mouth cancer. However, just as with the surgeon, not all radiotherapists are created equal! A radiation therapist who does not employ physics, proper treatment planning, modern equipment and/or associates with other head and neck cancer disciplines, may offer as much variability in head and neck cancer treatment as that of the surgeon. In such situations, excessive morbidity is usually the rule.

Just as quality of life is important in determining the treatment modality for small oral cancers, so is the patient's age. Radiotherapy produces prolonged immunological and tissue aberrations that can give rise to the development of other head and neck cancers. Usually these cancers occur 10–30 years after having received head and/or neck irradiation. The pendulum would thus seem to favour surgery over radiotherapy in the younger patient. Interestingly, a patient aged 73 has a statistical probability of living 10 or more years. Although some head and neck oncologists feel that oral carcinoma in the young represents a more malignant disease, a recent review of a group of oral cavity patients less than 40 years old revealed good survival following surgery alone (Mendez et al 1985). However, utilization of irradiation in the young patient seemed to be much less effective than expected from comparison with studies in which older oral cavity cancer patients were treated with irradiation therapy alone.

Another area of concern in selecting primary surgery for oral cavity cancer is the staging upon which subsequent therapy is selected. Both Snow and Spittle relate survival statistics regarding treatment based upon an anatomical TNM staging system, i.e. American Joint Committee on Cancer (AJCC) or International Union against Cancer (IUCC). The inadequacy of TNM staging accurately to categorize head and neck tumours is not necessarily revealed in comparing surgery and radiotherapy of T1 or T2 oral cavity cancers. Experienced head and neck oncologists, such as our authors, realize that the present TNM staging system does not provide a reliable method for assessing the three-dimensional spread of tumour (Byers et al 1978). Ulcerated and infiltrating tumours have been shown to have a far poorer prognosis than superficial tumours. Prognosis for survival appears to be more dependent upon

operative and pathological staging than the inaccurate preoperative clinical TNM staging. This fact alone may explain why an M.D. Anderson study reported 89% surgical survival versus only a 64% radiotherapy cure rate, with T1 and T2 floor of mouth cancers (Guillamondegiu et al 1980). Surgery provides a specimen which can be histologically examined for perineural invasion, adequacy of resection margins, extracapsular lymph node spread, tumour emboli and differentiation. All these factors appear to be important to patient prognosis, although none of them are taken into account by current tumour staging criteria. The development of the STNMP (site-tumor-mode-metastases-pathology) system proposed by the German Austrian Association for Head and Neck Tumours might be more appropriate than the TNM system in determining patient prognosis and treatment (Platz et al 1982). In general, biopsy and radiotherapy is a wait-and-see situation. Clinically evaluating patients for recurrence following irradiation therapy, especially when interstitial implants are utilized, is difficult, regardless of the examiner's experience (Cummings 1987). Frequently persistent oedema or nocturnal pain are the only indications that the irradiated patient has a recurrence. In these cases tumour detection is hidden within the radiation-induced fibrosis. Computerized tomography (CT) and/or magnetic resonance imaging (MRI), although quite helpful in pretreatment analysis of oral cavity tumours, has not been that useful for this author in determining recurrence before clinical detection (Schaefer et al 1982). It would appear from this brief analysis that primary surgical therapy would be important in patients with more invasive cancers, regardless of its T classification. Likewise a T1 cancer located more toward the midline, or extending anteriorly or posteriorly out of the oral cavity, would suggest a more aggressive tumour and thus cause me to favour primary surgical therapy over radiotherapy (Panje et al 1980).

Examining primary surgery for larger oral cavity tumours reveals that curative results with ablation are considerably better than those obtained by radiation therapy (Chu et al 1978, Guillamondegui et al 1980). Likewise, Razak et al (1982) have shown that recurrence of stage III and IV disease after initial treatment (regardless of modality) renders the patient unlikely to benefit from further sequential treatment

and salvage. Radiation following postoperative recurrences resulted in 12.6% salvage rate. In this
study, surgery (when compared to radiation) as the
initial modality of therapy had a better survival rate
at all stages and 48% of those patients with resectable
recurrences were salvaged by surgery. On the other
hand, the most important prognostic factor in the
management of head and neck squamous cell cancer,
including oral cavity malignancy, is the status of
the cervical nodes. Control of subclinical regional
metastasis has been shown to be quite effective with
irradiation (Fletcher 1972). However, cancerous
cervical nodes over 3 cm in diameter appear to be
better managed by excision with subsequent irradiation therapy for subclinical disease (Kraus &
Panje 1982). Thus, it appears that some type of
multimodality therapy is indicated for treating oral
cavity cancer with regional metastasis. Both Snow
and Spittle have indeed suggested just this.

A case for primary surgery seems today overwhelmingly justified for initial management of stage
III and IV oral cancer. Primary surgery offers the
best chance for local control, provides a pathological
specimen, as well as microscopic evidence of complete tumour removal. Initial surgery produces
immediate removal of the primary neoplasm (source
of metastasis), less chance for postoperative wound
complications and, because of the advances in reconstructive surgery, provides a milieu for better
postoperative speech and swallowing rehabilitation.
Radiotherapy can be given postoperatively with as
good a result as when given preoperatively. Disadvantages of primary surgery includes orofacial
mutilation and potential for delay of subsequent
multimodality therapy. Initial surgical removal of
oral cavity cancer provides a 'natural' tumour specimen for histopathological examination. Recent
information obtained from the microscopic controlled
excision of primary epithelial malignancies of the
upper aerodigestive tract have demonstrated a significant improvement in local control and projected
survival (Davidson & Haghighi, to be published).
Induction radiotherapy and/or chemotherapy,
although quite successful in shrinking and in some
cases eradicating T3 and T4 cancers, does so by
producing cell kill throughout the tumour and not
from the periphery inward as suggested by some
radiological experiments. These experiments showed

that radiation is most cancercidal in a well-oxygenated
environment and thus local recurrence should be
less when the tumour is treated before surgery. This
scenario, at least clinically, has not been the case
(Lindberg et al 1974). In practice, histological
examination of tumour specimens following irradiation and/or chemotherapy reveals the presence
of isolated islands of viable cancer cells throughout
the original tumour. This finding alone substantiates
the clinical reality that, unless the surgeon excises
the original 'pretreatment' tumour volume regardless of initial radiotherapy and/or chemotherapy
response, a high incidence of local and distant failure
occurs (Barrs et al 1979). In the Iowa study completed by Schuller et al (1979), it was suggested that
the reason for such a high incidence of distant
metastasis and no improvement in survival with
combined preoperative irradiation and surgery over
that of surgery alone was because original tumour
margins were obscured by irradiation response: the
surgeon either seeded tumour cells or left islands of
tumour behind. Thus it would seem more rational
first to excise the tumour before additional therapy,
since a similar volume of tissue will need to be removed regardless of when the neoplasm is removed,
this avoids histological artifacts produced by radiation
therapy or chemotherapy and physically improves
the surgeon's ability to remove the tumour specimen.
adequately.

Another reason for considering initial surgery for
T3 and T4 oral cavity cancers is the fact that the
tumour remains in situ when being initially treated
with either irradiation and/or chemotherapy. During
additional time the cancer remains in the host,
lymphatic field alteration and changes produced in
local tumour resistance might explain the increased
incidence of metastases associated with delayed
surgical excision (Bartelink et al 1982, DeSanto et
al 1982).

Radiation therapy adversely effects wound healing.
This is especially true when operating upon the oral
cavity, with its moist and contaminated environment. In general, removal of oral cavity cancers
following preoperative irradiation, especially if given
to curative doses, accentuates the problems of
mandible conservation, fistulization, type of reconstruction and wound dehiscence, infection and
carotid blow-out (DeSanto & Thawley 1987).

Chemotherapy also adversely effects wound healing but appears to be limited to a two-week perioperative period.

The fear of orofacial mutilation following oral cancer surgical treatment produces the most opposition to surgery. The fact that oral dysfunction increases with the extent of resection also encourages radiotherapist and chemotherapist to reserve surgery for their failures. It is promoted that utilizing radiation therapy and/or chemotherapy and withholding surgery for recurrences produces some cures without surgery. Of course, if no surgery is utilized, better cosmesis, oral function and increased cost-effectiveness is often realized. Although this case can be argued more rationally for T1 and T2 cancers, the local recurrence rate following curative irradiation for T3 and T4 floor of mouth is approximately 75% (Guillamondegui et al 1980). Surgical salvage of recurrent irradiated oral cavity cancers requires larger excisions than the original size of the tumour. I have found that up to three times the original cancer volume is required to excise adequately recurrent cancer after irradiation failure (Panje 1984). It is hypothesized that a larger excision than the orginal tumour is because of the time interval, or disease-free interval, between radiation therapy and subsequent surgery. During this time interval, usually 6–24 months, residual islands of tumour can grow unchecked by the usual tissue barriers to tumour spread. Over 90% of surgical salvaged patients will require extensive reconstructive surgery, prolonged hospitalization and necessarily increased costs (Panje 1987). Likewise, oral dysfunction and facial mutilation are excessive, despite newer more sophisticated reconstructive techniques. The cure rate for salvage surgery remains disappointingly low as compared with an overall 56–65% cure rate for primary surgical treatment of T3 and T4 cancers. Thus it would seem prudent to use initial surgery in a planned, combined manner with either postoperative irradiation and/or chemotherapy. In this way, a smaller resection is required, more successful oral functional reconstruction is obtained and a higher cure rate achieved.

Another argument against primary surgical therapy of oral cavity cancer is that of potential postoperative delay in administering irradiation and/or chemotherapy. Professor Snow alludes to this problem in that several studies have demonstrated a decreased disease-free interval and increased local-regional failure when radiation therapy was delayed greater than six weeks following surgery. However, these studies are misleading in that longer term studies, both retrospective and prospective, demonstrate that adding radiation therapy to surgical therapy did not increase survival over that group which had surgery alone (Schuller et al 1987, Panje et al 1987, Eisbach & Kraus 1977).

CONCLUDING REMARKS

Treatment of oral cavity cancer presents unique considerations when compared to other upper aerodigestive tract sites. Unlike laryngeal cancer, in which salvage or delayed surgery is frequently as defunctionalizing as primary surgical therapy, the T1 and T2 oral cavity tumour can often be removed without noticeable, or minimal, oral dysfunction of facial mutilation. However, delayed surgery of the oral cavity often presents a formidable undertaking with significant patient disability and decreased survival.

Snow and Spittle have both produced excellent arguments concerning primary surgical therapy of oral cavity cancer. In essence, both surgery and radiation therapy play equally important roles in managing oral cavity cancers. Either surgery or radiation therapy are equally effective in treating T1 and T2 neoplasms. Selection of primary surgery for smaller oral cavity cancers appears to be more dependent upon surgical capability, potential for oral dysfunction and patient factors such as age, oral hygiene, and oral habits. The side effects of radiation therapy of smaller oral cancers seem to be minimal with the advent of newer radiotherapeutic devices and techniques used in conjunction with patient cooperation and multidisciplinary care. The larger T3 and T4 oral cancers appear to be better managed by primary surgical therapy with subsequent radiotherapy and/or chemotherapy. Survival results and biological rationale seem to outweigh the disadvantages of oral facial mutilation and possibility of delaying combined therapy. Dr Spittle's closing remarks seem very appropriate to managing patients with larger head and neck cancers. 'The patient should be offered the best treatment available for his malignancy, whether or not this is primary

surgery. At the same time, greater effort should be concentrated on prevention and early diagnosis.'

REFERENCES

G B Snow

Ali S, Tiwari R M, Snow G B 1985 False-positive and false-negative neck nodes. Head and Neck Surgery 8: 78–82

Ariyan S 1979 The pectoralis major myocutaneous flap. A versatile flap for reconstruction of the head and neck. Plastic and Reconstructive Surgery 63: 73–81

Arriagada R, Eschwege F, Cachin Y, Richard J M 1983 The value of combining radiotherapy with surgery in the treatment of hypopharyngeal and laryngeal cancers. Cancer 51: 1819–1825

Bartelink H, Breur H, Hart G, Annyas A A, van Slooten E A, Snow G B 1983 The value of postoperative radiotherapy as an adjuvant to radical neck dissection. Cancer 52: 1008–1013

Beahrs O H 1973 Fators minimizing mortality and morbidity rates in head and neck. American Journal of Surgery 126: 443–451

Beahrs O H, Barber K W 1962 The value of radical dissection of structures of the neck in the management of carcinoma of the lip, mouth and larynx. Archives of Surgery 85: 49–56

Becker J M, Tiwari R M, Snow G B 1986 Surgical management of T1 and T2 tongue carcinomas. Submitted for publication in Clinical Otolaryngology.

Bocca E, Pignataro O, Sasaki C 1980 Functional neck dissection. Archives of Otolaryngology 106: 524–527

Byers R M, Bland K I, Borlase B, Luna M 1978 The prognostic and therapeutic value of frozen section determinations in the surgical treatment of squamous carcinoma of the head and neck. American Journal of Surgery 136: 525–528

Cachin Y, Eschwege F 1975 Combination of radiotherapy and surgery in the treatment of head and neck cancers. Cancer Treatment Review 2: 177–191

Cachin Y, Sancho-Garnier H, Micheau C, Marandas P 1979 Nodal metastasis from carcinomas of the oropharynx. Otolaryngology Clinics of North America 12: 145–154

Callery C D, Spiro R H, Strong E W 1984 Changing trends in the management of squamous carcinoma of the tongue. Amererican Journal Surgery 148: 449–454

Carpenter R J III, De Santo L W, Devine K D et al 1976 Cancer of the hypopharynx: analysis of treatment and results in 162 patients. Archives of Otolaryngology 102: 716–721

Carter R L, Tanner N S B, Clifford P, Shaw H J 1980 Direct bone invasion in squamous carcinomas of the head and neck: Pathological and clinical implications. Clinical Otolaryngology 5: 107–116

Cohen I K, Theogarj S D 1975 Nasolabial flap reconstruction of the floor of the mouth after extirpation of oral cancer. American Journal of Surgery 130: 479

Cummings B J 1984 Radiotherapy aspects of malignant disease of the oral cavity. In: van der Waal I, Snow G B (eds) Oral oncology. Martinus Nijhoff, Boston, p 187–217

Daniel R K, Taylor G I 1973 Distant transfer of an island flap by microvascular anastomoses. Plastic and Reconstructive Surgery 52: 111–117

Decroix Y, Ghossein N A 1981 Experience of the Curie Institute in treatment of cancer of the mobile tongue. I. Treatment policies and results. Cancer 47: 496–502

Fletcher G H 1972 Elective irradiation of subclinical disease in cancers of the head and neck. Cancer 29: 1450–1454

Franklin J D, Shack R B, Stone J D, Madden J J, Lynch J B 1980 Single-stage reconstruction of mandibular and soft tissue defects using a free osteocutaneous groin flap. American Journal of Surgery 140: 492–498

Frazell E L, Lucas J C 1962 Cancer of the tongue. Cancer 15: 1085–1099

Fu K K, Ray J W, Chan E K, Phillips T L 1976 External and interstitial radiation therapy of carcinoma of the oral tongue. American Journal of Roentgenology 126: 107–115

Goffinet D R, Fee W E Jr, Goode R L 1984 Combined surgery and postoperative irradiation in the treatment of cervical lymph nodes. Archives of Otolaryngology 110: 736–738

Guillamondegui O M, Jesse R 1976 Surgical treatment of advanced carcinoma of the floor of the mouth. American Journal of Roentgenology 126: 1256–1259

Guillamondegui O M, Oliver B, Hayden R 1980 Cancer of the anterior floor of the mouth, selective choice of treatment and analysis of failures. American Journal Surgery 140: 560–562

Harrold C C Jr 1969 Cancer of the tongue: Some comments on surgical treatment. In: Gainsford J C (ed) Symposium on cancer of the head and neck: Total treatment and reconstructive rehabilitation, vol II. CV Mosby, St Louis, p 185–190

Henk J M 1985 Management of the primary tumour. In: Henk J M, Langdon J D (eds) Malignant tumours of the oral cavity. E Arnold, London

Hibbert J, Marks N J, Winter P J, Shaheen O H 1983 Prognostic factors in oral squamous carcinoma and their relation to clinical staging. Clinical Otolaryngology 8: 197–203

Hintz B, Charynler K, Chandler J R, Sudarsanam A, Garciga C 1979 Randomized study of control of the primary tumor and survival using preoperative radiation, radiation alone, or surgery alone in head and neck carcinomas. Journal of Surgical Oncology 12: 75–85

Hirata R M, Jacques D A, Chambers R G, Tuttle J R, Mahoney W D 1975 Carcinoma of the oral cavity: an analysis of 478 cases. Annals of Surgery 182: 98–1033

Jesse R H 1981 Modified neck dissection with and without radiation. In: Kagan A R, Miles J W (eds) Head and neck oncology, controversies in cancer treatment, G K Hall, Boston, p 247–254

Jesse R H, Lindberg R D 1975 The efficacy of combining radiation therapy with a surgical procedure in patients with cervical metastasis from squamous cancer of the oropharynx and hypopharynx. Cancer 35: 1163–1166

Jesse R H, Fletcher G H 1977 Treatment of the neck in patients with squamous cell carcinoma of the head and neck. Cancer 39: 868–872

Johnson M J T, Leipzig B, Cummings C W 1980

Management of T1 carcinoma of the anterior aspect of the tongue. Archives of Otolaryngology 106: 249–251

Johnson J T, Barnes E L, Myers E N, Schramm V L Jr, Borochovitz D, Sigler B 1981 The extracapsular spread of tumors in cervicalnode metastasis. Archives of Otolaryngology 107: 725–729

Jones T A, Stell P M 1985 The preservation of shoulder function after radical neck dissection. Clinical Otolaryngology 10: 89–92

Joseph D L, Shumrick D L 1973 Risks of head and neck surgery in previously irradiated patients. Archives of Otolaryngology 97: 381–384

Kalnis I K, Leonard A G, Sako K, Razack M S, Shedd D P 1977 Correlation between prognosis and degree of lymph node involvement in carcinoma of the oral cavity. American Journal of Surgery 134: 450–454

Larson D L, Lindberg R D, Lane E et al 1983 Major complications of radiotherapy in cancer of the oral cavity and oropharynx: a 10-year-old retrospective study. American Journal Surgery 146: 531–536

Lee J G, Litton W B 1972 Occult regional metastasis: Carcinoma of the oral tongue. Laryngoscope 82: 1273–1280

Lee E S, Wilson J S P 1973 Carcinoma involving the lower alveolus. British Journal of Surgery 60: 85–107

Leipzig B, Hokanson J A 1982 Treatment of cervical lymph nodes in carcinoma of the tongue. Head and Neck Surgery 5: 3–9

Leipzig B, Cummings C W, Chung C T, Johnson J T, Sagerman R H 1982 Carcinoma of the anterior tongue. Annals of Otolaryngology 91: 94–97

Lldstad S T, Bigelow M E, Remensnyder J P 1983 Squamous cell carcinoma of the mobile tongue. American Journal of Surgery 145: 443–449

Looser K G, Shah J, Strong E W 1978 The significance of 'positive' margins in surgically resected epidermoid carcinomas. Head and Neck Surgery 1: 107–111

Mantravadi R V P, Haas R E, Liebner E J, Skolnik E M, Applebaum E L 1983 Postoperative radiotherapy for persistent tumor at the surgical margin in head and neck cancer. Laryngoscope 93: 1337–1340

Marchetta F C, Sako K, Murphy J 1971 The periosteum of the mandible and intraoral carcinoma. American Journal of Surgery 122: 711–713

Marchetta F C, Sako K, Razack M S 1977 Management of 'localized' oral cancer. American Journal of Surgery 134: 448–449

Marcus R B Jr, Million R R, Cassissi N J 1979 Postoperative irradiation for squamous cell carcinomas of the head and neck: analysis of time-dose factors related to control above the clavicles. International Journal of Radiation Oncology Biology Physics 5: 1943–1949

Marks J E, Lee F, Freeman R B, Zivnuska F R, Ogura J H 1981 Carcinoma of the oral tongue: a study of patient selection and treatment results. Laryngoscope 91: 1548–1559

McCraw J B, Dibbel D G, Carraway J H 1977 Clinical definition of independent myocutaneous vascular territories. Plastic and Reconstructive surgery 60: 341–352

McGregor J B, Morgan G 1973 Axial and random pattern flaps. British Journal of Plastic Surgery 26: 202–213

McGregor I A, McGrouther D A 1978 Skin-graft reconstruction in carcinoma of the tongue. Head and Neck Surgery 1: 47–51

McGuirt W F, Loevy S, McCabe B F, Krause C J 1977 The risks of major head and neck surgery in the aged population. Laryngoscope 87: 1378–1382

McGuirt W F, McCabe B F, Krause C J 1979 Complications of radical neck dissection: a survey of 788 patients. Head and Neck Surgery 1: 481–487

McQuarrie D G 1986 Oral cancer. In: McQuarrie D G, Adams G L et al (eds) Head and neck cancer. Year Book Medical Publishers, Chicago

Meikle D, Hibbert J, Winter P J, Tong D, Shaheen O H 1985 Interstitial irradiation for squamous carcinoma of the oral cavity. Clinical Otolaryngology 10: 171–176

Mendenhall W M, Million R R, Cassisi N J 1980 Elective neck irradiation in squamous cell carcinoma of the head and neck. Head and Neck Surgery 3: 15–20

Mendelson B C, Woods J E, Beahrs O H 1976 Neck dissection in the treatment of carcinoma of the anterior two-thirds of the tongue. Surgery, Gynecology and Obstetrics 143: 75–80

Micheau C, Sancho H, Gerard-Marchant R 1978 Prognostic des adenopathies cervicales metastatiques en fonction des facteurs anatomopathologiques. Nuovo Archivio italiano di otologia VI 1: 5–14

Million P R 1974 Elective neck irradiation for TxN0 squamous carcinoma of the oral tongue and floor of mouth. Cancer 34: 149–155

Panje W, Cutting C 1980 Trapezius osteomyocutaneous island flap for reconstruction of the anterior floor of mouth and mandible. Head and Neck Surgery 3: 66–71

Pierquin B, Chassagne D, Baillet F 1971 The place of implantation in tongue and floor of mouth cancer. Journal American Medical Association 215: 961–963

Schuller D E, McGuirt W F, Krause C J, McGabe B F, Pflug B K 1979 Increased survival with surgery alone vs combined therapy. Laryngoscope 89: 582–594

Schuller D E, Reiches N A, Hamaker R C et al 1983 Analysis of disability resulting from treatment including radical neck dissection of modified neck dissection. Head and Neck Surgery 6: 551–558

Snow G B 1984 Surgical treatment of malignant tumors of the oral cavity. In: van der Waal I, Snow G B (eds) Oral oncology. Martinus Nijhoff, Boston, p 155–186

Snow G B, Kruisbrink J J, van Slooten E A 1976 Reconstruction after mandibulectomy for cancer. Archives of Otolaryngology 102: 207–210

Snow G B, Annyas A A, van Slooten E A, Bartelink H, Hart A A M 1982 Prognostic factors of neck node metastasis. Clinical Otolaryngology 7: 185–192

Snow G B, Balm A J M, Arendse J W et al 1986 Prognostic factors in neck node metastases. In: Larson D L et al (eds) Treatment of metastatic cancer in the head and neck. MacMillan Publishing Company, New York

Soutar D S, Scheker L R, Tanner S B, McGregor I A 1983 The radial forearm flap: a versatile method for intraoral reconstruction. British Journal of Plastic Surgery 36: 1–8

Spiro R H, Strong E W 1971 Epidermoid carcinoma of the mobile tongue: treatment by partial glossectomy alone. American Journal of Surgery 122: 707–710

Spiro R H, Gerold F P, Strong E W 1981 Mandibular 'swing' approach for oral and oropharyngeal tumors. Head and Neck Surgery 3: 371–378

Strong E W, Henschke U K, Nickson J J, Frazell E L, Tollefsen R, Hilaris B S 1966 Preoperative X-ray therapy as an adjunct to radical neck dissection. Cancer 19: 1509–1516

Strong M S, Vaughan C W, Kayne H L et al 1978 A randomized trial of preoperative radiotherapy in cancer of the oropharynx and hypopharynx. American Journal of Surgery 136: 494–500

Teichgraeber J, Bowman J, Goepfert H 1985 New test series for the functional evaluation of oral cavity cancer. Head and Neck Surgery 8: 9–20

Terz J J, Lawrence W Jr 1981 Ineffectiveness of combined radiation and surgery in the management of malignancies of the oral cavity, larynx and pharynx. In: Kagan A R, Miles H W (eds) Head and neck oncology, controversies in cancer treatment. G K Hall Boston, p 111–123

Terz J J, King E R, Lawrence W Jr 1981 Preoperative irradiation for head and neck cancer. Results of a prospective study. Surgery 89: 449–453

Tiwari R M, Snow G B 1983 Role of myocutaneous flaps in reconstruction of the head and neck. Journal of Laryngology and Otology 97: 441–458

Vandenbrouck C, Sancho H, Le Fut R, Richard J M, Cachin Y 1977 Results of a randomized clinical trial of preoperative irradiation versus postoperative in treatment of tumors of the hypopharynx. Cancer 39: 1445–1449

Vandenbrouck C, Sancho-Garnier H, Chassagne D, Saravane D, Cachin Y, Micheau C 1980 Elective versus therapeutic radical neck dissection in epidermoid carcinoma of the oral cavity, results of a randomized clinical trial. Cancer 46: 386–390

Vegers J W M, Snow G B, van der Waal I 1979 Squamous cell carcinoma of the buccal mucosa. A review of 85 cases. Archives of Otolaryngology 105: 192–195

Vikram B 1979 Importance of the time interval between surgery and postoperative radiation therapy in the combined management of head and neck cancer. International Journal Radiation Oncology Biology Physics 5: 1837–1840

Vikram B, Strong E W, Shah J et al 1980 Elective postoperative radiation therapy in stages III and IV epidermoid carcinoma of the head and neck. American Journal of Surgery 140: 580–584

Westbury G 1981 Carcinoma of the tongue. In: Rob C, Smith R, Wilson J S P (eds) Operative surgery, head and neck. Butterworths, London, p 664–671

White D, Byers R M 1980 What is the preferred initial method of treatment for squamous carcinoma of the tongue? American Journal of Surgery 149: 553–555

Whitehurst J O, Droulias C A 1977 Surgical treatment of squamous cell carcinoma of the oral tongue. Archives of Otolaryngology 103: 212–215

Williams R G, Murtagh G P 1973 Mortality in surgery for head and neck cancer. Journal of Laryngology and Otology 87: 431–440

M F Spittle

Aygun C, Salazar O M, Sewchand W et al 1984 Carcinoma of the floor of the mouth; A 20-year experience. International Journal of Radiation Oncology, Biology, Physics 10: 619–625, 1984.

Beahrs O M, Myers M H (eds) 1983 Manual for staging of cancer, 2nd edn. J P Lippincott Philadelphia, p 25–36

Belli J A, Disans G J, Bonte F J 1962 Radiation response of mammalian tumour cells. Journal of the National Cancer Institute 38: 673–682

Callery C D, Spiro R H, Strong E W 1984 Changing trends in the management of squamous carcinoma of the tongue. American Journal of Surgery 148: 449–454

Caterall M 1977 The results of randomized and other clinical trials of fast neutrons from the Medical Research Council cyclotron, London International Journal of Radiation Oncology, Biology, Physics 3: 247–253

Ensley J, Crissman J, Kish J et al 1986 The impact of conventional morphologic on response rate and survival in patients with advanced carcinoma of the head and neck treated initially with Cisplatin containing compounds. Cancer 57: 711–717

Jesse R H, Barkley H T, Lindberg R D, Fletcher G H 1970 Cancer of the oral cavity: Is elective neck dissection beneficial? American Journal of Surgery 120: 505–508

Klopp C T, Alfordd T C, Bateman J et al 1950 Fractionated intra-arterial cancer chemotherapy with methyl bis amine hydrochloride. A preliminary report. Annals of Surgery 132: 811–832

Kramer S 1975 Methotrexate and radiation therapy in the treatment of advanced squamous carcinoma of the oral cavity, oropharynx, supraglottic larynx and hypopharynx. Canadian Journal of Otolaryngology 4: 213–218

Larson D L, Lundberg R D, Lane E, Goepfert H 1983 Major complications of radiotherapy in cancer of the oral cavity and oropharynx. American Journal of Surgery 146: 531–536

McCraw J B, Magee W P, Kalworic H 1979 Uses of the trapezius and sternomastoid myocutaneous flaps in head and neck reconstruction. Plastic and Reconstruction Surgery 63: 49–57

Marks J E, Lee F, Smith P G, Ogura J H 1983 Floor of mouth cancer; Patient selection and treatment results. Laryngoscope 93, 475–480

OPCS 1985 Cancer statistics registrations 1982 HMSO, London, p 1

Rooney M, Stanley R, Weaver A et al 1983 Superior results in complete remission rate and overall survival of patients with head and neck cancer treated with cisplatinum combination chemotherapy. Proceedings of ASCO 2: C-620

Sharer L A, Horton C E, Adamson J E et al 1976 Intraoral reconstruction in head and neck cancer surgery. Plastic Surgery 3: 495–509

Spaulding M, Ziegler P, Sundquist N et al 1986 Induction therapy in head and neck cancer. Cancer 57: 1110–1114

Spittle M F 1984 Experience with Novantrone as a single agent in breast cancer. Proceedings of the 1st UK Novantrone Symposium: Media Medica, Paris

Stell P M, McCormick M S 1985 Cancer of the head and neck: are we doing any better? Lancet ii: 1127

Union Internationale Contre le Cancer 1978 TNM classification for malignant tumours. UICC, Geneva

Vogl S E, Komisar A, Kaplan B H et al 1986 Sequential methotrexate and 5 Flourouracil with bleamycin and cisplatin in the chemotherapy of advanced squamous cancer of the head and neck. Cancer 57: 706–710

Wang C C 1981 Twice daily radiation therapy for carcinomas of the head and neck. International Journal of Radiation Oncology, Biology, Physics 7: 1261–1262, 1981.

W R Panje

Barrs D M, DeSanto L W, O'Fallon W M 1979 Squamous cell carcinoma of the tonsil and tongue-base region. Archives of Otolaryngology 105: 479

Bartelink H, Breur K, Hart G et al 1982 Radiotherapy of lymph node metastasis in patients with squamous cell carcinoma of the head neck region. International Journal of Radiation Oncology, Biology, Physics 8: 893

Barton R T, UcMakli A 1977 The treatment of squamous cell carcinoma of the floor of the mouth. Surgery, Gynecology and Obstetrics 145: 2127

Berkett P R, Miller G F 1979 Mucosal tattooing in oral cavity carcinoma. Otolaryngology, Head and Neck Surgery 87: 775

Byers R M et al 1978 The prognostic and therapeutic value of frozen sections in the determination of surgical treatment of squamous cell carcinoma of the head and neck. American Journal of Surgery 136: 525

Chu W, Litwin S, Strawitz J G 1978 The comparison of resection and radiation in the control of cancer within the mouth. Surgery, Gynecology and Obstetrics 146: 38

Cummings C W 1987 Controversy in the management of tumors of the oral cavity. In: Thawley S E, Panje W R (eds) Comprehensive management of head and neck tumors. Saunders, Philadelphia, p 60–611.

Davidson T, Haghighi P Parallel histologic sections (MOHS) for head and neck mucosal. Cancer, to be published

DeSanto L W, Thawley S E 1987 Surgical therapy. In: Thawley S E, Panje W R (eds) Comprehensive management of head and neck tumors. Saunders, Philadelphia, p 699–755

DeSanto L W, Holt J J, Beahr O H, O'Fallon W M 1982 Neck dissection: Is it worthwhile? Laryngoscope 92: 502

Eisbach K J, Krause C J 1977 Carcinoma of the pyriform sinus, a comparison of treatment modalities. Laryngoscope 87: 904

Fletcher G H 1972 Elective irradiation of subclinical disease in cancers of the head and neck. Cancer 29: 1450

Fuller D, Zaggy M A, Verdolini K 1987 Speech and swallowing rehabilitation for head and neck tumor patients. In: Thawley S E, Panje W R (eds) Comprehensive management of head and neck tumours. Saunders, Philadelphia p 100–131

Guillamondegiu O M, Oliver B, Haden R 1980 Cancer of the floor of the mouth: Selective choice of treatment and analysis of failure. American Journal of Surgery 140: 560

Kraus E M, Panje W R 1982 Factors influencing survival in head and neck patients with giant cervical lymph node metastasis. Otolaryngology 3: 53–56

Lindberg R D, Jesse R H, Fletcher G H 1974 Radiotherapy before or after surgery? In: Neoplasia of head and neck. Chicago, Year Book Medical Publishers, p 47–85

Mendez P Jr, Maves M D, Panje W R 1985 Squamous cell carcinoma of under the age of 40. Archives of Otolaryngology 111: 762–764

Panje W R 1986 Improved surgical salvage therapy of upper aerodigestive tract carcinoma. Bicentennial Meeting Ireland—Royal College of Surgeons, Dublin, Ireland, July 1984. Presented UCLA Research Club Meeting

Panje W R 1987 Immediate reconstruction of the oral cavity. In: Thawley S E, Panje W R (eds) Comprehensive management of head and neck tumors. Saunders, Philadelphia, p 563–595

Panje W R, Smith B, McCabe B F 1980 Epidermoid carcinoma of the floor of the mouth. Surgical therapy vs combined therapy vs radiation therapy. Otology, Head and Neck Surgery 88: 714

Panje W R et al 1987 Tumors of the oral cavity In: Thawley S E, Panje W R (eds) Comprehensive management of head and neck tumors, Saunders, Philadelphia, p 714

Platz H et al 1982 Carcinomas of the oral cavity: Analysis of various pretherapeutic classifications. Head and Neck Surgery 5: 93

Razack M S et al 1982 The role of initial modality in treatment of squamous cell carcinoma of the tongue. Journal of Surgical Oncology 19: 136

Schaefer S D, Merkel M, Diehl J et al 1982 Computed tomographic assessment of squamous cell carcinoma of oral and pharyngeal cavities. Archives of Otology 106: 688

Schuller D E, McGuirt W F, Krause C J, McCabe B F, Pflug B K 1979 Increased survival with surgery alone vs combined therapy. Laryngoscope 89: 582–594

Schuller D et al 1987 In: Thawley S E, Panje W R (eds) Comprehensive management of head and neck tumors. Saunders, 590–594

Strong M S, Vaughan C W, Healy G B et al 1979 Transoral management of localized carcinoma of the oral cavity using the CO_2 laser, Laryngoscopy 89: 897

Westbury G 1981 Carcinoma of the tonue. In: Rob C, Smith R, Wilson J S P (eds) Operative surgery, head and neck. Butterworths, London, p 664–671

19

The management of the patient with cervical node metastases from an occult primary

A.G.D. Maran

Background

In the 1940s and 1950s, the literature was richly endowed with articles on branchogenic carcinoma. Hayes Martin set out four postulates that made it almost impossible to diagnose branchogenic carcinoma ever again (Maran et al 1950). He, very correctly, made the point that these cases were almost certainly cervical node metastases from primaries in the head and neck. His four postulates were that:

1. The cervical tumour must occur in a line from anterior to the tragus to the anterior border of the sternocleidomastoid muscle.

2. The histological appearance must be consistent with an origin from tissue known to be present in branchial vestigia.

3. The patient must have survived and been followed by periodic examination for 5 years, without development of any other lesion which could possibly have been the primary lesion.

4. There was histological demonstration of cancer developing in the wall of an epithelial lined cyst situated in the lateral aspect of the neck.

Since then, there have only been 15 reliable reports of branchogenic carcinoma (Black & Maran 1978).

In the 1960s and 1970s, branchogenic carcinoma articles were replaced by articles on metastatic cervical cancer from occult primaries. In the 1980s, however, there have been very few articles on this subject and certainly little new has been added to the management of these patients. On the contrary, most writers have retreated from listing an enormous catechism of investigation because it is now not such an apparently vital problem.

Definitions

This subject has created a marsh of information that is to clarity what Schoenberg was to the melodic line. Most papers are not comparable because they start from different points: some use the point when the patient presented with an undiagnosed lump in the neck suspected of being cancer, others use as a starting point the patient with a histologically proven cancer of the neck with no obvious primary. Even in this latter group, however, there is no consistency in defining the term 'obvious'. In some it is prior to history, examination and investigation and in others it is prior to endoscopy and biopsy. Nowadays, after endoscopy and biopsy, few patients presenting with a metastatic neck node would have an 'unknown' primary, but an undiscovered one.

Comess et al (1967) defined what is unknown:

1. No history of prior malignancy or surgical ablation of any indeterminate lesion.

2. No history of symptoms related to a specific organ.

3. No clinical or laboratory evidence of a primary neoplasm proved or not.

4. One or more cervical masses proved histologically to be cancer.

This is a very tight and correct definition but it fails to provide for two of the other features that confuse the literature, namely:

1. Are supraclavicular nodes in the series, as well as deep jugular nodes? If primaries from outside the aerodigestive system are included, it makes meaningful analysis impossible.

2. Are tumours other than squamous cell carcinoma included, e.g. adenocarcinoma and melanoma? One of the most outstanding articles in the literature

on this subject included 29 adenocarcinomas and 11 melanomas (Spiro et al 1983).

Figures measuring the number of primaries that later come to light are often meaningless because of the fact that metachronous primaries are not uncommon in patients with one head and neck tumour. The author recalls one of his cases who presented with a metastatic carcinoma in a neck node and 5 years later had a carcinoma in the temporal bone removed. It would, of course, be manifest nonsense to presume that that original neck node came from the temporal bone primary. Similarly, it is meaningless to provide lists of primaries discovered either earlier or later, or above or below the clavicles.

It does seem apparent that the number of undiagnosed primaries is getting less in departments handling a large volume of head and neck tumours.

If one considers the biology of cancer as it affects the head and neck, it would seem reasonable only to accept primaries that developed within 18 months of the node being discovered as relating to the original node. To allow anything other than this is to open the floodgates of conjecture that surround branchogenic carcinoma.

There is also a geographical variation in most head and neck cancers. In south-east Asia, a Chinese with a neck node is presumed to have nasopharyngeal carcinoma, even without symptoms or signs, and the nasopharynx must be biopsied and rebiopsied if necessary to prove this. In Scotland, which has the highest prevalence of lung cancer per head of population in Europe, 5% of these patients will manifest a node in the neck at some stage during the disease and so bronchoscopy and bronchial cytology must be performed and repeated frequently if initially negative. In southern Europe, where there is a 14 times greater incidence of laryngopharyngeal cancer than in northern Europe, the most likely site is, of course, the hypopharynx.

The present state of the art

Batsakis (1979) reviewed the major series in the subject and listed the following items of consensus.

1. It is not known whether initial biopsy influences survival of patients who subsequently undergo curative resection. The data presented by Razack et al (1977) would indicate there is no adverse affect.
2. There is a predominance of males.
3. The peak age is between 50 and 69.

4. The commonest nodes affected are in the upper deep jugular chain.
5. Patients with a metachronous regional node involvement have a better prognosis than those with synchronous primary cancer and regional lymph nodes.
6. Squamous cell carcinoma is the most common histological type.
7. The discovery of a hidden primary tumour decreases with the passing of time.
8. Most primaries below the clavicle manifest themselves during the first year.
9. The upper respiratory tract and oral cavity are the sites of origin for the majority of apparently occult metastases that are eventually classed as determinate secondaries.
10. The majority of detected primary neoplasms below the clavicles are from the lungs or gastrointestinal tract.
11. The prognosis for the patient with a subsequently located primary neoplasm is apparently worse than those patients in whom the primary remains undiscovered.
12. Patients with the involved lymph nodes limited to the upper one half of the neck have a better prognosis than those with lower node metastases.
13. The prognosis is better in patients with a single node in the upper part of the neck
14. Patients with supraclavicular node metastases have a very poor prognosis and almost all have primary neoplasms below the clavicle.
15. Survival of patients with multiple or bilateral lymph nodes is generally brief.
16. Metastatic adenocarcinoma has a poor prognosis.
17. There is no prognostic significance attached to the histological type when the node is in the lower half of the neck.
18. The site of adenopathy may provide a clue to the location of the primary lesion.
To this one might add that, (a) when the condition occurs in those under 30, it has a universally bad prognosis and (b) the metastatic neck node is usually over 4 cm, if in the upper part of the neck.

INVESTIGATIONS

This section will relate to the investigation of a patient who presents with a neck lump that may, or may not be, carcinoma and with no other signs or symptoms.

History

The age and sex of the patient are obviously important because those under the age of 25 are unlikely to have a carcinomatous deposit in the neck and males are more likely than females to have carcinomas arising from the upper respiratory tract. The vast increase in smoking in females in the UK, however, may well alter this ratio. One enquires of the usual symptoms of hoarseness, dysphagia, pain or weight loss, but it is likely that, if the patient had any of these symptoms, he would present with them. It is important to get the patient to relate any curious feelings that he has developed in his tongue, because base of tongue tumours do not often present as such but can subtly alter speech and swallowing patterns. Although trismus is an easily recognizable sign by all, mild trismus is worth enquiring about as is the occurrence of febrile illness, unexplained tiredness or anaemia.

Head and neck examination

This takes the usual form and most would now use the nasal endoscope, the nasopharyngoscope and the flexible laryngoscope if indicated.

We will presume for the purposes of this section that no primary is obvious on clinical examination.

Fine-needle aspiration biopsy

It is now our custom to perform this on all neck masses. This is not the technique that one advises for universal use, because there must be somebody to do the cytology expertly. Good cytologists do not exist in every pathology department and it is usually not rewarding to send these specimens to the general pathology department. One must have a cytologist who is interested and who achieves a greater than 95% accuracy rate over a wide range of pathology. False negatives must be interpreted in the light of clinical suspicion, but false positives would cast grave doubt on the technique and it has been the author's good fortune never to have been in receipt of one of these. Not only does the cytologist need to be good, but the technique of the aspirator needs to be practised. It has been our experience in this

department that, if anyone unused to the technique does the aspirate, then the report often suggests there is no adequate cytological material for examination.

Radiology

There has been more nonsense talked about the use of radiology in this clinical problem than in most other subjects in the head and neck. The author has added to this lunacy by listing radiological investigations in the past, which have proved to be expensive, time wasting and of little or no yield (Stell & Maran 1979). It was formerly our custom to carry out chest X-ray, base-of-skull views, barium swallow, meal, enema and an i.v.p. We stopped short of thyroid and parotid scans in the absence of masses and also sialograms and sinus X-rays.

It is now our opinion that no imaging, except a chest X-ray and, occasionally, a base-of-skull view, is helpful. Primaries that are not seen, or palpable, are rarely shown up by any form of imaging, including CT scanning or nuclear magnetic resonance.

Most head and neck surgeons will remember cases where radiology has confused the issue, resulting in delay and expense.

Laboratory investigations

Few laboratory investigations are worth carrying out in the search for a carcinoma, apart from the serum titre of IgA to the viral capsid antigen (VCA) of the Epstein–Barr virus (EBV). The production of antibodies to the various EBV-specific antigens is influenced by many factors other than the availability of EBV specific antigens. In pretreatment cases of stage 1 nasopharyngeal carcinoma, the false negative rate may be as high as 12% and the diagnostic titre of IgA anti-VCA is set at greater than 1:5. The false positive rate is about 10%, which reflects the presence of other tumours (Ho 1978).

Endoscopy

It is normal to carry out a quadruple endoscopy, namely nasopharyngoscopy, laryngoscopy, oesophagoscopy and bronchoscopy. We formerly listed the commonly accepted seven or eight biopsy sites, but it is now our custom, if no primary tumours are identifiable, only to curette the nasopharynx with an adenotome, to remove the ipsilateral tonsil and have many sections cut and to biopsy the ipsilateral piriform sinus after stretching it to open up the apex. Bronchial cytology completes the investigation. If the cytology is negative and the fine-needle aspiration biopsy is positive, then the bronchoscopy is repeated with a flexible bronchoscope and the cytology repeated.

Biopsy

If fine-needle aspiration biopsy is negative, then one proceeds to open biopsy.

Core biopsies with a Vin Silverman needle may be requested by some pathology departments. Patients with a metastatic cancer of the neck from an occult primary are really facing such poor prognosis that the increased implantation risk is not important.

Open biopsy

Here one has to face the question of excision or incisional biopsy. Hayes Martin made eloquent pleas that no cervical node biopsy be performed till after a thorough search for the primary. Unfortunately, his pleas still go unheeded where surgeons are not practised in the art of head and neck surgery. As recently as 1973, Jesse (Jesse et al 1973) pointed out that 53% of his series of 210 had been biopsied prior to presentation. McGuirt et al (1979) have shown that there is an increased incidence of local recurrence if there has been previous biopsy, but this was not supported by Razack et al (1977).

It is curious that there is such a high recurrence rate, because excisional biopsy has been performed for metastatic cancer by general surgeons for years prior to head and neck surgery attaining its present excellence of practice. It is not clear in most papers how many recurrences had incisional and how many excisional biopsies. It is the author's personal experience in dealing with 74 patients who presented with incisional biopsies, that none lived for 5 years, whereas 34 patients who presented with excisional biopsy had a survival rate that was the same as a matched unbiopsied group. It could be argued that, if the original surgeon carried out an incisional biopsy, then not only was local recurrence likely because of implantation of tumour into a fresh

wound, but he possibly carried out the incisional biopsy because the node was bigger and more fixed, in which case the patient had a very bad prognosis anyway. Furthermore, if an excisional biopsy is well done, then to spill tumour means that there is tumour in the lymphatic trunks, which suggests that more than one node is involved and indicates a very much reduced survival (Kalnins et al 1977).

The other very curious pathological point that demonstrates the unique tumour–host dynamic is why these few patients have enormous metastases from an inapparent primary tumour. Spiro et al (1983) listed 45% of his cases as N1 and 86% as N2 or N3. Although it is generally accepted that nodes over 3 cm in size have extranodal spread and thus a very reduced prognosis, Snow et al (1982) found that 20% of nodes in his series that were over 1 cm had extranodal spread. In Spiro's series, 23% had to have an extended radical neck dissection, which is the experience of most head and neck surgeons. It shows that these unfortunate patients have tumours that are far more aggressive than the normal nodal metastases from a recognized primary.

BRANCHIOGENIC CARCINOMA

This concept must be raised again in line with the evidence on the so-called branchial cysts. It is now considered that branchial cysts have little to do with the branchial apparatus (Maran & Buchanan 1978). They are cysts of squamous epithelium within lymph nodes and there is no reason that these cannot go on to become carcinomatous. The squamous epithelium is heterotopic tissue and so liable to abnormal biological behaviour. Hayes Martin's postulates that were referred to at the beginning of this chapter, made it virtually impossible ever to diagnose branchiogenic carcinoma. If the concept of a carcinoma arising in squamous epithelium in a lymph node is accepted, then it could account for those few cases that never have a primary discovered after initial work-up or within 2 years. It does not rule out the possibility of metachronous primary. Some patients do have long survivals when the so-called metastatic node is removed from the neck. It surely is odd to postulate that, by removing a metastases the primary becomes dormant. This reverses the normal pathological concept of dormancy, which usually applies to metastases and not primaries.

Treatment Policy

The patient arriving, presenting with a node and having a negative work-up

In this instance, it is our custom to carry out a fine-needle aspiration biopsy and, if this is negative, to go on to an open excisional biopsy and frozen section. If this proves to be carcinoma, or if the FNAB is positive, then we proceed to radical neck dissection; if extracapsular spread is shown, or if there is more than one node positive, then we follow this with postoperative radiotherapy.

The patient presenting with a node which is histologically positive for cancer

If the patient has a fine-needle aspiration biopsy and it is positive, then we search for a primary; if it is undiscovered we proceed as above. If they present having had an excisional biopsy that is positive, we carry out a search for the primary tumour and, if none is discovered, we give radiotherapy to the neck. If he has had an incisional biopsy; then we carry out an extended radical neck dissection, excision of neck skin and appropriate reconstruction.

What is quite unacceptable, is to do a biopsy, not carry out a search, but give postoperative radiotherapy. Should we perhaps mute our criticisms of the expensive searches that were promulgated in the 60s and 70s and continue to teach our colleagues that they must not biopsy or irradiate without searching?

The other unacceptable practice is the modified neck dissection. It is now generally accepted that this is a reasonable procedure to carry out in the N0 neck where it carries no more of a recurrence rate and less morbidity than a radical neck dissection. In the N1 neck, however, it carries with it a higher recurrence rate and, since most of the patients presenting with a metastatic neck cancer and unknown primary present with very large nodes, then they must have a full classical neck dissection.

The evaluation of the circumscribed neck mass remains a considerable challenge to physicians in general and surgeons in particular. Much can be learned about the circumscribed neck mass by the use of such time-tested activities as detailed history taking and a complete and comprehensive physical examination. This is much simpler for otolaryngologists and those in other disciplines who specialize in head and neck surgery, simply because of their familiarity with the anatomy of the head and neck and with the specialized instruments utilized in the evaluation of these anatomical sites.

Had I been asked to write this chapter several years rather than several months ago, this task, as well as the reality of the evaluation, would have been considerably more difficult. The use of CT scanning and fine-needle aspiration biopsy has added immeasurably to what we can learn in certain cases in which we have not achieved a diagnosis by history and physical examination. Only with accurate diagnosis can one make a rational plan of management. Therefore, one's ability to help the patient, particularly those with malignant disease, is really directly related to how accurate we are in our diagnosis.

The differential diagnosis of a mass in the neck requires a familiarity with many different entities, some normal, but most abnormal. A classification of these conditions is presented in Table 19.1 (Feldman 1985). In addition to the abnormal conditions listed, several normal structures should be added, such as a torturous carotid bulb, the transverse process of second cervical vertebra in persons with a very thin neck and the greater cornu of the hyoid bone. These normal structures in certain individuals can, and have, been interpreted as abnormal (Suen & Myers 1981).

History-taking remains of paramount importance in the evaluation of the neck mass. In children, the inflammatory neck mass most often will have a rather short history and usually pain, swelling and redness accompany the appearance of the mass. In

Table 19.1 Differential diagnosis of a lump in the neck

Cervical masses in children
I Congenital:
  1. Branchial cleft cyst
  2. Cystic hygroma (lymphangioma)
  3. Haemangioma

  4. Thyroglossal duct cyst
  5. Laryngocoele
  6. Teratoma
II. Inflammation:
  1. Non-specific lymphadenitis with lymphoid hyperplasia (overwhelming majority)
III. Neoplasms:
  A. Benign (see above)
  B. Malignant
    1. Lymphoma/leukaemia
    2. Rhabdomyosarcoma
    3. Neuroblastoma

Cervical masses in adults
I. Congenital:
  1. Branchial cleft cyst
  2. Thyroglossal duct cyst
II. Inflammation:
  A. Lymph nodes
    1. Non-specific lymphadenitis with lymphoid hyperplasia
    2. Specific lymphadenitis—cat scratch disease, toxoplasmosis.
    3. Granulomatous lymphadenitis—tuberculosis, sarcoidosis, fungal disease
  B. Thyroid
    1. Thyroiditis
III. Neoplasms
  A. Benign
    1. Thyroid—follicular adenoma, Hurthle cell adenoma
    2. Salivary glands—benign mixed tumour (pleomorphic adenoma), papillary cystadenoma lymphomatosum (Warthin's tumour), monomorphic adenoma, benign lymphoepithelial lesion
    3. Soft tissue—lipoma, neurilemoma, carotid body, tumour
  B. Malignant, primary (approx 20%)
    1. Lymph nodes—malignant lymphoma
    2. Thyroid—papillary carcinoma, follicular carcinoma, medullary carcinoma, undifferentiated (small cell, giant cell, spindle cell) carcinoma
    3. Salivary glands—mucoepidermoid carcinoma, malignant mixed tumours, acinic cell carcinoma, adenoid cystic carcinoma
    4. Soft tissue—rare
  C. Malignant, secondary (80% plus): histological type and origin
    1. Squamous cell carcinoma—upper aerodigestive tract (most frequent source), lung, larynx, skin oesophagus, uterine cervix, salivary gland
    2. Adenocarcinoma—lung, breast, thyroid, salivary glands, gastrointestinal tract including pancreas, genitourinary tract (kidney, prostate), uterus, ovary
    3. Malignant lymphoma—any lymph node or extranodal site
    4. Small cell undifferentiated carcinoma—lung, oesophagus, larynx
    5. Melanoma—skin, mucous membranes (oral cavity, upper respiratory tract) ear, eye
    7. Seminoma—testis

From: Feldman P S 1985 Pathologic and cytologic diagnosis of a lump in the neck. In: Chrethien P et al (eds) Head and neck cancer, vol I. B C Decker, Philadelphia Pa, p 282 children with a mass in the lateral neck, it is important to inquire about whether there is a cat as a pet in the home, since cat scratch fever presents in such a way. A mass in the anterior triangle of the neck, which appears only at the time of an upper respiratory tract infection, would make one consider a branchial cleft cyst, just as intermittent enlargement of a mass in the midline of the neck would make one think of thyroglossal duct cyst.

It is important in certain masses, such as the branchial cleft and thyroglossal duct cyst and dermoid cyst, that the mass, if it has been present for some time, should be growing at the same rate as the patient rather than more rapidly. Rapid growth would make one think of a neoplasm. Neoplasms in children are fortunately unusual and are usually painless. The appearance of a mass in the area of the thyroid gland in a child is most commonly a thyroid cancer rather than a benign tumour and, even if the history is short term, an aggressive effort to establish a diagnosis is important.

In children and teenagers, the recent occurrence of a mass or bilateral masses in the anterior cervical triangle should alert one to the possibility of a nasopharyngeal carcinoma, or a lymphoma and, again, diagnosis should be aggressively sought. Mesenchymal tumours, such as fibromatosis or fibrosarcoma, rhabdomyosarcoma and neuroblastoma, are fortunately rare. However, the occurrence of a painless mass with an indolent course in this area, although circumscribed, should arouse the examiner's curiosity that this may well represent a malignant neoplasm.

The age of the patient is an important item. A mass in the lateral neck in patients over 40 years of age must be considered neoplastic until proven otherwise. Most of these neoplasms are malignant and metastatic from an anatomical site in the head and neck. Certainly, a lymphoma or primary neoplasm in this area must also be considered.

The sex of the patient is of some importance in the sense that cancer of the upper aerodigestive tract occurs more frequently in men than in women. However, with the social acceptance of the use of tobacco and alcohol in women, we should no longer exclude the possibility of carcinoma in the female with a mass in the neck.

Race may be an item of some importance. For instance, a Black patient with a mass in the neck would not be thought of as having metastatic malignant melanoma to the lymph node, since melanomas are rare in the Black races. Conversely, the mass in the neck in a Chinese patient should certainly rouse the suspicion of the possibility of metastasis from a carcinoma arising in the nasopharynx.

The patient with a mass in the neck, who has a history of tobacco and alcohol abuse, should certainly raise the examiner's index of suspicion of the possibility of squamous cell carcinoma of the mucosal surfaces, since this is the milieu in which such cancers develop. The presence of other symptoms which occur in squamous cell carcinoma of the upper aerodigestive tract, such as hoarseness, haemoptysis, epistaxis, stridor, unilateral sore throat, especially with otalgia, difficulty swallowing and weight loss, should be sought. The presence of such symptoms should be carefully evaluated in the physical examination and an effort should be made in the diagnostic evaluation to rule out the possibility of cancer arising in the areas to which such symptoms could be ascribed.

The duration of the presence of the mass of the neck is of importance. The patient who has had a mass in the neck which has been noticed for many years is more likely to have a congenital anomaly, or benign neoplasm, than a malignant or metastatic tumour. The history of a change in size is of importance, since progressive increase in size should arouse suspicion of malignancy. Fluctuation in size would be more consistent with an inflammatory lesion or inflammation in a congenital anomaly, such as branchial cleft cyst associated with an upper respiratory tract infection.

Many patients who have a mass in the neck are treated with antibiotics. Certainly, some inflammatory masses in the neck, such as reactive lymph node hyperplasia occurring during upper respiratory tract infection, will decrease in size with antibiotics. Granulomatous inflammatory masses, such as tuberculosis and sarcoid, do not usually decrease in size with antibiotics. A more problematic situation is that of lymphoma. A mass in the neck which is lymphoma may be treated by a practitioner with antibiotics, mistaking this for an inflammatory mass. Lymphoma may temporarily decrease in size when an antibiotic is administered. This should not lull the physician into a false sense of security, and such masses should be re-evaluated.

Pain is an important symptom in differential diagnosis, since most acute inflammatory masses present with pain. Primary and metastatic malignant tumors are not usually painful, unless they are large enough to cause pressure on, or infiltration of, the neural structures.

The size of a mass is of importance, particularly in evaluating lymph nodes. Lymph nodes may be single or multiple, whether this be inflammation, lymphoma or metastatic tumour. If one is concerned that the mass represents metastatic tumour, then the presence of additional symptomatology should be included. The consistency of the mass is important, since a very firm or hard mass is more likely to represent benign or malignant tumour than inflammation. Lymphoma is characteristically described as a mobile 'rubbery' mass, although this is not always the case. Masses which have a doughy consistency may represent lipoma. Tumours which are firm and fixed deeply or fixed to the skin usually denote malignancy.

The location of the mass is another important differential feature. Most masses in the midline of the neck, other than the immediate area of the thyroid gland, usually represent benign conditions, e.g. congenital anomalies such as thyroglossal duct or dermoid cysts. Masses in the submental space may represent inflammatory lymph nodes or dermoid cysts. Metastasis to the submental space is rare from sites other than carcinoma of the lip, which should be readily apparent. The submandibular space may be difficult to evaluate, since most of the problems in this area represent inflammation. This may be of submandibular gland origin or may be lymph nodes closely associated with the gland, which may be inflamed secondary to inflammatory disease of the skin, face, teeth or intraoral structures. Lymph nodes in this area may also be associated with chronic granulomatous disease, such as actinomycosis, toxoplasmosis or sarcoidosis. It may be difficult on the basis of history and physical examination alone to distinguish these conditions from lymphoma or metastatic squamous cell carcinoma

Masses in the anterior triangle may be congenital, e.g. branchial cleft cyst, or inflammatory, e.g. hyperplastic lymph nodes from conditions such as tonsillitis, or neoplastic, e.g. metastatic tumour from the upper aerodigestive tract. A mass in the anterior triangle, which is unilateral, asymptomatic and relatively immobile, without associated symptoms, may be a carotid body, or glamus vagale tumour. The oral cavity must be examined in such cases to rule out the possiblility of parapharyngeal space involvement. Such cases may have associated symptoms due to involvement of cranial nerves 10, 11 and 12.

Metastatic cancer from the upper aerodigestive tract metastasizes most commonly to the superior deep jugular lymph nodes. These ordinarily occur in people 40 years and older and may be single or multiple, mobile or fixed, and usually occur in patients who have a history of tobacco and alcohol abuse. The great need here is to examine the mucosal surfaces of the upper aerodigestive tract in order to ascertain the location of the primary cancer. This is not always possible in metastatic squamous cell carcinoma of the neck and such cases are considered to have an 'occult' primary cancer. More often, this is an 'undiscovered', rather than occult, primary as different levels of intensity and expertise are utilized in trying to seek the point of origin for such malignant tumours.

Masses found in the posterior triangle of the neck may be inflammatory, such as tuberculosis, which can occur both singly and multiply and occasionally are accompanied by draining sinuses in the skin. The mass in the posterior triangle in an oriental person should certainly bring to mind the possibility of a primary carcinoma of the nasopharynx. The posterior triangle is also a characteristic site for lymphoma.

A mass in the supraclavicular fossa may represent a primary benign tumour, such as lipoma, but more often metastasis from structures above the clavical, such as thyroid gland, and from below the clavical, most commonly from lungs, breast, stomach, testis, and prostate.

Physical examination remains a matter of paramount importance in the diagnosis of the circumscribed mass in the neck. At the time of the physical examination, important clues as to the nature of the condition may be acquired and, when correlated with the history, can be useful in achieving a working diagnosis. As part of the evaluation, a mass of the neck should always be measured and the size recorded. It is important to note the exact anatomical location and drawings should be utilized in order to record this information.

Notes should be taken about any inflammation in the overlying skin. This may be an inflammatory response, although the so-called peau d'orange effect of infiltration of skin by cancer may look much like inflammation. Whether the mass is mobile or fixed to underlying structures is also of great importance in differential diagnosis.

If a vascular tumour, such as a paraganglioma, is suspected, then the mass should be palpated for the presence of a thrill and auscultation may reveal a bruit. The thyroid is usually relatively easy to evaluate and a mass which moves on swallowing in this area is usually within the thyroid gland. If, in addition to the thyroid mass, there is palpable cervical lymphadenopathy, vocal cord paralysis, or difficulty in swallowing, then there is an increased possibility of malignancy. The palpation of a midline mass which moves with swallowing, or protruding tongue, would certainly be consistent with the diagnosis of thyroglossal duct cyst. The midline mass which does not move with swallowing may also be a thyroglossal duct cyst, but one must also consider dermoid cyst and cavernous haemangioma.

In the evaluation of a mass in the lateral cervical area in the adult one must be suspicious of metastatic squamous cell carcinoma. Evaluation in such a situation must not be limited to the neck but should include a detailed examination of both the cutaneous and mucosal surfaces of the head and neck. The otolaryngologist is in a particularly advantageous position to identify the primary tumour responsible for cervical lymph node metastasis because of his ability to examine the intraoral cavity, as well as such less accessible sites as base of tongue, tonsil, nasopharynx, larynx and the hypopharynx. In addition, the areas of the major/minor salivary glands, nasal cavity and the ears may yield a primary lesion that would be difficult for a general physician or surgeon to evaluate and identify.

Occasionally, even after a detailed examination, no primary tumour will be found. It is the newer modalities of diagnostic tests that are of value in achieving a diagnosis in such cases.

Adjuncts to diagnosis

In achieving a diagnosis in inflammatory diseases, routine evaluations, such as complete blood count and skin tests for tuberculosis, histoplasmosis, or other fungal infections, may be of importance. In a patient who has a supraclavicular mass in the face of an established primary in an anatomical site below the clavicles, such as lung or breast, very little additional evaluation is necessary. However, if such a primary site has not been established, then additional evaluation and search for primary cancer in the lung, oesophagus, or the gastrointestinal tract, may be of value. Certainly, radioisotope scanning is helpful in the patient who has a mass which is in the area of the thyroid gland. Routine radiographical studies of the nose and paranasal sinuses and a barium swallow to identify a primary tumour in the oesophagus may be of value.

CT scan

No doubt the most important step in diagnostic imaging in the head and neck has come with computerized tomography (CT scan). Magnetic resonance imaging (MRI), a newer modality which does not require ionizing radiation, may also become important in the future. However, this technique is not readily available in many institutions and its advantage in diagnosis over the more available CT scan is still under study. The use of CT scanning should be tailored to the specific complaint of the patient and the clinical problem. In my own practice, there are precise indications for the use of CT scanning in the evaluation of the circumscribed mass in the head and neck. One of the most common indications for CT scanning is in the patient whose neck is anatomically difficult to evaluate. This usually occurs in the patient who has a short and very stocky neck, or thick muscular neck, which makes accurate palpation difficult. The CT scan can often identify a structural abnormality which escapes the hands of the examiner. There are also patients with quite thin necks in whom there is a prominent, although asymetrical, structure such as the hyoid bone, torturous carotid artery, prominent carotid bulb, or a prominent transverse process of the 2nd cervical vertebra, which may concern the patient and may make the less experienced examiner mistake this for a tumour. Such anatomical variations can be displayed on a CT scan and offer credence to the impression that no tumour is present.

Patients who have a circumscribed mass in the neck, which presents with a parapharyngeal component, usually have a vascular tumour such as a paraganglioma. These can be imaged with CT scan utilizing contrast, in which case the vascular lesion is quite distinctly seen. This may be diagnostic of a vascular lesion and further information may then be obtained with an arteriogram.

In the presence of what appears to be metastatic tumour in the patient who has a known primary in the mucosal surface of the head and neck, the mass in the neck is usually considered nodal metastasis. It is usually not necessary to use a CT scan to evaluate this situation. However, in the event that a CT scan is obtained, any enhanced or non-enhanced mass in the lymph node-bearing area of the neck, which has a central low density, irrespective of size, should be considered as a nodal metastasis.

An important study of this application of CT scanning was reported by Friedman et al (1985). Fifty consecutive patients at the University of Illinois, who underwent radical neck dissection, were studied in order to find surgical confirmation by CT scanning. All CT scans were obtained with contrast utilizing a GE A800 scanner. They found that the overall accuracy of CT diagnosis was 90% and the majority of patients in the study had clinically positive nodes, as well as positive CT and pathological findings. All patients who had clinically positive nodes confirmed on pathology were correctly diagnosed by CT. A clinically negative neck in patients who were at high risk for nodal metastasis was confirmed by CT and pathological study in nine patients. There was another group of five patients who were clinically negative, but CT positive and pathologically positive. These patients had occult nodal metastasis which were accurately diagnosed by CT scanning. The smallest node which was positive pathologically and diagnosed by CT was 1 cm. Comparison of clinical with CT accuracy indicates CT is superior in correctly evaluating nodal disease. In this study the clinical examination was correct in 82% of patients, whereas the CT was correct in 90%.

Such information is important in proper diagnosis and staging of patients with head and neck cancer. The value of improved diagnostic acumen in nodal disease was considered to benefit patients with occult metastasis. In a high-risk group of patients, Friedman at el noted that 39% had occult disease based on clinical staging. With the information supplied by CT scanning the figure decreased to only 10%. This now raises a question as to the value of elective treatment of the neck. CT scanning may be utilized in a patient who has a clinically established metastasis in one side of the neck in order to determine whether there are CT positive nodes in the opposite side, which is of importance in treatment planning.

Occasionally, patients present with a circumscribed neck mass which is suspected to be metastatic cancer, with no apparent site of primary tumour. The use of the CT scan of the nasopharynx and oropharynx have, in some cases, revealed the primary carcinoma when there was no sign of tumour following endoscopic examination under general anaesthetic. Patients may also present with other symptoms suggestive of primary tumour in the upper aerodigestive tract, such as atypical facial pain in the distribution of the third division of the trigeminal nerve or referred otalgia. In some of these patients CT has shown deeply infiltrating cancer in the absence of visible mucosal disease (Mancuso 1985). Both groups of patients are most likely to have primary sites in the nasopharynx, tongue base or tonsil, depending on the spectrum of clinical signs and symptoms.

The occurrence of tumours arising from the upper aerodigestive tract, not discoverable on examination under anaesthesia, is an unusual circumstance. In such cases, CT scanning should be used as an integral part of the diagnostic evaluation in head and neck neoplasms. The approach to evaluation is dictated by clinical circumstances. The patient presenting with cervical nodes suspected to be metastatic cancer should undergo a thorough examination of the upper aerodigestive tract. The diagnosis of metastasis may have already been established, either by open biopsy or fine-needle aspiration. If the pathological diagnosis is squamous cell carcinoma, then a detailed examination of the nasopharynx is carried out by CT scanning. If the nasopharynx is normal, then sections may be made through the regions of the tonsillar pillar and the tongue base. If these are normal then the rest of the neck should also be examined. Patients who have the facial pain mentioned above require a detailed examination of the nasopharynx and skull base (Kalovidouris et al 1984). The CT study then serves as a guide to the endoscopist who can perform endoscopy under anaesthesia and obtain a biopsy from the area in question on CT scan. This eliminates the need for the so called 'blind biopsy' during endoscopy.

Fine-needle aspiration biopsy

The actual diagnosis of the circumscribed mass in the neck has, in the past, required surgical removal of the mass. In most cases this is quite appropriate, since removal for most congenital or inflammatory masses, whether acute or chronic, and benign neoplasms is a diagnostic and therapeutic exercise.

Where malignant tumours of the neck are suspected, whether primary or metastatic, opening the neck to obtain tissue to establish a diagnosis should never be the first step in diagnosis. This approach is usually not in the patient's best interest. Opening of normal tissue planes and partially, or completely, excising the malignant neoplasm has often been thought to have been associated with local and systemic dissemination of the disease.

More than 50 years after Dr Hayes Martin published the landmark-paper on needle aspiration biopsy, there has been a renewed interest in this diagnostic technique (Martin & Ellis 1930). Fine-needle aspiration biopsy has played an increasingly important role in establishing a diagnosis without the need to open the neck. Eighty per cent of the malignant tumours found in the neck are metastasic. In 85% of these patients the primary malignant tumour originates above the clavical, in 10% from a distant primary and in 5% the primary is unknown (Feldman 1985). Approximately 20% of the malignant tumours in the neck arise from thyroid gland, salivary glands and soft tissue.

The technique of needle aspiration biopsy is quite simple. A small area of skin overlying the mass is anaesthetized and a 22-gauge needle is attached to a specialized syringe holder. The needle is inserted through the skin and suction applied to the syringe while the tip of the needle is moved within the confines of the mass (Young 1985). Suction is released before the needle is withdrawn so that the tissue sample remains within the needle. The needle and syringe are disconnected and the sample is expressed onto a slide, which is fixed and prepared according to the Papanicolaou cytology method.

The specific diagnosis of the cell type obtained in needle aspiration suggests the likely nature of the mass and so indicates the direction of further investigation or treatment. If aspiration yields uniform or abnormal lymphocytes, appropriate excisional biopsy for suspected diagnosis of lymphoma can be undertaken. It is essential for the pathologist to examine the tissues in order to give an accurate histological diagnosis, since the trend now is towards tailoring treatment of lymphoma to cell types. Establishing the diagnosis of lymphoma obviates the need for endoscopic procedures and random biopsies.

If the aspiration is positive for squamous cell carcinoma, endoscopic procedures can then be scheduled and other unnecessary studies can be avoided. Certainly, fine-needle aspiration biopsy of the thyroid gland has markedly changed the management of a mass of the thyroid, as the patient who has an aspirate negative for malignancy may be treated with suppression therapy rather than immediate surgery.

In most patients with a clinically malignant neck mass, the diagnosis of malignancy has been established by needle aspiration biopsy before general anaesthetic is administered. If the preoperative evaluation has failed to detect the primary site in a patient whose needle aspiration is positive for squamous cell, or poorly differentiated carcinoma, 'panendoscopy', including laryngoscopy, hypopharyngoscopy, oesophagoscopy, bronchoscopy with tracheal bronchial washings, are carried out. Careful examination of the nasopharynx is by direct inspection and palpation. It is particularly important to palpate the base of the tongue and tonsil. This endoscopic evaluation is carried out to find the as yet undetected primary and also to search for other possible synchronous primary cancers in the upper or lower aerodigestive tract.

If a primary tumour is found on visualization, or palpation, then directed biopsies are indicated. This aspect of management has been made more precise with the advent of CT scanning. The rate of positive diagnosis should, one hopes, increase with more frequent use of scanning in such cases. Differentiation of the tumour may act as a guide to the site of the primary, with poorly differentiated tumours lesions arising more commonly in nasopharnyx, base of tongue and tonsil.

If needle aspiration biopsy is not diagnostic or suggestive, then open biopsy of the neck is indicated. In cases where the cytologist indicates malignancy, but cannot be more specific, open biopsy should also be made. In the past, open biopsies made in patients with suspected squamous cell carcinoma, in which a primary cannot be found, were then subjected to frozen section diagnosis and, if positive for squamous cell carcinoma, radical neck dissection carried out. This general plan of management still is accepted as the standard of care in most institutions.

CONCLUSIONS

The introduction and general use of CT scanning and fine-needle aspiration biopsy as an adjunct to the important approach of detailed history-taking and physical examination has made the management of the circumscribed mass of the neck much more precise. It may be that, in the future, nuclear magnetic resonance and other imaging techniques may make the evaluation even more precise.

INTRODUCTION

Management of the single, circumscribed neck mass remains a diagnostic dilemma. This adjudicator attempts to provide a set of guidelines which can be followed where appropriate to the particular clinical problem.

For the purposes of the discussion, the problem lump under consideration is asymptomatic, is lateral to the midline of the neck and is exclusive of thyroid, or thyroid track, masses. It is also to be assumed that every facility is available for clinical examination, including either a fibreoptic telescope (Storz-Hopkins), flexible nasopharyngoscope, or laryngoscope (Olympus). Furthermore, this undiagnosed mass is at least partially mobile and, therefore, resectable and, if malignant, potentially curable. A past history of skin lesions of the head and neck may be extremely important and will necessitate research of the details.

The two authors approach the subject quite differently: E. N. Myers in the broad sense where all possible diagnoses are considered, whereas A. Maran limits the diagnostic field to cancer, which is the commonest practical problem in 80% of cases. The age, sex and race of the patient, together with the clinical features of the neck mass, are the determining factors in deciding which investigation should be undertaken. Thus it is not possible to lay down a clinical protocol to be followed in all cases. In general, management will proceed as follows.

INVESTIGATIONS

Full blood examination is considered routine. The ESR is optional. In young patients, tests for heterophil antibodies (e.g. the Paul Bunnell) are more useful than those for specific EBV antibodies, since positivity of the former is temporary and usually indicative of active infection.

The Mantoux test is of limited value, since patients with atypical tuberculosis may have a weakly positive test, but a strong positive result is suggestive of *Mycobacterium tuberculosis*, especially if the patient has a suspect ethnic background.

Tests for toxoplasmosis vary in mode according to the laboratory (Hoeprich 1977). A high and rising titre of IgM antibodies demonstrated by the indirect fluorescent antibody test is strong evidence of the infection. In a recent analysis of the cause of cervical adenopathy in 203 patients in Singapore (Chua 1986), Chua found an incidence of 7.4% with toxoplasmosis, whereas histoplasmosis occurs only sporadically throughout the world and is virtually absent in Australia. In affected areas (e.g. central USA), serological tests and special staining and culture of exudates are undertaken for diagnosis (Hoeprich 1977).

The serum titre of IgA to the EBV is of value as a single measurement since it has been shown that patients suffering from nasopharyngeal cancer (NPC) have an approximate 10-fold elevated titre against viral capsid antigen (VCA), as also occurs in Burkitt's lymphoma. This can be used as a screening test in high-risk populations, since patients with high IgA/VCA antibodies have a 38-times higher chance of suffering from asymptomatic NPC (Simmons & Shanmugaratnam 1982). A high titre, together with positive histology for squamous cell carcinoma on aspiration biopsy cytology (ABC) indicates the need for a nasopharyngeal biopsy.

In homosexual patients, the serum titre of antibody to HIV virus may be of interest, but it is more likely that a patient suffering from AIDS would have acquired some additional infective process as the primary cause of a neck lump.

Radiology

Chest X-ray is routine in all cases. I am in agreement with Maran that other conventional radiological studies (sinus X-rays, barium swallow, etc.) are of limited value unless directed by symptoms. A skull base view should be ordered if clinical examination of the nasopharynx is unsatisfactory.

The question of CT scanning as a routine is contentious and there I am in agreement with Myers. CT scanning helps enormously in certain instances, where the clinical nature of the neck lump is uncharacteristic of a nodal mass and aspiration needle biopsy may be difficult. CT is diagnostic of parapharyngeal tumours and chemodectomas, thereby avoiding the necessity of aspiration or open-neck biopsy and directing the need for angiography. As

Myers states, it is also useful in the short, thick, or fat neck, which is difficult to evaluate clinically. Aspiration needle biopsy may be undertaken during CT scanning as an adjunct to obtaining a specimen under difficult conditions.

Ideally, CT scanning of the neck should be undertaken in all head and neck cancer patients. Myers has pointed out that CT will demonstrate occult metastatic cervical nodes in 10% of clinically negative necks, thereby improving clinical staging accuracy and indicating the need for appropriate surgical or radiotherapy treatment (Stevens et al 1985). However, it can also be argued that the investigation is expensive and hardly cost-effective in all cases.

It would seem to this author that, in the diagnostic processing of a neck lump, initial CT scanning should be undertaken only for specific reasons, as discussed previously. However, in the event of positive confirmation of squamous cancer in the neck mass by ABC but failure to find a primary site on clinical examination, then CT scanning of the entire head and neck should be undertaken. This may provide evidence to direct examination under anaesthetic (e.u.a.) and biopsy of the primary site, which may avoid the necessity of repeating the procedure following subsequent CT scanning.

Aspiration biopsy cytology (ABC)

Both authors employ this technique near routinely, so that there is unanimous opinion concerning its value. Both stress the importance of having a cytologist who is familiar and experienced in the technique and who is available to provide the services on the premises using a Franzen pistol grip syringe attachment and a choice of 20–25 gauge needles (Linsk & Franzen 1983). A probable answer as to the nature of the pathology can usually be provided within a few minutes in 80% of cases and will distinguish between chronic inflammation, squamous carcinoma, adenocarcinoma, thyroid carcinoma, melanoma, lymphoma or anaplastic malignancy. In cysts of the branchial type, aspiration via a wider gauge needle is both diagnostic and therapeutic and will defer the urgency of excisional procedure. To date there has been no evidence that ABC may cause seeding of malignant cells and local recurrence in the aspiration tract.

In a minority group, ABC will fail to provide a diagnosis. Occasionally, it is impossible to obtain adequate material if the tumour mass is hard or fibrotic. A core biopsy may then be undertaken, using either a Silverman needle or a mechanical drill. Critics of needle biopsy point out that excisional biopsy is usually necessary anyway and will always confirm the diagnosis. It is still an advantage to know the probable nature of the neck mass as positive evidence of metastatic cancer directs an extremely thorough search for the primary.

Panendoscopy

The situation arises where, either there is no definitive information concerning the nature of the neck mass, or the ABC is suggestive of lymphoma or metastatic cancer. There is general agreement that a panendoscopy should be undertaken with preliminary visual examination of the nasopharynx, followed by manual palpation of that area and the ipsilateral tonsil, tongue base and pharyngeal wall. Blind biopsy should be taken of the nasopharynx and elsewhere if there is any suggestion of thickening or induration. Enucleation tonsillectomy is an advantage for the histopathological differentiation of lymphomas and should be undertaken if there is any suggestion of unilateral enlargement. Finally, oesophagoscopy should be undertaken, followed by bronchoscopy and lavage for bronchial washings, even despite a negative plain chest X-ray.

MANAGEMENT OF THE NECK MASS

When there is still no evidence of a primary tumour in the upper aerodigestive tract, the surgeon should proceed to excisional biopsy of the neck mass. The pathologist requires a whole fresh lymph node for accurate identification of the lymphoma type and, also, fresh material may be required for culture. The pathologist and bacteriologist need to work closely together in this area. There is general agreement that incisional biopsy is undesirable as spillage of tumour cells in the process may jeopardize the results of potentially curative treatment. Several studies have highlighted the poor prognosis of patients undergoing incisional biopsy. This finding, of course, should be considered against the background of a generally poor prognosis for all such patients and the fact that, probably, those with the largest neck lumps were subjected to an incisional type of biopsy.

The incision in the neck should be planned as part of the usual incision used for a full neck dissection. The excised neck mass is sent for frozen section and provisional identification of the pathology. Both authors are in agreement that, when the diagnosis is metastatic cancer and the primary tumour is most likely in the upper aerodigestive tract, the surgeon should proceed to a full neck dissection, with or without preservation of the accessory nerve. Clearly, the extent of the neck dissection will depend on the features of the presenting neck lump in terms of its size, fixation and involvement of adjacent structures. It is unlikely that any such lump will be suitable for a true functional neck dissection.

Occasionally, the excisional biopsy frozen section will provide an unexpected pathological diagnosis in the form of metastatic thyroid cancer, adenocarcinoma or melanoma. Again, each situation will require management according to the site and extent of the neck disease.

Metastases of thyroid origin are usually papillary or follicular and it is unlikely that any form of incontinuity resection of neck nodes and thyroid will be contemplated. Furthermore, it is unlikely that the thyroid gland itself will have been investigated in terms of thyroid function tests, scanning or tracheal involvement. There will have been no opportunity for discussion with the patient concerning the possible sequelae of complete thyroid lobectomy, or total thyroidectomy.

In the circumstance of the neck lump being relatively remote from the thyroid lobe of origin, it may be preferable to close the neck and, subsequently, further investigate the thyroid status and allow time for consideration of the various options of treatment, including total thyroidectomy. In the event of the neck lump being adjacent to the suspect thyroid lobe, then it is probably better to take the opportunity of the surgical exposure and proceed to carry out a complete thyroid lobectomy, together with the isthmus of the gland, taking every precaution to preserve the recurrent laryngeal nerve.

Metastases from adenocarcinomas of the upper aerodigestive tract are rare. Adams (McQuarrie et al 1986) points out that metastases in the lower neck are most likely from infraclavicular primaries, so that there is no point in proceeding to a full neck dissection. Metastases in the upper neck adjacent to the major salivary glands are most likely from those sources, so that it would seem logical in this situation to complete the neck dissection, incorporating submandibular gland or the superficial parotid.

Finally, cervical metastases from an unknown malignant melanoma site have a very poor prognosis. A complete excisional biopsy may be sufficient under the circumstances, or, at the most, a limited or functional type neck dissection may be undertaken, realizing that treatment will be essentially palliative.

Unfortunately, a proportion of cases are referred secondarily after incisional biopsy at other centres. Ideally, a radical neck dissection should be undertaken, incorporating excision of the neck scar on the assumption that there are residual neck metastases and that there may be seeding in the incision. The type of neck dissection will need to be tailored according to the circumstances and surgical excision may be impractical, since tethering, diffuse spread or fixation may have occurred in the interval between referral. Radiotherapy alone then becomes the only alternative. Occasionally, wide skin excision and skin replacement with a deltopectoral flap will be necessary.

Pathology—bacteriology of excisional node biopsy

Frozen section examination of the excisional biopsy specimen usually confirms the findings of a positive ABC, but may provide additional information in the event of an inconclusive or negative report. The pathologist can usually provide sufficient information for the surgeon to proceed with definitive treatment. In the event of lymphoma, fresh tissue is required for immunological marker studies and also for glutoraldehyde fixation for electron-microscopy, which aids in the differentiation between undifferentiated malignancies, e.g. lymphoma, anaplastic carcinoma or melanoma.

Aspiration biopsy cytology, or fresh node examination may provide evidence of a chronic inflammatory process, which will initiate an alternative pathway of investigation. Fresh lymph node material is forwarded to microbiology for culture, and special staining of paraffin sections is undertaken to demonstrate acid-fast bacilli and fungi. There is no special stain or immunohistochemical feature which is specific for sarcoid.

The identification of chronic infective agents depends on successful culture of fresh lymph node tissue with special techniques. The differentiation between tuberculosis and atypical *Mycobacterium* infection is made on the basis of growth patterns and biochemical characteristics, whereas fungal identification depends on histological features with special staining and confirmation by culture.

Postoperative irradiation

Opinions are divided on the question of post-neck dissection radiotherapy and whether the field should encompass all potential primary sites. Pathological examination of the neck dissection specimen provides evidence as to the multiplicity of nodes involved and of extracapsular spread, these being the usual indications for postoperative irradiation. There appears to be no reason for the same policy not being followed in this situation, but the question arises as to whether all necks should be irradiated when the primary remains undiscovered?

In the event of there being a single confined nodal metastasis, then a policy of observation seems appropriate. Otherwise, the answer is probably in the positive, since statistics suggest that the prognosis is better when the primary remains undiagnosed. It has to be assumed, in most cases, that the primary will be somewhere in the upper aerodigestive tract and therefore it would seem logical to undertake total neck irradiation in the majority of cases, but sparing the nasopharynx for reasons of morbidity, unless there is an indication to direct treatment to that site, e.g. an Asian patient with or without a high IgA/EBV serum titre. There will still be considerable morbidity from deprivation of mucus secretion and soft tissue fibrosis.

SUMMARY

1. The age, sex and race of the patient, together with the physical characteristics of the neck lump, provide strong evidence for a provisional diagnosis in the evaluation of the asymptomatic lateral neck mass.

2. These features direct the need for biochemical and radiological investigations. Only f.b.e. and chest X-ray are mandatory. CT scanning is valuable.

3. Aspiration biopsy cytology will provide a diagnosis in 80% of cases, is cost-effective and is a strong indication of subsequent management.

4. Manual e.u.a., panendoscopy and excisional node biopsy remain necessary in the majority of cases for confirmatory diagnosis.

5. Approximately 10% of patients with metastatic cervical node cancer will have an undiscovered primary source. In general, management should be sequential radical neck dissection and postoperative radiotherapy.

REFERENCES

A G D Maran

Batsakis J G 1979 Tumours of the head and neck: clinical and pathological considerations, 2nd edn. Williams and Wilkins, Baltimore

Black B, Maran A G D 1978 Branchiogenic carcinoma. Clinical Otolaryngology 3: 27

Comess M, Behars O, Dockerty M 1967 Cervical metastases from occult carcinoma. Surgery, Gynaecology and Obstetrics 104: 607

Ho J H C 1978 An epidemiological and clinical study of nasopharyngeal carcinoma. International Journal of Radiation Oncology, Biology, Physics 4: 181

Jesse R H, Perez C A, Fletcher G H 1973 Cervical node metastases—unknown primary carcinoma. Cancer 31: 854

Kalnins K, Leonard A G, Sako K, Razack M S, Shedd D P 1977 Correlation between prognosis and degree of lymph node involvement in carcinoma of the oral cavity. American Journal of Surgery 134: 450

McGuirt W F, McCabe B F, Krause C J 1979 Complications of radical neck dissection: a survey of 788 patients. Head and Neck Surgery 1: 481

Maran A G D, Buchanan D 1977 Branchial cysts, sinuses and fistulae. Clinical Otolaryngology 3: 77

Martin H, Morfit H M, Ehrlich H 1950 The case for branchiogenic cancer (malignant branchioma). Annals of Surgery 132: 867

Razack M S, Sako K, Marchetta F C 1977 Influences of initial neck node biopsy on the incidence of recurrence in the neck and survival in patients who subsequently undergo curative resectional surgery. Journal of Surgical Oncology 9: 347

Snow G B, Annyas A A, Van Slooten E A, Bartelink H,

Hart A A M 1982 Prognostic factors of neck node metastases. Clinical Otolaryngology 7: 185

Spiro R H, De Rose G, Strong E W 1983 Cervical nose metastases of occult origin. American Journal of Surgery 146: 441

Stell P M, Maran A G D 1979 Head and neck surgery. Heinemann, London

E N Myers

Feldman P S 1985 Pathologic and cytologic diagnosis of a lump in the neck. In: Chrethien P et al (eds) Head and neck cancer, vol I. B C Decker, Philadelphia P A, p 282

Friedman M, Grybauskas V, Mafee M, Skolnik E, Miller M 1985 Computerized tomography in the diagnosis of head and neck diseases: a clinical approach. In: Chretien P et al (eds) Head and neck cancer, vol I. B C Decker, Philadelphia P A, p 109

Kalovidouris A, Mancuso A A, Dillon W 1984 A CT clinical approach to the V, VII, IX–XII cranial nerves and cervical sympathetics. Radiology 151: 671–676

Mancuso A 1985 Computed tomography and magnetic resonance imaging in the detection and staging of head and neck cancer. In: Chretian P et al (eds) Head and neck cancer, vol I. B C Decker, Philadelphia P A, p 120

Martin H E, Ellis E B 1930 Biopsy by needle puncture and aspiration. Annals of Surgery 92: 169–181

Suen J Y, Wetmore S J 1981 Cancer of the neck. In: Suen J Y, Myers E M (eds) Cancer of the head and neck. Churchill Livingstone, New York, p 189

Young J E 1985 The unknown primary: operative evaluation. In: Chrethien P et al (eds) Head and neck cancer, vol I. B C Decker, Philadelphia P A, p 286

H S Millar

Chua C L 1986 The value of cervical lymph node biopsy—a surgical audit. Australian and New Zealand Journal of Surgery 56: 335–339

Hoeprich P D 1977 Infectious diseases, 2nd edn. Harper and Row, London

Linsk J A, Franzen S 1983 Clinical aspiration cytology. J B Lippincott, Philadelphia

McQuarrie D G et al 1986 Head and neck cancer. Year Book Medical Publishers, Chicago

Simmons M H, Shanmugarathnam K 1982 The biology of nasopharyngeal carcinoma. In: Biology of human cancer UICC Report no 16, Geneva

Stevens M H, Harnsberger H R, Mancuso A A et al 1985 Computed tomography of cervical lymph nodes. Archives of Otolaryngology 111: 735–739

20

Is needle biopsy of value in the routine examination of head and neck tumours?

A.P. Freeland

One dilemma which faces the head and neck surgeon is whether to use needle biopsy as part of the routine management of head and neck tumours. The technique to be discussed and strongly supported in this chapter is fine-needle aspiration (FNA), also called aspiration biopsy cytology (ABC), which is a cytological examination and must be distinguished from wide-bore needle biopsy, which is a histological technique.

Historical background

In 1930, Martin & Ellis published their experience in using needle biopsy to obtain material for examination. They used wide-bore needles and the specimen obtained was suitable for histology rather than cytology, because a core of tissue was aspirated. Their technique led to complications, one of which was seeding of tumour cells along the needle tract and so fell into disuse in the USA

Cytological studies from aspirates were undoubtedly pioneered in Scandinavia and large series began to be reported in the mid-1960s. Eneroth & Zajicek (1966) reported their FNA results on 368 mixed salivary tumours (pleomorphic adenomas) and Franzen & Zajicek (1968) reviewed 3479 consecutive breast aspirates. More recently, renewed interest has been shown in other countries and encouraging results have been reported, particulary in the USA by workers such as Frable & Frable (1982).

Why has this technique not, therefore, had universal acclaim and why is it not commonly used, particularly in the UK, as part of the routine examination of head and neck tumours? Clinical examination of cervical metastases is notoriously unreliable, since false positive and false negative rates are estimated to be between 20–30% (Sako et al 1964). Open biopsy, whether incisional or excisional, of neck nodes is not acceptable (McGuirt & McCabe 1978). It is all the more perplexing, therefore, given the reported accuracy of FNA, why it is not a routine technique in the management of head and neck tumours. It is proposed to discuss FNA under three headings: accuracy, complications and cost.

ACCURACY OF FINE-NEEDLE ASPIRATION

Accuracy is primarily dependent on two factors: the acquisition of a good sample and the expertise in its interpretation. These aspects will be discussed before considering the reported accuracy from different sites within the head and neck.

Technique

The technique used by Feldman et al (1983), which is a modification of the one described by Franzen & Zajicek (1968), is, with minor differences, the one preferred by the author. A syringe holder, such as the Cameco is of great value since aspiration can be done with one hand while the other fixes the mass between thumb and forefinger. Many authors use a 20 ml syringe, but we find a 10 ml one adequate and favour a 22-gauge needle. Most wide-bore histological needles, such as the Vim-Silverman and Tru-Cut, are of 14-gauge and allow a core of tissue to be removed rather than a few cells.

Once the mass has been immobilized with one hand, the needle is inserted through antiseptically prepared skin into the midpoint of the mass. When the needle is in the lession, the plunger of the syringe-holder is pulled back to create a negative pressure.

The negative pressure is kept constant and the needle withdrawn slightly and reinserted into different areas of the mass in turn, often in five different directions to maximize sampling of the whole mass. The aim is only to fill the needle with a sample of cells and, when material is seen at the junction of the needle and the syringe, the aspiration is discontinued and the negative pressure is slowly released while the tip of the needle remains in the mass. Once all the pressure is released, the needle is gently withdrawn and a swab placed on the puncture site.

Preparation of smears

The syringe and needle are detached from one another and the syringe is filled with air and reattached to the needle. The needle bevel is placed in contact with a clean, dry, glass slide and a small drop of aspirate is gently expressed onto the slide. Using another slide held at 45°, a smear is produced in the same way as a blood film. Four slides are prepared, two are rapidly air dried and two are immediately fixed with 95% ethyl alcohol spray. Staining is carried out in the laboratory with Papanicolaou and May-Grunwald Giemsa stains. The rest of the contents of the needle are then ejected into a bottle containing transport medium (1 ml of human AB serum, 14 ml Eagle's culture medium and 125 mg of heparin) for further cytology and immunocytochemical studies. The ideal arrangement is for the cytologist to be in the clinic to examine the prepared slides and, if they are inadequate, to ask for a further aspirate. This may involve a little wait for the patient, but usually a second aspirate will provide a definite answer.

Occasionally, a cyst is aspirated and, although cells from the cyst fluid may be examined, it is important to reaspirate the collapsed cyst to obtain material from its wall or residual tumour mass.

It needs to be re-emphasized that only small quantities of aspirate within the needle lumen are required. If too much blood or fluid enter the syringe, the resulting dilution of cells may make cytology inaccurate. There is no disgrace in being asked by the cytologist for a better specimen and close co-operation ensures a reliable service. It is suggested (Crucioli 1985, personal communication) that the following is a reasonable course of action:

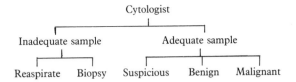

It is essential to regard an adequate sample that is suspicious as being malignant until proved otherwise, if necessary with an open biospy.

Fine-needle aspiration benefits the patient, the clinician and the laboratory. The patient benefits from having a safe outpatient procedure, which leaves no scar and can be repeated, but, above all, there is no worrying wait for the result of a biopsy to be interpreted. The clinician benefits from an early diagnosis. It is a technique that can be used for screening and as a check after radiotherapy. The laboratory benefits, since time and money are saved, and it is a test that can be done in the outpatient department, or in the operating room and can often be checked for accuracy against future histology, which improves the expertise of the cytologist.

Salivary gland pathology

Most surgeons regard a lump in the parotid gland, that is not apparently inflammatory, as a neoplasm until proved otherwise by histological examination and consider the only way to provide the necessary material is to perform a superficial or total parotidectomy. A safe margin of normal parotid tissue around the mass is necessary to prevent seeding, most of all from pleomorphic adenomas, which are the commonest of all parotid tumours. Careful dissection and preservation of the facial nerve is required in the surgery of benign parotid tumours, but the excision of malignant tumours may be compromised by facial nerve preservation. FNA can provide a preoperative, accurate assessment as to whether the lesion is benign or malignant and allow possible facial nerve resection to be discussed with the patient.

Frable & Frable (1982) reported the technique on 227 salivary glands and quote a 99% specificity for the presence of tumour and a 92% for the absence. There were 94 tumours and the exact tumour type was correct in 85% of cases. There were 133 other non-neoplastic conditions. Qizilbash et al (1985) reported the results of FNA in 160 major salivary gland lesions and quoted the overall accuracy as being 98%. There were 146 good samples, the other 14 were acellular, or inadequate. Of the 146, 122 were benign and were made up of 47 tumours and 75 other lesions, 24 were malignant, 10 being primary tumours and 14 metastatic. There were no false positives and three false negatives in this series. The benign group were all correctly called benign and the actual tumour type was accurate in 91.4% of cases. The accuracy was 86.6% in the non-neoplastic group. The benign tumours consisted of 35 pleomorphic adenomas, of which 33 were correctly diagnosed by smears which were quite characteristic. There were 4 monomorphic adenomas, of which 3 were correctly diagnosed, as were 7 out of 8 adenolymphomas. The malignant group consisted of 3 adenoid-cystic carcinomas, which were all correctly diagnosed, as were 2 acinic cell carcinomas, 1 undifferentiated and 1 adenocarcinoma. There were three mucoepidermoid carcinomas, of which only 1 was correct on FNA. However, the other 2 cases were called malignant and were, in fact, poorly differentiated at the eventual histological examination. The metastatic group included 3 false negatives. One of 9 squamous cell carcinoma metastases was called benign due to a sampling error. One malignant lymphoma and 1 Hodgkin's disease metastasis were also called benign due to inexperience. These authors summarized the results of other workers in their accuracy of correct tumour typing for benign lessions, examples being Frable (1983) 98%, Webb (1973) 95.8% and Persson & Zettergren (1973) 97.4%. They also quote the vast series of Eneroth & Zajicek (1966), who correctly diagnosed benign mixed tumours (pleomorphic adenomas) 92.4% of the time.

The figures quoted are, of course, from enthusiastic experts, but on a much smaller scale Slack et al (1985) reported the results of FNA in 10 salivary gland lesions. They were all correctly diagnosed as benign and of the 8 neoplasms, 6 were correctly diagnosed for tumour type.

The accurary of FNA in salivary gland pathology, as judged by the figures above, suggests an extremely useful technique, making it possible to plan with the patient the type of treatment necessary, including the possibility of having to resect the facial nerve in malignant disease. If this is known in advance, planned reconstruction of the nerve can be undertaken at the same time. It also allows for preoperative planning of possible interstitial radiation to the tumour bed at the end of the procedure, rather than the usual difficulties of not knowing whether this might be necessary until the results of frozen section diagnosis at the time of surgery are available. It is also evident from the series of Qisilbash et al (1985) that nearly two-thirds of their benign group were not tumours and it is reasonable to speculate that FNA prevented at least some of their patients from having unnecessary exploratory surgery.

It would seem, therefore, that the accuracy of FNA in salivary gland pathology is not in question.

Cervical lymph nodes

Since most metastatic cervical lymph nodes arise from primary disease within the head and neck, the correct initial management is to look for the primary site, usually by panendoscopy. In most cases, the primary site will be found and, if biopsy demonstrates squamous cell carcinoma, then palpable ipsilateral nodes are likely to be the same and no further node investigation is necessary. However, it is not uncommon for an extensive hunt for a primary tumour to be unrewarding and the temptation exists to biopsy the palpable neck nodes for a histological clue as to the whereabouts of the primary tumour. McGuirt & McCabe (1978) showed very clearly that open biopsy of a neck node may cause an increased chance of recurrence and metastasis and it also makes definitive surgery in the form of radical neck dissection more complex due to the necessity for wide excision of the biopsy site. The presence of a cervical metastasis and an unknown primary is an ideal situation for FNA. The technique is also of great value in assessing postirradiation or postsurgical necks which may be very difficult to palpate accurately. Aspiration of areas of induration or vague masses can alleviate the clinical worry that there may be residual or recurrent disease. Open biopsy in this situation is likely to produce a wound-healing problem. FNA may also be used to investigate contralateral neck masses, which may have a significance in treatment planning and prognosis.

However, is FNA accurate in the above situations? Frable & Frable (1982) reported 649 lymph node aspirates and quoted the specificity for absence of tumour as 98% and 95% for the presence. They point out, however, that it is not a good technique for the primary diagnosis of malignant lymphoma. Felman et al (1983) report specimens as unsatisfactory, negative, suspicious, or positive for malignancy and they say that a negative result is highly significant, since they had only 1 false negative out of 172 samples. FNA was positive for malignancy in 108 neck masses and, of these, 72 had histological confirmation which was not available for the other 36, who had radiotherapy carried out on the basis of the cytological report. Fifty-five aspirates were negative for malignancy and, of these, 21 were examined histologically and all but 1 were benign. There were 9 aspirates that were reported as suspicious and all were biopsied; of these, 6 turned out to be malignant and 3 benign. These authors justify the role of FNA in suspicious areas of the neck by stating that clinical evaluation alone, in assessing N0 neck masses, fails to identify 15–45% of metastases. Their overall accuracy of FNA for squamous cell carcinoma from head and neck sites was 99%. Since 60% of their suspicious aspirates were positive when an open biopsy was performed, they strongly suggest this action if the cytologist is suspicious. Unsatisfactory specimens mean nothing and clinical judgement has to be used to decide whether to re-aspirate, observe, or biopsy.

Gertner et al (1984) quote an overall accuracy for FNA of lymph nodes from 138 patients as 85.4%, but if those with lymphoma are excluded, the accuracy for malignant nodes is 92% and 100% for benign nodes.

The accuracy of FNA is clearly more than adequate as an adjunct to clinical examination of cervical lymph nodes. Hopefully, its increased use will avoid the temptation to excise or incise cervical nodes. It needs to be stressed again that unsatisfactory samples add nothing to the clinical management and suspicious samples must be replaced, or an open biopsy planned. Finally, although a negative result is highly significant, if it is at variance with the clinical impression, then further investigation should be carried out.

The solitary thyroid nodule

The solitary thyroid nodule may present a major diagnostic problem, for althoug a toxic, hot nodule, or a thyroid cyst may be relatively easy to diagnose, the difference between a colloid nodule, or a benign follicular adenoma and thyroid carcinoma may be extremely difficult to determine clinically. It is common practice to apply certain criteria, including age, sex, previous radiation exposure, recent growth, firmness, irregularity, fixation to surrounding structures and lymphadenopathy to identify the malignant nodule (Blum 1978, Burrow 1981). However, a large number of patients operated on using these criteria turn out to have benign lesions and, therefore, possibly unnecessary surgery. Lowhagen et al (1981) quote their huge experience with FNA in the diagnosis of the solitary thyroid nodule at the Karolinska Hospital, Stockholm during the last 25 years and state that about 2500 aspirates are being performed annually in thyroid disease. Their main object is to distinguish the different types of malignancy and also to decide which patients should be subjected to surgery and which can be managed in other ways. They recognize that about 10% of all thyroid tumours cannot be identified specifically by cytology and need surgical exploration for histological evaluation. Eighty per cent of their aspirates show the patients to have colloid goitres. They recognize that the identification of a solitary nodule containing Hashimoto's disease can be difficult since lymphocytic thyroiditis may be difficult to distinguish from the lymphocytic infiltrate of carcinoma. With regard to malignant thyroid tumours, they summarize a number of other reports and there seems to be a false negative rate of about 10% with virtually no false positive cases. Between three and four patients with solitary nodules out of every five seen are spared surgery due to the results of cytological examination. Despite this very high success rate, they emphasize the use of sound clinical judgement as to whether a patient should be explored surgically. They counter the 10% false negative rate by saying that, although aspiration cytology might be negative and the nodule clinically suspicious, they would explore the thyroid glands of those under the age of 25 or ever the age of 60 in whom the risk of malignancy may be as high as 60%. This means they only treat patients between 25 and 60 years conservatively (with thyroxine and observation), in which case the risk of missing carcinoma is negligible. FNA is most accurate with papillary carcinoma, especially those with lymph node involvement. Medullary and anaplastic carcinoma can also readily be identified. However, FNA cannot distinguish between malignant and benign follicular tumours and histology is therefore very necessary in these cases.

An interesting evaluation was made by Belanger et al (1983), who carried out FNA on 63 consecutive, unselected patients with a solitary cold nodule of the thyroid gland who were all submitted to surgery. This study compares preoperative cytology with eventual histology in all these patients. The cytologist was not told the clinical findings or impressions. Histological examination showed that, of the 63 thyroid nodules, 13 were malignant and 50 benign. Cytology of the 13 malignant nodules showed 9 to be malignant, 2 to be suspicious and 1 as an indequate specimen. The other aspirate was read incorrectly as benign. It is reasonable to assume that the two read as suspicious might have been read as malignant if further aspirates had been performed and the authors also thought this is possible with the inadequate specimen, which would adjust their accuracy rate to 92%. This was in comparison with their clinical suspicions which suggested only 8 of the 13 tumours were malignant. FNA in the benign group showed that 42 out of the 50 specimens (84%) were correctly diagnosed, whereas only 39 of the 50 (72%) were correct on clinical assessment alone. Six aspirates in this group were inadequate and, if they had been repeated, the accuracy might have been greater. They conclude that all nodules with a malignant, suspicious, or inadequate cytological report should be operated on. They feel that FNA would certainly save unnecessary surgery if it were backed up with sound clinical judgement.

Local experience in Oxford is similarly encouraging and FNA is significantly adding to the confidence in the decision to operate. In the year ending December 1985 there have been 95 solitary thyroid nodules examined by FNA (Dudley 1986, personal communication), including 15 cysts, 4 toxic nodules and 3 which showed autoimmune thyroiditis; 73 were operated on and FNA compared with histology obtained from surgery; 66 were benign and 7 malignant. There was 1 false positive and 1 false negative, producing and overall accuracy rate of 97.3%. Inadequate specimens in this study were 12% for the first 6 months and only 4% for the second

showing there is a learning curve for this technique.

It seems clear that the role for FNA in the management of solitary thyroid nodules is well established.

COMPLICATIONS OF FINE-NEEDLE ASPIRATION

The major doubt about FNA is the possibility of tumour seeding along the needle tract, particularly with such lesions as pleomorphic adenomas of the salivary glands. Seeding has certainly occurred along Vim-Silverman wide-bore needle tracts in parotid carcinoma (Yamaguchi et al 1979) and from the pleura (Schachter & Basta 1973). Six cases of seeding to the perineum from prostate aspiration have also occurred (Desai & Woodruff 1974). Crile & Vickery (1952) reported a thyroid carcinoma implant to the skin of the neck and Peacock & Byars (1958) reported seeding from biopsy of a mixed parotid tumour (pleomorphic adenoma). The monograph by Zajicek (1974) covers the subject well.

On the other hand, there are no reports of seeding occurring from the use of FNA in salivary glands, nor from any other head and neck site, though it has occurred from the thorax (Sinner & Zajicek 1976). Great effort has been made to investigate seeding from FNA. Engzell et al (1971) followed 157 patients with pleomorphic adenoma for 10 years. They all had FNA prior to surgical excision. There were no recurrences in the skin, or at the needle puncture site. Qisilbash et al (1985) tattooed the needle puncture site in patients with pleomorphic adenomas and subsequent histological examination of the skin around the tattoo and the tract, which was excised with the main specimen, failed to find tumour cells. However, this tumour type is well known occasionally to recur many years later. Frable (1983) also found no recurrence in pleomorphic adenomas from FNA seeding.

Another theoretical complication of FNA is of tumour cells being released into the blood stream by the needle piercing blood vessels. This might result in distant metastases and reduced survival rate. There is no experimental evidence for blood vessel spread in rabbits where FNA has been used (Engzell et al 1971). Survival studies in renal and breast carcinoma, where FNA has been part of the management, failed to show any decrease in survival compared with control groups (Von Schreeb et al 1967, Franzen & Zajicek 1968).

The technique is otherwise virtually free of any serious complication, although occasional vasovagal episodes, blood vessel punctures and haematomas are reported (Feldman et al 1983).

The potential benefit of avoiding open neck biopsies, of detecting early recurrence and better treatment planning for thyroid nodules and salivary gland lesions far outweigh the theoretical, non-proven complication of tumour seeding by the technique of FNA.

THE ECONOMICS OF FINE-NEEDLE ASPIRATION

Fine-needle aspiration is sophisticated enough to guide treatment policies because of its accuracy. There are obvious financial advantages to health services in all countries if unnecessary surgery can be avoided. The solitary cold thyroid nodule is a case in point. Inflammatory lesions of the salivary glands are another situation where a non-surgical policy can be identified by FNA whereas clinically they can mimic rapidly growing malignant tumours. Benign tumours of the salivary glands in the elderly may reasonably be observed rather than operated upon if FNA is employed. There are, of course, many other examples of potential operation-saving instances if FNA is used expertly along with good clinical judgement.

The actual cost of FNA was discussed by Frable & Frable (1982), who compared FNA of a neck node as an outpatient procedure with excision biopsy as an inpatient. In 1982 the materials used for FNA cost less than $1 and $75 was the total charge to the patient. This is in comparison with $2310 for neck node biopsy in hospital. They also point out that, because the node biopsy contaminates the field, the definitive surgical procedure is, by necessity, more complex.

The financial savings are, of course, considerable, but it is more difficult to quantify the saving in alleviation of patient anxiety. An example of this may be seen in many breast clinics, where women with breast masses are examined and told their diagnosis after the FNA is interpreted by the cytologist attending the clinic. The relief of knowing a breast mass is innocent is enormous and, if malignant, treatment planning and counselling can be given straight away.

SUMMARY

Although this chapter has been drawn largely from the experience of experts, close co-operation by interested surgeons and cytologists can achieve equally excellent results and help establish FNA as an accurate, safe, cheap and major advance in the management of head and neck tumours.

Treatment planning, with informed input from the patient, is frequently hampered by having to await the outcome of an open biopsy, or a biopsy obtained at endoscopy; identification of the treatment options can usually be made confidently as soon as the histological verification of, for example, a neck mass has been made. The options can then be discussed intelligently with the patient.

The need to secure the histological diagnosis as early as possible is particularly important when acute problems, such as increasing airway obstruction, are emerging. Frequently, the patient's problem cannot be discussed adequately in an interdisciplinary head and neck oncology conference until the histology of the lesion is known; this is particularly true when dealing with masses in the neck, in the salivary glands and in the thyroid gland. Whether a mass is developmental, inflammatory, benign or malignant is always of concern and has significant implications in treatment planning.

DEVELOPMENT OF FINE-NEEDLE ASPIRATION BIOPSY

There is nothing new about needle aspiration biopsy. The concept was introduced by Martin & Ellis (1930); an immediate flurry of interest ensued, but thereafter the concept lay fallow for a decade or two. Several European scientists resurrected interest in the technique and this culminated in a report by Eneroth et al (1967) on the use of fine-needle aspiration biopsy (FNA) in 1000 salivary gland tumours.

Since that time, the use of the technique has been reintroduced into the USA by several investigators, including Koss et al (1984), Frable & Frable (1982) and others. The technique enjoys widespread usage in many head and neck oncology centres; each year increasing numbers of favourable reports are appearing in the literature.

RATIONALE OF FINE-NEEDLE ASPIRATION BIOPSY

The reliability of the FNA technique makes it a most useful adjunct in the workup and evaluation of the patient with a mass in the head and neck. Frable & Frable (1982) have demonstrated a specificity for the absence of tumour in lymph nodes to be 98% and for the presence of tumour to be 95%. It is of interest that these investigators found all of the false positives to be in relation to malignant lymphoma. In salivary gland tumours the specificity for the presence of tumour was 92%, with identification of the exact tumour type in 85% of patients. There was a 99% specificity for the absence of tumour. In thyroid disease the sensitivity for tumour was 92% with zero false negatives. This experience has been essentially confirmed by Sismanis et al (1980) and Gertner et al (1984) and others.

The cost-effectiveness of FNA compared with open excisional biopsy is unquestioned; Frable & Frable (1982) found that excisional biopsy was 30 times more expensive in their institution than an FNA. With the escalating cost of health care, any cost-saving manoeuvre that can be safely introduced is a rational choice.

The non-invasive nature of FNA makes it readily acceptable to patients; the fact that diagnostic information can be obtained without 'undergoing an operation' appeals to even the most stoical patient! Core-needle biopsy has always been a source of concern regarding the possibility of seeding into the needle tract; such as occurrence has been documented by Yamaguchi et al (1979). Seeding into the tract of a fine needle has not been reported and must be extremely rare, if it has ever occurred. Seeding therefore is not a concern after FNA.

PREREQUISITES FOR SUCCESS

Initially, it might be thought that no special equipment is needed to carry out FNA successfully and consistently. However, it is essential to be able to hold the aspirating syringe in one hand while creating the greatest possible vacuum within the syringe (e.g. Cameco Syringe Pistol). This allows the mass to be defined with the fingers and thumb of the other hand so that the needle tip can accurately be introduced into, and held within, the tumour mass while suction is maintained. It is essential that the mass be traversed on multiple occasions (at least more than three) by the needle tip so that adequate cell samples may be obtained.

If FNA is utilized only occasionally, the reliability of it will be extremely low. If reliability is to be achieved, FNA must be carried out frequently and on a continuing basis. Ordinarily, it is to be recommended that no decisions be made on the basis of the first 50 patients evaluated—this will allow the surgeon and the pathologist to develop the necessary degree of confidence. Thereafter, the results of FNA may be introduced confidently into the decision-making process.

The input of a committed, interested pathologist, of course, is what makes FNA a reliable method of histological diagnosis. Without question, it is more difficult for the pathologist to make the diagnosis from a few clumps of cells than when he is presented with larger portions of tissue. On the other hand, the clumps of cells taken from several areas of the tumour by multiple puncture are likely to be more representative than a biopsy taken from one area of the tumour. Without question, however, an interested and enthusiastic pathologist and surgeon can quickly develop the needed expertise and reliability. The surgeon must be prepared to give all the available clinical information to the pathologist and also be willing to study the prepared smears along with the pathologist if maximal reliability is to be maintained.

APPLICATION

Neck masses

Neck nodes

This histological identity of neck nodes that have become palpable is of great importance in planning, even when the patient is known to have a primary carcinoma in the adjacent mucous membrane; this is particularly true in the presence of contralateral nodes, when a decision regarding the need for bilateral radical neck dissection and/or adjuvant radiotherapy has to be made. A decision to advise either of these treatments cannot be made lightly; whereas, in the presence of histological verification, the decision making becomes easier for the surgeon and acceptance of the subsequent advice easier for the patient. Identification of the cell type, without resorting to incisional biopsy, is an additional

advantage, because the risk of seeding into the wound and having to plan for re-excision of the scar at the time of definitive surgery is eliminated.

Cancers of base of tongue

Most tumours of the mucosal lining of the upper air and food passages can readily be sampled by cup forceps biopsy, carried out either under topical or general anaesthesia; cancers of the base of the tongue, however, frequently present as submucosal masses so that a surface biopsy may not be contributory. Fine-needle aspiration of such a mass is frequently possible and may be carried out without difficulty or use of anaesthesia. In patients with an already compromised airway, this approach may be of particular benefit as tracheostomy usually can be avoided.

Salivary gland masses

Without knowing the histology of a salivary gland mass, it is extremely difficult to discuss the treatment plan with a patient; since open incisional biopsy is not an option in this organ site, because of the high risk of tumour seeding, treatment has often been empirical; routine superficial lobectomy of the parotid gland for what turns out to be an inflammatory node must certainly be recognized as overtreatment. Although the pathologist has more difficulty in determining the particular tumour cell type than determining whether the lesion is malignant or benign, the knowledge that the tumour is, in fact, malignant makes pretreatment planning much less difficult.

Thyroid masses

Fine-needle aspiration biopsy of a thyroid mass almost always gives information that proves to be extremely useful. On some occasion, FNA may identify a cyst and may, on occasion, eliminate the need for further treatment entirely. The knowledge that a lesion has been shown to be malignant rather than benign makes it possible to discuss the patient's needs and the treatment options confidently. In the past, the empirical performance of a partial thyroidectomy for a mass that later turned out to be a benign cyst or adenoma was more treatment than was necessary; tailoring the treatment to fit the needs of each patient is always our responsibility.

Base of the skull

Lesions of previously inaccessible areas, such as the infratemporal fossa or the ptyeragopalatine fossa, can successfully be sampled if the tip of the needle is monitored by X-ray or CT (Abemayor et al 1985). The careful placement of the fine needle causes minimal morbidity and often yields extremely useful information that cannot otherwise be obtained except by a major surgical exploration.

SUMMARY

The advent of FNA has been one of the most important and significant events of the past decade in the management of head and neck cancers; it has placed treatment planning on a more solid footing and made it easier for patients to understand and accept the treatment option most suited to their circumstances.

The place of FNA in the management of head and neck cancer is assured for the foreseeable future.

A. P. Freeland's paper is a well-planned assessment of the technique of fine-needle aspiration cytology (FNA), as applied to the diagnosis of swellings in the head and neck region. There is also little to criticize in its general appraisal of the subject and conclusions relating to its use and cost effectiveness. However, confusion in the use of terminology and in the correct final conclusion for its use in certain clinical situations suggests some inexperience on the part of the author.

The use of the word 'biopsy' in the title of the paper is misleading and should be either 'biopsy or cytology' to distinguish two differing techniques, or simply 'fine-needle aspiration cytology' if it is intended to discuss the value of a cytological aspirate only. Again, the term aspiration biopsy cytology in the first paragraph compounds this confusion. Any aspiration biopsy technique implies the study of tissue by histopathological methods, such specimens always requiring a wide-bore needle in contrast to a cytology technique, for which the 21–23-gauge fine needle is required. The two are quite separate methods and should be so considered.

The author dismisses the wide-bore needle aspiration technique for obtaining a tissue specimen for histology using the Vim Silverman needle (14-gauge) as being too risky owing to the danger of seeding and gives references for the occasional case reported. He also alleges that the technique of tissue core aspiration, advocated by Martin and Ellis in 1930, has been abandoned for the same reason. Not so. This technique of aspiration biopsy using an 18-gauge needle to obtain a core of tissue for histological diagnosis has remained in use, notably at Memorial Hospital, New York, up to the present time, although with diminished enthusiasm for salivary neoplasms. It is there felt that the theoretical risk of seeding, or displacing malignant cells into lymphatics or blood vessels, is no greater than the manipulations involved in other biopsy techniques (Spiro 1986).

In his introduction, the author also states that open biopsy is unacceptable, without further qualification. Those with experience in head and neck surgery must occasionally make use of open biopsy as a last resort when needle biopsy fails (i.e. in lymphoma), or as a preliminary to a frozen section examination when a decision may be taken for immediate surgical resection or early irradiation.

The description given of the technique of fine-needle aspiration cytology is mainly correct. The author rightly emphasizes the need for close co-operation between clinician and cytologist—more correctly the cytopathologist—to the extent that, if the latter is readily available, he should be invited to carry out the aspiration himself—and the ease with which second, or if necessary, third aspirates can be taken and a rapid report given within an hour or two.

The paragraphs dealing with salivary gland pathology cover the experience in the literature in relation to parotid tumours. However, the author's conclusion that 'the accuracy of f.n.a.c. in salivary gland pathology is not in question' does not fit the facts. Even from the published results of Eneroth & Zajicik (1966), both experienced cytopathologists, it would seem that there is an 8% margin of error in diagnosing pleomorphic adenomas. In less experienced hands, this could be more serious. Given an experienced assessment, valuable information regarding the clearly benign or malignant nature of a tumour may be obtained. Ultimately, however, an exploration with superficial parotidectomy and histological assessment of the specimen is needed to determine specific therapy, especially in relation to the facial nerve. It is really essential to know whether one is dealing with a benign tumour, a high- or low-grade mucoepidermoid, or a poorly differentiated adenocarcinoma. No mention is made of the submaxillary salivary gland, where needle cytology may also be used to confirm a suspicion of malignancy.

In dealing with the diagnosis of cervical lymph node enlargement, the author is on better ground, although he should avoid the word 'accuracy' in relation to FNA when he really means the 'value' of FNA. Certainly, aspiration cytology is a first line of investigation when cancerous lymph node enlargement is suspected and open biopsy a last resort, except where there are grounds for suspecting lymphoma.

The value of fine-needle aspiration cytology in the cold thyroid nodule is very similar to that in parotid tumours. Even for the experienced cytopathologist there will be a definite margin of error, but a clear diagnosis of differentiated or undifferentiated carcinoma will be valuable to the clinician. Where a benign adenoma is indicated, surgical resection may still be the best advice and should not be termed unnecessary.

No mention is made of the value of FNA in other head and neck sites, such as the tongue base and certain areas around the skull base, such as the infratemporal fossa, the pterygopalatine fossa and even on occasions the upper jaw area and orbit.

Most authorities believe that the dangers of seeding or releasing cells into the blood vessels (or lymphatics) is negligible using the FNA technique. It has never yet been demonstrated in the last 13 years of routine experience in the head and neck clinics of the Royal Marsden Hospital. Haematoma is occasionally noted, but can usually be avoided by performing aspiration while the patient is sitting up and with immediate pressure for a few minutes after withdrawal of the needle.

M. S. Strong's paper again uses incorrect titles for the introduction of the subject and further confuses the issue by implying that Martin & Ellis (1930) described the same technique as Eneroth (1967), Frable & Frable (1982) and others. 'Fine needle aspiration biopsy' is quite incorrect. Needle (thick) aspiration biopsy is the technique described by Martin & Ellis and still in use at Memorial Center, New York to obtain a tissue core for histological examination. 'Fine needle aspiration cytology' is the more modern, and now more popular, technique described by Eneroth, Franzen, Frable et al. It is time this semantic confusion is ended.

Dr Strong, in fact, discusses fine-needle aspiration cytology, or cytopathology, and the word biopsy is inappropriate in this context. His presentation of the rationale of FNA accuracy in experienced hands, the very rare possibility of seeding along the needle track and its cost effectiveness is concise and factual. Emphasis on technical expertise and the need for clinician and cytopathologist to work closely together is appropriate.

The paragraphs dealing with the clinical application of FNA rightly emphasize the ease and rapidity of obtaining a diagnosis so that no time is lost in proposing an effective plan of treatment. An ability to determine accurately the presence of a benign or malignant lesion is of great value by this method, even although 100% accuracy in identifying the precise tumour type may need to await confirmation by histological analysis, as in thyroid or parotid tumours, and is alone a considerable clinical aid.

The author also properly draws attention to the value of FNA at other sites such as the tongue base, the pterygopalatine fossa and the infratemporal fossa, where punch biopsy techniques are often impracticable.

The authors of both papers draw attention to the FNA technique as a recent major advance in the management of head and neck tumours. In view of its proven value as detailed by Scandinavian workers in the 1960s it is surprising that it has taken about 20 years for general acceptance. Its greatest application must certainly be nodal swellings in the neck, with the exception of lymphoma and a few other rare neck swellings. Its accuracy will be in proportion to its frequency of use and the experience of the team involved. Its results must always be interpreted alongside a good history of the condition, with properly determined clinical features and results of other investigations.

REFERENCES

A P Freeland
Belanger R, Guillet F, Matte R, Havrankova J, d'Amour P 1983 The thyroid nodule: evaluation of fine needle biopsy. The Journal of Otolaryngology 12: 2 109
Blum M 1978 Management of the solitary thyroid nodule—a selective approach. Thyroid Today 1: 1
Burrow G N 1981 Aspiration needle biopsy of the thyroid. Annals of Internal Medicine 94: 536
Crile G, Vickery A L 1952 Special use of the Silverman biopsy needle in office practice and at operation. American Journal of Surgery 82: 83
Desai S G, Woodruff L M 1974 Carcinoma of the prostate: Local extension following perineal needle biopsy. Urology 3: 87

Eneroth C M, Zajicek J 1966 Aspiration biopsy of salivary gland tumours: III. Morphologic studies on smears and histologic sections from 368 mixed tumours. Acta Cytologica 10: 440
Engzell U, Eposti P L, Rubio C et al 1971 Investigation on tumour spread in connection with aspiration biopsy. Acta Radioligica; Therapy, Physics, Biology 10: 385
Feldman P S, Kaplan M J, Johns M E, Cantrell R W 1983 Fine needle aspiration in squamous carcinoma of the head and neck. Archives of Otolaryngology 109: 735
Frable M A, Frable W J 1982 Fine needle aspiration biopsy revisited. Laryngoscope 92: 1414
Frable W J 1983 Thin needle aspiration biopsy. W B Saunders, Philadelphia

Franzen S, Zajicek J 1968 Aspiration biopsy in diagnosis of palpable lesions of the breast: Critical review of 3479 consecutive biopsies. Acta Radiologica; Therapy, Physics, Biology 7: 241

Gertner R, Podoshin L, Fradis M 1984 Accuracy of fine needle aspiration biopsy in neck masses. Laryngoscope 94: 1370

Lowhagen T, Willems J S, Lundell G, Sundblad R, Granberg P O 1981 Aspiration biopsy cytology in the diagnosis of thyroid carcinoma. World Journal of Surgery 5: 61

McGuirt W F, McCabe W F 1978 Significance of node biopsy before definitive treatment of cervical metastatic carcinoma. Laryngoscope 88: 594

Martin H E, Ellis E B 1930 Biopsy by needle puncture and aspiration. Annals of Surgery 92: 169

Peacock E E, Byars L T 1958 Management of tumours of the parotid salivary gland. North Carolina Medical Journal 19: 1

Persson P S, Zettergren L 1973 Cytologic diagnosis of salivary gland tumours by aspiration biopsy. Acta Cytological 17: 351

Qizilbash A H, Sianos J, Young J E M, Archibald S D 1985 Fine needle aspiration biopsy cytology of major salivary glands. Acta Cytologica 29: 503

Sako K, Pradier R N, Marchetta F C et al 1964 Fallibilty of palpation in the diagnosis of metastases to cervical nodes. Surgery, Gynecology and Oncology 118: 989

Schachter E N, Basta W 1973 Subcutaneous metastasis of an adenocarcinoma following a percutaneous pleural biopsy. American Review of Respiratory Disease 107: 283

Sinner W N, Zajicek J 1976 Implantation metastasis after percutaneous transthoracic needle aspiration biopsy. Acta Radiologica; Diagnosis 17: 473

Slack R W T, Croft C B, Crome L P 1985 Fine needle aspiration cytology in the management of head and neck masses. Clinical Otolaryngology 10: 93

Von Schreeb T, Arner O, Skousted G et al 1967 Renal adenocarcinoma. Is there a risk of spreading tumour cells in diagnostic puncture? Scandinavian Journal of Urology and Nephrology 1: 270

Webb A J 1973 Cytologic diagnosis of salivary gland lesions in adult and paediatric patients. Acta Cytologica 17: 51

Yamaguchi K T, Strong M S, Shapshay S M et al 1979 Seeding of parotid carcinoma along Vim-Silverman needle tract. Journal of Otolaryngology 8: 49

Zajicek J 1974 Aspiration biopsy cytology: cytology of supradiaphragmatic organs. In: Wied G L (ed) Monographs in clinical cytology, vol 4. S Karger, Basel, p 21–23, p 62–63

M S Strong

Abemayor E, Ljung B M, Larson et al 1985 CT-directed fine needle aspiration biopsies of masses in the head and neck. Laryngoscope 95: 1382–1386

Eneroth C M, Franzen S, Zajicek J 1967 Cytologic diagnosis on aspirates from 1000 salivary-gland tumors. Acta Otolaryngologica (suppl) 244: 167–171

Frable M A S, Frable W J 1982 Fine needle aspiration biopsy—revisited. Laryngoscope 92: 1414–1418

Gertner R, Bodoshin L, Fradis M 1984 Accuracy of fine needle biopsy in neck masses. Laryngoscope 94: 1371–1374

Koss L G, Woyke S, Olszewski W 1984 Aspiration biopsy, cytology interpretation and histologic basis. Igaku-Shoin, New York

Martin H E, Ellis E G 1930 Biopsy by needle puncture and aspiration. Annals of Surgery 92: 169–181

Sismanis A, Strong M S, Merriam J 1980 Fine needle aspiration biopsy diagnosis of neck masses. Otolaryngologic Clinics of North America 13: 421–429

Yamaguchi K T, Strong M S, Shapshay S M, Soto E 1979 Seeding of parotid carcinoma along Vim-Silverman needle tract. The Journal of Otolaryngology 8: 49–52

H J Shaw

Spiro R H 1986 Salivary neoplasms—overview of 35 years experience. Head and Neck Surgery 8: 177–184

21

Adjuvant chemotherapy for head and neck cancer—an unproven form of treatment

P. Clifford

Prior to the discovery of radiotherapy by Roentgen in 1895, excisive surgery was the only form of treatment for a cancer. Surgery entails the ablation of part of the body and even modern techniques, (visceral transposition, musculocutaneous flaps and free pedicle grafts) will not fully restore function and correct disfiguration. Though amputation of a leg with a compound fracture of the femur may be life-saving, one cannot consider such a measure as curative and to speak of surgical cures is nonsensical.

RADIOTHERAPY

Lederman (1981) has described the development of radiotherapy from 1895 to 1939. Catterall (1975) pioneered the use of fast neutrons in England and Sealy & Cridland (1984) have used a radiosensitizing drug, misonidazole, with and without hyperbaric oxygen, in an attempt to improve results by overcoming the resistance of hypoxic cells to external irradiation.

External supravoltage radiotherapy is, at present, the single most effective non-surgical modality for use against cancer. Radiation damages both proliferating and non-proliferating normal and malignant cells and, though radiation may be classified as a non-cycle specific agent, in fact its effects are maximal during mitosis and the late G_2 phase of the cell cycle and minimal during the latter part of the S phase (Sinclair 1968). Steel & Peckham (1979) discussed the concept of additive cytotoxicity by combination of radiotherapy and chemotherapy.

Because of the failures of surgery used with pre-operative or postoperative radiotherapy to salvage many patients with advanced head and neck cancer (stage III and IV), clinical oncologists turned to chemotherapy, which had achieved spectacular results in the curative treatment in choriocarcinoma, lymphomas, acute lymphocytic leukaemia and other cancers, (Zubrod 1972, Clifford 1976) and chemotherapy has now become a recognized therapeutic modality.

Surgical oncologists in some centres in England, France and America denigrated the role of chemotherapy in head and neck cancer, having an understandable bias in favour of surgery (Cachin 1982, McElwain 1979). In the past, chemotherapy has been used as an 'adjuvant' to enhance the effects of radiotherapy, or as a palliative to relieve symptoms after the other two modalities had failed. The majority of patients with squamous carcinoma of the head and neck are in an age group where morbidity is more important than mortality and to subject such patients to the discomforts and malaise associated with chemotherapy is not always in the best interests of the patient. The failures of radiotherapy have not, until recently, been cured by chemotherapy and, if the relief of pain is the principle reason for using palliative chemotherapy, one of the morphine group of drugs which can be given without unpleasant side effects, is probably a more caring and appropriate treatment.

Stell et al (1983) reported a trial in which patients with stage III and IV squamous carcinoma of the head and neck were randomly allotted to receive chemotherapy and radiotherapy or radiotherapy alone. The chemotherapy regime, devised by Price & Hill (1977), was a kinetically based multidrug schedule which included vincristine, hydrocortisone, methotrexate and 5-Fu followed, after an interval, with hydroxyurea-6-mercaptopurine and cyclophosphamide. Radiation in both arms of the trial was given as megavoltage in a dose of 4000–6000

Gy over a 4–6 week period. This trial was never concluded as it was thought that the chemotherapy prejudiced survival. The conclusions were based on frequent protocol violations and were not calculated by an independent statistician. The adverse effects, which led to Stell abandoning the study after only 86 patients had been entered, may have been due to the use of a chemotherapy protocol unsuitable for combination with relatively large fractions of radiotherapy. Using a similar chemotherapy protocol, Price et al (1975) considered the regimen safe and effective and this opinion was confirmed by Price & Hill (1981) and by Hill et al (1984).

Stell's results have been widely quoted by clinicians, surgically orientated, who instinctively objected to the introduction of a new treatment modality in a field where radiotherapy had only recently become acceptable.

CYTOTOXIC DRUGS EFFECTIVE IN SQUAMOUS CARCINOMA OF THE HEAD AND NECK

Carter (1977) has reviewed various chemotherapy studies on squamous carcinoma of the head and neck and considers that the eight drugs listed in Table 21.1 have shown significant antitumour effect. None of these drugs acts specifically against malignant cells; all body cells are affected. Since this table was compiled, cisplatin (cisdiammine-dichloroplatinum II), discovered by Rosenberg in 1965, has been shown to show a similar response. Studies of the eight drugs listed in Table 21.1 have shown that some of these agents differed in their antitumour activity according to the type of cancer being treated.

Table 21.1 Drugs showing a 'positive response' (50% reduction in tumour, measured in two diameters) when tested as a single agent in squamous carcinoma. This must not be confused with 'cure' or total tumour remission for years

Methotrexate	
Bleomycin	
Cyclophosphamide	
5-Fluorouracil	Tested by
Hydroxyurea	Carter 1977
Vinblastine	
Adriamycin	
Nitrogen mustard	
Cisplatin	

In some instances, the biological effect of the drug could be enhanced if used in combination with two or three other drugs.

Alkylating agents

The work of Kennaway and Haddow in London and Gillman and Phillips in New York and Washington pioneered the development of a group of drugs referred to as the alkylating agents (HN_2 nitrogen mustard, Mustargen). These were the first cytotoxic chemotherapeutic drugs and later developments in this group of chemicals have led to the production of cyclophosphamide, chlorambucil, melphalan and busulphan. The alkylating agents are reactive compounds which intercalcate the twin strands of DNA, produce breaks in the DNA molecule and thus interfere with cell division. The interference with the intracellular enzyme system blocks the transcription of RNA. Similar effects are produced by ionizing radiation and so this group of drugs is referred to as 'radiomimetic'. The alkylating agents are cycle non-specific and the differences in activity among the various drugs relates to differences in absorption, site and rate of metabolism and tissue affinity, rather than the basic differences in the mode of action.

Cyclophosphamide is a bifunctional alkylating agent, which differs from other drugs in this group in that it requires metabolic activation, initially in the liver, to become cytotoxic. Consequently, the drug is unsuitable for local administration, but it has been widely used in various multidrug protocols, some in the treatment of head and neck squamous carcinomas and other areas of the body. Cyclophosphamide is well tolerated in low doses, but toxic side effects are dose-dependent, i.e. small doses given over a period of time may be associated with nausea, vomiting, alopecia, myelosuppression and haemorrhagic cystitis.

Methotrexate

This antimetabolite has long been considered the single most effective drug in the treatment of head and neck cancer. The drug is unique amongst the anticancer drugs in that it has a specific antidote (citro vorum factor, or folinic acid). This has allowed the use of large doses of methotrexate, which would normally be lethal unless followed by folinic acid rescue. In the body, the drug is in part metabolized in the liver and in part excreted by the kidneys. The amount of folinic acid necessary to counteract the effect of the drug remaining in circulation after 24 hours depends on the efficacy of hepatic and renal function. Calvert (1985) has described the use of:

1. Low dose methotrexate (less than $100 \, mg/m^2$).

2. Moderate dose methotrexate with folinic acid rescue, i.e. doses between 100 and $1000 \, mg/m^2$ followed by folinic acid rescue.

3. High dose methotrexate with folinic acid rescue. Doses as high as $5000 \, mg/m^2$ may be used. Calvert has reviewed the relevant literature on this drug using different dosage schedules and concludes that there is no doubt about the drug's effectiveness as an antitumour agent. The optimum dosage and periods of administration have not yet been defined.

Adriamycin

An antitumour antibiotic thought to act by intercalcation of the DNA double helix. The drug has shown a degree of activity against some solid tumours and leukaemias, but its use in tumours of the head and neck has been limited because of toxicity associated with its administration. These include myelosuppression, mucositis, alopecia and general malaise. Long-term administration can lead to cardiomyopathy.

Hydroxyurea

An antimetabolite, which effects the synthesis of DNA. The drug has not been widely used in treating head and neck carcinoma because of associated myelosuppression.

Bleomycin

An antibiotic, isolated from *Streptomyces verticillis*, was found to have an activity against a variety of squamous cell carcinomas. Maximum antitumour effect is evident in the late G_2 premitotic phase. The reported overall response rates vary from 45–60% and, at present, the drug is mainly used in multidrug combinations because of its phase-specific effect. Bleomycin has a wide range of toxic side effects:

skin reactions, colicky abdominal pains and fevers and, in large doses, the danger of pulmonary fibrosis is serious when the total dose exceeds 500 mg.

The vinca alkaloids

Vincristine, vinblastine and vindesine are alkaloids derived from the African periwinkle plant and their place in chemotherapy protocols is due to their effectiveness at inhibiting spindle formation prior to mitosis (Livingstone et al 1973). Cells in cycle are arrested at a phase in which they will be most sensitive to the effects of bleomycin. The main toxic side effects of these drugs are peripheral neuritis, which may cause para-aesthesia, loss of tendon reflexes and stocking distribution sensory loss. Constipation or incontinence may follow an autonomic neuropathy. Myelosuppression and alopecia have also been reported. Neurotoxicity is the most serious side effect of vincristine, whereas the dosage of vinblastine is limited mainly by myelotoxicity. Vindesine is intermediate in its range of toxicity. Very little has been recorded on the effectiveness of this drug used as a single agent in squamous carcinoma of the head and neck.

5-Fluorouracil

The use of this drug in the treatment of squamous carcinoma of the head and neck has been summarized by Livingstone & Carter (1970). The drug, a cycle-specific antimetabolite, pyramidine analogue, has been in use for over 20 years, mainly in multidrug protocols for the treatment of breast and gastrointestinal cancers. It is well tolerated apart from mucositis and a dose-dependent myelosuppression.

Cisplatin (cisdiammine-dichloro-platinum II)

An active antitumour agent affecting the synthesis of DNA, cisplatin was found to have quite exceptional properties both in its clinical antitumour effect and in a wide spectrum of toxicities. Administration is associated with severe vomiting and, unless assisted with hyperhydration (Hayes et al 1977), the risk of nephrotoxicity and renal failure is high. Other side effects include anaemia, peripheral neuropathy and high-frequency deafness (Prestayko et al 1980). The drug has been clinically used in doses varying

varying from 120 mg/m^2 to 20 mg/m^2. Toxicity, and the measures necessary to combat these side effects, are related to dosage. As with all the other drugs, prior treatment with radiotherapy or other drug combinations reduces response rate. Wittes et al (1979) achieved complete tumour response and 6 partial responses in 26 patients heavily pretreated with radiotherapy. This drug has been used in combination with bleomycin. Hong et al (1979) found, using a combination of cisplatin 120 mg/m^2 after prehydration and sequential mannitol diuresis, that it had a very significant antitumour effect in a treatment protocol which utilized the two-drug combination prior to surgery and radiotherapy. This report conflicts with the results of Morton et al (1983), who compared the palliative effects of bleomycin and cisplatin in the palliation of patients with unresectable squamous carcinomas. These authors concluded that there was no significant synergistic effect when bleomycin was given with cisplatin. Bleomycin was found to be ineffective as a palliative drug, but the results in those patients treated with cisplatin were encouraging. Three patients out of a total of 86 initially classified as unresectable had tumour regression to a point where surgery was feasible and multiple pulmonary metastases cleared completely in one further patient. Desai et al (1985) have described the use of a combination of cisplatin, methotrexate and bleomycin in a protocol in which patients who show a complete response after two courses of chemotherapy proceed to surgery, but if the response is not complete, the patients then receive radiotherapy and subsequently surgery.

Interest has recently been shown in two new platinum compounds: JM8 (diamine-1, 1-cyclobutane dicarboxylato platinum II) and JM9 (cis-dichloro-trans-dihydroxy-bis [isopropylamine] platinum IV) (Prestayko et al 1980).

MULTIDRUG (POLYDRUG) CHEMOTHERAPY AND THE IMPORTANCE OF PHARMACODYNAMICS

Kinetic studies by Skipper et al (1967) and Schabel (1969, 1975) influenced the work of Holland (1971) and Frei (1972), who improved the treatment results in leukaemia by using multidrug combinations.

The drugs listed in Table 21.1 may be classified as cycle non-specific, cycle specific or phase specific (Zubrod 1972). Livingstone et al (1973) noted that vincristine in adequate concentrations arrests cells in cycle in the late metaphase.

Bleomycin, a truly radiomimetic drug, has a maximal cytotoxic effect on cells at mitosis and in the S phase of the cell cycle.

Methotrexate is most cytoxic during the late G$_2$ and S phase. The antimetabolite, cycle specific 5-FU, given sequential to methotrexate, results in more than a simple additive cytotoxicity. The work of Bertino and the Yale group over the past five to seven years (studies reviewed by Bertino & Mini 1984) indicate that the sequential administration of 5-FU after prior administration of methotrexate results in a significant inhibition of thymidilate synthesis. This increase in tumour cell kill only occurs when methotrexate precedes 5-FU administration. Less than additive effects are noted with the reverse sequence. Pitman et al (1983) have confirmed the value of administering 5-FU sequential to methotrexate in the treatment of patients with squamous carcinoma of the head and neck.

By regarding radiotherapy as a cycle non-specific agent and vincristine, bleomycin and methotrexate as cycle specific agents, a drug protocol which would lead to a constant percentage tumour cell kill on the Schabel model was designed. Details of these two

Table 21.2 VBM regimen

Time (h)	Regimen
00	Vincristine 2 mg (i.v. stat)
06	Bleomycin 30 mg (i.m. stat)
24	Methotrexate 200 mg in 1000 ml saline (24 h infusion)
48	Folinic acid (Leucovorin) 15 mg (i.v. stat)
Followed by 9 mg leucovorin i.m. 6-hourly 5 doses	

Table 21.3 VBMF

Time (h)	Drug
00	Vincristine sulphate 2.0 mg i.v.
06	Bleomycin 30 mg i.v.
24	Methotrexate 200 mg i.v. infusion in 1 litre N saline
48	Completion of methotrexate infusion folinic acid 50 mg i.v. followed by 9 mg 6-hourly × 6
54	5-fluorouracil 500 mg i.v. stat.

drug regimes, VBM and VBMF, are outlined in Tables 21.2 and 21.3.

THE KING'S COLLEGE HOSPITAL (KCH) PILOT STUDIES

Prior to 1974, patients all stages of squamous carcinoma of the head and neck were treated initially with external supravoltage radiotherapy from a cobalt source to a total tumour dose of 6–6.500 rad. Surgery was reserved for those considered to have residual disease six weeks after completing radiotherapy.

In an attempt to improve results, from 1974, patients with squamous carcinomas of the head and neck stage III and IV were treated at KCH with the synchronous combination of vincristen, bleomycin and methotrexate given as four pulses during the administration of 6 Gy over a 10-week period. The chemotherapy/radiotherapy protocol was based on the Schabel (1975) model, which showed that total tumour cell kill could be achieved in some laboratory tumour cell systems by the use of 'cycle non-specific' and 'phase and cycle specific' cytotoxic drugs in a kinetically designed protocol.

In the protocol (Fig. 21.1) radiotherapy was used as the cycle non-specific agent, used synchronously with a combination of cycle and phase-specific agents (Table 21.2), previously described by Clifford (1975, 1976).

O'Connor et al (1982) reported the 7-year results of this prospective pilot study of 198 patients with stage III and IV squamous carcinomas of the head and neck (i.e. T1 or T2 with clinical positive nodes and T3 and T4 irrespective of nodal status). Radiotherapy is divided into three equal courses; the total dose aimed at was 60–66 Gy (1.8/2 Gy fractions daily). Usually, three or four courses of VBM were given, one before the first subcourse of radiotherapy and the others immediately after each subcourse. The intervals between each subcourse of radiation produced a median reduction of 4.5% in TDF (RET rate NSD) below the standard course of 30 x 20 Gy in 6 weeks.

Results

Survival and recurrence-free data were fully documented. The crude actuarial survival probability was 41% at 60 months (198 patients). The probability of remaining totally recurrence-free (disease-

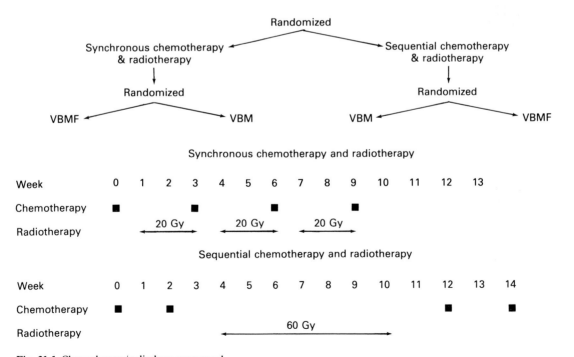

Fig. 21.1 Chemotherapy/radiotherapy protocol.

free deaths excluded) was 52% at 60 months. The presence of positive nodes (N+) adversely affected both survival and non-recurrence (30% versus 61% and 46% versus 67% respectively at 30 months). The reduced survival in patients with N+ disease was in part due to systemic metastases. Maintained local remission of disease above the clavical was observed in 122 out of a total of 198 patients (62%). Salvage surgery was performed in 28 patients and 11 were rendered free of local disease during the period of follow-up. Such patients would be counted in the crude actuarial survival probability curves, but not in the recurrence-free disease curves where surgical salvage is counted as a treatment failure.

Comparative results

In a comparative study on the efficacy of combined radiotherapy and VBM chemotherapy regimen, O'Connor et al (1979), used a historical control for comparative purposes. In the 5-year period 1974–1979, 179 patients with stage III and IV squamous carcinoma of the head and neck were treated with supravoltage radiotherapy alone at KCH. In this control group, disease-free survival was estimated at 21% and the total crude survival as 24.5% at 50 months from commencement of treatment.

In the pilot study group treated with radiotherapy and chemotherapy, the crude computer recorded actuarial survival curves was 56% against 24.5% in the historial control group. The probability of disease-free survival in patients treated with combined regime was 56.5% against 21.9% in the control group.

Thus the addition of synchronous chemotherapy showed a statistical improvement in treatment results ($P<0.000001$ and $P<0.001$) (O'Connor et al 1979).

The advantages of combined treatment have recently been reported from Italy. Workers in Genoa, Rosso (1986) and Barbari (1986) in Bologna have reported the advantageous results achieved using sychronous VBM with radiotherapy.

POSTCRICOID AND CERVICAL CARCINOMA

The management of squamous carcinoma of the postcricoid area and cervical oesophagus is one of the most formidable problems which may face a

head and neck surgeon and is associated with many hazards for the patient. Using VBMF synchronously (Table 21.3) with radiotherapy, Clifford (1979) and Grant & Clifford (1985) reported on the value of the combined treatment.

SOUTH EAST CO-OPERATIVE ONCOLOGY GROUP (SECOG)

In the light of the results achieved in the KCH pilot study, using synchronous VBM and VBMF with radiotherapy, a group of clinicians (radiotherapists, otolaryngologists and pathologists from 10 centres in the south-east of England) met in 1979 and set up the South-East Co-operative Oncology Group (SECOG). It was designed to establish a multicentre randomized trial to compare the results achieved using synchronous chemotherapy with chemotherapy given before and after radiotherapy.

The conditions for entering patients to the trial, the registration and randomization, have been described (SECOG Steering Committee 1982). It was considered essential that the conduct of the trial and the assessment of results should be under the control of a totally independent statistician. Entry into this trial (SECOG I) was closed in February 1984, at which time 270 patients with stage III and IV squamous carcinoma of the head and neck had been registered. Once a patient had been registered and randomized, NO withdrawals were permitted. No patients were lost to follow-up. 267 were con-

Table 21.4 The SECOG I trial—267 patients. Causes of death within six months of entry into trial

Carcinoma	
Disseminated disease	8
Local disease including carotid rupture	20
General medical condition	
Cardiovascular disease	1
Bronchopneumonia	6
Gastric haemorrhage	1
Legionnaire's disease	1
Cirrhosis of liver	1
Treatment-related causes	
Drug toxicity	2
Incorrect nasogastric intubation	1
Postoperative	2
Total	43

sidered suitable for analysis. There were no serious problems with drug toxicity. The results showed, of the 267 patients registered, 43 died within 6 months of entry into the trial, but only 5 of these deaths were related to treatment causes (see Table 21.4).

Results have been analysed by site. The addition of 5 FU to VBM produced a significant improvement in disease-free survival ($P<0.04$), though not in overall survival. Synchronous chemotherapy was similarly better than sequential chemotherapy, but the difference was not statistically significant ($P=0.1$). These results await publication. (SECOG I trial results 1986).

A new study, termed SECOG II, started in February 1984, in which patients are randomized into three arms, one pure radiotherapy and the other two arms are radiotherapy and chemotherapy given synchronously or sequentially with VBM or VBMF, also randomly allocated. To ensure a statistical balance, randomization takes into account the disease site and the treatments previously allocated to each institution.

The assessment of results

False facts are highly injurious to the progress of science, for they often long endure; but false views, if supported by some evidence, do little harm, as everyone takes a salutary pleasure in proving their falseness.

Charles Darwin, *The Descent of Man (1871)*

Bradford Hill (Medical Research Council 1948) introduced the randomized clinical trial. This outlined how a protocol which would provide statistically valid answers to questions inherent in any trial should be formulated. Peto et al (1977) have described the design and analysis of randomized clinical trials. Haybittle (1985) has outlined some of the difficulties in analysis of trial results because of the biological variability and inherent differences in trial arms. Bias in the presentation of results can be avoided by adhering to certain well-defined rules (Evans & Pollock 1985a, 1985b).

CONCLUSIONS

The results using synchronous VBM and VBMF have produced a significant increase in the disease-free survival rates by which patients are cured of their cancers without resort to surgery and this can only be viewed as a highly significant advance.

In reporting trial results, it is erroneous to equate a patient who is alive, having undergone excisive surgery, with a patient who is alive without surgery; a patient without a larynx or tongue to a patient with a larynx and tongue. The most important curve in assessing the success or otherwise of a particular treatment is the probability of disease-free survival. This curve, of course, excludes all patients who have undergone surgery.

Hibbert (1983) suggested that the use of chemotherapy impaired the possibility of survival, but this statement has not been borne out by other workers. Clifford (1979) included, in a report, 23 patients who had undergone salvage surgery after failure of primary treatment with radiotherapy and synchronous VBM. In the SECOG I trial, in which the results of treating 267 patients were analysed, 91 patients have undergone salvage surgery. The addition of chemotherapy to the primary treatment did not, in the experience of the particulars of the SECOG trial, prejudice healing or treatment results beyond that normally expected in patients who have had prior radiotherapy (H.R. Grant—personal communication, 1986).

The range of chemotherapeutic drugs available for treating head and neck cancer is rapidly expanding with newer compounds which have less systemic toxicity, but increased anticancer effects, particularly when used in combinations. So, the place of chemotherapy in the armoury of modalities of value in treating cancer can no longer be regarded as unproven.

'Establishing a definitive role for chemotherapy in the treatment of head and neck cancer remains an elusive task' (Taylor 1981).

Chemotherapy for malignant disease has been available for about 40 years. About 15 years ago it began to make great contributions to the treatment of lymphomas and combinations of various agents are now clearly effective in these diseases. More recently, there has been a spate of interest in chemotherapy for solid epithelial tumours. There is little evidence that chemotherapy is very effective in squamous carcinoma of the head and neck. This can, in part, be explained by cellular kinetic data, which show that most carcinomas of the upper respiratory and digestive tract have kinetics which are relatively unfavourable to the action of chemotherapy because about 75% of cells are in the resting phase of the cycle and are thus not accessible to the agent (Cachin 1982).

Chemotherapy can be used in one of two ways: in combination with radiotherapy or surgery, or for the sole treatment of advanced/recurrent disease which is no longer amenable to surgery or radiotherapy. The latter is sometimes called palliative treatment, but who it palliates is far from clear—certainly no evidence has been produced that it palliates these patients' symptoms. But we are concerned here with adjuvant treatment, which can be divided into three types:
1. Induction chemotherapy
2. Simultaneous chemotherapy and radiotherapy (radiosensitizers)
3. Maintenance chemotherapy.

DESIGN OF CHEMOTHERAPY TRIALS

All, save for a few backwoodsmen, acknowledge that new treatments must be subjected to clinical trials. The design of trials will therefore be discussed first. A new drug must pass through three levels of trial:

Phase I studies

These studies are usually carried out under the surveillance of drug companies and are used to establish safe doses, toxicity, etc.

Phase II studies

These have as their end-point the response of the tumour. The criteria for response are now internationally agreed: a partial response is a reduction of more than 50% of the sum of two perpendicular diameters and a complete response is disappearance of all clinical evidence of the disease (Miller et al 1981). The alternative, i.e. that the disease progresses, is usually not reported, but is in fact what happens to most patients. Even if all tumours were readily accessible for measurement and even if all observers were scrupulously unbiased and honest, the inter-and intraobserver error in measuring a tumour are obviously enormous. Phase II studies do not usually contain a control arm, so that it is impossible to assess whether the patient survives any longer than he would have done without treatment. Because responders generally live longer than non-responders, it is generally assumed that response indicates prolonged survival, but there is no logical reason to accept this. Responders and non-responders are biologically different—the former are known to be in better general condition, for example. They would thus have survived longer than non-responders in any case. A phase II trial does *not* show that responders live longer than they otherwise would have done if they had not received chemotherapy. Convincing evidence has been produced that indeed they do not (Oye & Martin 1984): Figure 21.2 shows the survival of responders and non-responders from a trial of 5-FU in metastatic colorental cancer. The impressive improvement

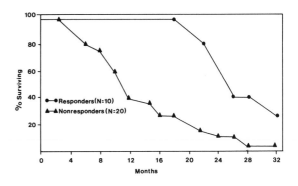

Fig. 21.2 Fluorouracil in metastatic colorectal cancer. Comparison of survival of responders and non-responders.

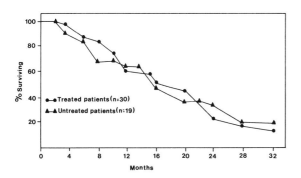

Fig 21.3 Fluorouracil in metastatic colorectal cancer. Comparison of survival of treated and untreated patients. (Reproduced with permission of Mr R K Oye and Editor of *Journal of the American Medical Association*.)

for responders disappears completely when the two groups are combined and compared with untreated controls, which unusually were available in this study (Fig. 21.3).

In addition to the uncertainties of bias in measurement of a tumour, particularly a metastasis, it is also necessary to consider the composition and kinetics of a tumour. There are numerous different types of cell in a tumour: malignant cells in various phases (mitosis, G_2, S phase, G_2 etc.), inflammatory cells, etc. From a cell kinetic standpoint, any gross measurements of a change in tumour size, particularly over a period as short as 4 weeks, have no meaning since we do not know what we are measuring. Indeed, increase in size of a tumour may not be bad: it may indicate widespread cell death with a brisk inflammatory response (Watson 1981).

Phase II studies require few patients, are easy to mount and are often financed by drug companies. The sponsors quite often insist on certain patients being excluded, notably those in poor general condition. Since response (and survival too) are dictated by general condition more than by any other single factor, exclusion of patients in poor general condition will guarantee a good result. Since reports of phase II studies very seldom indicate how many eligible patients were untreated in the same period, the applicability of the regimen to the generality of patients cannot be assessed.

There are three agents thought to be effective in squamous carcinoma of the head and neck: methotrexate, bleomycin and cisplatin. These have all been available for many years, have all been subjected to numerous phase II studies, singly or in combination, and have been shown to induce response rates of about 25%. It is astonishing that oncology journals continue to grind out phase II trials ad nauseam—83 of 84 trials summarized in the most recent issue of the EORTC Cancer Chemotherapy Annual were phase II studies. There is surely an overwhelming case for oncologists to turn their attention now to what matters most: the *survival* of the patient.

Phase III trials

These are a considerable challenge. These trials have a control arm—usually an untreated group—and the end point is survival. Unlike response, this end point is known with absolute accuracy, and is the 'hardest' of all data. To quote a historian in a different context: 'There is no appeal from the verdict of a date'. Sadly, phase III trials are rarely carried out mainly because of the sheer size of a trial required to achieve a significant result. Stage III and IV head and neck cancer has a 5-year survival of about 40%. The maximum improvement in survival which could be achieved by currently available chemotherapy is 10%. Although a significant result *might* be achieved in a relatively short time with relatively few patients, a huge number is required to ensure that a non-significant result is truly non-significant and not due to the sample size being too small. A trial of this sort demands 1000 patients, and 8–10 years to complete. A recent trial of adjuvant chemotherapy and radiotherapy in pharyngeal cancer did indeed take 8 years to complete and the answer was non-significant. The effect on the morale of the participating clinicians can be imagined

Pleas are repeatedly heard for using other end points, such as 'control' disease-free survival, 'quality of life', etc. All these are important, but are difficult to define, liable to subjectivity in measurement and are less important than survival, which is and must remain the gold standard for measurement of the efficacy of treatment.

ADJUVANT CHEMOTHERAPY

One question which needs to be answered clearly is what adjuvant chemotherapy is meant to achieve, in the light of the causes of failure in head and neck cancer. In the author's series, 40% of patients were alive at 5 years. A further 15% died before 5 years of intercurrent disease, or a second tumour, so that only 45% die of their disease. Although induction chemotherapy is often used only for patients with advanced disease, there is much evidence that this form of treatment is more likely to be effective (if it is effective at all) in patients with smaller tumours. Logically, therefore, induction chemotherapy should be considered for all patients. Unfortunately, this would expose more than half the patients to a potentially dangerous form of treatment from which they will not benefit: worse, some patients who would have been cured by surgery or radiotherapy alone might be killed by the addition of chemotherapy.

The commonest cause of failure is recurrence at the primary site, or in the nodes of the neck. Induction chemotherapy given before radiotherapy might reduce the size of the tumour and thus improve local control. Twenty-five years ago preoperative radiotherapy was enthusiastically advocated on the same premise: sadly it proved to be a false dawn. In a controlled trial, patients given preoperative radiotherapy had the same survival as patients submitted to surgery alone (Strong et al 1978). A recent trial of radiotherapy, with or without preceding cisplatinum, produced a similar result: 86% of the patients given cisplatin showed a response, but the survival at 1 year was identical to that of patients treated by radiotherapy alone (Haas et al 1985).

Secondly, chemotherapy given at the same time as radiotherapy might act as a radiosensitizer, but, sadly, this combination often has an unacceptably high morbidity.

Thirdly, chemotherapy might retard or prevent the development of a distant metastasis, but this is not a common cause of failure in head and neck cancer.

The possibility that chemotherapy might actually reduce survival is seldom seriously considered, but there are good grounds from controlled trials for believing that it might. There are also theoretical grounds for concern: cytotoxic agents are mutagens and may well hasten the appearance of more malignant variants (Kerbel & Davies 1982). A final difficulty is that most patients given chemotherapy do *not* respond and are therefore subject to a 2–3 months delay, which will *reduce* survival and they will enter surgery in a worse condition.

Induction chemotherapy followed by radiotherapy

The most impressive trial published of induction chemotherapy is a multicentre study of 638 patients randomized to radiotherapy alone, or radiotherapy preceded by methotrexate every 3 days for 15 days. The group given chemotherapy had a modest increase in survival, which disappeared when the survival was adjusted for T and N stage, age, performance, status, etc. The authors considered that this schedule should not be adopted for routine clinical use (Fazekas et al 1980).

The most recent (1984) EORTC Cancer Chemotherapy Annual summarizes 33 reports of induction studies: 31 were phase II studies. More than half the reports did not record long-term survival rates. They are thus of little value. Only 2 studies had untreated controls and measured survival. The first was a trial of intra-arterial methotrexate and radiotherapy which increased survival significantly from 25% to 43% in stage II/IV disease (Arcangeli et al 1983). The second trial of the much-publicized VBM kinetic regimen was carried out by ourselves. The results were disastrous: no patient with a carcinoma of the mouth or pharynx treated with VBM followed by radiotherapy survived beyond 18 months, and the reduction of survival in this group was significant (Stell et al 1983). Other randomized prospective trials similar to ours on patients with advanced disease assigned randomly to radiotherapy alone, or radiotherapy plus chemotherapy, also did not produce an increase in survival (Stolwijk et al 1983, Rossa et al 1984). Similar disappointing results with this regimen in palliative studies have been reported by Tannock et al (1982).

In the year since the résumé referred to in the last paragraph, quite a few trials have been reported of induction chemotherapy. The result has almost always been the same, i.e. that chemotherapy induces a response of varying degree, but long-term survival is unaffected (Taylor et al 1985, Vogl et al 1982, Cruz et al 1982). A typical example is the study, quoted by Haas, of cisplatin + 5-FU: a response rate of 86%, but a 1-year survival of 56% in the radiotherapy alone arm and 53% in the chemotherapy plus radiotherapy arm (Haas et al 1985).

Many regimens tested in phase II trials have been of combinations of two or more drugs, no doubt inspired by the success of polychemotherapy in treatment of the lymphomas. Sadly, the very few phase III trials of multiple agents against single agents have all shown that adding agents merely increases toxicity but not survival (Jacobs et al 1983, Cachin et al 1977, Campbell et al, in press).

Induction chemotherapy and surgery

Very few trials of this method have been published. One large trial has been published by the NCI and is referred to below (under maintenance chemotherapy). In brief, the results showed no benefit from adjuvant cisplatinum and bleomycin plus surgery. A second trial has recently been completed by the EORTC of preoperative intra-arterial methotrexate in oral carcinoma. At the time of writing, the results have not been published, but it is believed that they showed increased survival for the chemotherapy plus surgery group, which did not quite reach significant levels.

Simultaneous chemotherapy and radiation therapy

The radiation sensitizer, misonidazole, has produced mixed results: response rates appear to be improved with the combination of misonidazole plus radiation over radiation alone, but neurotoxicity has prevented the use of higher dosage and any improvement in survival is questionable (Taylor 1983).

Most authors have found that the simultaneous use of radiation with bleomycin, or methotrexate-containing combinations, produces increased toxicity but no gain in response rate or duration (Taylor et al 1985, Cachin et al 1977, Ansfield et al 1970). In contrast, O'Connor & Clifford have reported good 5-year results with 4 courses of bleomycin, vincristine and methotrexate given before, during and after irradiation. They observed severe weight loss and mucositis, but claimed a greater than 30% increase of survival compared with historical controls (O'Connor et al 1979). All trials are open to criticism, but historical trials more than most. The historical group would have contained 'all-comers', i.e. including the 20% or so of patients who would be unfit for the demanding combined synchronous regimen. This group would be excluded from the treated group, producing a mighty inbuilt bias.

Laboratory studies have shown that cisplatin may act as a hypoxic cell radiosensitizer, interfere with repair of sublethal and potentially lethal radi-ation damage and enhance radiation lethality of mammalian cells. As an adjuvant to radiotherapy it is usually given in combination sequentially with radiotherapy, but two recent reports suggest that it can be used concurrently, with acceptable toxicity. Complete remission was achieved in 7 of 8 in one series and a high rate of complete regression (15/18–83%), with a low incidence of early regional relapse (7%) in another ECOG study. However, Fu (1985) felt that the value of cisplatin, used as a single agent concurrently with radiotherapy, must await the results of further clinical trials.

The use of cisplatin as a radiation sensitizer in an uncontrolled trial during full-course radiation therapy was said to produce 'very promising results of a high response rate', although survival rates are not quoted (AL-Sarraf et al 1983).

Maintenance chemotherapy

At the present time, no randomized trials have been carried out of standard treatment followed by maintenance chemotherapy. Maintenance regimens have been built into a very few trials of induction chemotherapy, the most impressive being an NCI study (Jacobs et al 1984) of cisplatin and bleomycin: 462 patients with resectable stage III and IV carcinoma of the mouth, hypopharynx and larynx were randomized to three arms:

1. Standard surgery followed by irradiation
2. Induction chemotherapy followed by standard therapy
3. Induction therapy, followed by maintenance chemotherapy for 6 months. The 2-year survivals were 59%, 56% and 58% respectively, i.e. chemotherapy, either as induction or maintenance, was of no value whatsoever in this large, well-controlled series.

SUMMARY

The most frequently studied method of adjuvant chemotherapy is induction chemotherapy followed by radiotherapy. There is overwhelming evidence from many studies showing that a high rate of response can be achieved. Survival, the only important outcome, has rarely been studied: when it has, adjuvant chemotherapy has been found wanting.

The purpose of this chapter is to make an assessment and a statement as to the effects of the use of adjunctive chemotherapy in the treatment of malignant neoplasia in the area of the head and neck. The question to be answered is, 'Has adjunctive chemotherapy been a worthwhile modality?'

Chemotherapy has been a hope of doctors and their patients for centuries (Burchenal 1977). This hope sputtered, with very little attention or success, until the introduction of nitrogen mustard in 1946 by Rhoads (Rhoads 1946). Since that time, a significant amount of scientific investigation, experimentation and clinical trial has been devoted to this subject. This has produced an astounding advance in the treatment of certain leukaemias, lymphosarcomas, Hodgkin's disease, ovarian cancer, embryonal rhabdomyosarcoma and multiple myeloma. There has also been significant success achieved in certain types of Wilms' tumours, neuroblastomas, osteogenic sarcomas and some lung, brain, testicular and breast cancers (Greenspan 1982).

The chemotherapeutic thrust against cancer in the head and neck has been almost completely disappointing. In the early stages, the meagre and sporadic regressions of the cancer accomplished more misery and death than was expected. The programmes were critically analysed and new concepts were applied. It became obvious that many of the doctors using chemotherapy were inexperienced. Their cases were being picked at random and were almost all advanced and hopeless. All of the patients were malnourished and caught up in the dying process. New drugs and the use of multiple drugs entered the methodology of treatment at that time. A great volume of empirical knowledge was accumulated, and this caused a revitalization of the whole programme, which was becoming better organized. It was recognized that co-operative efforts throughout the United States, with large numbers of cases, was essential in establishing meaningful protocols. All of these creative acts became functional and still the clinical effects on cancers in the area of the head and neck were discouraging (Watne 1984).

It was, therefore, necessary again to devise new concepts and one of these concepts was adjunctive chemotherapy. (De Vita 1977, Spaulding et al 1980,

1982). The incorporation of this symbiotic programme was a logical development and an outgrowth of the overall failures with chemotherapy and surgery, with the hope that, by combining the modalities of treatment with the standard, recognized programmes, one might not only enhance the management of these cancers, but even improve the cure rate (Bosi 1983, Cachin 1982).

The assessment of all of the work in this direction has now left little question that adjunctive chemotherapy, when combined with conventional surgical excision, or sugical excision and postoperative radiotherapy, does not increase the cure rate in cancer of the head and neck (Holoye et al 1984, Huang et al 1985, Stolwijk et al 1985, Taylor et al 1985). Almost every investigator has been specific and negative in statements concerning the lack of success in enhancing the cure rate. Their statements concerning the futility of adjunctive chemotherapy under the circumstances of its present administration with the use of the drugs employed, the methods of administration of those drugs and the selection of patients for treatment did not accomplish what had been hoped for. This leads directly to the proposition that this phase of adjunctive chemotherapy has been answered and a continuation of this type of treatment must be carried out within entirely new perspectives and different motivations. In the meantime, new protocols have been established to continue the search for something more meaningful in the use of adjunctive chemotherapy in the area of the head and neck (Schuller et al, in press). Ultimately, it is believed that these programmes can be enhanced by including genetics, immunology and a more sophisticated variety of biological engineering. These ambitions will require decades of experience before the truth is known.

There is more to the failures in chemotherapy than is immediately apparent. In order to evaluate where we have been and where we are going in this field, it is necessary to ask the question as to who originally were, and who now are, the chemotherapists and what was the nature of the programme. In the early stages of this form of treatment, there were no specialists in chemotherapy. Many surgeons became interested and experimented with drugs and a modality of administration on their hopeless patients and their surgical failures. Some internists and general practitioners also became involved. Almost all of the trials at that time were selected at random and were exclusively carried out on hopeless and terminally ill cases. The results were understandably unsatisfactory and, at times, disastrous. From this rather alarming starting-point, chemotherapy has grown into a full-fledged science and specialty. One can hardly expect any of the original results to be acceptable at this time. Objectively, they supply the important data as to what programmes were unsuccessful and what were the pernicious effects, and suggested new ideas for treatment. As the scientific knowledge of chemotherapy expanded and the clinical experience broadened, a group of dedicated specialists have taken over the responsibility of treatment of these serious problems. It is now recognized that this field of therapy is complex, is very scientific and is still evolving, and certainly is not an arena for the dilettante.

Attempts to 'outsmart' a cancer and anticipate its pernicious potentials by performing elective surgical procedures or elective irradiation to the regions of high vulnerability have added a small increment of control in advanced cases. An analysis of this control feature has been challenged by some investigators, but has not caused combined or composite treatment to be abandoned when it seems appropriate for stage III and stage IV cancers. It has caused modifications, however, in radicality and introduced a variety of nuances into the management programme. Unrestrained radicality in the area of the head and neck is no longer acceptable.

The problem of how to treat cancer in the head and neck has obviously not been unequivocally solved by any of these modifications and, in some instances, it has even become confused. At times it seems as if there is excessive imagination, unfounded hope and unjustified trials. The most serious contributor to this unsteady and provocative situation is the uncertainty one must face when dealing with a potentially life-threatening disease. In spite of these imponderables, it is fair to state that the local control of cancer has improved, longevity has been slightly extended, distant spread has become more manifest in the patients who live longer, and the method of dying from cancer of the head and neck has been modified.

The basic concept of surgical removal of all of the cancer cells from the body at the primary site and, when appropriate, from the regional lymph node system is still the paramount method of treatment. This concept is, of course, not applicable to all cancers, for a variety of reasons. Irradiation has attempted to accomplish the same thing as surgery by killing the cancer cells in situ. Unfortunately, in both irradiation and surgery, in a significantly high percentage of cases, these efforts are doomed to failure at their incipiency. The failures are due to human and biological factors that cannot be dictated or controlled in all instances. The human factors are mistakes in judgement and technically inadequate operations on the primary cancer and failure to control regional metastasis. Biologically, the tumour may have deceptive extensions at the primary site or to the regional lymph nodes, or even wide dissemination. These foci may be microscopic and indiscernible in the beginning, and have therefore not been included in the initial therapeutic programme. When they become grossly discoverable, salvage of the patient, by all modalities combined, is problematical or hopeless. Herein lies the rationale and the necessity for either a supplementary or a complementary programme of chemotherapy. One of the tantalizing aspects of chemotherapy is that it has been able to create substantial reasons for its continuing investigation and use. Just when it would appear to have exhausted its value in certain aspects of therapy, a new discovery arises from the ashes. A case in point is the very impressive response rates now being obtained from the use of cisplatin, fluorouracil, bleomycin, methotrexate and other drugs, of 60–80% partial regression and 30–60% total regression of the neoplasm. Even though all of these cases ultimately developed recurrences, one is very favourably stimulated by the fact that large volumes of cancer cells are being killed by these drugs (Wolf et al 1984).

Another indicator in chemotherapy is the division of cases into responders and non-responders. Those patients who have a complete remission of their tumour, on the whole, do better in treatment programmes than those that do not respond. Certainly, this group contains undiscovered secrets about the potential for cure and the methodology of management and have suggested a programme of selection for treatment. The responders are given every therapeutic assistance in the form of adjunctive surgery or irradiation or both, in an 'all out' programme for control or cure. This aggressive treatment, with this particular group of responders, appears to have the best chance of improving local control of the primary cancer, of delaying metastasis and, conceivably, altering the method of dying. Whether it will cause an improvement in the overall cure rate remains to be seen.

Another group of partial responders has been identified. The gross volumetric reduction in size of their neoplasms may be insignificant, or spectacular. There often is some simultaneous improvement in gross symptomatology. Although response rates in all patients are only temporary, the group of partial responders stimulates the therapist to carry on with modifications in the regimen with the hope that improvements will ultimately put some of these patients in with the group that has attained a complete remission. The precise drugs to be used, the timing of administration and the selection of patients in this group are still variable factors, and still being modified.

There is another group that does not respond in any way to any of the chemotherapeutic agents. The biological implications of this refractory group of patients are not understood, but it has definite clinical significance. It is this particular group that has the gravest prognosis, the most serious aspects of management and the highest immediate and protracted futility. It further highlights the complexity of the cancer problem in that the ultimate solution is more than the application of a chemotherapeutic drug which will act miraculously in all cases.

Although the conclusions of the authors who have studied adjunctive chemotherapy are quite definite, in that chemotherapy is not successful under these circumstances, they do not necessarily take a defeatist position (Mead & Jacobs 1982). The entire subject is so vast that results only speak for the concepts that are used. Secondary effects and revelations from all of these trials have suggested new principles of management: new trials, with different therapeutic programming and a continued use of chemotherapeutic agents with fresh concepts.

A variety of preoperative and postoperative chemotherapeutic programmes have been studied (Gad-El-Mawla et al 1984). There is no evidence at this time that the use of chemotherapy in any of those protocols, which include gross metastasis, cures more cancer cases than the conventional methods of management. In the preoperative trials of chemotherapy, there was no support for the concept that a smaller, more conservative type of operation could be performed because of gross shrinkage of the neoplasm, nor was there any significant improvement in control of the neoplasm at the primary site in the follow-up examinations.

In the postoperative trials with chemotherapy there was no improvement in survival in stages III and IV cancers, but there was an apparent reduction in the incidence of regional and systemic metastasis (Jacobs et al 1983, 1984). This was suggested by a delay in the clinical appearance of those metastases. This prolongation of the interval of relapses led to the supposition that chemotherapy may be affecting disseminated microscopic metastases in a favourable way. It is well recognized that chemotherapy is effective against micrometastases in laboratory mice and it had been hoped that this might behave similarly in humans. This led directly to the concept of 'maintenance chemotherapy', which would be sustained over a period of months or years (Johnson et al 1985). Whether it will prove to be a satisfactory palliative programme or, guardedly, a curative programme must be established by trial, the actuarial analysis of large numbers of controlled cases followed for a period of 5–10 years. The incipient phase of this investigation has already begun.

A not-so-subtle aspect of the use of chemotherapy today is the psychological effect of the administration of these drugs on the patient, the surgeon, the family group and the chemotherapist. Their emotional reactions are always positive in the beginning. The patient does not feel forsaken and is buoyed up by the proposition of a different form of treatment that possibly might help him. The surgeon who has failed in his efforts to control the cancer is unhappy and eager to share this failure with another physician, the chemotherapist. The family group is reassured that something is being done that might prove helpful. The chemotherapist is practising his art and craft and is guardedly optimistic or pessimistic. All of this might be classified as a manifestation of human compassion within the framework of the mores of modern scientific medical management.

The most important question is whether it is the right treatment and what are the ultimate dividends.

At its best, it creates hope and some measure of palliation. At its worst, it makes a patient, already suffering from the burden of cancer, more uncomfortable, depletes the quality of life and may, indeed, even shorten his life. There is obviously no simple answer to all of the questions generated by this act. Each patient must be assessed individually and each patient must make his decision concerning the use of this treatment within the framework of support of his doctor and his family.

In conclusion, one can state that adjunctive chemotherapy in the treatment of cancer in the head and neck has not improved local control at the primary site, has not prevented regional or systemic metastasis and has not enhanced the cure rate over conventional treatment by surgery and irradiation. Any continuation of its use under the circumstances that have been studied would have to be done for reasons other than expected statistical improvements. There are obvious reasons to support chemotherapy in a continuum of modified and creative investigations. The alternatives of lack of interest, or the abandonment of chemotherapy, are unacceptable at the present time. We must also continue controlled protocols to attempt to exploit the known and, as yet, undiscovered 'killing power' of chemotherapy by new concepts and trials for the benefit of the patient.

REFERENCES

P Clifford

Barbari E 1986 Abstract 19. The proceedings of the 1st International IST Seminar, Genoa (in press)

Bertino J R, Nini E 1984 Sequential methotrexate/5-fluoroacil: a review of laboratory studies and clinical results. Cancer Topics 4: 11–126

Cachin Y 1982 Adjuvant chemotherapy in head and neck cancer. Clinical Otolaryngology 7: 121–132

Calvert A H 1985 In: Henk J M, Langdon J D (eds) Chemotherapy in malignant tumours of the oral cavity. Edward Arnold, London

Carter S K 1977 Seminars in Oncology 4: 413

Catterall M, Sutherland I, Belley D K 1975 First results of random clinical trial on fast neutrons compared with X-or gamma rays in the treatment of advanced tumours of the head and neck. British Medical Journal ii: 653–656

Clifford P 1975 Combined modality therapy in head and neck cancer. In: R G Chambers et al (eds) Cancer of the head and neck. 67–72

Clifford P 1976 Prospectives in head and neck oncology. Journal of Laryngology & Otology 90: 221–251

Clifford P 1979 The role of cytotoxic drugs in the surgical management of head and neck malignancies. Journal of Laryngology & Otology 93: 1151–1180

Desai P, Vyas J J, Charma S et al 1985 The impact of combined therapeutic modalities in head, neck and oesophageal cancer. Seminars in Surgical Oncology 1: 116–131

Evans M, Pollock A V 1985a British Journal of Surgery 72: 256–260

Evans M, Pollock A V 1985b Journal of the Royal Society of Medicine 78: 937–940

Frei B III 1972 Cancer Research 32: 2593–2607

Grant H R, Clifford P 1985 European Journal of Surgical Oncology 11: 37–40

Haybittle J L 1985 Guide to clinical trials analysis. Cancer Topics 5:9: 102–103

Hayes D M, Cvitkovic E, Golbey R B, Krakoff I H, Scheiner E, Helson L 1977 High dose cisplatinum diammine-dichloride amelioration of renal toxicity by mannitol diuresis. Cancer 39: 1372–1381

Hibbert J 1983 Editorial. Clinical Otolorolaryngology 8: 3–6

Hill B T, Shaw H J, Dalley V M, Price L A 1984 24-hour combination chemotherapy without cisplatin in patients with recurrent or metastatic head and neck cancer. American Journal of Clinical Oncology 7(4): 335–340

Holland J F 1971 Cancer Research 31: 1319–1329

Hong W K, Bhuthani R, Shapshay et al 1979 Proceedings of the American Society of Clinical Oncology 19: 321

Lederman M 1981 The early history of radiotherapy—1859–1939. International Journal of Radiation Oncology, Biology & Physics 7: 639–648

Livingstone R B, Carter S K 1970 Single agents in cancer chemotherapy. IFI Plenum, New York

Livingstone R B, Bodey G P, Gottlieb J A, Frei E 1973 Kinetic scheduling of vincristine and bleomycin in patients with lung cancer and other malignant tumours. Cancer Chemotherapy Reports 57: 219–224

McElwain T A 1979 Some traps and pitfalls in cancer chemotherapy. Clinical Oncology 5: 1–2

Medical Research Council 1948 British Medical Journal ii: 769–782

Morton R P et al 1983 Clinical Oncology 9: 359

O'Connor A D, Clifford P, Dalley V M, Durden-Smith D J, Edwards V G, Hollis B A 1979 Advanced head and neck cancer treated by combined radiotherapy and VBM cytotoxic regimen—4 year results. Clinical Otolaryngology 4: 329–337

O'Connor D, Clifford P, Edwards W G et al 1982 Long term results of VBM and radiotherapy in advanced head and neck cancer. International Journal of Radiation Oncology, Biology and Physics 8: 1525–1531

Peto R, Rike M C, Armitage P et al 1977 Design and analysis of randomised clinical trials requiring prolonged observation of each patient. British Journal of Cancer 35:1–47

Pitman S W, Kowal C D, Bertino J R 1983 Seminars in Oncology 10 (suppl 2): 15

Prestayko A W 1980 Antitumour, toxic and biochemical properties of cisplatinum and eight other platinum complexes. In: Cisplatin. Academic Press, New York

Price L S, Hill B T, Calvert A H, Shaw H J, Hughes K B 1975 A kinetically based multidrug treatment for cancer of the head and neck. British Medical Journal 3: 10

Price L A, Hill B T 1977 A kinetically based logical approach to the chemotherapy of head and neck cancer. Clinical Otolaryngology 2: 339–345

Price L A, Hill B T 1981 Safe and effective combination chemotherapy with cisplatinum for squamous cell cancer of the head and neck. Cancer Treatment Reports 64 (suppl): 141–145

Rosenberg B, Van Camp L, Krigas T 1965 Inhibition of cell division in *Escherichia coli* by electrolysis products from a platinum electrode. Nature 205: 698

Rosso R 1986 Abstract A 20. The proceedings of the 1st International IST Seminar, Genoa (in press)

Schabel F M Jnr 1969 The use of tumour growth kinetics in planning 'curative' chemotherapy of advanced solid tumours. Cancer Research 29: 2384–2389

Schabel F M Jnr 1975 Cancer 35: 15

Sealy R, Cridland S 1984 The treatment of locally advanced head and neck cancer with misonidazole, hyperbaric oxygen and irradiation—an interim report. International Journal of Radiation Oncology, Biology and Physics 10: 1721–1723

SECOG Steering Committee 1982 SECOG head and neck trial. Letter to the Editor. Lancet ii: 708–709

SECOG I Trial Results 1986 A randomized trial of multidrug chemotherapy and radiotherapy in advanced squamous cell carcinoma of the head and neck. European Journal of Surgical Oncology 12: 289–295

Sinclair W K 1968 Radiation Research 33: 620

Skipper H E, Schabel F M, Wilcox W S 1967 Cancer Chemotherapy Reports 51: 125

Steel G G, Peckham M J 1979 International Journal of Radiation Oncology, Biology and Physics 5: 85–91

Stell P M, Dalby J E, Strickland P, Fraser J G, Bradley P J, Flood L M 1983 Sequential chemotherapy and radiotherapy in advanced head and neck cancer. Clinical Radiology 34: 463–467

Wittes R E, Cvoilkovic E, Shah K 1979 Cis-dichlorodiamine-platinum (II): the treatment of epidermoid cancer of the head and neck. Cancer Treatment Reports 61: 359

Zubrod C G 1972 Proceedings of the National Academy of Science USA 69: 1024

Zubrod C G 1972 In: Holland J F, Frei E III (eds) Cancer medicine. Lea & Febiger, Philadelphia, P 627–632

P M Stell

Al-Sarraf M, Jacobs J, Kinzie J et al 1983 Combined modality therapy utilizing single high intermittent dose of cisplatinum and radiation in patients with advanced head and neck cancer. Proceedings American Society of Clinical Oncology Abstracts: 159

Ansfield F J, Ramirez G, Davis H L Jnr, Korbitz B C, Vermund H, Gollin F F 1970 Treatment of advanced cancer of the head and neck. Cancer 25: 78–82

Arcangeli G, Nervi C, Righini R, Creton G, Mirri M A, Guerra A 1983 Combined radiation and drugs: the effect of intra-arterial chemotherapy followed by radiotherapy in head and neck cancer

Cachin Y 1982 Adjuvant chemotherapy in head and neck carcinoma. Clinical Otolaryngology 5: 121–132

Cachin Y, Jortray A, Sancho H et al 1977 Preliminary results of a randomised EORTC study comparing radiotherapy and concomitant bleomycin, to radiotherapy alone in epidermoid carcinomas of the oropharynx. European Journal of Cancer 13: 1389–1395

Campbell J B, Dorman E B, Morton R P, Rugman F, Wilson J A, Stell P M 1987 Cisplatinum in combination is no

better than cisplatinum alone for advanced head and neck cancer. Clinical Otolaryngology (in print)

Cruz A B, Perkins M, Bradley J et al 1982 Concurrent chemotherapy and radiation therapy of selected head and neck squamous cell carcinomas using bleomycin and hydroxyurea: a southwest oncology group study. Journal of Surgical Oncology 20: 233–237

Fazekas J T, Sommer C, Kramer S 1980 Adjuvant intravenous methotrexate or definitive radiotherapy alone for advanced squamous cancers of the oral cavity, oropharynx, supraglottic larynx or hypopharynx. International Journal of Radiation Oncology, Biology and Physics 6: 533–541

Fu K K 1985 The value of DDP used as a single agent concurrently with radiotherapy awaits results of further clinical trials. In: Wittes R E (ed) Head and neck cancer. John Wiley & Sons, New York, p 235

Haas A, Toohill R J, Cox J D et al 1985 Randomized study of 5-fluorouracil (5-FU) and cisplatinum (DDP) with standard therapy for treatment of locally advanced head and neck cancer. International Journal of Radiation, Oncology, Biology and Physics 11, Suppl 1: 89

Jacobs C, Meyers F, Hendrickson C, Kohler N, Carter S 1983 A randomized phase II study of cisplatin with or without methotrexate for recurrent squamous cell carcinoma of the head and neck. Cancer 52: 1563–1569

Jacobs C, Wolf G T, Makuch R W, Vikram B 1984 Adjuvant chemotherapy for head and neck squamous carcinomas. Proceedings American Society of Clinical Oncology Abstracts: 182

Kerbel R S, Davies A J S 1982 Facilitation of tumour progression by cancer therapy. Lancet ii: 977–978

Miller A B, Hoogstraten B, Staquet M, Winker A 1981 Reporting results of cancer treatment. Cancer 47: 207–214

O'Connor A D, Clifford P, Dalley V M, Durden-Smith D J, Edwards W G, Hollis B A 1979 Advanced head and neck cancer treated by combined radiotherapy and VBM cytotoxic regimen—four-year results. Clinical Otolaryngology 4: 329–337

Oye R K, Martin F 1984 Reporting results from chemotherapy trials. Journal of The American Medical Association 252: 2722–2725

Rosso R, Merlano M, Sertoli M R et al 1984 Multidrug chemotherapy (vincristine, bleomycin and methotrexate (VBM)) with radiotherapy in stage III-IV squamous cell carinoma of the head and neck. Cancer Treatment Reports 68:7: 1019–1021

Stell P M, Dalby J E, Strickland P, Fraser J G, Bradley P J, Flood L M 1983 Sequential chemotherapy and radiotherapy in advanced head and neck cancer. Clinical Radiology 34: 463–467

Stolwijk C, Van den Broek P, Wagener D J Th, Levendag P C, Kazem I 1983 Randomized adjuvant chemotherapy trial in advanced head and neck cancer. Clinical Otolaryngology 8: 285

Strong M A, Vaughan C W, Kayne H L et al 1978 A randomized trial of preoperative radiotherapy in cancer of the oropharynx and hypopharynx. The American Journal of Surgery 136: 494–500

Tannock I, Sutherland D, Osoba D 1982 Failure of short course multiple drug chemotherapy to benefit patients with recurrent or metastatic head and neck cancer. Cancer 49: 1358–1361

Taylor S G IV 1981 In: Pinedo H M (ed) Cancer chemotherapy. Amsterdam, Elsevier, p 292

Taylor S G 1983 Head and neck cancer. In: Pinedo H M, Chebner B A (eds) Cancer chemotherapy/5. The EORTC cancer chemotherapy annual. Elsevier, Amsterdam, p 291–306

Taylor S G, Applebaum E, Showel J L et al 1985 A randomized trial of adjuvant chemotherapy in head and neck cancer. Journal of Clinical Oncology 3: 672–678

Watson J V 1981 What does 'response' in cancer chemotherapy really mean?. British Medical Journal 283: 34–37

Vogl S E, Lerner H, Kaplan B H et al 1982 Failure of effective initial chemotherapy to modify the course of stage IV (MO) squamous cancer of the head and neck. Cancer 50: 840–844

J Conley

Bosi G J 1983 Adjuvant chemotherapy in the management of stage III and IV tumours of the head and neck. CA-A Cancer Journal for Clinicians 33: 139–144

Burchenal J H 1977 The historical development of cancer chemotherapy. Seminars of Oncology 4: 135–146

Cachin Y 1982 Adjuvant chemotherapy in head and neck carcinoma. Clinical Otolaryngology 7: 121–132

De Vita V T 1977 Adjuvant therapy: An overview. In: Salmon S E, Jones S E (eds) Adjuvant therapy of cancer. Elsevier North Holland Biomedical Press, Amsterdam

Gad-El-Mawla N, Abul-Ela M, Mansour M D, MacDonald J S 1984 Preoperative adjuvant chemotherapy in relatively advanced head and neck cancer. American Journal of Clinical Oncology (CCT) 7: 195–198

Greespan E M (ed) 1982 Clinical interpretation and practice of cancer chemotherapy. Raven Press, New York, NY

Holoye P Y, Grossman T W, Toohil R J et al 1984 Randomized study of adjuvant chemotherapy for head and neck cancer. Otolaryngology—Head and Neck Surgery 93: 712–717

Huang P Y, Grossman T W, Toohil R J et al 1985 Randomized study of adjuvant chemotherapy for head and neck cancer. Annals of Surgery 200: 195–199

Jacobs C, Meyers F, Hendrickson D, Kohler N, Carter S 1983 A randomized Phase II study of cisplatin with or without methotrexate for recurrent squamous cell carcinoma of the head and neck. Cancer 52: 1563–1569

Jacobs C, Wolf G T, Makuch R W, Vikram B 1984 Adjuvant chemotherapy for head and neck squamous carcinomas. Proceedings: American Society of Clinical Oncology Abstracts 182

Johnson J T, Myers E N, Strodwa C N et al 1985 Maintenance chemotherapy for high-risk patients. Archives of Otolaryngology 3: 727–729

Mead G M, Jacobs C 1982 Changing role of chemotherapy in treatment of head and neck cancer. The American Journal of Medicine 73: 582–595

Rhoads C P 1946 Nitrogen mustard in treatment of neoplastic disease. Journal of the American Medical Association 131: 656–658

Schuller D E, Wilson H E, Hodgson S E, Mattox D, McCracken J D 1987 Preoperative reductive chemotherapy: A phase III Southwest Oncology Group Study. Cancer (in press)

Spaulding M B, Klotch D, Grillo J, Sanani S, Lore J M 1980 Adjuvant chemotherapy in the treatment of advanced tumours of the head and neck. American Journal of Surgery 140: 538–541

Spaulding M B, Kahn A, De Los Santos R, Klotch D, Lore J M 1982 Adjuvant chemotherapy in advanced head and neck cancer: An update. American Journal of Surgery 144: 432–436

Stolwijk C, Wagener D J T, Van den Brock P et al 1985 Randomized neo-adjuvant chemotherapy trial for advanced head and neck cancer. Netherlands Journal of Medicine 28: 347–351

Taylor S G IV, Applebaum E, Showel J L et al 1985 A randomized trial of adjuvant chemotherapy in head and neck cancer. Journal of Clinical Oncology 3: no 5 (May) 672–679

Watne A L 1984 Treatment alternatives: head and neck cancers. Cancer (Dec. 1 Supplement) 54: 2673–2681

Wolf G T, Makuch R W, Baker S R 1984 Predictive factors for tumour response to preoperative chemotherapy in patients with head and neck squamous cancer. Cancer 54: 2869–2877

Index